Autism and Child Psychopathology Series

Series Editor
Johnny L. Matson
Baton Rouge, Louisiana, USA

More information about this series at http://www.springer.com/series/8665

Autism and Child Psychopathology Series

Johnny L. Matson
Michael L. Matson
Editors

Comorbid Conditions in Individuals with Intellectual Disabilities

Springer

Editors
Johnny L. Matson
Department of Psychology
Louisiana State University
Baton Rouge
Louisiana
USA

Michael L. Matson
Center for Research Disability
Consultants, LLC
Baton Rouge
Louisiana
USA

ISSN 2192-922X ISSN 2192-9238 (electronic)
Autism and Child Psychopathology Series
ISBN 978-3-319-15436-7 ISBN 978-3-319-15437-4 (eBook)
DOI 10.1007/978-3-319-15437-4

Library of Congress Control Number: 2015933017

Springer Cham Heidelberg New York Dordrecht London

Printed on acid-free paper

Springer International Publishing AG Switzerland is part of Springer Science+Business Media (www.springer.com)

Contents

About the Editors

Johnny L. Matson, Ph.D., is Professor and Distinguished Research Master and Director of Clinical Training in the Department of Psychology at Louisiana State University, Baton Rouge, LA, USA. He has also previously held a professorship in psychiatry and clinical psychology at the University of Pittsburgh. He is the author of more than 800 publications including 41 books. He also serves as Founding Editor-in-Chief of three journals; *Research in Developmental Disabilities* (Elsevier), *Research in Autism Spectrum Disorders* (Elsevier), and *Review Journal of Autism and Developmental Disorders* (Springer).

Michael L. Matson, M.S.W. received his master's degree in social work from Tulane University and his bachelor's degree in psychology from Louisiana State University. He works in the research and training program of Disability Consultants, LLC. Michael is the former Managing Editor of the journals *Research in Developmental Disabilities* (Elsevier), *Research in Autism Spectrum Disorders* (Elsevier) and *Review Journal of Autism and Developmental Disorders*. He is the author of four books and 15 journal articles.

Contributors

Hilary L. Adams Department of Psychology, Louisiana State University, Baton Rouge, LA, USA

Marta Badia Institute on Community Integration (INICO), Department of Personality, Assessment & Psychological Treatments, University of Salamanca, Salamanca, Spain

Lauren D. Berkovits Department of Psychology, University of California, Los Angeles, CA, USA

Lynn M. Breau Psychology Services, Glenrose Rehabilitation Hospital, Edmonton, Alberta, Canada

Amanda Faith Casey Department of Human Kinetics, St. Francis Xavier University, ANtigonish, NS, Canada

Lisa L. Christensen Department of Psychology, University of California, Los Angeles, CA, USA

Dimitrios Patikas Department of Physical Education and Sport Science at Serres, Aristotle University, Thessaloniki, Greece

Peter A. Girolami Kennedy Krieger Institute/Johns Hopkins University School of Medicine, Baltimore, MD, USA

Rachel L. Goldin Department of Psychology, Louisiana State University, Baton Rouge, LA, USA

Melissa L. González Kennedy Krieger Institute/Johns Hopkins University School of Medicine, Baltimore, MD, USA

Megan A. Hattier Department of Psychology, Johns Hopkins School of Medicine, Baltimore, MD, USA

Sarah Helps London, UK

Max Horovitz Keystone Behavioral Pediatrics, Jacksonville, FL, USA

Matthew J. Konst Department of Psychology, Louisiana State University, Baton Rouge, LA, USA

Alison M. Kozlowski Kennedy Krieger Institute, Baltimore, MD, USA

Meir Lotan Faculty of Health Sciences, Department of Physical Therapy, Ariel University Center of Samana, Ariel, Israel

Johnny L. Matson Department of Psychology, Louisiana State University, Baton Rouge, LA, USA

Danessa Mayo Department of Psychology, Loma Linda University, Loma Linda, CA, USA

Joav Merrick Division of Pediatrics, Hadassah Hebrew University Medical Center, Jerusalem, Israel

Kentucky Children's Hospital, University of Kentucky, Lexington, USA

Center for Healthy Development, School of Public Health, Georgia State University, Atlanta, GA, USA

Pedro Montoya Research Institute on Health Sciences—IUNICS, University of the Balearic Islands, Balearic Islands, Spain

Cameron L. Neece Department of Psychology, Loma Linda University, Loma Linda, CA, USA

Begoña Orgaz Faculty of Psychology, Department of Basic Psychology, Psychobiology, and Methodology of Behavior Sciences, University of Salamanca, Salamanca, Spain

Lauren W. Rasmussen Adjunct Professor of Neuropsychology, Louisiana State University, Baton Rouge, LA, USA

Roy Rasmussen Department of Human Kinetics, St. Francis Xavier University, ANtigonish, NS, Canada

Inmaculada Riquelme Research Institute on Health Sciences—IUNICS, Department of Nursing and

Physiotherapy, University of the Balearic Islands, Balearic Islands, Spain

Tessa Taylor Lizard Centre, Eastwood, South Australia, Australia

Lauryn M. Toby Neurobehavioral Unit—Outpatient Clinic, Department of Behavioral, Psychology Kennedy Krieger Institute, Johns Hopkins University School of Medicine, Baltimore, MD, USA

Nicole Turygin Department of Psychiatry, Indiana University School of Medicine, Indianapolis, IW, USA

Lindsey W. Williams Department of Psychology, Louisiana State University, Baton Rouge, LA, USA

Part I
Overview

Chapter 1
Scope and Prevalence of the Problem

Hilary L. Adams and Johnny L. Matson

Introduction

Intellectual disability (ID) is characterized by deficits in cognitive, adaptive, and behavioral functioning (American Association on Intellectual and Developmental Disabilities 2010; Matson and Shoemaker 2009; Soenen et al. 2009). Nonetheless, a variety of other problems often occur among individuals with ID. Although a commonly held belief of the past was that persons with ID could not have psychopathology, this idea has since been refuted (Matson et al. 2012). At present, dual diagnosis, generally defined in the field as the presence of ID and a co-occurring mental illness (Matson and Sevin 1994; Reiss and Valenti-Hein 1994; Werner and Stawski 2012), is an increasingly popular topic. The general consensus in this area is that individuals with ID are at risk for comorbid psychopathology (Bhaumik et al. 2008; Borthwick-Duffy 1994; Chaplin 2004; Einfeld et al. 2011; Horovitz et al. 2011; Morgan et al. 2008; Whitaker and Read 2006). Further, psychopathology appears to be relatively stable in this population (Horovitz et al. 2011). Some experts suggest that psychopathology is the most common and serious complication that co-occurs with ID (Tonge and Einfeld 2003).

Additionally, challenging behavior (CB) is also frequently exhibited and is sometimes included in psychopathology research among this population (Matson and Rivet 2008). CB includes a variety of disruptive and/or dangerous behaviors that range from self-injurious behavior (SIB) to aggression and property destruction (Matson and Neal 2009). At present, the relationship between CB and psychopathology is still unclear (Myrbakk and von Tetzchner 2008).

Furthermore, feeding disorders among individuals with ID are also common. These include but are not limited to food refusal, food selectivity, pica, and rumination (Kuhn and Matson 2004). Additionally, sleep problems among individuals with ID occur frequently (Doran et al. 2006; van de Wouw et al. 2012), seemingly at high-

H. L. Adams (✉) · J. L. Matson
Department of Psychology, Louisiana State University, Baton Rouge, LA, USA
e-mail: Hilary.1.adams@gmail.com

J. L. Matson, M. L. Matson (eds.), *Comorbid Conditions in Individuals with Intellectual Disabilities,* Autism and Child Psychopathology Series,
DOI 10.1007/978-3-319-15437-4_1

er rates than among the general population (e.g., 8.5–34.1 % across reviewed studies, see van de Wouw et al. 2012). These problems include but are not limited to night waking, waking early, low sleep efficiency, delayed sleep onset, and sleep apnea.

Beyond criteria-based syndromes or disorders, persons with ID may face additional difficulties that affect their quality of life (QOL) and limit their opportunities for integration into society. Issues include medical problems that are more common among individuals with ID than the general population, such as epilepsy (Bowley and Kerr 2000; Matson and Sevin 1994), and troubles frequently faced by the general population, such as obesity and dementia (Evenhuis 1997). Motor skills may also be affected among this population (Hartman et al. 2010; Simons et al. 2008), decreasing the likelihood of both independent movement and the ability to complete activities of daily living.

Fortunately, increased attention has been given to the needs of individuals with ID (Hatton 2002). The present chapter aims to provide prevalence estimates and brief overviews of the existing knowledge about the aforementioned disorders and additional problems that a population with ID may face. In-depth explanations of each issue are provided in the following chapters. Additionally, discussions of related topics with growing bodies of research are included, such as assessment of psychopathology and other issues, risk factors, and implications of the co-occurring incidence of issues beyond the presence of ID.

Prevalence Rates

Although experts agree that individuals with ID commonly exhibit psychopathology and additional problems, prevalence rates vary widely. Discussion of the factors that may affect prevalence rates is crucial in order to illuminate shortcomings of the reported estimates and to urge professionals to use caution when considering these statistics as they stand. As such, in the following section, explanations of factors affecting prevalence rates for this particular population are provided, followed by the prevalence rates themselves.

Factors Influencing Reported Prevalence Rates

Assessment of Comorbidity in Intellectual Disability Assigning diagnoses is an inherent component in determining prevalence rates of disorders. Among individuals with ID, diagnostic assessment is complicated by a number of factors. As such, prevalence rates may differ between studies based on their assessment method and the influence of additional complicating components.

With much of assessment of psychopathology based on self-report, the ability to conceptualize and communicate emotions is a skill that is important for accurate recognition of disorders (Cooper et al. 2003; Costello and Bouras 2006). However, self-report measures may be difficult or impossible for persons with ID to complete due to the presence of communication skill deficits (Bhaumik et al. 2008;

Deb et al. 2001; Hatton 2002). Although not considered a definitive symptom of ID, communication problems are common among this population (Bott et al. 1997; Bradshaw 2001). As a result, clinicians should consider both severity of cognitive disability and communication ability when choosing a diagnostic assessment technique.

For instance, for some persons with mild or moderate ID, measures designed for typically developing (TD) individuals may be appropriate and sufficient, as many of these individuals can adequately describe their mental states (Hatton 2002). Further, persons with mild ID seem to have similar clinical presentations, including suicidal ideation, as TD individuals, and thus generally can be assessed using standard practice with few adjustments (Bouras and Drummond 1992; Hurley 2006). For example, if using standard self-report measures among this population, language should be adapted to a developmentally appropriate level, and the interviewer should be ready to clarify or rephrase while avoiding use of leading questions (Cooper et al. 2003).

An alternative frequently used for diagnostic assessment among this population is the informant-report measure, in which a caregiver or relative provides information about the individual's behavior (Costello and Bouras 2006). The quality of this information depends upon a number of factors including the relationship between the caregiver and the person with ID (e.g., experience with the person, time spent together) and the qualifications of the caregiver (e.g., experience with persons with ID, quality of observations, ability to recognize change in behavior or function; Cooper et al. 2003). Additionally, more prominent symptoms that present significant challenges for caregivers are more likely to be reported than behavior that is less noticeable or problematic (Cooper et al. 2003). That is, SIB or physical aggression are likely to have increased implications for the caregiver and thus may be reported as the primary concern, whereas social withdrawal or loss of interest do not present danger and consequently are more likely to be ignored. As such, informant-report measures should not be used in isolation to determine diagnoses. Instead, self-report and informant-report techniques should be used in conjunction with other sources of information, such as behavioral observations and historical records.

Behavioral observations conducted by an experienced professional are critical. For individuals with severe or profound ID, reliable and valid structured observation measures that assess behavior allow professionals to interpret behavior as communicative of internal state and experience (Adams and Oliver 2011). Research is mixed on whether or not maladaptive behaviors are observable signs of psychopathology (i.e., so called "behavioral equivalents"), but behavioral observations are nonetheless an essential component of any assessment. Further, caregivers who are asked to report symptoms often find items that address observed behavior easier to answer than items that include psychiatric terminology (Bouras and Drummand 1992).

Additionally, historical information may also play a role in diagnostic decisions. This component allows the assessor to consider change in functioning over time. Further, if good historical data are available, this information may also help to determine age of onset of symptoms, which is necessary for certain diagnoses that generally begin in early development.

Manifestations of Disorder and Application of Standardized Criteria "Diagnostic overshadowing" may be another cause of imprecise prevalence rates, in that symptoms related to psychopathology may be inaccurately attributed to ID, resulting in underestimates of disorder among this population (Costello and Bouras 2006). Developmental factors may contribute to the presentation of such symptoms, but symptoms cannot be fully attributed to ID (Cooper et al. 2003). Hatton (2002) provided a helpful example, noting that problems with self-care actually attributable to negative symptoms of psychosis could be overlooked as deficits inherent to ID. Further, symptoms that are perceived as minimally problematic, such as internalizing symptoms, may be overshadowed by more serious problems, like CB in the form of aggression toward others.

Additionally, there is some concern that symptoms of psychopathology are being missed among this population because they are manifested differently than in TD individuals (Costello and Bouras 2006; Deb et al. 2001). Similarly, some criteria require sophisticated intellectual abilities in order to understand concepts (e.g., hopelessness, guilt) related to symptoms. For these and other reasons, applicability of standard diagnostic criteria (e.g., DSM, ICD), designed for TD individuals, may not be appropriate to use and has not been extensively tested without modifications on a population with ID (Hatton 2002).

Diagnostic criteria have been developed specifically for use with individuals with ID, such as the Diagnostic Criteria for Psychiatric Disorders for Use with Adults with Learning Disorder/Mental Retardation (DC-LD; Royal College of Psychiatrists 2001), which are intended for diagnosis of adults that have moderate to profound ID (Cooper 2003). When developing the criteria, the task force conducted a literature review that focused on clinical presentation of psychopathology among this population. However, they found that the research available on this topic was very limited, and thus used a "combined evidence-based and pragmatic consensus approach" to determine criteria (Cooper et al. 2003, p. 47; Hatton 2002).

In the subsequent field-testing, psychiatrists separately diagnosed 709 clinical cases based on clinical judgment and then based on the DC-LD (Cooper et al. 2003). They found agreement between clinical judgment and DC-LD diagnoses in 96.3 % of the sample. The criteria are not intended for children or adolescents and may be less appropriate for application to individuals with mild ID than existing criteria for TD individuals. Nevertheless, development of criteria specifically for an ID population is promising, and further work should be conducted in order to provide refinement of and empirical support for proposed criteria. An appropriate taxonomy system would allow for better clinical management and service planning among this population, as well as allow valid comparisons between research studies (Cooper et al. 2003).

Furthermore, some behaviors commonly exhibited by persons with ID (e.g., stereotypic behavior, CB) do not appropriately fit into current diagnostic criteria, which could indicate that such standardized criteria may not be as applicable (Costello and Bouras 2006; Tonge and Einfeld 2003). Researchers have not yet clarified whether some behaviors commonly exhibited by individuals with ID are symptoms of psychopathology or independent behavior problems unrelated to mental disorder (Hatton 2002; McIntyre et al. 2002). Thus, some researchers have specified whether or not prevalence rates included CB or strictly delineated, standardized, and criteria-based diagnoses in their results (e.g., Cooper et al. 2007a).

Procedural Differences and Limitations Additional complicating matters in determining accurate prevalence rates of comorbidity in ID are procedural differences or limitations among studies (Cooper et al. 2007a; Costello and Bouras 2006; Deb et al. 2001; Dekker and Koot 2003; Morgan et al. 2008; Vereenooghe and Langdon 2013; Whitaker and Read 2006). These issues range from conceptual issues, such as the application of a diagnostic system, to a population for which it may not be appropriate, to methodological issues, such as utilizing unrepresentative samples.

One such issue in determining prevalence rates of psychopathology in ID is the question of what merits inclusion. General terms, such as "mental disorder," may be operationally defined differently for each individual study. Even with procedural details included, results are difficult to compare among studies. As a result, a consensus is challenging to determine. To resolve this issue, and to allow for greater generalization of findings, some authors recommend using the term "mental health problem" to characterize symptoms, signs, or abnormal traits that are generally associated with psychopathology (Costello and Bouras 2006). This broader term may encompass clusters of symptoms, generally called syndromes/disorders, or a significantly severe, disabling, or distressing behavior that may be present on its own.

Methodological Limitations Beyond these conceptual issues, methodological problems may also be present among these studies. For instance, many prevalence findings are based on samples of individuals that have accessed services, which may reflect a population with more prevalent or severe comorbidity than occurs in the overall population of people with ID (Whitaker and Read 2006). Biased sampling like this, with results based on institutional or clinic samples that likely have higher rates than an overall population with ID (Costello and Bouras 2006), may skew estimates (Cooper et al. 2007a; Deb et al. 2001).

Additionally, many researchers have utilized record reviews or case files to determine prevalence rates. In some instances, this type of study may limit the reliability and/or validity of results, should insufficient information be available regarding diagnostic procedures (e.g., training of the person assigning the diagnosis, assessment measures utilized, diagnostic criteria used; Cooper et al. 2007a; Dekker and Koot 2003). Also, inaccurate prevalence rates may result from the use of screening measures rather than full diagnostic assessments (Costello and Bouras 2006; Deb et al. 2001; Emerson 2003), particularly in terms of inflating estimates based on checklists of symptoms rather than comprehensive analyses. Taking these issues into account, the standard for sampling for an epidemiological study, applied in order to avoid bias, is the use of population-based, representative samples (Dankner and Dykens 2012), along with the use of comprehensive assessment to determine diagnosis.

Overall Prevalence Statistics

Overall, research suggests that individuals with mild ID can have the same range of mental illness as their TD counterparts and at comparable or higher prevalence rates (Hatton 2002). However, persons with more severe ID may have somewhat different clinical presentations, posing a greater challenge to classification systems and a barrier to assessment (Hatton 2002), thus rendering prevalence study results general estimates lacking conclusive statistics. Additionally, overall prevalence rates of mental health issues may be misleading because researchers sometimes include CB and Autism Spectrum Disorder (ASD), both of which commonly co-occur with ID (Matson and Neal 2009; Matson and Shoemaker 2009), in their results. As such, studies that include these common problems may result in inflated rates of overall psychopathology prevalence (Allen et al. 2012; Emerson et al. 1999). Consequently, comparisons with the general population may be inaccurate in terms of these overarching statistics. Studies that differentiate between disorders (i.e., separate CB and ASD from other diagnoses, consider prevalence of individual diagnoses separately) may be more valuable for comparisons (e.g., Cooper et al. 2007a).

Nonetheless, rates of overall psychopathology are included in this discussion because numerous researchers have investigated this topic. Rates separated by disorder are provided and likely deserve more consideration. Additionally, these rates appear to differ based on age; as such, prevalence rates are presented for adults separately from children and adolescents.

Prevalence Among Adults When making comparisons between an ID population and the general population, most researchers have assessed prevalence of psychopathology among samples with wide age ranges or among adults separately (Cooper et al. 2007a). A better method is to focus on either adults or children and adolescents when examining psychopathology among individuals with ID, as prevalence and other factors (e.g., clinical presentation) appear to differ somewhat with age. A discussion of studies that used adult samples will be provided first. Among adults with ID, review articles cite prevalence rates of psychopathology ranging from 7 to 97 % (Cooper et al. 2007a), with most prevalence statistics in the 30–50 % range (O'Brien 2002). To illustrate the variance among methodologies and results, the following brief summaries of these components for a small sample of studies, representative of the state of the field at present, are provided.

Morgan and colleagues (2008) found the rate of psychiatric morbidity of any type to be 33 % in their large sample of participants whose information they extracted from a registration database. Similarly, in their population-based sample of adults with ID seeking social, health, voluntary, or independent sector services per a register, Bhaumik and colleagues (2008) found that 33.8 % had an ICD-10-based psychiatric disorder. When behavior disorder was excluded from their analysis, 20.2 % of adult participants had a psychiatric disorder.

Deb and colleagues (2001) examined prevalence of comorbid disorders among a sample of 90 adults with ID. These authors used a standardized assessment, including interviews with participants and their caregivers, and ICD-10 criteria for diagnoses. They excluded Attention-Deficit/Hyperactivity Disorder (ADHD) and ASD from their analysis because they are childhood-onset disorders, and diagnosis cannot be determined without historical information, to which they did not have access. They found that only 14.4 % of their sample had a diagnosis. Using similar methodology, Cooper and colleagues examined point prevalence of clinical diagnoses based upon comprehensive assessments of a population-based sample of adults with ID (Cooper et al. 2007a). When they excluded CB and ASD from their analysis, they determined a prevalence rate of 22.4 % of co-occurring disorders. With CB and ASD included, that prevalence rate jumped to 40.9 %. Additionally, 29.1 % of the sample had one diagnosis, while 9.2 % had two diagnoses, 2.4 % had three diagnoses, and .2 % had four diagnoses.

Prevalence Among Children/Adolescents As aforementioned, using a sample with a wide range of ages is not advised. Instead, adults should be considered separately from children and adolescents, among whom researchers have found distinctions in various aspects of psychopathology and other issues. A discussion of studies that used child and adolescent samples is provided. For children and adolescents with ID, review articles cite prevalence rates of psychopathology ranging from 31 to 50 % (Emerson 2003). Similarly, several community-based studies of prevalence reported rates of diagnosable psychiatric problems ranging from 35 to 40 % among children and adolescents with ID (Emerson and Hatton 2007).

In their analysis, Emerson (2003) examined psychopathology in a population of children with ID using a standardized assessment and ICD-10 criteria and classifications of ID based on parent or teacher report. Their assessment consisted of two interviews (child and caregiver) and a teacher questionnaire. The authors found that 39 % of their sample had a diagnosis (19 % had one diagnosis, 16 % had two diagnoses, and 3 % had three or more diagnoses). With similar methodology and results, Dekker and Koot (2003) examined comorbid psychopathology among a sample of children and adolescents with borderline to mild ID. They utilized a standardized measure and DSM-IV criteria to assign diagnoses. Their results indicated that 38.6 % of their sample had a diagnosis of psychopathology, with 14.2 % having multiple diagnoses. In line with these statistics, Molteno and colleagues (2001) reported a prevalence rate of 31 % for psychopathology among their sample of children with ID from special educational facilities.

Prevalence Rates and Research by Disorder or Problem

In their studies in which overall prevalence of psychopathology was included, most researchers also reported statistics for each disorder in order to indicate which disorders were most commonly present among their samples. Among adults, Bhaumik and colleagues (2008) found behavior disorder most common (19.8 %), followed by ASD (8.8 %), depression (4.3 %), and bipolar affective disorder (3.0 %). Deb and colleagues (2001) found the greatest rates of schizophrenia (4.4 %) and phobic disorder (4.4 %) in their adult sample. In the study by Cooper and colleagues, the most common clinical diagnosis for adults with ID was CB (22.5%), followed by ASD (7.5%), affective disorder (6.6%), psychotic disorder (4.4%), and anxiety disorder (3.8%), with phobic disorder excluded from their analysis (Cooper et al. 2007a). Among children and adolescents in his sample, Emerson (2003) found 25% had a conduct disorder, 9.5% had an emotional disorder, 8.7% had an anxiety disorder, 7.6% had PDD, and 0.0% had a psychotic disorder.

As aforementioned, comparing overall prevalence rates can be misleading in that the high prevalence of CB and ASD in an ID population overshadows the lower rates of other types of psychopathology. As such, comparing rates for each disorder provides a more accurate and representative appraisal. The following sections delineate estimates based on type of disorder or problem and briefly discuss current and/or important topics in the research literature for each disorder.

Challenging Behavior As previously discussed, CB is common among persons with ID. Estimates of CB range from 10 to 17% (Allen et al. 2012; Emerson et al. 2001). CB may be included in overall prevalence rates regarding comorbidity, skewing the interpretation of psychopathology among this population (Allen et al. 2012). However, CB can occur without the presence of a form of psychosis, neurosis, or personality disorder, as displayed in CB that is environmentally driven (Allen et al. 2012). Such forms of CB are unlikely to respond to individual therapies that may specifically target psychiatric symptoms (e.g., psychotropic drug administration; Allen et al. 2012).

Although CB is not a defined disorder per se, and may occur without any psychiatric cause, it is important to consider in an examination of comorbid psychopathology for several reasons. First, CB may be triggered or exacerbated by a comorbid mental disorder among persons with ID (Emerson et al. 1999). Indeed, greater rates of psychopathology were associated with "more demanding" CB (i.e., requiring more resources to manage) in a study by Moss and colleagues (2000). In particular, depression and hypomania were significantly related to presence of CB, with four times and three times increased risk, respectively, compared to individuals without CB. In terms of manifestation of disorder, CB may be the atypical or currently unrecognized presentation of psychopathology among this population (Emerson et al. 1999). Nonetheless, the relationship between CB and psychopathology is yet unknown, with potential influences including type of psychopathology, type and severity of CB, degree of ID, and living conditions (Myrbakk and von Tetzchner 2008). Regardless, CB presents additional challenges for the individual and his or her family similar to that of diagnosed comorbid psychopathology. This may include increased financial burden and exclusion from the community (Moss et al. 2000), interference with education, training, and social development (Matson & Rivet, 2008), breakdown of relationships, and significant physical and psychological costs for the individual and his or her caregivers (James 2013).

Autism Spectrum Disorder Although it is recognized that ASD occurs among an ID population frequently, prevalence studies offer a wide range of estimated rates of this comorbidity. These numbers vary from 4 to 40% of people with ID having comorbid ASD (Matson and Shoemaker 2009). These comorbid conditions may interact and subsequently influence presence or severity of CB and/or additional psychopathology (Matson and Shoemaker 2009), worsening prognosis and increasing negative outcomes. Further, for individuals with ASD and ID, CB may hinder diagnosis of comorbid mental illness (McCarthy et al. 2010).

Much research has been conducted comparing individuals with ASD and ID and individuals with ASD alone. Compared to persons with ASD alone, persons with dual diagnosis may differ in terms of core symptoms of ASD as well as additional comorbid problems (Matson and Shoemaker 2009). As severity of ID increases, escalations in SIB (Murphy et al. 2009) and stereotypy (Goldman et al. 2009) may occur among individuals with comorbid ID and ASD. Nonetheless, some researchers suggest that presence of CB is independent from occurrence of comorbid psychopathology among individuals with both disorders (McCarthy et al. 2010). The relationship between ASD, psychopathology, and CB is not yet fully understood and warrants more empirical analysis.

Anxiety In a review article regarding comorbid anxiety and ID, prevalence estimates of anxiety disorders cited ranged from.63 to 57.3 %, while prevalence of anxiety symptoms ranged from 6 to 31 % (Bailey and Andrews 2003). More recently, Reid and colleagues (2011) examined prevalence of anxiety disorders among a large, population-based sample and determined that 3.8 % of their sample had an anxiety disorder (Reid et al. 2011). Most common anxiety disorders among this sample were generalized anxiety disorder (1.7 %) and agoraphobia (0.7 %).

Various qualities of anxiety as it is manifested in ID and symptoms of ID itself may cloud the diagnostic picture for professionals lacking experience in assessing dual diagnosis. For instance, fears appear to differ between TD adults and their counterparts with ID. Persons with ID appear to have fears representative of their developmental level, with one study showing that adult participants with ID had more similar fears to mental age-matched child participants without ID than chronological age-matched adult participants without ID (Duff et al. 1981). Furthermore, for individuals with severe or profound ID, symptoms that may appear to be associated with anxiety (e.g., shaking, sleep problems, exaggerated startle response) could also be related to other emotional problems, tardive dyskinesia due to long-term psychotropic medication use, or another developmental disorder (Matson et al. 1997).

Obsessive compulsive disorder (OCD) appears to be especially difficult to diagnose among individuals with ID. First, sophisticated communication skills are necessary to describe obsessions. Not only that, but as discussed, the conceptual understanding required to meet standard criteria may not be fully developed in a population with ID. As such, these individuals may not comprehend that their thoughts or actions are excessive or unreasonable, making it particularly hard for them to endorse symptoms included in criteria for TD persons (Bailey and Andrews 2003). Nonetheless, compulsions can generally be recognized with behavioral observations alone. Thus, diagnosis of OCD in this population may be based only on presence of compulsions and whether they interfere with daily life, as this is readily observable and more objective. Nevertheless, compulsions in this population must be differentiated from tics and stereotypy, which are commonly exhibited by individuals with ID, especially those who have comorbid ASD (Bailey and Andrews 2003).

Depression Mood disorders are frequently identified in individuals with ID (Hurley 2006). Prevalence of depression ranges from 4% (Cooper et al. 2007a; Meins 1993) to 8% (White et al. 2005) among adults with ID. In one sample of children with ID, depressive disturbance according to the Children's Depression Inventory (CDI; Kovacs 1992) was found among 11% of the group (Linna et al. 1999).

Notably, cognitive level may affect depressive symptomatology, although there is no consensus regarding this topic. Individuals with mild ID have been found to exhibit similar symptoms as a TD population with depression, whereas depression may manifest as "behavioral depressive equivalents," such as aggression, screaming, SIB, psychomotor change, irritability and anger, and loss of activities of daily living skills, among a population with more serious cognitive deficits (Davis et al. 1997; Marston et al. 1997). As such, diagnostic criteria designed for a TD population may be appropriate for application among persons with less severe cognitive deficits, whereas observational assessment with a focus on behavioral criteria may be more appropriate for individuals with more severe cognitive deficits (Hurley 2006). For the latter population, sadness, irritability, social withdrawal, regression in skills, sleep disturbance, diurnal variation, and aggression have been included in proposed modified criteria (Janowsky and Davis 2005). Nonetheless, results from some research groups do not support the idea of behavioral equivalents, as CB has not been correlated with depression among participants with varying levels of ID, and instead core depressive features proved appropriate (Tsiouris et al. 2003).

Sadness or depression could indicate later suicidal behavior in a population with ID (Merrick et al. 2006). Nonetheless, prevalence of suicide and suicide attempts are much less common among this population than among the general population (Hurley 2006; Merrick et al. 2006). For individuals with ID, risk factors for suicidal behavior include sexual abuse, family instability, stress, and lack of social support (Merrick et al. 2006). Additionally, suicidal thoughts, threats, and behaviors appear to be more common among individuals with less severe ID (i.e., mild or moderate compared to severe or profound; Merrick et al. 2006), so preventative treatment of sadness or depression is indicated to prevent the development of suicidal thoughts or behavior.

Psychosis and Schizophrenia There is some evidence that there is more psychosis, schizophrenia in particular, among persons with ID compared to the general population (Costello and Bouras 2006; Deb et al. 2001) with review articles suggesting a prevalence of 3% versus the estimated 1% in the general population (Melville 2003). In their large sample of information from a registration database, Morgan and colleagues (2008) found rates of schizophrenia among an ID population ranged from 3.7 to 5.1%, which they cited as at least three times higher than among the general population. Similarly, in their review of schizophrenia prevalence among adults with ID, Cooper and colleagues found point prevalence rates between 2.6 and 4.4% (Cooper et al. 2007a).

Compared to TD persons with schizophrenia, persons with ID seem to exhibit more negative symptoms (Welch et al. 2011) and use more psychiatric services (Morgan et al. 2008). However, much like the other disorders mentioned, reliable assessment of psychosis is difficult among individuals with severe or profound ID, as they are generally unable to communicate symptoms (e.g., hallucinations, delusions). Other behavior that may be socially inappropriate but observed among a population with ID, such as talking aloud to oneself or speaking one's thoughts aloud, may be misinterpreted as symptomatic of psychosis (Cooper et al. 2003). In addition to this qualitative difference, presence of schizophrenia may be a risk factor for suicide or self-harm beyond that found in TD individuals (Morgan et al. 2008).

Epilepsy Prevalence estimates for epilepsy suggest the seizure disorder occurs in 20–40% of people with ID, which is about 30 times higher than in the general population (Arshad et al. 2011; Espie et al. 2003). Presence of epilepsy appears to be affected by severity of ID, with one study suggesting that persons with severe ID were four times more likely to have epilepsy than those with mild or moderate ID (Arshad et al. 2011). Epilepsy in this population may also influence the development of psychopathology, although research on this topic is inconclusive at this time, and the manner in which this may occur remains speculative. Suggested influential factors in the development of psychopathology among individuals with comorbid ID and epilepsy include the impact of seizures upon the well-being and quality of life of the individual affected, as well as the role of atypical neural development (Arshad et al. 2011). Nevertheless, some researchers have found no increased risk of comorbid psychopathology among adults with ID and epilepsy, but rather decreased rates of schizophrenia, personality, and anxiety disorders among this group (Arshad et al. 2011).

As in a TD population, the primary intervention for epilepsy among individuals with ID is anti-epileptic drugs (Espie et al. 2003). Less psychopathology among the population with this specific comorbidity may be detected due to the calming and mood-stabilizing effects of anti-epileptic drugs (Landmark 2008).

Appropriate treatment of epilepsy in this population is important because, as discussed, the disorder may be a risk factor for psychopathology in some individuals with ID (Espie et al. 2003). Additionally, successful management of seizures may decrease caregiver burden and stress (Espie et al. 2003).

Comparisons With Prevalence Among Typically Developing Individuals

Beyond ascertaining prevalence estimates of comorbidity in ID, much research has been conducted to determine if ID is a risk factor for psychopathology. That is, does the presence of ID increase the likelihood that an individual will have a mental health problem beyond what may occur in a TD person? This question has been investigated for overall mental health and for individual disorders. Nonetheless, conclusive judgments regarding this topic may not yet be made, as researchers have discovered conflicting patterns in their examinations of this topic.

Research has been conducted that supports the pattern of prevalence that indicates individuals with ID have at least as high or higher rates of psychopathology than the general population (Cooper et al. 2007a; Costello and Bouras 2006). More specifically, Werner and Stawski (2012) suggested in their review that psychiatric illness is twice as common in a population with ID relative to a TD population, with cited estimates of 40 versus 19 %, respectively.

Another group of researchers suggested that major psychopathology occurs in over 40 % of young people with ID, a rate two to three times higher than that found among the general population (Tonge and Einfeld 2003). When reviewing existing literature, Emerson (2003) found that for a population of children with ID compared to a general child population, rates of conduct disorder, anxiety disorder, ADHD, and pervasive developmental disorder (PDD) were higher. Relatedly, Emerson and Hatton (2007) used semi-structured interviews of caregiver and child, as well as teacher questionnaires, in their comparison of psychopathology point prevalence between a TD group and a group of children and adolescents with ID. Of their 28 comparisons between groups, the participants with ID had greater point prevalence rates of psychopathology for 27 comparisons. Comparisons of ASD, hyperkinesis, and any conduct disorder were particularly different between groups. Finally, higher rates of depression were reported among school-age children and adolescents with ID than were reported among their TD counterparts (Hurley 2006).

Nonetheless, Deb and colleagues (2001) found that overall point prevalence of psychiatric illness defined by ICD-10 criteria, excluding behavior disorders, ASD, dementia, and alcohol problems, were similar to that found among the general population. Furthermore, with diagnoses separated, differences did not exist between a group of children with ID and a group of TD children in terms of rates of depressive disorder, eating disorder, and psychosis (Emerson 2003). There is some evidence that there is less depression in a population with ID than the general population (Costello and Bouras 2006), including a review article regarding depression among adults with ID that cited studies reporting equal or lower rates of the disorder as compared to the general population (Janowsky and Davis 2005).

Based on the inconsistencies in prevalence rates due to the aforementioned issues with conducting such analyses, differences in comparative study results are not surprising. In addition to the problems regarding assessing and diagnosing psychopathology among individuals with ID, comparative studies should use similar methodologies, definitions, and criteria between the group with ID and the control group in order to make accurate and reliable comparisons (Whitaker and Read 2006). This may include random sampling of the population as a whole and/or random sampling among individuals with ID, rather than using a sample based on convenience (e.g., clinic referrals; Whitaker and Read 2006), which may inflate rates of psychopathology among the group with ID, subsequently skewing comparisons. As such, further epidemiological studies that compare these two populations should aim to use as similar protocols, in terms of sampling, assessing, and assigning diagnoses, as possible.

Risk Factors for Comorbidity in ID

Various factors may influence the development of mental illness in a population with ID. Such persons may be at increased risk for difficult life situations and may be less resilient due to poor coping skills. They may have a reduced support network and fewer social relationships on which to rely. The severity of their disability and their communication deficits may also play a role in the manifestation of comorbid psychopathology.

Social and Environmental Factors

In their study, Emerson and Hatton (2007) found that children and adolescents with ID were more likely to experience particular social and environmental risk factors that may influence the development of psychopathology. These experiences included the following: lone parent family, income poverty, exposure to two or more negative life events, poor family functioning, primary caregiver has no educational qualifications, household with no paid employment, mother with potential mental health disorder, maternal self-rated physical health less than "good," exposure to three or more potential risk factors. When they statistically removed the influence of these social and environmental risk factors, the researchers found risk for development of psychopathology was significantly decreased.

Similarly, Cooper and colleagues discovered that endorsement of a higher number of life events within the past year was associated with mental ill health (Cooper et al. 2007a). Socioeconomic disadvantage may also play a role in the frequency of adverse life events experienced by this population (Gilmore et al. 2014). In their study of adolescents with ID, Taggart and colleagues (2010) found that the group with CB, hyperactivity, and mental health problems had poorer physical health and experienced a greater number of negative life events than the group without such problems. Finally, the results of another study suggested similar risk factors for children with ID, including the individual's physical health, family dysfunction, and parental psychopathology (Wallander et al. 2006).

Reducing exposure to these adverse situations subsequently reduces risk of development of psychopathology. As such, a multidisciplinary team should be involved in preventative intervention and care for a person with ID and his or her family or other caregivers. Additionally, treatment should target building resilience and teaching coping skills if exposure to the discussed social and environmental situations is inevitable.

Severity of Disability

Severity of cognitive deficits may be a risk factor for comorbid psychopathology among those with ID. But, at present, research is inconclusive regarding how cognitive ability may affect presence of co-occurring disorder, as researchers have published conflicting results (Costello and Bouras 2006). In their large sample, Morgan and colleagues (2008) found that persons with ID and comorbidity were more likely to have IQs in the borderline or mild range than in the severe or profound range. In contrast, Cooper and colleagues cited greater likelihood of mental illness among individuals at lower ability levels (Cooper et al. 2007a). Relatedly, Bhaumik and colleagues (2008) found that psychiatric service use increased as severity of impairment increased. Some experts suggest that psychopathology among individuals with more severe deficits may be less likely to be recognized because atypical behavior may be inaccurately attributed to ID rather than to mental illness (Borthwick-Duffy and Eyman 1990). Goodman and Graham (1996) found that IQ was the strongest predictor of psychiatric disorder among their sample, with an association discovered between lower IQ and more psychiatric problems. Considering this idea in a child sample, Einfeld and Tonge (1996) found less psychopathology among children with profound ID than their counterparts with less severe ID.

Relatedly, some researchers have examined whether ability to communicate, intrinsically linked to severity of ID, may be related to presence of comorbid disorders. In their study, Molteno and colleagues (2001) found that children with ID who lacked the ability to speak exhibited higher levels of psychopathology than their counterparts who could communicate vocally. Nonetheless, Cooper and colleagues suggested that higher prevalence rates of psychopathology among individuals with more severe cognitive deficits could not be accounted for by deficits in communication alone (Cooper et al. 2007a).

Presence of Multiple Diagnoses

The presence of multiple types of comorbid psychopathology may exacerbate symptoms and affect an individual's ability to function. For instance, in their study of children and adolescents with ID, Dekker and Koot (2003) found that young people with multiple DSM-IV diagnosis were 2.9 times more likely to be impaired in two or more domains of everyday functioning than their counterparts with one DSM-IV diagnosis. Further, having ID and ASD or Williams syndrome increases risk of comorbid anxiety (Dankner & Dykens).

Implications of Comorbidity in ID

Implications of having an ID are varied and numerous for the individual affected and his or her family or caregivers. The presence of comorbid psychopathology and related behavior problems among individuals with ID are related to further consequences for QOL (Horovitz et al. 2014) and community involvement (Maes et al. 2003). The risk factors discussed above may not only be associated with presence of psychopathology but also with severity of symptoms, which in turn may influence the degree to which a person and his or her support network is affected. Comorbidity in this population has effects not only on personal independence, school and social functioning, and QOL, but also increases stigmatization and prejudices, reducing the likelihood of full integration for these individuals (Wallander et al. 2003).

Service Use and Cost

Investigations into service use optimization and best fit for individuals with a dual diagnosis are lacking (Chaplin 2004), despite implications of findings in terms of policy change. Instead, research into the service domain has thus far primarily focused on utilization, including comparisons between ID and general populations. For instance, in their comparison of psychopathology among individuals with ID versus TD individuals, Morgan and colleagues (2008) noted that persons with ID and comorbid mental illness were more likely to have an in-patient admission and spent more days admitted than persons with TD and mental illness. Researchers have indicated that the majority of patients with ID in their sample were admitted for inpatient psychiatric care due to aggressive, disruptive, and/or SIB (Charlot et al. 2011).

In one of the few studies looking at outcomes of different service types for individuals with ID and mental illness using a meta-analysis of extant research, Chaplin (2004) discovered that specialist services had better outcomes than those of general services. This result may be related to his other finding that staff members working in general services feel unprepared to serve this population due to lack of training (Chaplin 2004). Knowledge and competence among practitioners serving persons with ID, as well as their attitudes toward service provision to meet mental health needs of this population, have much room for improvement (Werner and Stawski 2012). Poor training leads to inadequate care, making appropriate education critical for serving a population with dual diagnosis.

Because ID is a life-long disability, costs, beyond just financial, associated with the disability are especially high (Ouellette-Kuntz et al. 2005). With increased risk of comorbid psychopathology, persons with ID are also more likely to be prescribed medications that may have additional implications for health, including numerous negative side effects. These negative outcomes may include tardive dyskinesia (Matson et al. 2010), decreased mobility, and serious injury, among many others (Ouellette-Kuntz et al. 2005).

Restrictive Environment and Decreased Opportunity

Having ID and comorbid psychopathology has been found to result in a more restrictive living environment (e.g., not being able to live independently) and less opportunity to participate in community programs (e.g., work placement, outings; Myrbakk and von Tetzchner 2008; Tonge and Einfeld 2003). Moreover, dual diagnosis and/or presence of CB may result in administration of physical or pharmacological restraints (Matson and Boisjoli 2009).

Comorbidity often influences the choice of residential placement (Maes et al. 2003). In a study of young adults with ID and their families, McIntyre and colleagues (2002) found that presence of mental illness and behavior problems affected families' living arrangement decisions. Although deinstitutionalization has occurred in many countries, individuals with more severe deficits, comorbid psychopathology, and/or CB may still require the comprehensive and intensive supports and services provided in a more restrictive setting (Raitasuo et al. 1999; Xenitidis et al. 1999). Typical individuals requiring these environments generally have mild cognitive deficits but have been reported to have psychosis, a prior psychiatric diagnosis, affective symptoms (e.g., affect lability, depressive mood), and/or disruptive symptoms (e.g., instances of aggression; Raitasuo et al. 1999).

Additionally, dual diagnosis may affect learning environment. The presence of psychopathology in persons with ID appears to have a negative effect on learning in a school setting (Molteno et al. 2001). Comorbid psychopathology is likely to impede development of positive school adjustment in children and adolescents with ID (McIntyre et al. 2006). Stressors the students' caregivers experience are likely to become stressors for teachers, presenting challenges in the classroom (McIntyre et al. 2006). Dually diagnosed children and adolescents may not be able to adapt or cope easily to new academic and socio-behavioral demands that are presented when they transition into formal schooling (McIntyre et al. 2006). As such, students with dual diagnosis and/or CB may be segregated into "special schools" rather than integrated, inclusive learning environments (Molteno et al. 2001). To improve acclimation to school, and therefore provide the least restrictive learning environment, clinicians should consider teaching self-regulatory processes and prosocial behavior to children and adolescents with ID (McIntyre et al. 2006).

Implications for Families and Caregivers

As psychiatric and/or behavioral problems co-occur or increase among an individual with ID, caring for that person appears to be increasingly problematic and more of a burden, requiring greater levels of support (Douma et al. 2006; Irazábal et al. 2012; Maes et al. 2003; Unwin and Deb 2011). For some caregivers, receiving feedback that the person with ID for whom they care has additional diagnoses generates similar feelings of grief, loss, and helplessness as to when they were made aware of the person's ID diagnosis (Faust and Scior 2008). Moreover, severity of psychopathology may affect parents or caregivers more than severity of ID (Tonge and Einfeld 2003). Receiving the news of additional diagnoses may result in additional confusion and uncertainty about the future of the person with ID (Faust and Scior 2008). Relatedly, feelings of inadequacy in terms of coping with the situation increase as well (Maes et al. 2003). Although attitudes regarding acceptance of their child did not change as a result of increased problems in terms of additional disorders, parents reported less experience of fun and more difficulty relating to their children (Maes et al. 2003).

Moreover, both increased CB and greater severity of ID predict reduced family QOL (Unwin and Deb 2011). Parents or caregivers of these individuals may feel ill-equipped to provide adequate care and serve additional expected roles (Faust and Scior 2008). In addition to feelings of stress, they may also experience anxiety and anger, fear for their safety, and/or poor sleep (Faust and Scior 2008). Insufficient planning, delivery of information, and inadequate support for the caregiver may result in a need for more resource-intensive interventions (Wodehouse and McGill 2009), generating higher costs for the individual's family, the community, and society as a whole. Use of respite care services, expansion of social networks (e.g., by joining a support group), and provision of information about ID, comorbid disorders, and/or CB and their management may decrease parental stress and improve QOL (Maes et al. 2003). Such support may allow caregivers to remain in this role despite comorbid psychopathology and/or CB exhibited by the person with ID they support (James 2013). Consequently, the caregiver may be less likely to seek out-of-home placement for the individual with ID.

Summary

The present chapter provided a basic overview of the current research on the topic of comorbidity in ID. Overall, extant research suggests that some psychopathology and other problems occur among individuals with ID at greater rates than TD individuals. Although this subject has increased in popularity over the past few decades, much research needs to be conducted to elucidate the conflicting results discovered thus far. Consensuses regarding prevalence rates, manifestation or clinical characteristics of disorder, and risk factors have yet to be established due to conceptual and methodological differences across studies. Standardization of methods needs to occur so that researchers in this field can reach agreement on these topics. More consistent research results will have a major impact clinically in terms of both assessment and treatment of comorbidity among this population, subsequently allowing integration and improved QOL for children, adolescents, and adults with ID.

References

Adams, D., & Oliver, C. (2011). The expression and assessment of emotions and internal states in individuals with severe or profound intellectual disabilities. *Clinical Psychology Review, 31* (3), 293–306.

Allen, D., Lowe, K., Matthews, H., & Anness, V. (2012). Screening for psychiatric disorders in a total population of adults with intellectual disability and challenging behaviour using the PAS-ADD checklist. *Journal of Applied Research in Intellectual Disabilities, 25*(4), 342–349.

American Association on Intellectual and Developmental Disabilities (2010). *Definition of intellectual disability.* Retrieved from www.aamr.org.

Arshad, S., Winterhalder, R., Underwood, L., Kelesidi, K., Chaplin, E., Kravariti, E., & . Tsakanikos, E. (2011). Epilepsy and intellectual disability: Does epilepsy increase the likelihood of co-morbid psychopathology?.*Research in Developmental Disabilities, 32*(1), 353–357.

Bailey, N. M., & Andrews, T. M. (2003). Diagnostic Criteria for Psychiatric Disorders for Use with Adults with Learning Disabilities/Mental Retardation (DC-LD) and the diagnosis of anxiety disorders: a review. *Journal of Intellectual Disability Research, 47*(s1), 50–61.

Bhaumik, S., Tyrer, F. C., McGrother, C., & Ganghadaran, S. K. (2008). Psychiatric service use and psychiatric disorders in adults with intellectual disability. *Journal of Intellectual Disability Research, 52,* 986–995.
Borthwick-Duffy, S. A. (1994). Epidemiology and prevalence of psychopathology in people with mental retardation. *Journal of Consulting and Clinical Psychology, 62*(1), 17.
Borthwick-Duffy, S. A., & Eyman, R. K. (1990). Who are the dually diagnosed? *American Journal on Mental Retardation, 94,* 586–595.
Bott, C., Farmer, R., & Rohde, J. (1997). Behaviour problems associated with lack of speech in people with learning disabilities. *Journal of Intellectual Disability Research, 41*(1), 3–7.
Bouras, N., & Drummond, C. (1992). Behaviour and psychiatric disorders of people with mental handicaps living in the community. *Journal of Intellectual Disability Research, 36*(4), 349–357.
Bowley, C., & Kerr, M. (2000). Epilepsy and intellectual disability. *Journal of Intellectual Disability Research, 44*(5), 529–543.
Bradshaw, J. (2001). Complexity of staff communication and reported level of understanding skills in adults with intellectual disability. *Journal of Intellectual Disability Research, 45*(3), 233–243.
Chaplin, R. (2004). General psychiatric services for adults with intellectual disability and mental illness. *Journal of Intellectual Disability Research, 48*(1), 1–10.
Charlot, L., Abend, S., Ravin, P., Mastis, K., Hunt, A., & Deutsch, C. (2011). Non-psychiatric health problems among psychiatric inpatients with intellectual disabilities. *Journal of Intellectual Disability Research, 55*(2), 199–209.
Cooper, S. A. (2003). The diagnostic criteria for psychiatric disorders for use with adults with learning disabilities/mental retardation (DC-LD) papers. *Journal of Intellectual Disability Research, 47*(s1), 1–2.
Cooper, S. A., Melville, C. A., & Einfeld, S. L. (2003). Psychiatric diagnosis, intellectual disabilities and diagnostic criteria for psychiatric disorders for use with adults with learning disabilities/mental retardation (DC-LD). *Journal of Intellectual Disability Research, 47*(s1), 3–15.
Cooper, S. A., Smiley, E., Morrison, J., Williamson, A., & Allan, L. (2007a). Mental ill-health in adults with intellectual disabilities: Prevalence and associated factors. *The British Journal of Psychiatry, 190,* 27–35.
Cooper, S. A., Smiley, E., Morrison, J., Allan, L., Williamson, A., Finlayson, J., Jackson, A., & Mantry, D. (2007b). Psychosis and adults with intellectual disabilities. *Social Psychiatry and Psychiatric Epidemiology, 42*(7), 530–536.
Costello, H., & Bouras, N. (2006). Assessment of mental health problems in people with intellectual disabilities. *Israel Journal of Psychiatry and Related Sciences, 43*(4), 241–251.
Dankner, N., & Dykens, E. M. (2012). Anxiety in intellectual disabilities: Challenges and next steps. *International Review of Research in Developmental Disabilities, 42,* 57–82.
Davis, J. P., Judd, F. K., & Herrman, H. (1997). Depression in adults with intellectual disability. Part 1: A review. *Australian and New Zealand Journal of Psychiatry, 31*(2), 232–242.
Deb, S., Thomas, M., & Bright, C. (2001). Mental disorder in adults with intellectual disability. 1: Prevalence of functional psychiatric illness among a community-based population aged between 16 and 64 years. *Journal of Intellectual Disability Research, 45,* 495–505.
Dekker, M. C., & Koot, H. M. (2003). DSM-IV disorders in children with borderline to moderate intellectual disability. I: Prevalence and impact. *Journal of the American Academy of Child & Adolescent Psychiatry, 42,* 915–922.
Doran, S. M., Harvey, M. T., & Horner, R. H. (2006). Sleep and developmental disabilities: Assessment, treatment, and outcome measures. *Mental Retardation, 44*(1), 13.
Douma, J. C. H., Dekker, M. C., & Koot, H. M. (2006). Supporting parents of youths with intellectual disabilities and psychopathology. *Journal of Intellectual Disability Research, 50*(8), 570–581.
Duff, R., La Rocca, J., Lizzet, A., Martin, P., Pearce, L., Williams, M., & Peck, C. (1981). A comparison of the fears of mildly retarded adults with children of their mental age and chronological age matched controls. *Journal of Behavior Therapy and Experimental Psychiatry, 12*(2), 121–124.

Einfeld, S. L., & Tonge, B. J. (1996). Population prevalence of psychopathology in children and adolescents with intellectual disability: II epidemiological findings. *Journal of Intellectual Disability Research, 40*(2), 99–109.

Einfeld, S. L., Ellis, L. A., & Emerson, E. (2011). Comorbidity of intellectual disability and mental disorder in children and adolescents: A systematic review. *Journal of Intellectual and Developmental Disability, 36*(2), 137–143.

Emerson, E. (2003). Prevalence of psychiatric disorders in children and adolescents with and without intellectual disability. *Journal of Intellectual Disability Research, 47,* 51–58.

Emerson, E., & Hatton, C. (2007). Mental health of children and adolescents with intellectual disabilities in Britain. *The British Journal of Psychiatry, 191*(6), 493–499.

Emerson, E., Moss, S., & Kiernan, C. (1999). The relationship between challenging behaviour and psychiatric disorders in people with severe developmental disabilities. In N. Bouras & G. Holt (Eds.), *Psychiatric and behavioural disorders in developmental disabilities and mental retardation* (pp. 38–48). Cambridge: Cambridge University Press.

Emerson, E., Kiernan, C., Alborz, A., Reeves, D., Mason, H., Swarbrick, R., Mason, L., & Hatton, C. (2001). The prevalence of challenging behaviors: A total population study. *Research in Developmental Disabilities, 22,* 77–93.

Espie, C. A., Watkins, J., Curtice, L., Espie, A., Duncan, R., Ryan, J. A., Brodie, M. J., Mantala, K., & Sterrick, M. (2003). Psychopathology in people with epilepsy and intellectual disability; an investigation of potential explanatory variables. *Journal of Neurology, Neurosurgery & Psychiatry, 74*(11), 1485–1492.

Evenhuis, H. M. (1997). The natural history of dementia in ageing people with intellectual disability. *Journal of Intellectual Disability Research, 41*(1), 92–96.

Faust, H., & Scior, K. (2008). Mental health problems in young people with intellectual disabilities: The impact on parents. *Journal of Applied Research in Intellectual Disabilities, 21*(5), 414–424.

Gilmore, L., Campbell, M., Shochet, I., Garland, R., Smyth, T., Roberts, C., & West, D. (2014). Promoting resilience in children with intellectual disability: A randomized controlled trial in Australian schools. In S. Prince-Embury & D. H. Sakiofske (Eds.), *Resilience interventions for youth in diverse populations* (pp. 353–373). New York: Springer.

Goldman, S., Wang, C., Salgado, M. W., Greene, P. E., Kim, M., & Rapin, I. (2009). Motor stereotypies in children with autism and other developmental disorders. *Developmental Medicine & Child Neurology, 51*(1), 30–38.

Goodman, R., & Graham, P. (1996). Psychiatric problems in children with hemiplegia: Cross sectional epidemiological survey. *British Medical Journal, 312*(7038), 1065.

Hartman, E., Houwen, S., Scherder, E., & Visscher, C. (2010). On the relationship between motor performance and executive functioning in children with intellectual disabilities. *Journal of Intellectual Disability Research, 54*(5), 468–477.

Hatton, C. (2002). Psychosocial interventions for adults with intellectual disabilities and mental health problems: A review. *Journal of Mental Health, 11*(4), 357–374.

Horovitz, M., Matson, J. L., Sipes, M., Shoemaker, M., Belva, B., & Bamburg, J. W. (2011). Incidence and trends in psychopathology symptoms over time in adults with severe to profound intellectual disability. *Research in Developmental Disabilities, 32*(2), 685–692.

Horovitz, M., Shear, S., Mancini, L. M., & Pellerito, V. M. (2014). The relationship between Axis I psychopathology and quality of life in adults with mild to moderate intellectual disability. *Research in Developmental Disabilities, 35,* 137–143.

Hurley, A. D. (2006). Mood disorders in intellectual disability. *Current Opinion in Psychiatry, 19*(5), 465–469.

Irazábal, M., Marsà, F., García, M., Gutiérrez-Recacha, P., Martorell, A., Salvador-Carulla, L., & Ochoa, S. (2012). Family burden related to clinical and functional variables of people with intellectual disability with and without a mental disorder. *Research in Developmental Disabilities, 33*(3), 796–803.

Janowsky, D. S., & Davis, J. M. (2005). Diagnosis and treatment of depression in patients with mental retardation. *Current Psychiatry Reports, 7*(6), 421–428.

James, N. (2013). The formal support experiences of family carers of people with an intellectual disability who also display challenging behaviour and/or mental health issues: What do carers say? *Journal of Intellectual Disabilities, 17*(1), 6–23.

Kovacs, M. (1992). *The Child Depression Inventory (CDI)*. New York: Multi-health Systems.

Kuhn, D. E., & Matson, J. L. (2004). Assessment of feeding and mealtime behavior problems in persons with mental retardation. *Behavior Modification, 28*(5), 638–648.

Landmark, C. J. (2008). Antiepileptic drugs in non-epilepsy disorders. *CNS drugs, 22*(1), 27–47.

Linna, S. L., Moilanen, I., Ebeling, H., Piha, J., Kumpulainen, K., Tamminen, T., & Almqvist, F. (1999). Psychiatric symptoms in children with intellectual disability. *European Child & Adolescent Psychiatry, 8*(4), S77–S82.

Maes, B., Broekman, T. G., Došen, A., & Nauts, J. (2003). Caregiving burden of families looking after persons with intellectual disability and behavioural or psychiatric problems. *Journal of Intellectual Disability Research, 47*(6), 447–455.

Marston, G. M., Perry, D. W., & Roy, A. (1997). Manifestations of depression in people with intellectual disability. *Journal of Intellectual Disability Research, 41*(6), 476–480.

Matson, J. L., & Boisjoli, J. A. (2009). Restraint procedures and challenging behaviours in intellectual disability: An analysis of causative factors. *Journal of Applied Research in Intellectual Disabilities, 22*(2), 111–117.

Matson, J. L., & Neal, D. (2009). Psychotropic medication use for challenging behaviors in persons with intellectual disabilities: An overview. *Research in Developmental Disabilities, 30*, 572–586.

Matson, J. L., & Shoemaker, M. (2009). Intellectual disability and its relationship to autism spectrum disorders. *Research in Developmental Disabilities, 30*, 1107–1114.

Matson, J. L., & Rivet, T. T. (2008). Characteristics of challenging behaviours in adults with autistic disorder, PDD-NOS, and intellectual disability. *Journal of Intellectual and Developmental Disability, 33*(4), 323–329.

Matson, J. L., & Sevin, J. A. (1994). Theories of dual diagnosis in mental retardation. *Journal of Consulting and Clinical Psychology, 62*(1), 6.

Matson, J. L., Smiroldo, B. B., Hamilton, M., & Baglio, C. S. (1997). Do anxiety disorders exist in persons with severe and profound mental retardation? *Research in Developmental Disabilities, 18*(1), 39–44.

Matson, J. L., Fodstad, J. C., Neal, D., Dempsey, T., & Rivet, T. T. (2010). Risk factors for tardive dyskinesia in adults with intellectual disability, comorbid psychopathology, and long-term psychotropic use. *Research in Developmental Disabilities, 31*(1), 108–116.

Matson, J. L., Belva, B. C., Hattier, M. A., & Matson, M. L. (2012). Scaling methods to measure psychopathology in persons with intellectual disabilities. *Research in Developmental Disabilities, 33*(2), 549–562.

McCarthy, J., Hemmings, C., Kravariti, E., Dworzynski, K., Holt, G., Bouras, N., & Tsakanikos, E. (2010). Challenging behavior and co-morbid psychopathology in adults with intellectual disability and autism spectrum disorders. *Research in Developmental Disabilities, 31*(2), 362–366.

McIntyre, L. L., Blacher, J., & Baker, B. L. (2002). Behaviour/mental health problems in young adults with intellectual disability: The impact on families. *Journal of Intellectual Disability Research, 46*(3), 239–249.

McIntyre, L. L., Blacher, J., & Baker, B. L. (2006). The transition to school: Adaptation in young children with and without intellectual disability. *Journal of Intellectual Disability Research, 50*(5), 349–361.

Meins, W. (1993). Prevalence and risk factors for depressive disorders in adults with intellectual disability. *Journal of Intellectual and Developmental Disability, 18*(3), 147–156.

Melville, C. A. (2003). A critique of the diagnostic criteria for psychiatric disorders for use with adults with learning disabilities/mental retardation (DC-LD) chapter on non-affective psychotic disorders. *Journal of Intellectual Disability Research, 47*(s1), 16–25.

Merrick, J., Merrick, E., Lunsky, Y., & Kandel, I. (2006). A review of suicidality in persons with intellectual disability. *Israel Journal of Psychiatry and Related Sciences, 43*(4), 258.

Molteno, G., Molteno, C., Finchilescu, G., & Dawes, A. R. L. (2001). Behavioural and emotional problems in children with intellectual disability attending special schools in Cape Town, South Africa. *Journal of Intellectual Disability Research, 45*(6), 515–520.

Morgan, V. A., Leonard, H., Bourke, J., & Jablensky, A. (2008). Intellectual disability co-occurring with schizophrenia and other psychiatric illness: Population-based study. *The British Journal of Psychiatry, 193,* 364–372.

Moss, S., Emerson, E., Kiernan, C., Turner, S., Hatton, C., & Alborz, A. (2000). Psychiatric symptoms in adults with learning disability and challenging behaviour.*The British Journal of Psychiatry, 177*(5), 452–456.

Murphy, O., Healy, O., & Leader, G. (2009). Risk factors for challenging behaviors among 157 children with autism spectrum disorder in Ireland. *Research in Autism Spectrum Disorders, 3*(2), 474–482.

Myrbakk, E., & von Tetzchner, S. (2008). Psychiatric disorders and behavior problems in people with intellectual disability. *Journal of Intellectual Disability Research,*(4), 316–332.

O'Brien, G. (2002). Dual diagnosis in offenders with intellectual disability: setting research priorities: a review of research findings concerning psychiatric disorder (excluding personality disorder) among offenders with intellectual disability. *Journal of Intellectual Disability Research, 46*(s1), 21–30.

Ouellette-Kuntz, H., Minnes, P., Garcin, N., Martin, C., Lewis, M. E., & Holden, J. J. (2005). Addressing health disparities through promoting equity for individuals with intellectual disability. *Canadian Journal of Public Health, 96*(2), S8–22.

Raitasuo, S., Taiminen, T., & Salokangas, R. K. R. (1999). Characteristics of people with intellectual disability admitted for psychiatric inpatient treatment. *Journal of Intellectual Disability Research, 43*(2), 112–118.

Reid, K. A., Smiley, E., & Cooper, S. A. (2011). Prevalence and associations of anxiety disorders in adults with intellectual disabilities. *Journal of Intellectual Disability Research, 55*(2), 172–181.

Reiss, S., & Valenti-Hein, D. (1994). Development of a psychopathology rating scale for children with mental retardation. *Journal of Consulting and Clinical Psychology, 62*(1), 28.

Royal College of Psychiatrists. (2001). *DC–LD: Diagnostic criteria for psychiatric disorders for use with adults with learning disabilities/mental retardation, (occasional paper OP48).* London: Gaskell.

Simons, J., Daly, D., Theodorou, F., Caron, C., Simons, J., & Andoniadou, E. (2008). Validity and reliability of the TGMD-2 in 7–10-year-old Flemish children with intellectual disability. *Adapted Physical Activity Quarterly, 25*(1), 71–82.

Soenen, S., Van Berckelaer-Onnes, I., & Scholte, E. (2009). Patterns of intellectual, adaptive and behavioral functioning in individuals with mild mental retardation. *Research in Developmental Disabilities, 30*(3), 433–444.

Taggart, L., Taylor, D., & McCrum-Gardner, E. (2010). Individual, life events, family and socioeconomic factors associated with young people with intellectual disability and with and without behavioural/emotional problems. *Journal of Intellectual Disabilities, 14*(4), 267–288.

Tonge, B. J., & Einfeld, S. L. (2003). Psychopathology and intellectual disability: The Australian child to adult longitudinal study. In L. M. Glidden (Ed.), *International review of research in mental retardation* (pp. 61–91). San Diego: Academic.

Tsiouris, J. A., Mann, R., Patti, P. J., & Sturmey, P. (2003). Challenging behaviours should not be considered as depressive equivalents in individuals with intellectual disability. *Journal of Intellectual Disability Research, 47*(1), 14–21.

Unwin, G., & Deb, S. (2011). Family caregiver uplift and burden: Associations with aggressive behavior in adults with intellectual disability. *Journal of Mental Health Research in Intellectual Disabilities, 4*(3), 186–205.

van de Wouw, E., Evenhuis, H. M., & Echteld, M. A. (2012). Prevalence, associated factors and treatment of sleep problems in adults with intellectual disability: A systematic review. *Research in Developmental Disabilities, 33*(4), 1310–1332.

Vereenooghe, L., & Langdon, P. E. (2013). Psychological therapies for people with intellectual disabilities: A systematic review and meta-analysis. *Research in Developmental Disabilities, 34,* 4085–4102.

Wallander, J. L., Dekker, M. C., & Koot, H. M. (2003). Psychopathology in children and adolescents with intellectual disability: Measurement, prevalence, course, and risk. *International Review of Research in Mental Retardation, 26,* 93–134.

Welch, K. A., Lawrie, S. M., Muir, W., & Johnstone, E. C. (2011). Systematic review of the clinical presentation of schizophrenia in intellectual disability. *Journal of Psychopathology and Behavioral Assessment, 33*(2), 246–253.

Wallander, J. L., Dekker, M. C., & Koot, H. M. (2006). Risk factors for psychopathology in children with intellectual disability: A prospective longitudinal population-based study. *Journal of Intellectual Disability Research, 50*(4), 259–268.

Werner, S., & Stawski, M. (2012). Mental health: Knowledge, attitudes and training of professionals on dual diagnosis of intellectual disability and psychiatric disorder. *Journal of Intellectual Disability Research, 56*(3), 291–304.

Whitaker, S., & Read, S. (2006). The prevalence of psychiatric disorders among people with intellectual disabilities: An analysis of the literature. *Journal of Applied Research in Intellectual Disabilities, 19*(4), 330–345.

White, P., Chant, D., Edwards, N., Townsend, C., & Waghorn, G. (2005). Prevalence of intellectual disability and comorbid mental illness in an Australian community sample. *Australian and New Zealand Journal of Psychiatry, 39*(5), 395–400.

Wodehouse, G., & McGill, P. (2009). Support for family carers of children and young people with developmental disabilities and challenging behaviour: What stops it being helpful? *Journal of Intellectual Disability Research, 53*(7), 644–653.

Xenitidis, K. I., Henry, J., Russell, A. J., Ward, A., & Murphy, D. G. M. (1999). An inpatient treatment model for adults with mild intellectual disability and challenging behaviour. *Journal of Intellectual Disability Research, 43*(2), 128–134.

Part II
Psychological Disorders

Chapter 2
Challenging Behaviors

Max Horovitz

Introduction

Challenging behaviors (CB) are one of the most important comorbid conditions found in individuals with intellectual disability (ID). Given the debilitating nature of CB, and their frequent comorbidity with ID (Durand and Carr 1992; Loftin et al. 2008; Matson and Dempsey 2009; Matson et al. 2009b; Matson et al. 1997; Morrison and Rosales-Ruiz 1997), it should come as no surprise that a wealth of literature exists regarding CB in this population (Matson and Cervantes 2013; Matson et al. 2011). The purpose of this chapter is to review the definition, prevalence, and intervention of CB in individuals with ID.

Definition of CB

While an abundance of literature exists on the topic of CB, many researchers have different definitions for the term and no clear consensus exists (Didden et al. 2012; Medeiros et al. 2012). Further complicating matters is that CB are often given different labels by different researchers, such as maladaptive, aberrant, externalizing, or problem behaviors (Mudford et al. 2008). However, as research in this area has developed, a general consensus on using the term CB has emerged (Brylewski and Duggan 1999). Emerson et al. (2001) described CB as those that "present a significant challenge to carers and support agencies." He later went on to define them as "culturally abnormal behavior of such intensity, frequency or duration that the physical safety of the person or others is placed in serious jeopardy, or behavior which is likely to seriously limit or deny access to the use of ordinary community facilities" (Emerson 2005). Mudford et al. (2008) defined CB as "Any behavior

M. Horovitz (✉)
Keystone Behavioral Pediatrics, Jacksonville, FL, USA
e-mail: maxh13@gmail.com

J. L. Matson, M. L. Matson (eds.), *Comorbid Conditions in Individuals with Intellectual Disabilities*, Autism and Child Psychopathology Series,
DOI 10.1007/978-3-319-15437-4_2

performed to excess in frequency or intensity, and beyond the immediate resources available for effective treatment." Additionally, in a similar fashion to Emerson et al. (2001), they included any behaviors that might interfere with learning, safety, or community integration. Furthering these definitions, Holden and Gitlesen (2006) distinguished between more and less demanding CB. This distinction was based on the amount of support needed to manage the behaviors and the amount of interference caused by these behaviors. Together, these definitions reflect an evolving definition of what categorizes a behavior as CB.

Researchers have further debated the definition of CB as they relate to psychopathology. More specifically, some researchers have argued that CB in individuals with ID represent so-called "behavioral equivalents" of psychopathology (Hurley2006); Marston et al. (1997); Witwer and Lecavalier (2010). This argument has been made due to the fact that it can often be difficult to apply the diagnostic criteria of various forms of psychopathology to individuals with ID. As such, authors have argued that CB, such as aggression or self-injury, may represent observable signs of psychopathology, such as depression (Marston et al. (1997). However, other researchers have cautioned against such assumptions (Ross and Oliver (2003); Tsiouris et al. 2003; Witwer and Lecavalier 2010). Sturmey et al. (2010) examined the relationship between a measure of depression and hypothesized behavioral equivalents of depression in a sample of 693 adults with ID. They found little relationship between measured depressive symptoms and CB and concluded that there is little support for interpreting CB as symptoms of psychopathology, at least as related to depression. Other researchers have found similar results and made similar conclusions (Ross and Oliver 2003; Tsiouris et al. 2003; Witwer and Lecavalier 2010). While Sturmey et al. (2010) did find a relationship between some CB and symptoms of mania, they cautioned that such findings are still preliminary and recommended that clinicians continue to focus on core symptoms when making a diagnosis. It has been argued that CB may be a general indicator of overall impairment, rather than indicative of a specific form of psychopathology (Witwer and Lecavalier 2010).

While there has been some debate as how to best define the term CB, there is more agreement as to what behaviors actually fall under this category. In fact, most researchers define CB by the specific classes of behaviors being studied. The most frequently cited CB include self-injurious behavior (SIB), aggression towards others, stereotypy, destruction of property, inappropriate sexual behaviors, screaming, noncompliance, disruptions, and eating inedible objects (Emerson et al. 2001; Holden and Gitlesen 2006; Matson and Nebel-Schwalm 2007). Yet, even within these terms, ambiguity exists as to what specific behaviors fall under each of these categories. As such, a brief discussion will be given regarding the definitions and various topographies of the most frequently cited categories of CB.

Self-injurious Behavior (SIB)

SIBs can, in their simplest form, be defined as self-directed behaviors that either cause or have the potential to cause injury, such as tissue damage (Didden et al. 2012; Kress 2003; Schroeder et al. 1980; Tate and Baroff 1973). This definition does not include behaviors such as suicidal behaviors, sexual behaviors, or socially typical behaviors (Didden et al. 2012; Winchel and Stanley 1991). While the basics of this definition are typically agreed upon, researchers have argued whether additional factors should be included in the definition. For example, some authors have argued the importance of intent, arguing that deliberate intent is inherent to the definition of SIB (e.g., Glaesser and Perkins 2013; Klonsky and Muehlenkamp 2007; Winchel and Stanley 1991). Others have removed the requirement of intent, focusing only on observable behavior in an attempt to avoid making incorrect inferences (e.g., Rojahn et al. 2007; Tureck et al. 2013). Other definitions of SIB have included (or purposefully excluded) their repetitive nature, degree and type of damage caused, self-evidence, pathological nature, the presence of frustration or anxiety motivating the behaviors, their relationship to ID and ASD, and the various topographies typically included under the label of SIB (Matson and Turygin 2012; Oliver et al. 1987; Rojahn et al. 2001; Schroeder et al. 1980; Tureck et al. 2013). Additionally, Matson and Turygin (2012) stressed the need to differentiate the term SIB from the term self-injury that has been traditionally used in the mental health field and has been associated with disorders such as borderline personality disorder, depression, and sexual abuse. In a similar fashion to CB, researchers often define SIB by the individual topographies included under the term.

Researchers have described numerous behaviors as encompassing the term SIB. The Behavior Problems Inventory (BPI; Rojahn et al. 2001), an assessment of CB in individuals with ID, lists the following behaviors under the domain of SIB: self-biting, head-hitting, body-hitting, self-scratching, vomiting, self-pinching, pica, stuffing objects, nail-pulling, poking, aerophagia, hair pulling, over drinking, and teeth-grinding. Other behaviors that have previously been included under this term include face slapping, self-choking, eye poking, hand-mouthing, and finger sucking (Didden et al. 2012; Iwata et al. 1994; Kahng et al. 2002). In a review of behavioral interventions for SIB, Kahng et al. (2002) found head-banging/hitting to be the most frequently cited form of SIB, followed by biting, hand-mouthing, and body-hitting. In a review of various forms of SIB, Didden et al. (2012) emphasized additional factors that must be considered when discussing the various topographies of SIB, including range of severity, frequency of occurrence, and social basis for the behaviors.

Aggressive Behaviors

As with SIB, no single definition of aggressive behaviors exists; Didden et al. 2012). Rojahn et al. (2001) defined aggressive behaviors as "abusive, deliberate attacks against other individuals or objects." In a study on aggressive behaviors in children with an autism spectrum disorder (ASD), Farmer and Aman (2011 discuss a number of problems that arise when trying to define aggressive behaviors. Firstly, a variety of terms have been used to describe aggressive behaviors, in an attempt to avoid the negative social connotations inherent to the aggressive label; Crocker et al. 2006; Farmer and Aman 2011). Additionally, researchers have traditionally attributed intent to the definition of physical aggression (as in the definition above), which can be difficult when applied to the ID population. Individuals with ID have impaired cognitive ability and may have difficulty empathizing with or taking the perspective of another individual (Farmer and Aman 2011). Thus the assumption of intent may be somewhat misguided when used with the ID population. Because of this, Farmer and Aman (2011 recommended looking at the various subtypes and topographies of aggressive behaviors when attempting to create a definition. An additional roadblock to a clear operational definition of aggressive behaviors is that different researchers often include and exclude different topographies when studying aggressive behaviors; Cooper et al. 2009; Crocker et al. 2006). For example, some authors have included destruction of property under the label of aggressive behaviors (e.g., Rojahn et al. 2001; Sturmey et al. 2008; Vitiello and Stoff 1997), while others categorize such behaviors separately (e.g., Lowe et al. 2007). This has led to widespread difficulties in comparing studies of aggressive behaviors (Crocker et al. 2006). In an attempt to make a clear operational definition that takes these difficulties into consideration, Didden et al. (2012 defined aggressive behaviors as "behavior that (potentially) results in injury or harm in another person or in property destruction without consideration of whether the aggressive behavior is 'deliberately' exhibited or not." However, they concede that a distinction usually needs to be made between aggressive behavior directed at objects and aggressive behavior directed at other people. Additionally, they agree on the presence of subcategories of aggression, including physical aggression, verbal aggression, and possibly self-directed aggression (i.e., SIB). Other researchers have similarly agreed on the need to separately examine these subtypes of aggressive behaviors; Cooper et al. 2009; Szymanski 2002). Additional ways to categorize aggression include proactive versus reactive aggression and the type of reinforcement maintaining the aggression (Didden et al. 2009, Farmer and Aman 2011; Matson et al. 2012).

A number of behaviors have been included by researchers under the label aggressive behaviors. The aforementioned BPI (Rojahn et al. 2001), includes the following behaviors under the domain of Aggression/Destruction: hitting, kicking, pushing, biting, grabbing, pulling, scratching, pinching, spitting, verbally abusive, destroys, and cruel. Other behaviors that have previously been included under this term include using threatening gestures, throwing objects at others, ripping clothes, yelling or shouting at others, banging on objects, forcibly taking objects, taking food, using weapons against others, and choking (Lowe et al. 2007; Matson and Rivet 2008a; Sigafoos 1995).

Stereotyped Behaviors

Stereotyped behaviors are often overlooked as a class of CB; yet the consequences of such behaviors can be as significant as those of the others discussed in this chapter (Didden et al. 2012; Loftin et al. 2008; MacDonald et al. 2007; Matson et al. 1997). Such consequences include reduced opportunities for interaction, exclusion from general education settings, impaired adaptive functioning, increased use of psychotropic drugs, and stress for parents and caregivers (Durand and Carr 1992;

Koegel and Covert 1972; Loftin et al. 2008; Matson and Dempsey 2009; Matson et al. 2009a; Matson et al. 1997; Morrison and Rosales-Ruiz 1997). As with the other CB discussed in this chapter, some debate exists as how to best define stereotyped behaviors. This may be due, in part, to a lack of empirical evidence looking at the defining features of stereotyped behaviors (Rapp and Vollmer 2005). Rojahn et al. (2001) defined stereotyped behaviors as "peculiar or inappropriate voluntary acts which occur habitually and repetitively." Berkson (1983 provided additional criteria for behavior to be categorized as stereotyped, including persistence over time, lack of variability, resistance to environmental change, and abnormality for age-related development. This last point is critical, as stereotyped behaviors are frequently displayed by typically developing infants and toddlers (Foster 1998; MacDonald et al. (2007). However, the frequency and intensity of stereotyped behaviors are much higher in atypically developing children (Klonsky and Muehlenkamp 2007). Additionally, they continue to persist throughout life in atypically developing individuals, whereas they decrease with age in typically developing children (MacDonald et al. 2007; Matson and Horovitz 2010). In contrast to Berkson's (1983) definition, some have argued that a degree of variability may exist for some types of stereotyped behaviors (Rapp and Vollmer 2005). Other factors that may be considered when defining stereotyped behaviors include the degree of repetitiveness, periodicity, time spent engaging in the behaviors, the context in which the behaviors occur, function of the behaviors, and the salience of the behaviors (MacDonald et al. 2007; Rapp and Vollmer 2005; Ross et al. 1998; Tierney et al.1978).

It should be noted, that of the CB discussed in this chapter, stereotyped behaviors are the only included in the diagnostic criteria for multiple DSM-5 diagnoses (American Psychiatric Association 2013). Stereotyped behaviors are the essential feature of stereotypic movement disorder. The DSM-5 definition of stereotyped behaviors includes their repetitive nature, lack of apparent purpose, and interference in social, academic, or other activities. Coding of stereotypic movement disorder includes specifiers indicating the presence or absence of SIB and the association with any known medical, genetic, neurodevelopmental, or environmental factors. In addition to being the essential feature of stereotypic movement disorder, stereotyped behaviors are one of the core features of ASD (American Psychiatric Association 2013). The DSM-5 places stereotyped motor movements in the same class as other restricted, repetitive behaviors/interests, including insistence on sameness, inflexible adherence to routines, unusual fixated interests, and hyper- or hyporeactivity to sensory input. Given that stereotyped behaviors are a core feature of both of these disorders that are commonly diagnosed comorbidly with ID, it should be expected that stereotyped behaviors are frequently evinced by individuals with ID.

A number of behaviors have been included by researchers under the label of stereotyped behaviors. Perhaps of all the categories of CB discussed, stereotyped behaviors have the most variability, as any unusual, repetitive behavior can be classified under this label. The aforementioned BPI (Rojahn et al. 2001) includes the following behaviors under the domain stereotyped behavior: rocking, sniffing objects, spinning, waving arms, head-rolling, whirling, body movements, pacing, twirling, hand movements, yelling, sniffing self, bouncing, spinning, running, finger movements, manipulating, sustained finger movements, rubbing self, gazing, posturing, clapping, grimacing, and hand-waving. Other topographies reported in the literature include repetition of words or phrases, unprovoked laughing or giggling, and echolalia (MacDonald et al. 2007).

Prevalence

Many researchers have examined the prevalence of CB in individuals with ID and factors that may increase the risk for the presence of CB. However, due to the tremendous variability in how to best define, significant variability has been seen by researchers on this topic. Emerson et al. (2001) identified a number of additional difficulties that have affected research on the prevalence of CB in individuals with ID: (1) many prevalence studies have focused on specific categories of CB (e.g., SIB), rather than CB as a whole; (2) studies have often focused on subpopulations of people with ID (e.g., those who are institutionalized), rather than the general population of individuals with ID; and (3) the few studies that have looked at CB in general have often failed to collect detailed data on specific forms of CB. Fortunately, the highlighting of these difficulties has led to more methodologically sound studies on the prevalence of CB in recent years. This section will first review various studies on the prevalence of CB in general, particularly those that have taken large-scale approaches and have attempted to address the methodological issues discussed above. This will be followed by findings on the prevalence of specific high-frequency categories of CB (i.e., SIB, aggressive behaviors, and stereotyped behaviors). Finally, risk factors associated with prevalence, both of CB in general and of specific categories of CB, will be discussed.

A number of large-scale population studies have been conducted looking at the prevalence of CB in the ID population. Emerson and colleagues (2001) conducted a total population study in two areas of England. They found CB to be present in 10–15 % of individuals with ID that were screened. Additionally, they found that 5–10 % of individuals with ID exhibited more demanding CB, meaning at least one of the following criteria were present: (1) engaging in the CB at least once a day; (2) the CB usually prevented the person from taking part in program or activities appropriate to their level of ability; (3) the CB usually required physical intervention by staff; or (4) the CB usually led to major injury. In order to be included in this study, less demanding CB had to be perceived as being, or potentially being, significantly difficult to manage. In addition to the findings on more and less demanding CB, Emerson and colleagues (2001) found that most participants engaged in multiple forms of CB (e.g., SIB and aggressive behaviors) and that many engaged in multiple topographies of the same category of CB (e.g., multiple forms of SIB).

A similar total population study was completed in Hedmark, Norway, examining 904 children and adults receiving at least a minimum of care for ID (Holden and Gitlesen 2010, 2006). They found the overall prevalence of CB to be 11.1 %. Using similar criteria to define more and less demanding CB, they found that 7.3 % of the participants engaged in less demanding CB, while 3.8 % engaged in more demanding CB. Holden and Gitlesen (2006) found that individuals with more demanding CB engaged in an average of 2.1 forms of CB, while individuals with less demanding CB engaged in an average of 1.7 forms. They also found that individuals with more demanding CB engaged in a higher number of specific topographies than did people with less demanding CB.

Lundqvist (2013) criticized previous prevalence studies, citing the fact that few studies used a psychometrically sound assessment instrument to determine the presence and frequency of CB. Additionally, Lundqvist (2013) argued that many prevalence studies, in defining what will be considered to indicate the presence of CB, have required the presence of at least one behavior problem considered to be severe. However, less severe problem behaviors may be overlooked by such a definition, despite their clinical significance. For example, the previously discussed studies by Emerson et al. (2001) and Holden and Gitlesen (2006) excluded CB that were not considered to cause significant impairment, despite the use of the high- and low-demand categories. Lundqvist (2013) therefore examined the prevalence of CB in 915 individuals with ID in Örebro, Sweden, using the previously discussed BPI (Rojahn et al. 2001). Lundqvist (2013) found that 62 % of participants engaged in at least one behavior problem on the BPI. However, this number dropped to 18 % if the behavior was required to be rated as severe. This number dropped to 11.8 % if the behavior was required to be rated as severe on a daily basis, meeting criteria similar to the high-demand CB discussed above. These distinctions, in addition to those previously discussed, may help to explain the wide variety of prevalence rates reported in the literature.

Prevalence of Specific Categories of CB

SIB While studies on the prevalence of SIB have been numerous, rates of prevalence have varied greatly, particularly due to the samples included in such studies and the ways in which SIB has been defined (Didden et al. 2012). Emerson et al. (2001) found the prevalence of SIB to be 4 % of the total population of individuals with ID studied. Holden and Gitlesen (2006) found a similar rate, at 4.4 %. They found SIB to occur at similar rates in those engaging in high- and low-demand SIB. However, they found biting and scratching to be two specific topographies that were more common in the high-demand group. As previously discussed, Lundqvist (2013) applied a broader definition to CB, resulting in much higher overall rates of prevalence. As such, he found an overall prevalence rate of 30.9 % for SIB. This meant that 30.9 % of participants were reported to have engaged in at least one form of SIB, regardless of severity or frequency. However, when applying a stricter definition more in line with that of other researchers, this rate dropped to 8.4 %. More demanding forms of SIB were found to occur in 6 % of participants. Lundqvist (2013) found that, of those exhibiting at least one behavior problem, the mean number of SIB topographies was 1.93, and the maximum number of SIB topographies engaged in by one individual was 9. Other researchers have cited slightly higher prevalence estimates, ranging from 10–12 % of individuals with ID (Didden et al.

2012). Factors associated with the prevalence of SIB, such as gender and age, will be discussed further below.

Aggressive Behaviors Emerson et al. (2001) found the prevalence of aggressive behaviors to be 7 % of the individuals investigated. It should be noted that Emerson et al. (2001) categorized aggressive and destructive behaviors separately. They found destructive behaviors to have a prevalence of 4–5 %. Holden and Gitlesen (2006) again found a similar rate at 6.4 %. In contrast to SIB, they found aggressive behaviors to be more frequent in those engaging in high-demand CB. In particular, they found hitting others, hitting others with objects, and biting to occur more frequently in the high-demand group. Additionally, the use of weapons, such as a knife or chair, was more common in the more demanding group. Similar to Emerson et al. (2001), Holden and Gitlesen (2006) categorized aggressive and destructive behaviors separately. They found a prevalence rate of 2.3 % for destructive behaviors. While such behaviors were more frequent in the high-demand group, this difference was not significant. Lundqvist (2013), using his broader definition of CB, found an overall prevalence rate of 34.4 %. He found 11.9 % participants to engage in severe aggressive behaviors. More demanding forms of aggressive behaviors were found to occur in 6.7 % of participants. Of those exhibiting at least one behavior problem, the mean number of aggressive behavior topographies was 3.06, with a maximum of 21.

Stereotyped Behaviors Less research is available on the prevalence of stereotyped behaviors. Neither Emerson et al. (2001) nor Holden and Gitlesen (2006) specifically examined the prevalence of stereotyped behaviors. Lundqvist (2013) found an overall prevalence rate of 41.3 % for stereotyped behaviors. However, only 6.1 % of participants were reported to engage in severe stereotyped behaviors and only 0.8 % of participants were reported to engage in more demanding stereotyped behaviors. This drop may be due to the fact that stereotyped behaviors do not typically have the same likelihood of causing significant injury when compared to SIB and aggressive behaviors and are often viewed as less problematic (Murphy et al. 2009). Other researchers have argued that as many as 50 % of individuals with ID may engage in at least one stereotyped behavior (Didden et al. 2012).

Risk Factors Associated With Prevalence of CB

Researchers have found a number of factors to be associated with higher and lower rates of CB. Such factors include gender, age, level of intellectual impairment, ASD, seizure disorders, genetic syndromes, comorbid psychopathology, level of adaptive behavior functioning, sensory impairments, medical problems, and institutionalization (Didden et al. 2012; Emerson et al. 2005; Holden and Gitlesen 2006; Lundqvist 2013; McClintock et al. 2003). While findings on the effects of these factors have been at times contradictory, some trends have been observed in the literature. A brief discussion will be given on the relationship between these factors and rates of CB.

Gender Many researchers have examined the relationship between gender and prevalence of CB, with often-conflicting findings. Emerson et al. (2001) found that approximately two-thirds of the individuals identified as engaging in CB were male. No statistical comparisons were made, however, limiting the interpretability of this finding. McClintock et al. (2003) conducted a meta-analysis looking at risk factors associated with SIB, aggression, stereotyped behaviors, and destruction of property. While they found no relationship between gender and SIB, they found that males were significantly more likely to engage in aggressive behaviors. However, they cited the need for caution when interpreting this finding, given that only two studies examining this relationship were found. Not enough studies were found by the researchers to examine the relationship between gender and other forms of CB, such as stereotyped behaviors. Lundqvist (2013) similarly found no relationship between gender and SIB, while also finding no relationship between gender and stereotyped behaviors. However, he found a different pattern in regards to gender and aggressive/destructive behaviors. Lundqvist (2013) found that women evinced significantly more aggressive/destructive behaviors and women's aggressive/destructive behaviors were rated as more problematic than men's. These findings were found to be particularly true of hitting, kicking, biting, scratching, being verbally abusive, and being cruel to others. In contrast to these findings, Holden and Gitlesen (2006) found no significant relationship between gender and prevalence, although a slightly higher nonsignificant percentage of males were found to engage in CB (14.3 % compared to 9.1 %). Additionally, they found no relationship between gender and any specific type of CB (e.g., aggression towards others). Finally, no relationship existed for either less demanding or more demanding CB. These conflicting findings call to the need for more rigorous studies examining the relationship between gender and CB (McClintock et al. 2003).

While none of the aforementioned studies found a relationship between gender and stereotypic behaviors, Hattier et al. (2011) found males with ID and ASD to engage in significantly more stereotyped behaviors than females. However, it is possible that this finding relates more to ASD than ID specifically.

Age Similar to gender, findings on the relationship between age and CB have often been conflicting. Emerson et al. (2001) found that approximately two-thirds of individuals identified as engaging in CB were adolescents or young adults. However, this finding was again not evaluated statistically and the authors cautioned against interpreting this finding. Holden and Gitlesen (2006) more rigorously examined the relationship between age and CB. They found more demanding CB to increase between the ages of 10 and 20 years, peak between the ages of 20 and 40 years, and then decrease later in life. They found less demanding CB to be fairly evenly distributed under 60 years of age. In general, they found CB to be rare in those above 60 years. CB were shown to be present in young children, with approximately 20 % of those under 10 years showing less demanding CB.

Lundqvist (2013) examined the relationship between age and specific categories of CB. He found SIB and stereotyped behaviors to be fairly constant across age groups, with a nonsignificant peak between the ages of 40 and 49 years. Aggressive and destructive behaviors were found to be significantly higher in those aged 40–59 years, when compared with younger ages. Additionally, a peak was seen among those aged 70 years and older. However, further analysis revealed that this peak only applied to males. In reviewing the relationship between age and SIB in individuals with ASD, Didden et al. (2012) found insufficient evidence to make clear conclusions.

Level of ID Findings on the relationship between level of ID and CB have been more consistent. In general, researchers have found overall rates of CB to increase as level of intellectual impairments increases (Emerson et al. 2001); Holden and Gitlesen 2006); Lundqvist 2013); McClintock et al. 2003); Murphy et al. 2009); Oliver et al. 1987); Rojahn et al. 2001). That is, those with lower levels of intellectual functioning are likely to engage in more CB. However, this finding does not appear to hold true for all categories of CB. Both Emerson et al. (2001) and Holden and Gitlesen (2006) found aggressive behaviors to be more common in those with mild to moderate ID, while SIB was found to be more likely in those with severe and profound ID. Lundqvist (2013) found that all categories of CB investigated (i.e., SIB, stereotyped behaviors, and aggressive/destructive behaviors) increased with increasing severity level of ID. However, this difference was only statistically significant for SIB and stereotyped behaviors. Similarly, McClintock et al. (2003) found, in a meta-analysis, that individuals with severe and profound ID were significantly more likely to engage in SIB and stereotyped behaviors when compared to individuals with mild to moderate ID. Other researchers have similarly reported the finding that SIB and stereotyped behaviors are more prevalent in those with more severe intellectual impairment (Didden et al. 2012); Oliver et al. 1987; Rojahn et al. 2001). McClintock et al. (2003) found a nonsignificant relationship between severity of ID and aggressive behaviors. More research on the relationship between aggressive behaviors and level of intellectual impairment appears warranted.

ASD Another consistent finding in the literature is the impact of ASD on rates of CB in individuals with ID. Researchers have consistently found that those with ID and ASD exhibit more CB than those with either condition alone (Didden et al. 2012); Holden and Gitlesen 2006); Matson and Rivet 2008a; Matson and Rivet 2008b); McCarthy et al. 2010); Tureck et al. 2013). Holden and Gitlesen (2006), for example, found that 35.8 % of participants with autism and ID exhibited CB, compared to the 11.1 % reported for the overall sample of individuals with ID. They did not, however, find the presence of an ASD to be particularly associated with more demanding CB.

Lundqvist (2013) found the prevalence of SIB, stereotyped behaviors, and aggressive/destructive behaviors to all be significantly greater in those with an ASD diagnosis. Similar findings were obtained by Mclintock et al. (2003) in a meta-analysis. Lundqvist (2013) found rates of SIB and stereotyped behaviors to increase with the presence of ASD and increasing severity level of ID, with each factor independently contributing to the increase. Interestingly, while the presence of ASD was associated with higher levels of aggressive/destructive behaviors in those with mild to moderate ID, there was no association between ASD and aggressive/destructive behaviors in those with severe or profound ID. McClintock et al. (2003) found both expressive and receptive communication deficits to be significantly associated with SIB, while only receptive communication deficits were significantly associated with aggressive behaviors.

In addition to the presence of an ASD, more severe symptoms of ASD have also been found to be associated with higher rates of CB in those with ID (Matson et al. 2009; Matson and Rivet 2008b); Matson et al. 2009). Similar to the findings of Lundqvist (2013), Matson and Rivet (2008b) found this relationship to be stronger in regards to SIB and stereotyped behaviors than to aggressive behaviors, at least in those with severe to profound ID. However, they did find communication impairments specifically to be significantly related to aggressive behaviors in this population.

Epilepsy Findings on the relationship between epilepsy and CB in those with ID have been limited, although researchers have shown the possibility of a significant relationship. While Holden and Gitlesen (2006) found no relationship between epilepsy and CB, Lundqvist (2013) found those with epilepsy to be more likely to engage in SIB and stereotyped behaviors. No significant relationship was found with regard to epilepsy and aggressive behaviors. Smith and Matson (2010) looked at CB in those with ID alone, those with autism and ID, those with epilepsy and ID, and those with all three conditions. Those with all three conditions exhibited significantly more CB than those with ID alone or ID and only one of the comorbid conditions studied.

Genetic Syndromes A number of genetic syndromes have been associated with CB in individuals with ID. Holden and Gitlesen (2006) found CB to be independent of genetic conditions. Other researchers, however, have found such relationships. Lundqvist (2013) found that those with Down syndrome were less likely to exhibit SIB or stereotyped behaviors than those without the syndrome. Additionally, those with Fragile X syndrome were found to be more likely to engage in stereotyped behaviors. Other researchers have cited a link between Fragile X syndrome and higher rates of SIB and stereotyped behaviors (Didden et al. 2012); Hall et al. 2008). Didden et al. (2012) noted that some genetic conditions may predispose an individual to engage in CB and may be associated with syndrome-specific forms of CB. For example, SIB is a characteristic symptom of Lesch-Nyhan disease (Anderson and Ernst 1994), while stereotyped behavior is characteristic of Rett disorder (Didden et al. 2012). More systematic comparison of prevalence rates between those with and without these conditions is still needed.

Other factors A number of other factors may also affect rates of CB in individuals with ID. These include comorbid psychopathology, level of adaptive behavior functioning, placement (e.g., residential settings, community settings, etc.), sensory impairments, and medical problems (Baghdadli et al. 2003); Didden et al. 2012); Holden and Gitlesen 2006); Emerson et al. 2001); Lowe et al. 2007); Lundqvist 2013); Matson and LoVullo 2010). While comorbid psychopathology may increase the risk for CB, particularly SIB and aggressive behaviors (Lundqvist 2013); Matson and LoVullo 2008), some researchers have argued that this may be an artifact of other variables and that CB occur independently of comorbid psychopathology (McCarthy et al. 2010). Some researchers have suggested that deficits in adaptive functioning may be related to CB (e.g., Baghdadli et al. 2003; Emerson et al. 2001); however, evidence of this relationship is limited at this time (Didden et al. 2012). Rates of SIB appear to be higher amongst those living in institutional settings when compared to residential settings (Didden et al. 2012; Holden and Gitlesen 2006; Lowe et al. 2007), although the full nature of this relationship remains unclear. Other factors that may influence rates of CB include sensory impairments (e.g., visual impairments), medical problems, and sleep problems (Didden et al. 2012; Lundqvist 2013). It is clear that more research is needed investigating the relationship between these factors and rates of CB. Additionally, more research is needed investigating the role of interactions between these variables.

Treatment

The treatment of CB in individuals with ID is critical, given the numerous adverse consequences associated with them. CB may be associated with serious injury to self and others, long-term health problems, increased risk for hospitalization, placement in residential facilities, increased risk of psychotropic medication use, social and physical isolation, social stigma, restricted opportunities for learning, impaired ability to engage in appropriate or adaptive behaviors, financial strains, burnout of support staff and caregivers, and even death (Didden et al. 2012; Lundqvist 2013); Matson et al. 2008; Matson et al. 2012; Matson and Nebel-Schwalm 2007; Mudford et al. 2008). Given the wide array of negative consequences associated with CB, it follows that treatment of CB is often a priority in individuals with ID. Numerous studies have been conducted examining various treatment techniques for CB, ranging from single case designs to meta-analyses. In general, treatment studies fall under one of two broad categories: behavioral treatments and pharmacological treatments (Matson et al. 2011; Matson et al. 2012; Mudford et al. 2008). While other forms of treatment have been proposed and advocated, the majority lack evidence and are often contraindicated (see Jacobson et al. 2005 for a more in-depth review). Of note, much of the literature on treatment of CB is not specific to the ID population; rather, most studies describe treatment in individuals with ID and/or an ASD. Thus, some caution is needed in interpreting these studies solely for the ID population. The current section will review behavioral and pharmacological treatments of CB, the various techniques involved, and the research behind them.

Behavioral Treatments

Most behavioral treatments of CB in individuals with ID are based on principles of operant conditioning and employ reinforcement-based procedures (Cooper et al. (2007); Rodriguez et al. 2012). While punishment-based procedures may be a component of behavioral treatments, reinforcement-based procedures are typically emphasized due to fewer negative side effects, fewer ethical and legal concerns, and the ability to teach adaptive replacement behaviors (Chowdhury and Benson 2011; Cooper et al. (2007). Punishment-based procedures are typically only employed when reinforcement-based procedures have proven ineffective (Chowdhury and Benson 2011; Matson et al. 2012). The majority of these procedures begin with identifying the function underlying a CB, a technique known as functional assessment (Iwata et al. 1994; Matson and Minshawi 2007; Matson and Nebel-Schwalm 2007; Mudford et al. 2008). Iwata et al. (1994) described a method of experimentally manipulating variables hypothesized to maintain CB, a technique now described as experimental functional analysis (Matson and Minshawi 2007; Vollmer et al. 2012). A number of other methods of functional assessment have been developed, including direct observation (Horovitz and Matson 2012; Sipes and Matson 2012), scaling methods (Durand and Crimmins 1988); Paclawskyj et al. 2000); Sipes and Matson 2012), ABC data collection (Sulzer-Azaroff and Mayer 1977), scatter plots (Touchette et al. 1985), and interview methods (O'Neill et al. 1997). At the heart of each of these methods is identifying the underlying variables maintaining the CB. The use of functionally based behavioral treatments reduces the likelihood of using punishment procedures and simplifies treatment protocols, removing extraneous components that are unnecessary (Pelios et al. 1999). While many of the original procedures were developed in the context of SIB (e.g., Iwata et al. (1994) all of these procedures have been broadened to include the other forms of CB discussed in this chapter. The rationale behind such techniques is that treatments are likely to be more effective if tailored to the hypothesized environmental variables (Matson et al. (2011). This hypothesis has been supported by several reviews of behavioral treatment for CB (e.g., Campbell 2003; Didden et al. 2006; Harvey et al. 2009.

Matson et al. (2011) conducted a review of 173 studies that used functional assessment procedures to identify the environmental variables maintaining various CB. They reported that the most frequently cited functions of CB included access to attention, alone (i.e., self-stimulatory, nonsocial, or automatic reinforcement), escape, and tangible functions. Access to attention and escape were the most frequently reported functions. Additionally, they found multiple functions to often maintain CB, with the most frequently reported pairs being attention plus escape and attention plus tangible. In some cases, several functions were identified or the function was ambiguous, perhaps suggesting automatic reinforcement or use of CB as a general communication strategy (Matson et al. 2011). The authors also described the relationship between specific categories of CB and various functions. In conclusion, they found clear evidence that environmental variables maintain the majority of CB. As such, behavioral techniques aimed at these environmental variables were recommended.

Mudford (2008) described three focuses of behavioral techniques after a function has been identified: (1) change antecedents to the behavior; (2) remove reinforcing contingencies found to maintain the behavior; and (3) strengthen competing or replacement behaviors. A number of techniques have been described to accomplish these goals. While the specific techniques may vary from behavior to behavior, and from one function of a behavior to another, the underlying bases of these techniques remain similar. Additionally, treatment of CB often involves a combination of techniques tailored to the individual's needs (Singh et al. 2011). In addition to the function of the behavior, behavioral treatments also require consideration of other factors, including the frequency of the behavior, the intensity of the behavior, and the specific topography of the behavior. For example, treatment for a child who engages in daily, low-intensity SIB would likely be different than treatment for a child who engages in less frequent, high-intensity SIB, even if both behaviors served a similar function. The current section provides a review of some of the most prominently researched behavioral techniques for treating CB, followed by a review of research on the effectiveness of behavioral treatments for CB. These techniques include differential reinforcement, functional communication training, noncontingent reinforcement (NCR), and extinction. While this is by no means a complete list, it represents some of the most commonly used behavioral techniques.

Differential Reinforcement

A number of treatment techniques fall under the umbrella of differential reinforcement. All differential reinforcement techniques are defined by reinforcing one behavior (e.g., asking for something appropriately) or class of behaviors while withholding reinforcement for another behavior (e.g., hitting others) or class of behaviors (Cooper et al. (2007). Four primary methods of differential reinforcement exist: differential reinforcement of incompatible behavior (DRI), differential reinforcement of alternative behavior (DRA), differential reinforcement of other behavior (DRO), and differential reinforcement of low rates (DRL)(Cooper et al. (2007). The reader is referred to Cooper et al. (2007) for a more thorough description of these individual techniques. The differential reinforcement technique chosen often depends on the specific topography of behavior being targeted, in addition to the frequency and intensity of the behavior.

Chowdhury and Benson (2011) conducted a review on the use of differential reinforcement procedures to reduce CB in adults with ID over the course of 30 years. They looked at a total of 31 studies, with the most frequently treated CB being SIB and aggression. Of the various differential reinforcement techniques, DRO (45 %) was the most frequently studied, followed by DRA (23 %), and DRI (13 %). Only one study employed a DRL technique, in combination with other behavioral techniques. Additionally, the authors found that 16 % of studies combined multiple differential reinforcement techniques. Overall, the majority of studies reviewed found differential reinforcement to be effective at reducing problem behaviors, although a handful of studies found these methods to only be successful when combined with additional behavioral strategies (e.g., punishment). The authors noted, however, that a number of methodological variables were omitted by the authors of these studies, somewhat limiting the interpretations that could be made. The authors concluded that considerable evidence exists demonstrating the effectiveness of differential reinforcement procedures for reducing CB in adults with ID; however, more research is needed exploring variables that may relate to their effectiveness. Additionally, they suggested more research into the feasibility of treatment implementation.

Functional Communication Training

The goal of functional communication training (FCT) is the development of appropriate communication skills that will effectively replace the use of CB (Cooper et al. 2007). Cooper et al. (2007) noted that functional communication training is a form of DRA, in that an alternative behavior (i.e., communication) is differentially reinforced compared to the CB. Carr and Durand (1985) were one of the first to describe the use of FCT in the treatment of CB. In their experiments, FCT involved identifying the functions of problem behaviors through functional assessment and using these identified functions to reinforce appropriate use of communication. They found such an intervention to reduce problem behaviors in a sample of four children.

Since this initial examination of the effectiveness of FCT, a wealth of research has been conducted examining FCT in the treatment of CB. Tiger, Hanley, and Bruzek (2008) conducted a review on FCT procedures. They found a total of 91 articles between the years 1985 and 2006 that examined FCT. While FCT was most frequently used in the treatment of aggression, SIB, and motor or vocal disruptions, the authors also found studies using FCT to treat inappropriate vocalizations, stereotyped behaviors, inappropriate sexual behaviors, self-restraint, and inappropriate communicative behaviors.

Tiger et al. (2008) provide a number of guidelines to increase the effectiveness of FCT, including conducting a functional assessment, considering strategies for generalization, considering the type of prompting used, and how to develop a schedule of thinning reinforcement. Cooper et al. (2007) noted a number of advantages and disadvantages of FCT. Advantages included a high chance for generalization and maintenance and high social validity. Disadvantages of FCT included the fact that most FCT treatments include some form of extinction that can be difficult to consistently implement, individuals may inappropriately engage in high rates of the newly learned communicative response to obtain reinforcement, it may not always be possible to reinforce the appropriate communicative response, and FCT does not attempt to alter the environment that initially developed the CB. Despite these possible disadvantages, a number of studies have demonstrated the effectiveness of FCT for reducing CB (Cooper et al. 2007; Mancil 2006; Tiger et al. 2008).

Noncontingent reinforcement

NCR is an intervention for CB in which an individual is provided reinforcement on a fixed-time or variable-time schedule, independent of the behaviors exhibited (Cooper et al. 2007). The rationale behind NCR is that CB will reduce in frequency, as the reinforcers maintaining these behaviors are available frequently and independently of the occurrence of the CB (Cooper et al. 2007). Cooper et al. (2007) provide recommendations for enhancing the effectiveness of NCR. They noted that the amount of reinforcement provided can alter the effectiveness of NCR and that the preferred reinforcer may change over time. Additionally, they recommended that NCR often be combined with extinction procedures. Other recommendations included the use of a functional assessment and considering the schedule of reinforcement and when to begin thinning the schedule.

Considerable research has supported the effectiveness of NCR in reducing CB in individuals with ID (Carr et al. 2000; Cooper et al. 2007; Tucker et al. 1998). The reader is directed to Tucker et al. (1998) and Carr et al. (2000) for in-depth reviews on the effectiveness of NCR procedures. Both reviews provide additional guidelines to implementing NCR, similar to those discussed above. Cooper et al. (2007) discussed some of the possible advantages and disadvantages of implementing NCR procedures. Advantages included ease of use, creation of a positive learning environment, possibility of reducing extinction bursts, and possible strengthening of appropriate alternative behaviors. Disadvantages noted included reduced motivation to engage in adaptive behaviors, possible strengthening of the CB due to chance pairings, and disruptions to learning.

Extinction

Extinction involves ceasing to reinforce a previously reinforced behavior (Cooper et al. 2007). As the behavior no longer is reinforced, the frequency of the behavior should decrease. As an example, take an individual who engages in SIB to obtain attention from caregivers. If the caregivers cease to provide attention for the SIB, the frequency of the behavior should decrease. Extinction can be used for behaviors that are maintained by positive reinforcement, negative reinforcement, or automatic reinforcement (Cooper et al. 2007). Each type of extinction requires identification of the variable maintaining the CB and subsequently withholding the reinforcing variable in the presence of the CB. With the implementation of extinction procedures usually comes an initial increase in the frequency of the CB, a pattern known as extinction burst (Cooper et al. 2007). Subsequent to this initial increase in frequency, the CB typically decreases steadily. However, after a certain period of decrease, the CB may show a brief increase known as spontaneous recovery (Cooper et al. 2007). Such an increase is typically brief if extinction procedures continue to be implemented.

Cooper et al. (2007) provide ten guidelines for using extinction effectively. These guidelines are (1) withholding all reinforcers maintaining the problem behavior; (2) withholding reinforcement consistently; (3) combining extinction with other procedures; (4) using instructions; (5) planning for extinction-produced aggression; (6) increasing the number of extinction trials; (7) including significant others in extinction; (8) guarding against unintentional extinction; (9) maintaining extinction-decreased behavior; and (10) understanding when not to use extinction. For example, extinction alone is unlikely to be recommended for the treatment of severe CB, due to their harmful nature. Numerous studies have demonstrated the effectiveness of extinction procedures (e.g., Anderson and Long 2002; Rincover 1978; Williams 1959). However, extinction procedures are rarely used as the sole intervention technique; rather, they are often combined with other reinforcement-based strategies that allow for the development of alternative, more adaptive skills.

Effectiveness of Behavioral Treatments

The above sections have discussed the effectiveness of some of the more commonly employed behavioral treatments for CB. A number of reviews have demonstrated the effectiveness of behavioral treatments as a whole in the treatment of CB in individuals with ID (Didden et al. 2006); Harvey et al. 2009); Hassiotis et al. 2009); Kahng et al. 2002). Harvey et al. (2009) conducted a meta-analysis on behavioral treatments for CB and found a number of factors that influenced the effectiveness of such treatments. Firstly, they found behavioral treatments to be more successful with SIB, stereotypy, socially inappropriate behavior, and destructive behaviors when compared to disruptive and aggressive behaviors. Additionally, severity of CB at the onset of treatment was negatively associated with the effectiveness of behavioral treatments. As previously discussed, most behavioral treatments aim to change antecedents, reduce or remove reinforcing contingencies maintaining behaviors, and/or strengthen competing response (Mudford et al. 2008). Harvey et al. (2009) found that strengthening of competing responses, in the form of skill replacement, had the highest independent effect sizes, although they urged the need for more research investigating this finding. Additionally, they found that, while overall all behavioral treatments investigated were effective, no one treatment technique (e.g., differential reinforcement or NCR) or combination of treatments was highly effective for all categories of CB. Thus, it is critical that treatment strategies be individually tailored to target the specific CB being treated. A similar review by Didden et al. (2006) additionally found higher effects for treatments that (1) were based on functional assessment results; (2) measured the reliability of data collection; (3) explicitly promoted stimulus generalization; and (4) were based on data collection designs that had internal validity. Didden et al. (2006) found no statistically significant differences between behavioral categories, although some trends in the data were observed.

Kahng et al. (2002) reviewed trends in the effectiveness of behavioral treatments specifically for SIB. They found the mean outcome of all reported treatments to be an 83.7% reduction in SIB from baseline to treatment, with a majority of treatments being successful at reducing SIB by at least 80%. They found reinforcement-based interventions to be much more common than punishment-based procedures, a trend that has become more pronounced over the past two decades. DRO procedures were the most frequently reported reinforcement procedure. While overall rates of effectiveness were not found to have increased since the 1960s, the authors reported a reduction in variability of effectiveness in more recent years. Finally, the authors stressed the need for more research on follow-up and generalizability.

Pharmacological Treatments

The use of psychotropic medications in the treatment of CB, while widespread in practice, has been highly controversial in the literature (Matson and Neal 2009); Matson et al. 2012). A number of factors must be considered when discussing the use of psychotropic medications to treat CB. Firstly, the evidence that psychotropic medications are effective in reducing CB must be considered. This will be discussed more in depth below. Additionally, one must take into account the potential for severe side effects (Mahan et al. 2010). This is especially critical, given that individuals with ID often have numerous comorbid medical conditions that require the prescription of additional medications, increasing the possibility of potential interactions and severe side effects (Mahan et al. 2010; Matson et al. 2012). The prevalence of psychotropic medication use in this population should also be considered, as evidence suggests overprescribing of psychotropic medications is common practice (Matson and Neal 2009; Matson et al. 2012). Additionally, the rationale behind the use of psychotropic medications must be sound. As discussed above, some researchers have argued that CB represent "behavioral equivalents" of psychopathology (Hurley 2006; Marston et al. 1997); Witwer and Lecavalier 2010). As such, the presence of CB has often been used to rationalize the provision of an Axis I diagnosis and subsequently the prescribing of psychotropic medication. However, there is a lack of empirical support for such practice (Ross and Oliver 2003; Tsiouris et al. 2003); Witwer and Lecavalier 2010; Matson et al. (2012) stress that psychotropic medications should be prescribed when a psychiatric condition has been clearly identified and the psychotropic medication prescribed is consistent with the condition identified. However, this is often not the case in practice (De Kuijper et al. 2010; Matson et al. 2012; Nøttestad and Linaker 2003); Matson et al. (2012) also conceded that, in cases of severe CB where behavioral treatments have proven ineffective, psychotropic medications may be warranted; however, they stressed the need for more rigorous investigation into the effectiveness of such use. The following sections will examine the prevalence of psychotropic medication use in this population and findings on effectiveness.

Prevalence of Psychotropic Medication Use

McGillivray and McCabe (2004) conducted a review of psychotropic medication use in 873 individuals with ID in Australia. This number represented 4.5 % of the total population of individuals with ID. Other researchers have found this number to be as high as 20–30 % in community settings (Nøttestad and Linaker 2003; Spreat et al. 1997). McGillivray and McCabe (2004) found males to be overrepresented at younger ages, while females were overrepresented at older ages. With regard to the number of psychotropic medications prescribed, they found the following: 62 % of the sample received, on average, one psychotropic medication; 25.9 % of the sample received, on average, two psychotropic medications; 8.8 % of the sample received, on average, three psychotropic medications; 2.8 % of the sample received, on average, four psychotropic medications; and 0.5 % of the sample received, on average, five psychotropic medications. Overall, the sample received an average of 1.54 psychotropic medications during the study period. The researchers also found that 79 individuals received a PRN (i.e., as needed) medication on at least one occasion. With regard to class of psychotropic medication prescribed, the authors found antipsychotic medications to be the most commonly prescribed (77.8 %), followed by antidepressants (21.0 %), anxiolytics (17.6 %), anticonvulsants/mood stabilizers (15.6 %), other (8.0 %), and psychostimulants (4.1 %). The most troubling finding by this study was the common use of intraclass polypharmacy, with multiple antipsychotic medications the most likely to be administered concurrently. Overall, intraclass polypharmacy was present in 53.8 % of the participants.

Robertson et al. (2000) examined many of these factors in the UK, with particular interest in community based or residential placement. The researchers found prescription of psychotropic medications to be much higher in residential settings when compared with village communities and community-based housing. This is similar to findings by other researchers who have estimated the use of psychotropic medication to be as high as 50 % in residential settings (De Kuijper et al. 2010; Nøttestad and Linaker 2003; Singh et al. 1997). It should be noted, however, that the process of deinstitutionalization alone does not appear to significantly reduce the use of psychotropic medications in individuals who previously lived in residential settings (Nøttestad and Linaker 2003). Robertson et al. (2000) also found the practice of intraclass polypharmacy, at least with respect to antipsychotic medications, to be more common in residential settings than in village communities or dispersed housing. Similar results were found with regard to the classes of psychotropic medications most frequently prescribed. Together, these studies provide insight into the widespread use of psychotropic medication in individuals with ID. Of additional concern is the fact that psychotropic medications are being prescribed at younger and younger ages, even as early as 2 years of age (Horovitz et al. 2012).

Effectiveness of Psychotropic Medication Use

The evidence for effectiveness of psychotropic medications for the treatment of CB is mixed. Currently, risperidone, an atypical antipsychotic medication, is approved by the Food and Drug Administration for the treatment of symptoms of ASD, including aggression, self-injury, and tantrums (Singh et al. 2011). While this approval is specific to ASD, it is relevant to the current discussion given the high comorbidity of ASD and ID. A number of small-scale studies have suggested the efficacy of various psychotropic medications, particularly risperidone, in the treatment of CB in individuals with ID (Deb and Unwin 2007); Gagiano et al. 2005); Horrigan and Barnhill 1997); McCracken et al. 2002); Read and Rendall 2007). For example, Gagiano et al. (2005) examined the use of risperidone in 77 individuals with ID and CB. They found that those who took risperidone for 4 weeks demonstrated significantly greater improvements on the Aberrant Behavior Checklist and BPI when compared to a placebo control group.

Yet, other researchers have at times found contradictory results. For example, Tyrer et al. (2008) examined the use of risperidone, haloperidol, and placebo in 95 individuals with ID and CB. They found rates of aggression to decrease substantially in all groups, with the placebo group showing the greatest improvement. What then, can explain these contradictory findings? Studies on the efficacy of psychotropic medication use in the treatment of CB have regularly been criticized for lack of methodological rigor, such as the use of double-blind procedures and use of appropriate control groups (Brylewski and Duggan 1999; Deb et al. 2014; Dinca et al. 2005; Matson and Neal 2009); Singh et al. 2010). Many of the contradictory findings may be due to differences in the methodological procedures employed by the researchers. As such, many authors have cautioned against making interpretations based on these limited studies (Dinca et al. 2005; Matson and Neal 2009); Singh et al. 2010).

Some attempts have been made at conducting larger scale reviews on the efficacy of psychotropic medications. Brylewski and Duggan (1999) conducted a systematic review of randomized controlled trials for antipsychotic mediation use in the treatment of CB. They were able to find only three truly controlled trials that could be included in their analyses and found no conclusive evidence as to their efficacy. Matson and Neal (2009) similarly conducted a review of studies looking at all classes of psychotropic medication in the treatment of CB. To be included in the initial review, studies were required to include participants with a primary diagnosis of ID prescribed psychotropic medications to treat CB. Of the 56 studies identified by such criteria, only 23 were reported to employ double blind, placebo-controlled procedures. Additionally, only 12 of these studies met more rigorous standards, such as random assignment, standardized doses, standardized evaluations, and appropriate statistical procedures. Only 3 of these 12 studies conducted follow-up assessment. Out of the 12 studies, 8 reported significant improvements with the use of psychotropic medications, when compared to the placebo control group. The authors noted that the four studies that showed no significant difference were the only four studies to use an objective observation in addition to rating scales. Additionally, all of the reportedly successful studies involved the atypical antipsychotic risperidone; conversely, of the four studies that found no effect, one examined risperidone and haloperidol, two examined the typical antipsychotic thioridazine, and one examined the antidepressant imipramine. The authors concluded that there is a staggering lack of evidence for the efficacy of psychotropic medication use when compared to behavioral techniques, especially when considering the high proportion of individuals who are prescribed psychotropic medications.

Of note, very few studies have directly compared the effectiveness of psychotropic medications and behavioral techniques (Campbell 2003). Most research on psychotropic medications has used placebo treatment as a control group, if anything. Heyvaert et al. (2012) conducted a meta-analysis of single-case and small-scale studies looking at treatment of CB in people with ID. In this review, the authors found behavioral treatments to have an overall positive effect, while they found no evidence for an overall positive effect of pharmacological interventions. However, they did not report on studies specifically comparing these two treatment modalities. On the other hand, a previous review by Heyvaert et al. (2010) found both behavioral and pharmacological treatments to demonstrate similar effectiveness. Taken together, the current literature provides some support for the effectiveness of psychotropic medication in treating certain CB, such as aggression and self-injury. However, this evidence is limited at best and clearly requires more rigorous exploration. Given the serious side effects associated with psychotropic medication use, it is critical that empirical evidence for the effectiveness of pharmacological treatments be more thoroughly tested to recommend their continued use in the treatment of CB.

Conclusions

CB are a serious comorbid condition affecting many individuals with ID. CB are associated with a number of negative consequences that affect the quality of life of individuals with ID (Durand and Carr 1992; Loftin et al. 2008; Matson and Dempsey 2009; Matson et al. 2009b; Matson et al. 1997; Morrison and Rosales-Ruiz 1997). The current chapter has reviewed what constitutes these CB and factors associated with their prevalence. More research on these risk factors may help in the implementation of strategies to prevent the occurrence of CB. Additionally, a better understanding of risk factors will aid in early identification of those at exhibiting CB, allowing intervention strategies to be implemented before CB become severe. A tremendous amount of research has been conducted on interventions for CB and a number of successful approaches have been discovered. Yet, more research is clearly needed. Many researchers, while reporting successful treatment techniques, often omit critical information, such as detailed methodological approaches and important demographic and background information. Such information is necessary to best understand what treatments are most likely to succeed with specific individuals. Additional research comparing specific treatment techniques, particularly comparing specific psychotropic medications to specific behavioral techniques, is needed. More research into the nature, prevalence, and treatment of CB will continue to lead to improvements in the quality of life of individuals with ID and their caregivers.

References

Anderson, C. M., & Long, E. S. (2002). Use of a structured descriptive assessment methodology to identify variables affecting problem behavior. *Journal of Applied Behavior Analysis, 35*, 137–154.

Anderson, L. T., & Ernst, M. (1994). Self-injury in Lesch-Nyhan disease. *Journal of Autism and Developmental Disorders, 24*, 67–81.

American Psychiatric Association. (2013). *Diagnostic and statistical manual of mental disorders* (5th ed.). Arlington, VA: American Psychiatric Publishing.

Baghdadli, A., Pascal, C., Grisi, S., & Aussilloux, C. (2003). Risk factors for self-injurious behaviours among 222 young children with autistic disorders. *Journal of Intellectual Disability Research, 47*, 622–627.

Berkson, G. (1983). Repetitive stereotyped behaviors. *American Journal of Mental Deficiency, 88*, 239–246.

Brylewski, J., & Duggan, L. (1999). Review: Antipsychotic medication for challenging behaviour in people with intellectual disability: a systematic review of randomized controlled trials. *Journal of Intellectual Disability Research, 43*, 360–371.

Campbell, J. M. (2003). Efficacy of behavioral interventions for reducing problem behavior in persons with autism: a quantitative synthesis of single-subject research. *Research in Developmental Disabilities, 24*, 120–138.

Carr, E. G., & Durand, V. M. (1985). Reducing behavior problems through functional communication training. *Journal of Applied Behavior Analysis, 18*, 111–126.

Carr, J. E., Coriaty, S., Wilder, D. A., Gaunt, B. T., Dozier, C. L., Britton, L. N., et al. (2000). A review of "noncontingent" reinforcement as treatment for the aberrant behavior of individuals with developmental disabilities. *Research in Developmental Disabilities, 21*, 377–391.

Chowdhury, M., & Benson, B. A. (2011). Use of differential reinforcement to reduce behavior problems in adults with intellectual disabilities: A methodological review. *Research in Developmental Disabilities, 32*, 383–394.

Cooper, J. O., Heron, T. E., & Heward, W. L. (2007). *Applied Behavior Analysis* (2nd ed.). Upper Saddle River, New Jersey: Pearson.

Cooper, S. A., Smiley, E., Jackson, A., Finlayson, J., Allan, L., Mantry, D., & Morrison, J. (2009). Adults with intellectual disabilities: Prevalence, incidence and remission of aggressive behaviour and related factors. *Journal of Intellectual Disability Research, 53*, 217–232.

Crocker, A. G., Mercier, C., Lachapelle, Y., Brunet, A., Morin, D., & Roy, M. E. (2006). Prevalence and types of aggressive behaviour among adults with intellectual disabilities. *Journal of Intellectual Disability Research, 50*, 652–661.

De Kuijper, G., Hoekstra, P., Visser, F., Scholte, F., Penning, C., & Evenhuis, H. (2010). Use of antipsychotic drugs in individuals with intellectual disability (ID) in the Netherlands: prevalence and reasons for prescription. *Journal of Intellectual Disability Research, 54*, 659–667.

Deb, S., Farmah, B. K., Arshad, E., Deb, T., Roy, M., & Unwin, G. L. (2014). The effectiveness of aripiprazole in the management of problem behaviour in people with intellectual disabilities, developmental disabilities and/or autistic spectrum disorder–A systematic review. *Research in developmental disabilities, 35*, 711–725.

Deb, S., & Unwin, G. L. (2007). Psychotropic medication for behaviour problems in people with intellectual disability: a review of the current literature. *Current Opinion in Psychiatry, 20*, 461–466.

Didden, R., Korzilius, H., van Oorsouw, W., Sturmey, P., & Bodfish, J. (2006). Behavioral treatment of challenging behaviors in individuals with mild mental retardation: Meta-analysis of single-subject research. *American Journal on Mental Retardation, 111*, 290–298.

Didden, R., Sturmey, P., Sigafoos, J., Lang, R., O'Reilly, M. F., & Lancioni, G. E. (2012). Nature, prevalence, and characteristics of challenging behavior. In J. L. Matson (Ed.), *Functional Assessment for Challenging Behaviors* (pp. 25–44). New York: Springer.

Dinca, O., Paul, M., & Spencer, N. (2005). Systematic review of randomized controlled trials of atypical antipsychotics and selective serotonin reuptake inhibitors for behavioural problems associated with pervasive developmental disorders. *Journal of Psychopharmacology, 19*, 521–532.

Durand, V. M., & Carr, E. G. (1992). An analysis of maintenance following functional communication training. *Journal of Applied Behavior Analysis, 25*, 777–794.

Durand, V. M., & Crimmins, D. B. (1988). Identifying the variables maintaining self-injurious behavior. *Journal of Autism and Developmental Disorders, 18*, 99–117.

Emerson, E. (2005). *Challenging behaviour: Analysis and intervention in people with severe intellectual disabilities*. Cambridge: Cambridge University Press.

Emerson, E., Kiernan, C., Alborz, A., Reeves, D., Mason, H., Swarbrick, R., et al. (2001). The prevalence of challenging behaviors: a total population study. *Research in developmental disabilities, 22*, 77–93.

Farmer, C. A., & Aman, M. G. (2011). Aggressive behavior in a sample of children with autism spectrum disorders. *Research in Autism Spectrum Disorders, 5*, 317–323.

Foster, L. G. (1998). Nervous habits and stereotyped behaviors in preschool children. *Journal of the American Academy of Child & Adolescent Psychiatry, 37*, 711–717.

Gagiano, C., Read, S., Thorpe, L., Eerdekens, M., & Van Hove, I. (2005). Short-and long-term efficacy and safety of risperidone in adults with disruptive behavior disorders. *Psychopharmacology, 179*, 629–636.

Glaesser, R. S., & Perkins, E. A. (2013). Self-injurious behavior in older adults with intellectual disabilities. *Social Work, 58*, 213–221.

Hall, S. S., Lightbody, A. A., & Reiss, A. L. (2008). Compulsive, self-injurious, and autistic behavior in children and adolescents with fragile X syndrome. *Journal Information, 113*.

Harvey, S. T., Boer, D., Meyer, L. H., & Evans, I. M. (2009). Updating a meta-analysis of intervention research with challenging behaviour: Treatment validity and standards of practice. *Journal of Intellectual and Developmental Disability, 34*, 67–80.

Hassiotis, A., Robotham, D., Canagasabey, A., Romeo, R., Langridge, D., Blizard, R., etc. (2009). Randomized, single-blind, controlled trial of a specialist behavior therapy team for challenging behavior in adults with intellectual disabilities. *American Journal of Psychiatry, 166*, 1278–1285.

Hattier, M. A., Matson, J. L., Tureck, K., & Horovitz, M. (2011). The effects of gender and age on repetitive and/or restricted behaviors and interests in adults with autism spectrum disorders and intellectual disability. *Research in Developmental Disabilities, 32*, 2346–2351.

Heyvaert, M., Maes, B., & Onghena, P. (2010). A meta-analysis of intervention effects on challenging behaviour among persons with intellectual disabilities. *Journal of Intellectual Disability Research, 54*, 634–649.

Heyvaert, M., Maes, B., Van Den Noortgate, W., Kuppens, S., & Onghena, P. (2012). A multilevel meta-analysis of single-case and small-n research on interventions for reducing challenging behavior in persons with intellectual disabilities. *Research in developmental disabilities, 33*, 766–780.

Holden, B., & Gitlesen, J. P. (2006). A total population study of challenging behaviour in the county of Hedmark, Norway: Prevalence, and risk markers. *Research in developmental disabilities, 27*, 456–465.

Horovitz, M., & Matson, J. L. (2012). In Vivo Assessment: Issues of Real-Time Data. In J. L. Matson (Ed.), *Functional Assessment for Challenging Behaviors* (pp. 143–158). New York: Springer.

Horovitz, M., Matson, J. L., & Barker, A. (2012). The relationship between symptoms of autism spectrum disorders and psychotropic medication use in infants and toddlers. *Research in Autism Spectrum Disorders, 6*, 1406–1411.

Horrigan, J. P., & Barnhill, L. J. (1997). Risperidone and explosive aggressive autism. *Journal of autism and developmental disorders, 27*, 313–323.

Hurley, A. D. (2006). Mood disorders in intellectual disability. *Current Opinion in Psychiatry, 19*, 465–469.

Iwata, B. A., Dorsey, M. F., Slifer, K. J., Bauman, K. E., & Richman, G. S. (1994). Toward a functional analysis of self-injury. *Journal of applied behavior analysis, 27*, 197–209.

Iwata, B. A., Pace, G. M., Dorsey, M. F., & Zarcone, J. R. (1994). The functions of self-injurious behavior: An experimental-epidemiological analysis. *Journal of Applied Behavior Analysis, 27*, 215–240. d

Jacobson, J. W., Foxx, R. M., & Mulick, J. A. (2005). *Controversial therapies for developmental disabilities: Fad, fashion, and science in professional practice*. New York: CRC Press.

Kahng, S., Iwata, B. A., & Lewin, A. B. (2002). Behavioral treatment of self-injury, 1964–2000. *American Journal on Mental Retardation, 107*, 212–221.

Klonsky, E. D., & Muehlenkamp, J. J. (2007). Self-injury: A research review for the practitioner. *Journal of Clinical Psychology, 63*, 1045–1056.

Koegel, R. L., & Covert, A. (1972). The relationship of self-stimulation to learning in autistic children *Journal of Applied Behavior Analysis, 5*, 381–387.

Kress, V. E. W. (2003). Self-Injurious Behaviors: Assessment and Diagnosis. *Journal of Counseling & Development, 81*, 490–496.

Loftin, R. L., Odom, S. L., & Lantz, J. F. (2008). Social interaction and repetitive motor behaviors. *Journal of Autism and Developmental Disorders, 38*, 1124–1135.

Lowe, K., Allen, D., Jones, E., Brophy, S., Moore, K., & James, W. (2007). Challenging behaviours: prevalence and topographies. *Journal of Intellectual and Developmental Disability, 51*, 625–636.

Lundqvist, L.-O. (2013). Prevalence and risk markers of behavior problems among adults with intellectual disabilities: A total population study in Örebro County, Sweden. *Research in developmental disabilities, 34*, 1346–1356.

MacDonald, R., Green, G., Mansfield, R., Geckeler, A., Gardenier, N., Anderson, J., … Sanchez, J. (2007). Stereotypy in young children with autism and typically developing children. *Research in Developmental Disabilities, 28*, 266–277.

Mahan, S., Holloway, J., Bamburg, J. W., Hess, J. A., Fodstad, J. C., & Matson, J. L. (2010). An Examination of Psychotropic Medication Side Effects: Does taking a greater number of psychotropic medications from different classes affect presentation of side effects in adults with ID? *Research in developmental disabilities, 31*, 1561–1569.

Mancil, G. R. (2006). Functional communication training: A review of the literature related to children with autism. *Education and Training in Developmental Disabilities, 41*, 213.

Marston, G. M., Perry, D. W., & Roy, A. (1997). Manifestations of depression in people with intellectual disability. *Journal of Intellectual Disability Research, 41*, 476–480.

Matson, J. L., & Cervantes, P. E. (2013). Comorbidity among persons with intellectual disabilities. *Research in Autism Spectrum Disorders, 7*, 1318–1322.

Matson, J. L., Cooper, C., Malone, C. J., & Moskow, S. L. (2008). The relationship of self-injurious behavior and other maladaptive behaviors among individuals with severe and profound intellectual disability. *Research in Developmental Disabilities, 29*, 141–146.

Matson, J. L., & Dempsey, T. (2009). The nature and treatment of compulsions, obsessions, and rituals in people with developmental disabilities *Research in Developmental Disabilities, 30*, 603–611.

Matson, J. L., Dempsey, T., & Fodstad, J. C. (2009a). Stereotypies and repetitive/restricted behaviors in infants with autism and Pervasive Developmental Disorder. *Developmental Neurorehabilitation, 12*, 122–127.

Matson, J. L., Dempsey, T., & Fodstad, J. C. (2009b). Stereotypies and repetitive/restrictive behaviours in infants with autism and pervasive developmental disorder. *Developmental Neurorehabilitation, 12*, 122–127.

Matson, J. L., Fodstad, J. C., & Rivet, T. T. (2009). The relationship of social skills and problem behaviors in adults with intellectual disability and autism or PDD-NOS. *Research in Autism Spectrum Disorders*, 258–268.

Matson, J. L., & Horovitz, M. (2010). Stability of autism spectrum disorders symptoms over time. *Journal of Developmental and Physical Disabilities, 22*, 331–342.

Matson, J. L., Kiely, S. L., & Bamburg, J. W. (1997). The effect of stereotypies on adaptive skills as assessed with the DASH-II and Vineland Adaptive Behavior Scales. *Research in Developmental Disabilities, 18*, 471–476.

Matson, J. L., Kozlowski, A. M., Worley, J. A., Shoemaker, M. E., Sipes, M., & Horovitz, M. (2011). What is the evidence for environmental causes of challenging behaviors in persons with intellectual disabilities and autism spectrum disorders? *Research in Developmental Disabilities, 32*, 693–698.

Matson, J. L., & LoVullo, S. V. (2008). A review of behavioral treatments for self-injurious behaviors of persons with autism spectrum disorders. *Behavior Modification, 32*, 61–76.

Matson, J. L., & Minshawi, N. F. (2007). Functional assessment of challenging behavior: Toward a strategy for applied settings. *Research in Developmental Disabilities, 28*, 353–361.

Matson, J. L., & Neal, D. (2009). Psychotropic medication use for challenging behaviors in persons with intellectual disabilities. *Research in Developmental Disabilities, 30*, 572–586.

Matson, J. L., Neal, D., & Kozlowski, A. M. (2012). Treatments for the challenging behaviours of adults with intellectual disabilities. *The Canadian Journal of Psychiatry/ La Revue canadienne de psychiatrie, 57*, 587–592.

Matson, J. L., & Nebel-Schwalm, M. (2007). Assessing challenging behaviors in children with autism spectrum disorders: A review. *Research in Developmental Disabilities, 28*, 567–579.

Matson, J. L., & Rivet, T. T. (2008a). Characteristics of challenging behaviours in adults with autistic disorder, PDD-NOS, and intellectual disability. *Journal of intellectual and developmental disability, 33*, 323–329.

Matson, J. L., & Rivet, T. T. (2008b). The effects of severity of autism and PDD-NOS symptoms on challenging behaviors in adults with intellectual disabilities. *Journal of Developmental and Physical Disabilities, 20*, 41–51.

Matson, J. L., Sipes, M., Horovitz, M., Worley, J. A., Shoemaker, M. E., & Kozlowski, A. M. (2011). Behaviors and corresponding functions addressed via functional assessment. *Research in developmental disabilities, 32*, 625–629.

Matson, J. L., & Turygin, N. C. (2012). How do researchers define self-injurious behavior? *Research in Developmental Disabilities, 33*, 1021–1026.

Matson, J. L., Wilkins, J., & Macken, J. (2009). The relationship of challenging behaviors to severity and symptoms of Autism Spectrum Disorders. *Journal of Mental Health Research in Intellectual Disabilities, 2*, 29–44.

McCarthy, J., Hemmings, C., Kravariti, E., Dworzynski, K., Holt, G., Bouras, N., & Tsakanikos, E. (2010). Challenging behavior and co-morbid psychopathology in adults with intellectual disability and autism spectrum disorders. *Research in Developmental Disabilities, 31*, 362–366.

McClintock, K., Hall, S., & Oliver, C. (2003). Risk markers associated with challenging behaviours in people with intellectual disabilities: A meta-analytic study. *Journal of Intellectual Disability Research, 47*, 405–416.

McCracken, J. T., McGough, J., Shah, B., Cronin, P., Hong, D., Aman, M. G., et al. (2002). Risperidone in children with autism and serious behavioral problems. *New England Journal of Medicine, 347*, 314–321.

McGillivray, J. A., & McCabe, M. P. (2004). Pharmacological management of challenging behavior of individuals with intellectual disability. *Research in developmental disabilities, 25*, 523–537.

Medeiros, K., Kozlowski, A. M., Beighley, J. S., Rojahn, J., & Matson, J. L. (2012). The effects of developmental quotient and diagnostic criteria on challenging behaviors in toddlers with developmental disabilities. *Research in developmental disabilities, 33*, 1110–1116.

Morrison, K., & Rosales-Ruiz, J. (1997). The effect of object preferences on task performance and stereotypy in a child with autism. *Research in Developmental Disabilities, 18*, 127–137.

Mudford, O. C., Arnold-Saritepe, A. M., Phillips, K. J., Locke, J. M., Ho, I. C. S., & Taylor, S. A. (2008). Challenging Behaviors. In J. L. Matson (Ed.), *Clinical Assessment and Intervention for Autism Spectrum Disorders*. London: Elsevier, Inc.

Murphy, O., Healy, O., & Leader, G. (2009). Risk factors for challenging behaviors among 157 children with autism spectrum disorder in Ireland. *Research in Autism Spectrum Disorders, 3*, 474–482.

Nøttestad, J. A., & Linaker, O. M. (2003). Psychotropic drug use among people with intellectual disability before and after deinstitutionalization. *Journal of Intellectual Disability Research, 47*, 464–471.

O'Neill, R. E., Horner, R., Albin, R., Sprague, J., Storey, K., & Newton, J. (1997). *Functional assessment and program development for problem behavior: A practical handbook*. Pacific Grove, CA: Brooks/Cole Publishing.

Oliver, C., Murphy, G. H., & Corbett, J. A. (1987). Self-injurious behaviour in people with mental handicap: A total population study. *Journal of Mental Deficiency Research, 31*, 147–162.

Paclawskyj, T. R., Matson, J. L., Rush, K. S., Smalls, Y., & Vollmer, T. R. (2000). Questions about behavioral function (QABF): A behavioral checklist for functional assessment of aberrant behavior. *Research in Developmental Disabilities, 21*, 223–229.

Pelios, L., Morren, J., Tesch, D., & Axelrod, S. (1999). The impact of functional analysis methodology on treatment choice for self-injurious and aggressive behavior. *Journal of Applied Behavior Analysis, 32*, 185–195.

Rapp, J. T., & Vollmer, T. R. (2005). Stereotypy I: A review of behavioral assessment and treatment. *Research in Developmental Disabilities, 26*.

Read, S. G., & Rendall, M. (2007). An Open-Label Study of Risperidone in the Improvement of Quality of Life and Treatment of Symptoms of Violent and Self-Injurious Behaviour in Adults with Intellectual Disability. *Journal of Applied Research in Intellectual Disabilities, 20*, 256–264.

Rincover, A. (1978). Sensory extinction: A procedure for eliminating self-stimulatory behavior in developmentally disabled children. *Journal of Abnormal Child Psychology, 6*, 299–310.

Robertson, J., Emerson, E., Gregory, N., Hatton, C., Kessissoglou, S., & Hallam, A. (2000). Receipt of psychotropic medication by people with intellectual disability in residential settings. *Journal of Intellectual Disability Research, 44*, 666–676.

Rodriguez, N. M., Fisher, W. W., & Kelley, M. E. (2012). Treatment Methods Commonly Used in Conjunction with Functional Assessment *Functional Assessment for Challenging Behaviors* (pp. 179–193). New York: Springer.

Rojahn, J., Matson, J. L., Lott, D., Esbensen, A. J., & Smalls, Y. (2001). The Behavior Problems Inventory: An instrument for the assessment of self-injury, stereotyped behavior, and aggression/destruction in individuals with developmental disabilities. *Journal of Autism and Developmental Disorders, 31*, 577–588.

Rojahn, J., Whittaker, K., Hoch, T. A., & Gonzàles, M. L. (2007). Assessment of self-injurious and aggressive behavior. In J. L. Matson (Ed.), *Handbook of assessment in persons with intellectual disability* (pp. 281–319). San Diego: Academic.

Ross, E., & Oliver, C. (2003). The assessment of mood in adults who have severe or profound mental retardation. *Clinical Psychology Review, 23*, 225–245.

Ross, L. L., Yu, D., & Kropla, W. C. (1998). Stereotyped behavior in developmentally delayed or autistic populations: Rhythmic or nonrhythmic? *Behavior Modification, 22*, 321–334.

Schroeder, S. R., Mulick, J. A., & Rojahn, J. (1980). The definition, taxonomy, epidemiology, and ecology of self-injurious behavior. *Journal of Autism and Developmental Disorders, 10*.

Sigafoos, J. (1995). Factors associated with aggression versus aggression and self-injury among persons with intellectual disabilities. *Developmental Disabilities Bulletin, 23*, 30–39.

Singh, A. N., Matson, J. L., Hill, B., Pella, R. D., Cooper, C. L., & Adkins, A. D. (2010). The use of clozapine among individuals with intellectual disability: A review. *Research in developmental disabilities, 31*, 1135–1141.

Singh, N. N., Ellis, C. R., & Wechsler, H. (1997). Psychopharmacoepidemiology of mental retardation: 1966–1995. *Journal of Child and Adolescent Psychopharmacology, 7*, 255–266.

Singh, N. N., Lancioni, G. E., Winton, A. S., & Singh, J. (2011). Aggression, tantrums, and other externally driven challenging behaviors *International handbook of autism and pervasive developmental disorders* (pp. 413–435). New York: Springer.

Sipes, M., & Matson, J. L. (2012). Scaling Methods of Functional Assessment. In J. L. Matson (Ed.), *Functional Assessment for Challenging Behaviors* (pp. 159–177). New York: Springer.

Smith, K. R. M., & Matson, J. L. (2010). Behavior problems: Differences among intellectually disabled adults with co-morbid autism spectrum disorders and epilepsy. *Research in Developmental Disabilities, 31*, 1062–1069.

Spreat, S., Conroy, J. W., & Jones, J. C. (1997). Use of psychotropic medication in Oklahoma: a statewide survey. *American Journal on Mental Retardation, 102*, 80–85.

Sturmey, P., Laud, R. B., Cooper, C., Matson, J. L., & Fodstad, J. C. (2010). Challenging behaviors should not be considered depressive equivalents in individuals with intellectual disabilities. II. A replication study. *Research in Developmental Disabilities, 31*, 1002–1007.

Sturmey, P., Seiverling, L., & Ward-Horner, J. (2008). Assessment of Challenging Behaviors in People with Autism Spectrum Disorders. In J. L. Matson (Ed.), *Clinical Assessment and Intervention for Autism Spectrum Disorders*. London: Elsevier.

Sulzer-Azaroff, B., & Mayer, G. R. (1977). *Applying behavior-analysis procedures with children and youth*. New York: Holt, Rinehart and Winston.

Szymanski, L. S. (2002), DC-LD (Diagnostic Criteria for Psychiatric Disorders for Use with Adults with Learning Disabilities/Mental Retardation). *Journal of Intellectual Disability Research, 46*, 525–527.

Tate, B. G., & Baroff, G. S. (1973). Aversive Control of Self-Injurious Behavior in A Psychotic Boy. In J. M. Stedman, W. F. Patton & K. F. Walton (Eds.), *Clinical studies in behavior therapy with children, adolescents and their families*. (pp. 352–360). Springfield, IL US: Charles C Thomas Publisher.

Tierney, I. R., McGuire, R. J., & Walton, H. J. (1978). Distributions of body-rocking manifested by severely mentally deficient adults in ward environments. *Journal of Mental Deficiency Research, 22*, 243–254.

Tiger, J. H., Hanley, G. P., & Bruzek, J. (2008). Functional communication training: A review and practical guide. *Behavior Analysis in Practice, 1*, 16–23.

Touchette, P. E., MacDonald, R. F., & Langer, S. N. (1985). A scatter plot for identifying stimulus control of problem behavior. *Journal of Applied Behavior Analysis, 18*, 343–351.

Tsiouris, J., Mann, R., Patti, P., & Sturmey, P. (2003). Challenging behaviours should not be considered as depressive equivalents in individuals with intellectual disability. *Journal of Intellectual Disability Research, 47*, 14–21.

Tucker, M., Sigafoos, J., & Bushell, H. (1998). Use of noncontingent reinforcement in the treatment of challenging behavior a review and clinical guide. *Behavior Modification, 22*, 529–547.

Tureck, K., Matson, J. L., & Beighley, J. S. (2013). An investigation of self-injurious behaviors in adults with severe intellectual disabilities. *Research in Developmental Disabilities, 34*, 2469–2474.

Tyrer, P., Oliver-Africano, P. C., Ahmed, Z., Bouras, N., Cooray, S., Deb, S., … Reece, B. (2008). Risperidone, haloperidol, and placebo in the treatment of aggressive challenging behaviour in patients with intellectual disability: a randomised controlled trial. *The Lancet, 371*, 57–63.

Vitiello, B., & Stoff, D. M. (1997). Subtypes of aggression and their relevance to child psychiatry. *Journal of the American Academy of Child & Adolescent Psychiatry, 36*, 307–315.

Vollmer, T. R., Roane, H. S., & Rone, A. B. (2012). Experimental functional analysis. In J. L. Matson (Ed.), *Functional Assessment for Challenging Behaviors* (pp. 125–141): Springer.

Williams, C. D. (1959). The elimination of tantrum behavior by extinction procedures. *The Journal of Abnormal and Social Psychology, 59*, 269.

Winchel, R. M., & Stanley, M. (1991). Self-injurious behavior: A review of the behavior and biology of self-mutilation. *The American journal of psychiatry, 148*, 306–317.

Witwer, A. N., & Lecavalier, L. (2010). Validity of comorbid psychiatric disorders in youngsters with autism spectrum disorders. *Journal of Developmental and Physical Disabilities*.

Chapter 3
Psychopathology: ADHD, Autism Spectrum Disorders, and Other Conditions Present in Early Childhood

Cameron L. Neece, Lisa L. Christensen, Lauren D. Berkovits and Danessa Mayo

Children and adolescents with intellectual disabilities (ID) have been shown to have the high risk of developing comorbid psychiatric and behavioral disorders. According to epidemiological studies of youth with ID, approximately 30–50% of cases have reported clinically significant emotional and behavior problems and/or other psychiatric disorders (Emerson 2003). Due to the large variability in assessment methods, clinical measures, classification systems, and referral sources, it is difficult to accurately calculate the true prevalence of comorbid disorders in children with ID (Borthwick-Duffy 1994). A large-scale study in the Netherlands attempted such an undertaking, and used structured clinical interviews to examine the prevalence, comorbidity, and impact of DSM-IV disorders among youth with ID (Dekker and Koot 2003). The study reported that a number of children with ID met criteria for comorbid anxiety disorders, mood disorders, and, most commonly, disruptive behavior disorder (Dekker and Koot 2003), suggesting that comorbid mental disorders are very common among children with ID. However, the prevalence of other mental disorders in children with ID can be often overlooked, as the diagnosis of ID may complicate the detection of other common mental health issues usually seen in typically developing children. "Diagnostic overshadowing" occurs when other clinical issues (e.g., behavior problems) are attributed to limited cognitive capacity despite any additional assessment, diagnosis, or treatment of the comorbid disorders (Jopp and Keys 2001; Reiss and Szyszko 1983). Thus, these prevalence estimates may actually be an underestimate of the true prevalence of psychopathology among children with ID.

C. L. Neece (✉) · D. Mayo
Department of Psychology, Loma Linda University, Loma Linda, CA, USA
e-mail: cneece@llu.edu

L. L. Christensen · L. D. Berkovits
Department of Psychology, University of California, Los Angeles, CA, USA

J. L. Matson, M. L. Matson (eds.), *Comorbid Conditions in Individuals with Intellectual Disabilities,* Autism and Child Psychopathology Series,
DOI 10.1007/978-3-319-15437-4_3

One of the current limitations in studies examining comorbid behavior disorders among children with ID is the lack of comparison groups. Currently, there is limited understanding of the relative risk of psychopathology among children with ID compared to typically developing children. A study by Dekker and colleagues (2002) in a sample of children ages 7–12 with and without ID reported that parents endorsed behavior problems scores in the borderline or clinical range in 49 % of children with ID compared to 18 % of children without ID. Similar rates of elevated behavior problems were indicated on teacher-reported scores for children with (46 %) and without ID (19 %). Emerson and Hatton's (2007) study on children aged 5–16 years old from the UK also reported elevated behavior problems scores for 36 % of children with ID and 8 % without ID. In comparison to the previous findings mentioned, our own studies indicated a lower relative risk ratio during childhood (1.60:1, Baker et al. 2010) and adolescence (1.74, Neece et al. 2013). However, it may be noteworthy to address that in both cases, the lower relative risk ratio reported may have been influenced by the elevated prevalence of ODD diagnosis found in the typically developing comparison groups.

Regarding differences in comorbid psychopathology as a function of intellectual functioning, children with mild to severe levels of ID have similar prevalence rates of comorbid psychopathology. However, one study found that the degree of psychopathology decreased over time more for persons with mild ID than for persons with severe ID (Einfeld et al. 2006). Nevertheless, there is currently limited information available on the developmental course of comorbid behavior and emotional disorders for children with ID due to the popular use of age-mixed samples in cross-sectional designs. To date, the deRuiter et al. (2007) study is one of the few studies that focus on the developmental trajectory of children with ID with comorbid behavior and emotional disorders. deRuiter and colleagues (2007) conducted three assessments over a 5-year period on a sample of children who were from ages 6 to 18 and conducted multilevel growth curve analyses to examine developmental trajectories. While the children with ID had higher levels of problem behaviors than typically developing children at all ages, the study also found that children with ID had greater decline in aggressive and attention problems over time. Limited research available on children with ID and comorbid emotional, behavioral, and other clinical disorders highlights the need for increased focus and in-depth understanding of prevalence rates for specific comorbid disorders and their developmental trajectories. The following sections provide a brief overview of several comorbid disorders that have been typically reported among children with ID.

Attention-deficit Hyperactivity Disorder in Children with ID

With respect to specific symptoms or diagnoses, disruptive behavior disorders appear to be the most prevalent co-occurring disorders among children and adolescents with ID (Baker et al. 2010; Dekker and Koot 2003; Neece et al. 2011, 2012, 2013. Dekker and Koot (2003) found that 25.1 % of their sample of 7- to 20-year-old youth with borderline to moderate ID met criteria for a disruptive behavior disorder, compared to 21.9% for any anxiety disorder, and 4.4% for any mood disorder. Likewise, Baker et al. (2010) reported that every disorder assessed in a sample of 5-year-old children was more prevalent for children with developmental delays than for those who were typically developing, with attention-deficit hyperactivity disorder (ADHD) most highly differentiating the two groups (risk ratio 3.21 to 1). A longitudinal follow-up (Neece et al. 2011) showed that children with ID continued to be at significantly higher risk for meeting ADHD diagnostic criteria at ages 6, 7, and 8 (risk ratios ranged from 3.10:1 to 4.07:1) and subsequently into adolescence (risk ratio: 3.38:1, Neece et al. 2012).

Among typically developing populations, ADHD is more common in males than females. According to the DSM-IV, the male-to-female ratios range from 4:1 (general population) to 9:1 (clinic settings) (APA 2000). However, other studies have found smaller ratios and the sex differences appear to decrease over time (2.5:1 in childhood and 1.6:1 in adulthood) (Kessler et al. 2006). Among children and adolescents with ID sex differences in the prevalence of ADHD may not appear. Some investigations have not found gender differences in ADHD among children meeting criteria for both ADHD and ID (Baker et al. 2010; Neece et al. 2011; Neece et al. 2013). Hastings et al. (2005) examined the associations between ADHD and gender in two samples of children with ID between the ages of 3 and 19. These researchers administered two measures of hyperactivity and one measure of attention. There was a gender difference for one of the three measures with boys rated as having more hyperactivity symptoms than girls on one measure of hyperactivity. However, on the second measure of hyperactivity and measure of inattention no gender differences were observed. Thus, sex differences may prove to be one way that ADHD in ID differs from ADHD in typically developing youth. A number of explanations have been offered for the lack of gender differences in psychopathology among youth with ID including gender differences based on chronological age versus mental age and the developmental differences in neurocognitive factors (see Einfeld et al. 2010 for detailed review).

Children with ADHD often have more than one psychiatric disorder. Among the children who participated in the large-scale Multimodal Treatment Study of Children with ADHD (MTA), only 31.8% of them had ADHD alone; the majority of children meeting diagnostic criteria for ADHD also met criteria for at least one other disorder (Jensen et al. 2001). Oppositional defiant disorder (ODD) is the disorder that most commonly co-occurs with ADHD (39.9% of children in the MTA study had ADHD + ODD). However, other diagnoses were also comorbid with ADHD, including anxiety (38.7%), conduct disorder (14.3%), and affective disorder (3.8%). Among children with ADHD and ID, comorbidity appears to be even more common than compared to typically developing children with ADHD (Baker et al. 2010; Neece et al. 2011; Neece et al. 2013; Simonoff et al. 2006). In our own work we have found that similar to previous findings with typically developing samples, ADHD and ODD are the two most common co-occurring disorders (Baker et al. 2010; Neece et al. 2011; Neece et al. 2013).

Regarding the symptom presentation, ADHD is a heterogeneous condition and individuals can obtain the same ADHD symptom count with very different symptom patterns, all of which result in the same diagnosis. Initial evidence examining the presentation of ADHD symptoms among children with ID indicates that they tend to meet criteria for ADHD in similar ways compared to typically developing children. In our own research we have found that the number of ADHD symptoms endorsed did not differ between youth meeting ADHD criteria in the ID and typically developing samples nor did the percent of youth meeting criteria for ADHD by the inattentive, hyperactive–impulsive, or combined subtype (Baker et al. 2010; Neece et al. 2013). Additionally, the underlying factor structure of ADHD symptoms (i.e., two broad factors representing inattentive–disorganized symptoms and the hyperactive–impulsive symptoms) appears to be very similar among youth with and without ID (Neece et al. 2013).

In terms of changes in ADHD symptoms over time, the course of ADHD across development appears to vary by subtype. Hyperactivity and overactivity are generally more pronounced in preschool and these symptoms tend to decline with time. In contrast, problems with inattention tend to emerge later in development (typically between ages 8 and 12) and become more pronounced with age as peers undergo rapid maturation of the prefrontal cortical structures and accompanying cognitive abilities at the same time that school demands intensify (Applegate et al. 1997; von Stauffenberg and Campbell 2007; Waschbusch et al. 2007; Willoughby 2003). Although there are changes in symptomotology across development, many children with ADHD have some form of impairment persisting into adulthood (Faraone et al. 2006). Among children with ID and ADHD, limited evidence suggests that the symptoms of ADHD may persist longer in this population (Xenitidis et al. 2010). Our own data indicate that the symptom trajectories of ADHD symptoms across middle childhood and adolescents (ages 5–13) are similar in children with and without ID; however, children with ID maintained higher levels of ADHD symptoms across time (Neece et al. 2011, 2013).

Finally, to meet criteria for ADHD, the child must have some evidence of clinically significant impairment in social, academic, or occupational functioning (APA 2013). In other words, it is not enough for the child to have clinical levels of inattention and/or hyperactive/impulsive symptoms but these symptoms must interfere with the child's daily life and overall functioning. Children with ADHD have been found to have more impairment across a variety of domains including behavioral functioning (Cunningham and Boyle 2002; Harvey et al. 2009), social functioning (Casey 1996), academic functioning (Barkley 1998; Barkley et al. 1990; Du-Paul and Stoner 1994), family functioning (Barkley et al. 2001; Johnston and Mash 2001; Pelham and Lang 1993; Taylor et al. 1991), and health outcomes (Biederman et al. 1994; Hartsough and Lambert 1985; Jensen et al. 1988; Szatmari et al. 1989).

Little research has examined functional impairment experienced by children and adolescents with ADHD and ID. Stein et al. (1995) compared children with ADHD (mean IQ = 101) to children with mild ID on measures of adaptive behavior. They found that the ADHD group had a mean Vineland Adaptive Behavior Scale (Sparrow et al. 1984) composite score of 73, which was well below what would be expected given their level of intellectual functioning. Additionally, the ADHD and mild ID groups were not significantly different from each other in terms of adaptive behavior (communication, daily living, and socialization domains). Our own investigation indicated that ADHD functioning predicted child functional impairment above and beyond the child's intellectual functioning (Neece et al. 2012) indicating that ADHD symptoms contribute to the child's functional impairment independent of his or her cognitive limitations.

Although there is evidence that the prevalence of psychopathology is elevated in children and adolescents with ID, questions remain about the validity of many of these diagnoses for this population. One critical problem in this area of research is that the base rate of most psychiatric symptoms among children and adolescents with ID has not been established and, therefore, the extent to which the symptoms of given disorders are intrinsic to ID is not clear. Thus, we do not know whether certain emotional and behavioral symptoms among youth with ID are solely an expression of impairments in intellectual functioning or if these disorders form a separate construct that accounts for variability in outcomes above and beyond the youth's cognitive abilities. Limited research has examined the validity of mental health disorders among children with ID, with the exception of ADHD for which these questions have begun to be examined. Two studies from our own lab have examined the clinical presentation, as well as the validity of ADHD, among adolescents with and without ID (Neece et al. 2012; Neece et al. 2013). In general, our findings indicated that the presentation of ADHD was similar among adolescents with and without ID and that similar "pre-pathway" influences were associated with ADHD regardless of cognitive functioning. This is a first step in establishing the validity of current diagnostic categories for children with ID.

Oppositional Defiant Disorder in Children with IDD

Like ADHD, ODD is also a disruptive behavior disorder and one of the most common forms of comorbid psychopathology for children and adolescents with ID (Dekker and Koot 2003; Emerson and Hatton 2007). The *Diagnostic and Statistical Manual of Mental Disorders*—Fifth Edition (DSM-5; American Psychiatric Association [APA] 2013) has defined ODD as "a pattern of angry/irritable mood, argumentative/defiant behavior, or vindictiveness lasting at least 6 months as evidenced by four symptoms from any of three categories, and exhibited during interactions with at least one individual who is not a sibling." In recognition of the complexity of this disorder, DSM-5 has divided the symptoms of ODD into three subgroups: angry/irritable mood, argumentative/defiant behavior, and vindictiveness. This revision was made to reflect research suggesting that ODD comprises both behavioral and emotional symptomatology, and to distinguish between these different domains. Additional revisions also reflect an understanding that some degree of oppositional and defiant behavior is normative, particularly for certain age groups (e.g. toddlers, adolescents). Accordingly, the text of DSM-5 provides guidelines regarding the frequency of symptoms for different age ranges, noting, for example, that for children ages 5 and younger the behavior should occur most days for at least 6 months.

While the diagnosis of ODD for children with typical development is complicated by the normative prevalence of behavior problems during various stages of development, the comorbidity between ID and ODD represents a particularly complex issue. There is considerable research to date illustrating an elevated rate of behavior problems among children with ID (Baker et al. 2002; Hastings et al. 2006; Neece et al. 2012; Whitaker and Read 2006). Thus, it may be difficult to determine the true prevalence of formally diagnosed behavior disorders such as ODD for children with ID, as a higher rate of behavior problems is already the norm. In that regard, the DSM-5 states that an individual's developmental level (as well as gender and culture) should be taken into account when considering whether the frequency of symptoms meets diagnostic criteria (APA 2013). This raises two problems. On the one hand, there may be considerable diagnostic overshadowing in which clinicians and researchers view all behavior problems as manifestations of the ID rather than an additional behavior disorder (Reiss et al. 1982). On the other hand, clinicians and researchers may fail to recognize the higher prevalence of behavior problems in individuals with ID and consequently, view all behavior problems as stemming from a comorbid diagnosis of ODD.

In this vein, there has been considerable uncertainty regarding the validity of ODD as a diagnosis for children with ID, and there is little research describing the clinical presentation of ODD for this population. One way to address the validity of ODD for children with ID is to consider the similarity between ODD in this population and ODD for typically developing youth. In comparing these two populations, researchers can determine whether the disorder appears the same for both groups and thus, whether the same diagnostic entity is being captured by this label. Diagnostic validity has historically been determined through clinical description, laboratory findings, exclusion of other disorders, follow-up studies, and family history (Robins and Guze 1970). More recently, researchers have also emphasized the importance of examining etiological factors, developmental course, outcomes, and treatment response (Andreasen 1995; Antshel et al. 2006). When examining whether a diagnosis is valid for a particular population, it is important to consider the convergence of these elements in the typical population and in the population of interest—whether the presentation, etiology, and sequelae of the disorder are the same for both groups. Likewise, it is important to consider sources of divergence and illustrate that the disorder in the population of interest diverges from other disorders or characteristics in that population.

Research suggests that youth with ID have an elevated rate of ODD compared to typically developing peers. The DSM-5 cites a prevalence rate of 1–11% for children with typical development, noting that the average is around 3.3%. Emerson and Hatton (2007) found a prevalence rate of 11.1% for children with ID; in contrast, they cited an ODD prevalence of 2.3% for children with typical development. Subsequent studies have also found considerably higher rates of ODD for children with ID, with prevalences ranging from 34 to 45% between ages 5 and 9 (Christensen et al. 2013). This is in contrast to rates of 20–28% for typically developing children. The notably higher rates described more recently may reflect differences in the methodology used by the researchers, including the use of maternal-report measures only. Likewise, the study by Christensen et al. (2013) examined a younger sample (point prevalences of ages 5 through 9), while earlier studies included youth in ages 5–16. Regardless, differences in prevalence between youth with ID and those with typical development remain consistent across studies, and researchers find that children with ID meet criteria for ODD at 2–5 times the rate of typically developing children.

Relatively few studies have examined other aspects of clinical presentation, and there continues to be a need for research in this area. However, one study by Christensen et al. (2013) found no differences between typically developing children and those with ID in terms of the gender distribution, age of onset, and stability of ODD over time. The results of this study are described in further detail below.

Within the typically developing population, there is some research suggesting that ODD is more prevalent among boys. Other studies have found no differences in prevalence by gender, and there is some evidence to indicate that such differences vary by reporter. For example, two groups of researchers (Maughan et al. (2004); Serra-Pinheiro et al. (2008)) found that significant gender differences in ODD were apparent for teacher-report data only. Similarly, the DSM-5 describes gender differences in ODD prior to adolescence (with slightly more boys than girls meeting criteria for the disorder; ratio of 1.4:1), but reports no gender difference in prevalence rates during adolescence (APA 2013). In this vein, recent research finds no gender differences in the prevalence of ODD for children with ID, and the gender distribution of ODD does not differ based on disability status (ID vs. TD; Christensen et al. 2013).

Research on the age of onset of ODD in typically developing children has also been somewhat inconsistent. While some studies cite the typical age of onset as 12–13 (Kessler et al. 2005; Nock et al. 2007), other studies find evidence for diagnoses as early as age 2–5 (Lavigne et al. 2001). The DSM-5 states that the first symptoms of ODD are often apparent during the preschool years, and typically no later than early adolescence. Christensen et al. (2013) examined the age of onset of ODD for children with and without ID. The authors categorized children as "early" or "late" onset, with children first meeting criteria for ODD at age 5 or 6 labeled as "early onset" and those first meeting criteria for ODD at age 7 or later as "late onset." Findings suggested that most children fell into the "early onset" category regardless of disability status, and no significant differences emerged between children with and without ID.

Finally, research suggests that 14–19 % of children with ID meet criteria for multiple psychiatric disorders, compared to only 3 % of typically developing children (Dekker and Koot 2003; Emerson 2003). Additional research has emphasized the comorbidity between ODD and ADHD. In this vein, findings suggest that about 40 % of typically developing children with ADHD meet criteria for ODD and vice versa (Jensen et al. 2001; Speltz et al. 1999). ODD also appears to be relatively stable over time, with approximately 50 % of typically developing youth continuing to meet criteria up to 4 years later (Speltz et al. 1999; Lahey and Loeber 1994).

Research on the stability of ODD for children with ID suggests that the diagnosis is relatively stable from year to year, with percent agreements of 50–67% (Christensen et al. 2013). More importantly, there appear to be no significant differences in stability over time between children with ID and those with typical development; when tracked from ages 5 to 9, most children in either group seem to have stable patterns of diagnosis (Christensen et al. 2013). In contrast, the comorbidity of ODD does appear to differ for children with and without ID. In particular, children with ID and ODD appear to meet criteria for another disorder at significantly higher rates than typically developing children with ODD. This also appears true for ADHD in particular, with 50–59% of children with ID meeting criteria for both ODD and ADHD compared to 12–24% of typically developing children (Christensen et al. 2013; Baker et al. 2010).

Overall, youth with ID appear to meet criteria for ODD at 2–5 times the rate of typically developing peers, and there is greater comorbidity with other psychiatric disorders. Otherwise, there appear to be no differences in the clinical presentation of ODD for children with and without ID, lending credence to the idea that ODD is the same disorder for both populations. Moreover, the elevated comorbidity of ODD for children with ID may be an artifact of the higher prevalence of most psychiatric disorders for youth with ID, and the increased prevalence of ADHD in particular (Baker et al. 2010).

Beyond the similarities in age of onset, gender distribution, and stability, research also suggests that youth with and without ID meet criteria for ODD in similar ways. In particular, Christensen et al. (2013) compared the symptom counts as well as specific DSM-IV-TR symptoms to determine whether children with ID meet criteria for ODD in the same manner that youth with typical development do. The authors found no significant differences in the total number of symptoms or in rank order correlations of the relative frequency with which items were endorsed. Finally, the authors found no group differences in the frequency with which particular items were endorsed, even when examined individually.

Autism Spectrum Disorders and ID

Autism spectrum disorder (ASD) is one of the most common neurodevelopmental disorders occurring in 1 out of 68 children (Centers for Disease Control and Prevention [CDC] 2014a) and is the second most common comorbid disorder with ID after ADHD (Strømme and Diseth 2000). According to the Diagnostic and Statistical Manual of Mental Disorders (5th ed.; DSM-5; American Psychiatric Association [APA] 2013), ASD is characterized by the following criteria: a) "Persistent deficits on social communication and social interaction across multiple contexts (i.e., deficits in social-emotional reciprocity; deficits in nonverbal communicative behaviors used for social interaction; deficits in developing, maintaining, and understanding relationships);" and b) "Restricted, repetitive patterns of behavior, interests or activities, as manifested by at least three of the following…(i.e., stereotyped or repetitive motor movements, use of objects, or speech; insistence on sameness, inflexible adherence to routines, or ritualized patterns of verbal or nonverbal behavior; highly restricted, fixated interests that are abnormal in intensity or focus; hyper- or hyporeactivity to sensory input or unusual interest in sensory aspects of the environment)." The DSM-5 (APA 2013) revisions sought to improve upon and address the diagnostic criteria for ASD, which also resulted in the creation of the new diagnosis of social communication disorder (SCD), which accounts for children who present with deficits in social functioning and communication but no repetitive patterns of behavior or interest (APA 2013).

A notable change in the ASD diagnostic criteria consists of the recognized high overlap between ASD and ID. The co-occurrence of ID in children with ASD (18–79%) has been repeatedly cited in several findings (CDC 2014a; Charman et al. 2011; Levy et al. 2010; Mannion et al. 2013; Matson and Nebel-Schwalm 2007). However, a smaller number of studies have reported on the comorbidity rate of ASD in children with ID (10–28%) (Bryson et al. 2008; De Bildt et al. 2005; Wing and Gould 1979). Differences in comorbid prevalence rates have been noted depending on the level of ASD severity. For children with autism, there is a higher prevalence rate of ID (66–70%) in comparison to those with pervasive developmental disorders-not otherwise (8–12%) and Asperger's disorder (0%) (Chakrabarti and Fombonne 2001, 2005). Among children with autism and comorbid ID, 50% had mild to moderate levels of ID, and 19.2% had severe ID. In order to make a comorbid diagnosis of ASD in youth with ID, the DSM-5 criteria states that "social communication should be below that expected for general developmental level" (e.g., few words or intelligible speech versus able to speak in full sentences or engage in communication; APA 2013).

Detecting comorbid ASD in children with ID is crucial for early intervention. Prior to school entry, children's learning and developmental difficulties are often not as apparent to parents until they enter the academic setting and their learning deficiencies are brought to parents' attention (Goin-Kochel et al. 2008). A study on parents' and caregivers' perceptions of their children's (age range 1.7–40.6 years) possible comorbid ID and ASD diagnosis revealed a 9% prevalence rate, which was significantly lower in comparison to the general clinical estimates of 18–79% for any ASD (Goin-Kochel et al. 2008). While some parents may have been unaware of their child's comorbid diagnoses, changes in prevalence rates by child age may also be a function of the diagnostic process. In general, ID is usually diagnosed in children over age 5 (Goin-Kochel et al. 2008), while ASD is usually diagnosed around ages 4 –6, but symptoms are apparent as early as 18–24 months old (CDC 2014a, 2014b; Levy et al. 2010; Maenner et al. 2013; Shattuck et al. 2009).

The diagnostic steps for identifying ASD in children consist of a developmental screening and a comprehensive diagnostic evaluation conducted by primary health care providers, child neurologists, and/or psychologists (CDC 2014b). Such evaluations can shed light on possible developmental delays and behavioral problems related to ASD. Collateral information from parent interviews is also helpful in diagnosing ASD in children with ID (Hartley and Sikora 2010). Among older youth with ID, presenting problems in social interactions, stereotyped language, pretend play, and narrow pattern of interests have been credited as important factors to help identify comorbid ASD (Hartley and Sikora 2010). However, this method can also run into the issue of parents either over- or under-reporting symptoms on children with ID and ASD. Therefore, the use of observational measures along with parent interviews/reports support the validity of a comorbid ASD diagnosis in youth.

Regarding the clinical presentation, boys are more likely to be diagnosed with ASD than girls (CDC 2014a), which is also true for children with ID and comorbid ASD, regardless of level of intellectual functioning (Bryson et al. 2008). Some studies have found that girls diagnosed with ASD tend to have more severe ASD symptoms and more severe ID (Charman et al. 2011; Lin et al. 2013), while other studies cite similar rates of severe ID in boys and girls (Bryson et al. 2008). In terms of ethnicity, ASD is most likely to be diagnosed in Caucasian children (1 in 63), followed by African-American (1 in 81), Asian/Pacific Islander (1 in 81), and Hispanic youth (1 in 93) (CDC 2014a). Among individuals with comorbid ID and ASD diagnoses, there is also a higher prevalence rate reported for Caucasians in relation to ethnic minority groups (Emerson 2012). The epidemiological outlook on children with ID and ASD over time is problematic. Longitudinal studies showed that youth with ID report high levels of comorbid psychopathology that was consistent over a 4–14-year period (Einfeld et al. 2006; Tonge and Einfeld 2000). Children with ASD and ID were also found to have more psychiatric outpatient care visits than children with ASD only, and are expected to have 2.7 times higher annual medical care costs than those with ASD only (Lin et al. 2013; Peacock et al. 2012). Peacock et al. (2012) concluded that comorbid ID and ASD diagnosis was associated with higher medical care costs (US$ 19,190 annual average) than children with ASD only (US$ 7,198), or other comorbid disorders such as ADHD (US$ 9,478) and epilepsy (US$ 11,847). Given that children with ID and ASD are likely to be high consumers of health care services over time, there is a significant need for more epidemiological and longitudinal research in order to clearly examine the developmental course and outcomes of children with ID and ASD over time.

Anxiety Disorders in Children with IDD

Anxiety disorders are diagnosed when an individual experiences excessive fear or anxiety and displays impaired functioning as a result. Anxiety disorders are one of the most common categories of mental illness among typically developing children, though prevalence estimates vary across studies (Cartwright-Hatton et al. 2006). The point prevalence estimates for some of the more common anxiety disorders are 0.5–3.0% for separation anxiety disorder, 0.3–2.5% for social phobia, and 0.4–2.5% for generalized anxiety disorder (e.g., Canino et al. 2004; Fleitlich-Bilyk and Goodman 2004; Roberts et al. 2007). However, each anxiety disorder develops differently throughout childhood and adolescence, with peaks in prevalence at varying stages of development. For example, separation anxiety disorder is most prevalent in preschool years (up to 4.9%) and declines rapidly in prevalence throughout elementary and middle school years (Compton et al. 2000). Social phobia is present at lower levels in early childhood but increases throughout development, particularly during late childhood and early adolescence (Canino et al. 2004). Generalized anxiety disorder tends to increase in girls but decrease in boys as children enter the later school-age years and progress through adolescence. Among typically developing children, anxiety diagnoses tend to be more prevalent in females than males by adolescence (e.g., Compton et al. 2000; Roberts et al. 2007). However, in studies of young children, no sex differences in prevalence are typically found for any of the anxiety disorders (e.g., Canino et al. 2004; Duchesne et al. 2007).

Children with ID have significantly higher prevalence rates of anxiety disorders than children with typical development. Among children and adolescents with ID, approximately 10–22 % meet criteria for any anxiety disorder at any given time, compared to just 3–7 % among youth with typical development (e.g., Dekker and Koot 2003; Emerson and Hatton 2007; Roberts et al. 2007). In fact, in one of these studies, specific phobia was the most prevalent DSM-IV disorder among children with ID (17.5 %) as assessed via the Diagnostic Interview Schedule for Children (DISC), though fewer children experience significant impairment due to their phobia (6.8 %; Dekker and Koot 2003). Five-year-old children with ID exhibit significantly higher rates of separation anxiety (17.6 %) than typically developing 5-year-old children (5.2 %), as measured using this same parent-interview measure (Green et al. 2014). However, later in childhood, children with TD and ID exhibit more comparable rates of separation anxiety. When analyzing parent reports of children's anxiety symptoms through written questionnaires, elementary-aged (i.e., 5–9 years) children with ID are more likely to fall within clinical levels of symptoms on the anxiety problems subscale of the Child Behavior Checklist (13.7–28.1 %) compared to children with typical development (6.0–14.8 %), with significant differences between the groups emerging by ages 8 and 9 (Green et al. 2014). Additionally, anxiety levels appear to be related to children's level of cognitive functioning. In one study, children with mild, moderate, and severe levels of ID exhibited high anxiety scores on the Developmental Behaviour Checklist, while children with profound ID exhibited significantly lower levels of anxiety (Einfeld and Tonge 1996). While anxiety may truly differ based on cognitive abilities (e.g., the cognitive symptoms of worrying as described in the criteria for many DSM anxiety diagnoses may be less likely to occur in individuals with low cognitive functioning), this finding also raises the possibility of under-recognition of children's anxiety due to children's language and communicative impairments impeding their ability to share their symptoms with caregivers.

In addition to exhibiting higher anxiety overall, children with ID also have higher co-occurrence of anxiety with other psychiatric disorders. Dekker and Koot (2003) found that twice as many children with ID and an anxiety disorder also met criteria for one or more co-occurring disruptive behavior disorders (42.5 %; i.e., ADHD, ODD, and conduct disorder), compared to typically developing children with anxiety disorders (20.6–20.9 %; e.g., Fleitlich-Bilyk and Goodman 2004). Green et al. (2014) also found significantly higher odds of children with ID meeting clinical significance for both anxiety and inattentive/hyperactive symptoms, in particular, and externalizing problems, overall. These odds proved to be above chance levels (at least twice the frequency as expected by chance), given the higher rates of clinical levels of anxiety and other psychiatric symptoms in this population, and may result in higher levels of impairment among these children. One possible explanation for this higher rate of comorbidity is that, given deficits in emotion regulation skills and communicative abilities, children with ID may be more likely to act out or be noncompliant when they are anxious. In contrast, the co-occurrence between anxiety and mood disorders is lower across both ID and TD populations (7.4–12.3 %) and is more similar across the two groups (e.g., Dekker and Koot 2003; Fleitlich-Bilyk and Goodman 2004).

The presentation of anxiety among children with ID appears to at least partially overlap with the presentation of anxiety among typically developing children. For example, similar to the comparable prevalence rates of anxiety across sexes for pre-adolescent children, studies examining sex differences in anxiety have not found consistent differences in prevalence among children with ID (Einfeld et al. 2011; Green et al. 2014). Relative equality in anxiety symptoms across genders was also seen when analyzing the amount and intensity of self-reported fears. In addition, though children with ID exhibit higher levels of anxiety, the growth in anxiety symptoms across development occurs at similar rates across the two groups. For example, Green et al. (2014) found similar, positive slopes when studying the development of anxiety symptoms in children with and without ID during elementary school years. With a focus on the types of fears experienced by children with ID, fears of failure and criticism were highest among adolescents (ages 14–18) as compared to younger children (ages 7–13), paralleling the increase of the prevalence of social phobia throughout development. However, while overall levels of anxiety may increase similarly in both groups, research suggests that different disorders may not follow the same trajectories in children with and without ID. For example, the higher rates of separation anxiety disorder in children with ID compared to typically developing peers at age 5 may indicate that separation anxiety disorder takes longer to decrease in children with ID, reaching comparable levels 1 year later (at age 6). Conversely, social phobia appears to increase similarly for both groups over time.

Overall, across multiple methods of measurement (i.e., DSM prevalence rates vs. ratings of clinical symptoms, parent interviews vs. rating forms), children with ID present with higher rates of anxiety symptoms and problems than their typically developing peers. Current evidence suggests a similar presentation of anxiety in children with ID, though higher comorbidities with externalizing symptoms and slightly different trajectories of specific anxiety symptoms are seen within this population.

Other Comorbidities

The developmental, emotional, and behavioral disorders discussed in this chapter appear to be more common among children with ID. However, other less common comorbid disorders have been noted, but currently there is limited information on these diagnoses such as mood disorders, eating and feeding problems, trauma, and other health conditions. Nevertheless, it is important to present the current information available in order to promote the development of additional research in these given areas.

Contemporary studies have shown some interest in the co-occurrence of mood disorders in children with ID. The clinical presentation of mood disorders such as depression and bipolar disorder in individuals with ID has been challenging to determine, especially among individuals with more severe ID (Masi et al. 1999). However, a key clinical symptom that has been noted among individuals with ID and comorbid mood disorders is self-injury and/or suicidal behaviors. Self-injury has been known to occur among individuals with ID (40 %), and with higher likelihood among those with severe ID and/or co-occurring ASD (Hill and Furniss 2006; Holden and Gitlesen 2006; Oliver et al. 2012). It is important to make the distinction that the function of self-injury is different for individuals with ID in comparison to typically developing children. For children with ID, the act of self-injury (e.g., head banging, hitting self, biting self, self-scratching) primarily includes physical (e.g., escape, relief, sensory stimulation), social (e.g., attention seeking, social reinforcement), to verbal functions (e.g., communication, desired outcome) (MacLean et al. 2010; O'Reilly et al. 2010). Conversely, self-injury for typically developing youth may serve as a way to attain emotional relief. It has also been observed that individuals with ID are more likely to engage in problem behaviors such as aggression and self-injury due to more severe ID symptomology (Kurtz et al. 2011; Kurtz et al. 2003). The prevalence rate of self-injury among children with severe ID is around 17–30 % (MacLean et al. 2010; Oliver et al. 2012). Among youth with ID from ages 13–17, the prevalence rates for suicidal ideation are 22–60 %, while suicidal behaviors range from 17–48 % (Ludi et al. 2012). In comparison, typically developing youth reported a much lower risk of suicidal ideation (14–16 %) and suicidal behaviors (7 %) (CDC 2012). Overall, the emerging studies on mood disorders in children with ID raise public awareness regarding the ongoing self-injury and suicide risk in the ID population.

Eating and feeding problems have also been known to occur among children with ID. Studies on feeding problems among children with ID indicate that it is a highly common issue (80–97 %), especially for children with more severe ID (Gal et al. 2011; Rezaei et al. 2011). In particular, children with ID are more prone to feeding problems related to lack of feeding skills, followed by disruptive behavior, under- and over-eating, and food selectivity (Rezaei et al. 2011). These studies highlight the need for general assessment of comorbid feeding problems among children with ID, along with family/parenting education on eating and feeding problems.

Further, despite the high suspected rates of abuse and trauma among individuals with disabilities, the research urgency to address abuse and trauma among children with ID has been minimal. Studies show that children with ID are twice as likely to be physically or sexually abused than typically developing children (Jones et al. 2012; Reiter et al. 2007). Specifically, children with ID have a 21 % risk of experiencing any history of violence, 27 % risk of physical abuse, 15 % risk of sexual abuse, 27 % risk of emotional abuse, and 8 % risk of neglect (Jones et al. 2012).

Compared to typically developing children, youth with ID tend to report higher rates of physical abuse (i.e., being forced to do something, being refused something essential for well-being), sexual abuse (i.e., sexual harassment, unwanted sexual touching), and emotional abuse (i.e., humiliation) (Reiter et al. 2007; Soylu et al. 2013). Sexual abuse among children with ID was also more frequent and repeated, was often under-reported, was more likely to involve someone familiar, and also involved more than one abuser (Soylu et al. 2013). These findings should serve as a call for immediate action against abuse and trauma among children and with ID.

Aside from psychiatric disorders, children with ID have also been found to have other lesser known comorbid health conditions. Obesity has been reported as a growing comorbid health concern among children with ID (Rimmer et al. 2010; Slevin et al. 2014). The prevalence of obesity among children with ID was higher compared to typically developing children (Slevin et al. 2014). Furthermore, children with ID endorsed more hours of low-level activity and had more fatty and sugary food intake (Maïano 2011). Neurological disorders have also been reported as co-occurring symptoms in children with ID. In particular, there is a 20–28 % prevalence risk of comorbid epilepsy in children with ID (Jelliffe-Pawlowski et al. 2003; Morgan et al. 2003; Nielsen et al. 2007b; Oguni 2013). Various studies also suggested 16–56 % prevalence rate of comorbid cerebral palsy among children with ID (Jauhari et al. 2012; Nielsen et al. 2007b; Zhang and Ji 2005). Visual (2–27 %) and hearing problems (4–17 %) were also noted and are prevalent with children who have moderate to severe ID (Jauhari et al. 2012; Nielsen et al. 2007a; Nielsen et al. 2007b). Lastly, children with ID present with a likelihood of having other comorbid physical health conditions such as gastrointestinal problems (7 %), malformations such as Down syndrome (2–7 %), and other congenital nervous system malformations (3–8 %) (Christianson et al. 2002; Dekker and Koot 2003; Petterson et al. 2007; Schrojenstein Lantman-de Valk et al. 1997; Zhang and Ji 2005). Overall, the diagnosis of ID puts children at great risk for developing co-occurring extensive physical and mental health issues that persist throughout their development.

Interventions and Clinical Implications

Comorbid psychiatric disorders in children with ID are complex and associated with a host of negative outcomes for children and their families. Children with ID and comorbid disorders show increased risk for lower academic functioning, adaptive functioning in the community, social functioning, and career opportunities (Borthwick-Duffy and Eyman 1990; Bromley and Blacher 1991; Eisenhower et al. 2005; Pearson et al. 2000; Seltzer and Krauss 2001). Parents of individuals with ID and comorbid disorders endorse elevated parenting stress (Baker et al. 2002; Baker et al. 2010; Blacher and McIntyre 2006; Herring et al. 2006; McIntyre et al. 2002) and an increased need for services (Douma et al. 2006). Families who undergo challenges in providing care for those with ID and comorbid disorders have an increased risk of seeking out-of-home placement for the individual (Blacher 1994; Bromley and Blacher 1991; McIntyre et al. 2002). For children with ID that live at home, most of them have unmet mental health needs that have a high social cost (Blacher et al. 1999). The annual cost of care for persons with ID and destructive behaviors was estimated around $3 billion. The individual, family, and societal cost of care for individuals with ID and comorbid psychiatric disorders highlight the overwhelming need for additional research on its causes and consequences.

Comorbid disorders among children with ID have been least understood and have not garnered the attention of most research on individuals with disabilities to date (Campbell and Malone 1991; McCarthy and Boyd 2002). General psychiatric and health care services lack adequate experience and knowledge in the assessment and treatment of individuals with ID (Sturmey et al. 2007). The limited clinical understanding of treatment and interventions for children with ID and comorbid disorders is a grave concern, and should serve as an impetus for continued research in such an underserved population.

Based on the overwhelming research presented, it is evident that children with ID are at great risk for developing a host of comorbid disorders. Since comorbid disorders tend to have negative long-term effects on various outcomes or children with ID and their families, they are an important target for early intervention (Baker et al. 2002; Baker et al. 2010; Blacher and McIntyre 2006; Eisenhower et al. 2005; Herring et al. 2006; McIntyre et al. 2002; Neece 2014; Pearson et al. 2000; Seltzer and Krauss 2001). Currently there are limited interventions specific to children with ID and comorbid disorders. Those that exist are generally based on existing interventions adapted for typically developing children. Given the increased needs of this population, these interventions have been largely unsuccessful with a few exceptions (Moree and Davis 2010). Additionally, most studies have taken an individual child-centered approach to treatment of comorbid emotional and behavioral problems in children with ID, with little consideration of family, school, cultural, or contextual factors that contribute to and maintain mental health problems in this population. Despite the absence of evidence-based treatments to serve this population, studies estimate that 2 – 14 % of youth referred for psychiatric care have ID, indicating that this population comprises a substantial subgroup of patients referred for psychiatric treatment (Sverd 2003; Sverd et al. 1995; Wozniak et al. 1997).

Regarding treatments for specific diagnoses, research examining the treatment of ADHD among children with ID is limited; however, the existing literature suggests that empirically supported treatments for typically developing children with ADHD, specifically stimulant medication and behavioral modification interventions, may also be effective in treating children with ID. Moreover, this research indicates that the combined use of stimulant medication and behavioral interventions can be beneficial for children with ID (Handen et al. 1996; Johnson et al. 1995).

Studies on psychosocial interventions for children with ID or low functioning ASD garner further support for behavioral and skill-based treatments (Eikeseth et al. 2012; Peters-Scheffer et al. 2010). Similarly, a range of treatments for ASD including behavioral skill-based treatments (e.g., applied behavior analysis [ABA], discrete trial teaching, pivotal response training [PRT]), cognitive (e.g., Social Stories, Learning Experiences: An Alternative Program for Preschoolers and Parents

[LEAP]), physiological (e.g., sensory integration), and other interventions (e.g., gluten-free diet, supplements) have also been used with children with co-occurring ID. Exploratory studies on adapted treatments for children with ID and ASD are emerging and tend to be skill-based, such as ABA, PRT, and low-intensity behavioral treatment. ABA is a form of behavioral intervention that has shown extensive improvements in children with ASD in the areas of communication, cognitive, and adaptive skills (Dawson and Faja 2008; Eldevik et al. 2009; Reichow and Wolery 2009; Schreibman 2000; Smith et al. 1997). PRT is another form of behavioral treatment approach that utilizes naturalistic situations to teach children to adopt more generalized skills, increase motivation, and with minimal prompting needed. Similarly, PRT has been used with children with ASD and targets increased skill generalization, self-management, and motivation (Bryson et al. 2007; Carter 2001; Koegel et al. 2003; Romaniuk and Miltenberger 2001). Low-intensity behavioral treatment is a modified version of standard ABA that was created to address the intervention barriers experienced by clinicians and parents (e.g., schedule availability, staff issues) (Peters-Scheffer et al. 2010). Compared to typically developing children, children with ASD and mild to severe ID reported greater developmental age and adaptive skills gain with low-intensity behavioral treatment (Peters-Scheffer et al. 2010, 2013). Specifically, children with ID and ASD showed significant improvements in attentiveness, communication, concentration, and more calm behavior. Parents of children with ID and comorbid ASD also reported a decrease in their child's challenging behaviors (Peters-Scheffer et al. 2010). The ongoing treatment outcomes for skill-based behavioral treatment is promising and suggests that it is an intervention that may be of great clinical interest in addressing comorbid ID and ASD symptoms. However, additional studies focused specifically on children with ID and ASD are needed in order to confirm the effectiveness of the intervention for this population.

There is also a need for research on the treatment of ODD in children with ID. There is some research on the use of evidence-based treatments for ODD with children with ID, specifically parent–child interaction therapy (PCIT). McDiarmid and Bagner (2005) completed a case study of a 3-year-old child with moderate ID who also met criteria for ODD. The authors found that after 14 sessions of PCIT, this child no longer met criteria for ODD, and they reported a significant reduction in parenting stress as well. Bagner and Eyberg (2007) extended these findings and conducted a randomized control trial of PCIT with 30 mother– child dyads. Children in this study ranged from ages 3 to 6, and each was diagnosed with ODD and either mild or moderate intellectual disability. The authors found significant changes in the parenting skills demonstrated by caregivers in the immediate treatment group (relative to the waitlist controls). More importantly, the authors also found evidence for improvement in the child's misbehavior as well as significant decreases in parenting stress.

Research into the treatment of anxiety disorders for children with ID consists largely of case studies applying behavioral or cognitive– behavioral approaches along with modifications for use with children with cognitive impairments. For example, several case studies describe using traditional in vivo exposure to treat children's anxiety symptoms, along with high levels of parent involvement, concrete presentation of concepts, and additional opportunities for behavioral practice through increased number of sessions or increased opportunities for exposure (Davis et al. 2008). However, limited additional research has been conducted regarding the ways to treat anxiety among individuals with ID. Cognitive – behavioral approaches have been studied in both individual cases as well as in larger, controlled studies; however, these have really only been examined in samples of adults with ID. Additionally, qualitative research has been conducted to explore client perceptions among adults with ID undergoing cognitive behavioral treatment for anxiety disorders or other psychiatric symptoms. Clients valued the process of talking to the therapist about areas of difficulty, as well as feeling validated and understood by the therapist, and noted increases in coping skills, self-expression, and daily living skills as a result of their treatments (Pert et al. 2013). Research has also been conducted on the use of mindfulness-based cognitive therapy for the treatment of anxiety and depression symptoms in adults with ID. Modifications applied to this treatment included the incorporation of caregivers into the treatment as active participants, in order to help them learn the skills and support skills participants need to develop. The participants exhibited a significant reduction in anxiety symptoms across a 9-week treatment, and improvements were maintained across an additional 6-week follow-up. However, this treatment appeared to be most effective for individual with mild levels of ID, as individuals with lower cognitive functioning (i.e., moderate ID) and their caretakers reported difficulty with the material and exhibited a higher dropout rate from the study. Thus, cognitive– behavioral techniques have been successfully applied to adults with cognitive impairments, though most studies have focused on, or exhibited greater outcomes for, adults with more mild levels of disability. A larger body of literature has examined interventions for anxiety in children with ASD; however, most of these studies have restricted samples to high-functioning individuals with ASD, excluding children with comorbid ASD and ID (e.g., Chalfant et al. 2007; Wood et al. 2009). Thus, the field has developed good models for ways to modify established treatments for use with populations with developmental disabilities. However, more focused research is needed regarding specific modifications necessary for children with ID, as well as carefully controlled studies to test the efficacy of these treatments.

In thinking about the future of intervention research for children with ID and comorbid psychopathology, a focus on families and other contextual factors may be particularly important. Our own and other longitudinal research with families of children at risk suggests that the relations between parenting stress and problematic child functioning involve mutually escalating cyclic interactions over time whereby elevations in parental stress predict increases in child problems which in turn predicts exacerbation of parental stress (Baker et al. 2003; Orsmond et al. 2003; Neece et al. 2012). The cyclic relationship between children's emotional, behavioral, and social problems and parenting stress highlights both variables as targets for intervention, although parent stress is rarely a direct focus within established intervention programs. Minimal research evidence is available concerning family-based interventions addressing behavior problems in children with IDD. A recent meta-analysis found only 19 studies representing 11 different family-based treatments, all of which were parent-training programs targeting parenting behavior rather than parenting stress (McIntyre 2013). Unfortunately, the majority of these studies had a small sample size (median $n=51$), lacked a control group, and did not include follow-up data or measure treatment integrity, limiting the conclusions that can be drawn from results. In research that has applied these parent-training programs to populations of children with ID, early results suggest that these programs may be effective in reducing negative parent–child interactions, parental stress, and child behavior problems (McIntyre 2008). However, the long-term effects of the intervention on parenting stress may not be as strong as the long-term effects on child behavior problems (Eyberg et al. 2001).

Interventions geared towards the needs of parents of children with ID have shifted their focus to examining the efficacy of mindfulness interventions (Bazzano et al. 2013; Neece 2014; Singh et al. 2007). Mindfulness is the complete awareness and attention of the here and now, devoid of judgment and worry about the future and the past (Stahl and Goldstein 2010). Mindfulness training has been shown to increase individuals' tolerance of negative emotions and sensations (Eifert and Heffner 2003), increase emotional acceptance (Linehan 1993), and decrease recovery time from negative emotional events (Kabat-Zinn 2009). Targeting the aforementioned processes has been theoretically shown to result in overall improvement in emotion regulation capacities and therefore lower perceived stress. A mindfulness-based intervention with parents of children with developmental disabilities reported decreased parenting stress, as well decreased aggression and increased social skills in children (Singh et al. 2007). Subsequently, a small randomized controlled trial examining the efficacy of mindfulness-based stress reduction (MBSR) for parents of young children with developmental delays found that parents who participated in MBSR reported significantly less stress and depression as well as greater life satisfaction than a waitlist-control group of parents (Neece 2014). Notably, the parents in the MBSR program reported decreased behavior problems (i.e., attention, ADHD-related symptoms) in their children at post-treatment. These preliminary findings suggest that MBSR and other mindfulness interventions may be effective in targeting parenting stress and well-being, as well as indirectly improving children's behavioral and emotional competence. However, further research is needed to determine its sustained effects on long-term parental well-being.

Advancement in the understanding of comorbid disorders in youth with ID should also accompany new implications for educational interventions and policy. According to the U.S. Individuals with Disabilities Education Act, all children with disabilities nationwide are entitled to a free and appropriate public education. This law applies to all children with ID and to children with mental health disorder in some states. However, under IDEA it is generally considered "best practice" to only classify children with one eligibility criteria, which is ID for children with dual diagnosis. The IDEA policy enforcement brings the question whether public schools are equipped to address or even offer differential services to children with ID and comorbid disorders. The purpose of an individualized educational plan (IEP) is to address children's education and learning needs and develop appropriate school services to facilitate their specialized learning. IEPs often lack individualization and do not sufficiently address the needs of the primary eligibility criterion (Ruble et al. 2010). Therefore, it is likely that secondary diagnoses (e.g. ADHD, ODD, anxiety) are also not being adequately assessed, discussed, and/or treated with educational accommodations.

Research Challenges, Clinical Implications, and Future Directions

Given the relatively recent recognition of comorbid psychopathology among children with ID, there have been several noteworthy research advancements; however, many challenges remain and much work remains to be done. First, assessing co-occurring mental disorders in children with ID has a number of challenges. Communication and cognitive delays among children with ID make traditional assessment tools less useful. These deficits may be particularly problematic in assessing internalizing disorders that rely on the individual to describe his/her internal experience (Davis et al. 2008). It may well be that certain disorders (e.g., generalized anxiety disorder) require some command of language in order for the child to represent internal emotional states. It may also be that symptoms of such disorders are expressed differently by nonverbal individuals (LoVullo and Matson 2009) and, in order to explicate such possibilities, research must better address the clinical presentation of disorders in this population with more developmentally refined and focused approaches to measurement that adopt multimodal, multi-method approaches (Lewis and Porter 2004). Nonetheless, the conditions under which comorbidity of behavioral and emotional problems are present require much further attention as this field of inquiry develops.

Second, although evidence is building supporting the validity of these comorbid disorders among children with ID, there continues to be a need for further investigation regarding the validity of specific mental health diagnoses for children with ID. A groundbreaking paper by Robins and Guze (1970) described a method for achieving diagnostic validity in psychiatric illnesses consisting of five phases: clinical descriptions, laboratory findings, exclusion of other disorders, follow-up study, and family study. Over the years researchers have expanded Robins and Guze's ideas and suggest that a psychiatric disorder is considered valid when a consistent pattern of data emerges in several domains, including clinical correlates (e.g., behavioral phenotypes), family history, treatment response, and developmental course and outcome (Antshel et al. 2006). More recently, a "second standard" of validation has emerged in which researchers must not only establish validation by clinical description and epidemiological criteria, but also by the mechanisms underlying the disorder (e.g., candidate genes) and fundamental levels of knowledge about the etiology of the disorder (Andreasen 1995). Limited studies have examined whether the same etiological factors contribute to the development of psychopathology among children with and without ID, although the little data that do exist further support the similarity of the disorders among children with ID and typical development. More specifically, regarding ODD, there is some research to suggest that factors such as child temperament—specifically, negative emotionality and fearlessness—and parent psychopathology contribute to oppositional and defiant behavior for children with and without ID (Christensen 2012). Additionally, research examining etiological factors related to ADHD in youth with ID have found similar patterns in terms of family history of ADHD, specific candidate genes, and neuropsychological deficits in predicting ADHD, regardless of whether the child has ID or not (Neece et al. 2012).

Further, there is a need for longitudinal research in order to better characterize the long-term outcomes of children with ID and comorbid psychopathology. For example, is the presence of ADHD associated with similar developmental consequences, including challenges in family functioning (e.g., more negative parenting behaviors, increased parenting stress, higher family conflict), social functioning (e.g., fewer friends, less reciprocal friendships, and peer rejection), and health outcomes (e.g., accident-proneness and injury) for children with and without ID? Regarding ODD, does this diagnosis confer the same risk for developing conduct disorder in children with ID as it does for typically developing children? Perhaps, the cognitive limitations of children with ID protect against future conduct problems by inhibiting the degree to which children with ODD are able to interact with peers or gain access to risky environments. Or might the intellectual challenges of this population place them at risk for greater conduct problems and increase the likelihood of negative outcomes such as incarceration and injury? Additional longitudinal research will help clinicians and investigators better determine prognoses for youth with ID and comorbid mental disorders.

With perhaps even more urgency, much research is needed in order to develop and examine the efficacy of treatments for these comorbid disorders in children with ID. Modifications made to traditional psychotherapy programs for typically developing children should be developed particularly for children with impaired cognitive functioning. Regarding cognitive behavioral therapy, it is often assumed that cognitive techniques would be less effective for these children, but it may be possible to utilize cognitive techniques with adjustments to help make techniques more concrete and utilize a range of modalities to help teach these concepts (e.g., incorporating visual, tactile, and/or motoric ways of engaging with the material) as seen for children with ASDs. Additionally, techniques to explain behavioral strategies to children and their families could be developed for children with ID, including the development of visual aids, interactive activities, and reminders to rehearse skills outside of session. Lastly, given the cognitive deficits within this sample, special efforts to help children with ID generalize skills outside of session should be made. Though the inclusion of family and caregiver involvement will likely be a large factor in this generalization, this assumption should be tested and validated. Additional strategies to generalize gains may include direct incorporation of treatment into children's educational services (e.g., training teachers to provide encouragement and reinforcement for coping strategies in the school environment).

Dual diagnosis is a highly significant problem for society. When ID is accompanied by a mental disorder or maladaptive behaviors there is increased likelihood of many negative outcomes for individuals with ID, families of individuals with ID, and the broader agencies that serve individuals with ID and their families. There is a compelling case for continued basic research examining the etiology and associated consequences of dual diagnosis, which will ultimately inform interventions to treat these conditions.

References

American Psychiatric Association. (2000). *Diagnostic and statistical manual of mental disorders, DSM-IV* (4th ed., Text Revision). Washington: American Psychiatric Association.

American Psychiatric Association. (2013). *Diagnostic and statistical manual of mental disorders* (5th ed.). Arlington: American Psychiatric Publishing.

Andreasen, N.C. (1995). The validation of psychiatric diagnoses: new models and approaches. *American Journal of Psychiatry, 152,* 161–162.

Antshel, K. M., Phillips, M. H., Gordon, M., Barkley, R., & Faraone, S. V. (2006). Is ADHD a valid disorder in children with intellectual delays? *Clinical Psychology Review, 26*(5), 555–572.

Applegate, B., Lahey, B. B., Hart, E. L., Biederman, J., Hynd, G. W., Barkley, R. A., et al. (1997). Validity of the age-of-onset criterion for ADHD: A report from the DSM-IV field trials. *Journal of the American Academy of Child & Adolescent Psychiatry, 36*(9), 1211–1221.

Bagner, D.M., & Eyberg, S. (2007). Parent-child interaction therapy for disruptive behavior in children with mental retardation: A randomized controlled trial. *Journal of Child Clinical and Adolescent Psychology, 36*(3), 418–429.

Baker, B. L., Blacher, J., Crnic, K. A., & Edelbrock, C. (2002). Behavior problems and parenting stress in families of three-year-old children with and without developmental delays. *American Journal on Mental Retardation, 107*(6), 433–444.

Baker, B. L., McIntyre, L. L., Blacher, J., Crnic, K., Edelbrock, C., & Low, C. (2003). Pre-school children with and without developmental delay: behaviour problems and parenting stress over time. *Journal of Intellectual Disability Research, 47*(4/5), 217–230. doi: 10.1046/j.1365-2788.2003.00484.x.

Baker, B. L., Neece, C. L., Fenning, R. M., Crnic, K. A., & Blacher, J. (2010). Mental disorders in five-year-old children with or without developmental delay: Focus on ADHD. *Journal of Clinical Child and Adolescent Psychology, 39*(4), 492–505.

Barkley, R. A. (1998). Attention-deficit/hyperactivity disorder. In E. J. Mash & R. A. Barkley (Eds.), *Treatment of childhood disorders* (2nd ed.) (pp. 55–110). New York: Guilford Press.

Barkley, R. A., DuPaul, G. J., & McMurray, M. B. (1990). Comprehensive evaluation of attention deficit disorder with and without hyperactivity as defined by research criteria. *Journal of Consulting and Clinical Psychology, 58*(6), 775–789.

Barkley, R. A., Edwards, G., Laneri, M., Fletcher, K., & Metevia, L. (2001). The efficacy of problem-solving communication training alone, behavior management training alone, and their combination for parent-adolescent conflict in teenagers with ADHD and ODD. *Journal of Consulting and Clinical Psychology, 69*(6), 926–941.

Bazzano, A., Wolfe, C., Zylowska, L., Wang, S., Schuster, E., Barrett, C., & Lehrer, D. (2013). Mindfulness Based Stress Reduction (MBSR) for parents and caregivers of individuals with developmental disabilities: A community-based approach. *Journal of Child and Family Studies,* 1–11.

Biederman, J., Milberger, S., Faraone, S. V., & Guite, J. (1994). Associations between childhood asthma and ADHD: Issues of psychiatric comorbidity and familiality. *Journal of the American Academy of Child & Adolescent Psychiatry, 33*(6), 842–848.

Blacher, J. (Ed.). (1994). *When there's no place like home: Options for children living apart from their natural families.* Baltimore: Paul H Brookes Publishing.
Blacher, J., Baker, B. L., & Feinfield, K. A. (1999). Leaving or launching? Continuing family involvement with children and adolescents in placement. *American Journal on Mental Retardation, 104*(5), 452–465. doi:10.1352/0895-8017.
Blacher, J., & McIntyre, L. L. (2006). Syndrome specificity and behavioural disorders in young adults with intellectual disability: Cultural differences in family impact. *Journal of Intellectual Disability Research, 50*(3), 184–198.
Borthwick-Duffy, S. A. (1994). Epidemiology and prevalence of psychopathology in people with mental retardation. *Journal of Consulting and Clinical Psychology, 62*(1), 17–27.
Borthwick-Duffy, S. A., & Eyman, R. K. (1990). Who are the dually diagnosed? *American Journal on Mental Retardation, 94*(6), 586–595.
Bromley, B. E., & Blacher, J. (1991). Parental reasons for out-of-home placement of children with severe handicaps. *Mental Retardation, 29*(5), 275–280.
Bryson, S. E., Koegel, L. K., Koegel, R. L., Openden, D., Smith, I. M., & Nefdt, N. (2007). Large scale dissemination and community implementation of pivotal response treatment: Program description and preliminary data. *Research and Practice for Persons with Severe Disabilities, 32*(2), 142–153. doi:10.2511/rpsd.32.2.142.
Bryson, S. E., Bradley, E. A., Thompson, A., & Wainwright, A. (2008). Prevalence of autism among adolescents with intellectual disabilities. *Canadian Journal of Psychiatry, 53*(7), 449–459.
Campbell, M., & Malone, R. P. (1991). Mental retardation and psychiatric disorders. *Hospital & Community Psychiatry, 42*(4), 374–379.
Canino, G., Shrout, P. E., Rubio-Stipec, M., Bird, H. R., Bravo, M., Ramirez, R., & ... Martinez-Taboas, A. (2004). The DSM-IV Rates of Child and Adolescent Disorders in Puerto Rico. *Archives of General Psychiatry, 61*(1), 85–93. doi:10.1001/archpsyc.61.1.85.
Carter, C. M. (2001). Using choice with game play to increase language skills and interactive behaviors in children with autism. *Journal of Positive Behavior Interventions, 3*(3), 131–151.
Cartwright-Hatton, S., McNicol, K., & Doubleday, E. (2006). Anxiety in a neglected population: Prevalence of anxiety disorders in pre-adolescent children. *Clinical Psychology Review, 26*(7), 817–833. doi:10.1016/j.cpr.2005.12.002.
Casey, R. J. (1996). Emotional competence in children with externalizing and internalizing disorders. In M. Lewis & M. S. Sullivan (Eds.), *Emotional development in atypical children* (pp. 161–183). Mahwah: Erlbaum.
Centers for Disease Control and Prevention [CDC]. (2012). Understanding suicide fact sheet. http://www.cdc.gov/violenceprevention/pdf/suicide_datasheet-a.pdf.
CDC. (2014a). Prevalence of autism spectrum disorder among children aged 8 years-autism and developmental disabilities monitoring network, 11 sites, United States, 2010. *Morbidity and Mortality Weekly Report. Surveillance Summaries, 63*(2), 1–21.
CDC. (2014b). Autism Spectrum Disorder (ASD): Screening and Diagnosis. http://www.cdc.gov/ncbddd/autism/screening.html.
Chakrabarti, S., & Fombonne, E. (2001). Pervasive developmental disorders in preschool children. *The Journal of the American Medical Association, 285*(24), 3093–3099. doi:10.1001/jama.285.24.3093.
Chakrabarti, S., & Fombonne, E. (2005). Pervasive developmental disorders in preschool children: Confirmation of high prevalence. *The American Journal of Psychiatry, 162*(6), 1133–1141. doi:10.1176/appi.ajp.162.6.1133.
Chalfant, A. M., Rapee, R., & Carroll, L. (2007). Treating anxiety disorders in children with high functioning autism spectrum disorders: A controlled trial. *Journal of Autism and Developmental Disorders, 37*(10), 1842–1857. doi:10.1007/s10803-006-0318-4.
Charman, T., Pickles, A., Simonoff, E., Chandler, S., Loucas, T., & Baird, G. (2011). IQ in children with autism spectrum disorders: Data from the Special Needs and Autism Project (SNAP). *Psychological Medicine, 41*(03), 619–627. doi:10.1017/S0033291710000991.
Christensen, L. L. (2012). Dual diagnosis: Intellectual disability and oppositional defiant disorder. UCLA: Psychology 0780. http://escholarship.org/uc/item/2mr74206.

Christensen, L., Baker, B.L., & Blacher J. (2013). Oppositional defiant disorder in children with intellectual disabilities. *Journal of Mental Health Research in Intellectual Disabilities, 6*(3), 225–244.

Christianson, A., Zwane, M., Manga, P., Rosen, E., Venter, A., Downs, D., & Kromberg, J. (2002). Children with intellectual disability in rural South Africa: Prevalence and associated disability. *Journal of Intellectual Disability Research, 46*(2), 179–186. doi:10.1046/j.1365-2788.2002.00390.x.

Compton, S. N., Nelson, A. H., & March, J. S. (2000). Social phobia and separation anxiety symptoms in community and clinical samples of children and adolescents. *Journal of the American Academy of Child & Adolescent Psychiatry, 39*(8), 1040–1046. http://doi.org/10.1097/00004583-200008000-00020.

Cunningham, C. E., & Boyle, M. H. (2002). Preschoolers at risk for attention-deficit hyperactivity disorder and oppositional defiant disorder: Family, parenting, and behavioral correlates. *Journal of Abnormal Child Psychology, 30*(6), 555–569.

Davis, N. O., & Carter, A. S. (2008). Parenting stress in mothers and fathers of toddlers with autism spectrum disorders: associations with child characteristics. *J Autism Dev Disord, 38*(7), 1278–1291. doi: 10.1007/s10803-007-0512-z.

Dawson, G., & Faja, S. (2008). Autism spectrum disorders: A developmental perspective. In T. P. Beauchaine & S. P. Hinshaw (Eds.), *Child and adolescent psychopathology* (pp. 575–613). Hoboken: Wiley.

De Bildt, A., Sytema, S., Kraijer, D., & Minderaa, R. (2005). Prevalence of pervasive developmental disorders in children and adolescents with mental retardation. *Journal of Child Psychology and Psychiatry, 46*(3), 275–286.

de Ruiter, K. P., Dekker, M. C., Verhulst, F. C., & Koot, H. M. (2007). Developmental course of psychopathology in youths with and without intellectual disabilities. *Journal of Child Psychology and Psychiatry, 48*(5), 498–507. doi:10.1111/j.1469-7610.2006.01712.x.

Dekker, M. C., Koot, H. M., van der Ende, J., & Verhulst, F. C. (2002). Emotional and behavioral problems in children and adolescents with and without intellectual disability. *Journal of Child Psychology and Psychiatry, 43*(8), 1087–1098.

Dekker, M. C., & Koot, H. M. (2003). DSM-IV disorders in children with borderline to moderate intellectual disability. I: Prevalence and impact. *Journal of the American Academy of Child & Adolescent Psychiatry, 42*(8), 915–922. doi:10.1097/01.CHI.0000046892.27264.1A.

Douma, J. C. H., Dekker, M. C., & Koot, H. M. (2006). Supporting parents of youths with intellectual disabilities and psychopathology. *Journal of Intellectual Disability Research, 50*(8), 570–581.

Duchesne, S., Vitaro, F., Larose, S., & Tremblay, R. E. (2007). Trajectories of anxiety during elementary-school years and the prediction of high school noncompletion. *Journal of Youth and Adolescence, 37*(9), 1134–1146. http://doi.org/10.1007/s10964-007-9224-0.

DuPaul, G. J., & Stoner, G. D. (1994). ADHD in the schools: *Assessment and intervention strategies.* New York: Guilford Press.

Eifert, G. H., & Heffner, M. (2003). The effects of acceptance versus control contexts on avoidance of panic-related symptoms. *Journal of Behavior Therapy and Experimental Psychiatry, 34*(3–4), 293–312. doi:10.1016/j.jbtep.2003.11.00.

Eikeseth, S., Klintwall, L., Jahr, E., & Karlsson, P. (2012). Outcome for children with autism receiving early and intensive behavioral intervention in mainstream preschool and kindergarten settings. *Research in Autism Spectrum Disorders, 6*(2), 829–835. doi:10.1016/j.rasd.2011.09.002.

Einfeld, S. L., & Tonge, J. (1996). Population prevalence of psychopathology in children and adolescents with intellectual disability: I. Rationale and methods. *Journal of Intellectual Disability Research, 40*(2), 91–98. doi:10.1111/j.1365-2788.1996.tb00610.x.

Einfeld, S. L., Piccinin, A. M., Mackinnon, A., Hofer, S. M., Taffe, J., Gray, K. M., Tonge, B. J. (2006). Psychopathology in young people with intellectual disability. *JAMA: Journal of the American Medical Association, 296*(16), 1981–1989. doi:http://dx.doi.org/10.1001/jama.296.16.1981.

Einfeld, S. L., Gray, K. M., Ellis, L. A., Taffe, J., Emerson, E., Tonge, B. J., & Horstead, S. K. (2010). Intellectual disability modifies gender effects on disruptive behaviors. *Journal Of Mental Health Research In Intellectual Disabilities, 3*(4), 177–189. doi:10.1080/19315864.2010.519098.

Einfeld, S. L., Ellis, L. A., & Emerson, E. (2011). Comorbidity of intellectual disability and mental disorder in children and adolescents: A systematic review. *Journal of Intellectual and Developmental Disability, 36*(2), 137–143. doi:10.1080/13668250.2011.572548.

Eisenhower, A. S., Baker, B. L., & Blacher, J. (2005). Preschool children with intellectual disability: Syndrome specificity, behaviour problems, and maternal well-being. *Journal of Intellectual Disability Research, 49*(9), 657–671.

Eldevik, S., Hastings, R. P., Hughes, J. C., Jahr, E., Eikeseth, S., & Cross, S. (2009). Meta-analysis of early intensive behavioral intervention for children with autism. *Journal of Clinical Child & Adolescent Psychology, 38*(3), 439–450. doi:10.1080/15374410902851739.

Emerson, E. (2003). Prevalence of psychiatric disorders in children and adolescents with and without intellectual disability. *Journal of Intellectual Disability Research, 47*(1), 51–58.

Emerson, E. (2012). Deprivation, ethnicity and the prevalence of intellectual and developmental disabilities. *Journal of Epidemiology and Community Health, 66*(3), 218–224.

Emerson, E., & Hatton, C. (2007). Mental health of children and adolescents with intellectual disabilities in Britain. *British Journal of Psychiatry, 191*(6), 493–499.

Eyberg, S. M., Funderburk, B. W., Hembree-Kigin, T. L., McNeil, C. B., Querido, J. G., & Hood, K. K. (2001). Parent-child interaction therarpy with behavior problem children: One an dtwo year maintenance of treatment effects in the family. *Child & Family Behavior Therapy, 23*(4), 1–20.

Faraone, S. V., Biederman, J., & Mick, E. (2006). The age-dependent decline of attention deficit hyperactivity disorder: A meta-analysis of follow-up studies. *Psychological Medicine, 36*(2), 159–165.

Fleitlich-Bilyk, B., & Goodman, R. (2004). Prevalence of Child and Adolescent Psychiatric Disorders in Southeast Brazil. *Journal of the American Academy of Child & Adolescent Psychiatry, 43*(6), 727–734. doi:10.1097/01.chi.0000120021.14101.ca.

Gal, E., Hardal-Nasser, R., & Engel-Yeger, B. (2011). The relationship between the severity of eating problems and intellectual developmental deficit level. *Research in Developmental Disabilities, 32*(5), 1464–1469. doi:10.1016/j.ridd.2010.12.003.

Goin-Kochel, R. P., Peters, S. U., & Treadwell-Deering, D. (2008). Parental reports on the prevalence of co-occurring intellectual disability among children with autism spectrum disorders. *Research in Autism Spectrum Disorders, 2*(3), 546–556. doi:10.1016/j.rasd.2007.11.002.

Green, S. A., Berkovits, L. D., & Baker, B. L. (2014). Symptoms and development of anxiety in children with or without intellectual disability. *Journal of Clinical Child and Adolescent Psychology: The Official Journal for the Society of Clinical Child and Adolescent Psychology, American Psychological Association, Division 53.* http://doi.org/10.1080/15374416.2013.873979.

Handen, B. L., McAuliffe, S., & Caro-Martinez, L. (1996). Stimulant medication effects on learning in children with mental retardation and ADHD. *Journal of Developmental and Physical Disabilities, 8*(4), 335–346.

Hartley, S. L., & Sikora, D. M. (2010). Detecting autism spectrum disorder in children with intellectual disability: Which DSM-IV-TR criteria are most useful? *Focus on Autism and Other Developmental Disabilities, 25*(2), 85–97. doi:10.1177/1088357609356094.

Hartsough, C. S., & Lambert, N. M. (1985). Medical factors in hyperactive and normal children: Prenatal, developmental, and health history findings. *American Journal of Orthopsychiatry, 55*(2), 190–201.

Harvey, E. A., Youngwirth, S. D., Thakar, D. A., & Errazuriz, P. A. (2009). Predicting attention-deficit/hyperactivity disorder and oppositional defiant disorder from preschool diagnostic assessments. *Journal of Consulting and Clinical Psychology, 77*(2), 349–354.

Hastings, R. P., Beck, A., Daley, D., & Hill, C. (2005). Symptoms of ADHD and their correlates in children with intellectual disabilities. *Research in Developmental Disabilities, 26*(5), 456–468.

Hastings, R. P., Daley, D., Burns, C., Beck, A., & MacLean, W. A. (2006) Maternal distress and expressed emotion: Cross-sectional and longitudinal relationships with behavior problems of children with intellectual disabilities. *American Journal on Mental Retardation, 111*(1), 48–61.

Herring, S., Gray, K., Taffe, J., Tonge, B., Sweeney, D., & Einfeld, S. (2006). Behaviour and emotional problems in toddlers with pervasive developmental disorders and developmental delay: Associations with parental mental health and family functioning. *Journal of Intellectual Disability Research, 50*(12), 874–882.

Hill, J., & Furniss, F. (2006). Patterns of emotional and behavioural disturbance associated with autistic traits in young people with severe intellectual disabilities and challenging behaviours. *Research in Developmental Disabilities, 27*(5), 517–528. doi:10.1016/j.ridd.2005.07.001.

Holden, B., & Gitlesen, J. P. (2006). A total population study of challenging behaviour in the county of Hedmark, Norway: Prevalence, and risk markers. *Research in Developmental Disabilities, 27*(4), 456–465. doi:10.1016/j.ridd.2005.06.001.

Jauhari, P., Bhargava, R., Bhave, A., Kumar, C., & Kumar, R. (2012). Comorbidities associated with intellectual disability among pediatric outpatients seen at a teaching hospital in Northern India. *Journal of Policy and Practice in Intellectual Disabilities, 9*(1), 10–16. doi:10.1111/j.1741-1130.2012.00327.x.

Jelliffe-Pawlowski, L. L., Shaw, G. M., Nelson, V., & Harris, J. A. (2003). Risk of mental retardation among children born with birth defects. *Archives of Pediatrics & Adolescent Medicine, 157*(6), 545–550. doi:10.1001/archpedi.157.6.545.

Jensen, P. S., Shervetter, R. E., Xenakis, S. N., & Bain, M. W. (1988). Psychosocial and medical histories of stimulant treated children. *Journal of American Academy of Child and Adolescent Psychiatry, 27*, 789–801.

Jensen, P. S., Hinshaw, S. P., Kraemer, H. C., Lenora, N., Newcorn, J. H., Abikoff, H. B., March, J. S., Arnold, L. E., Cantwell, D. P., Connors, C. K., Elliott, G. R., Greenhill, L. L., Hechtman, L., Hoza, B., Pelham, W. E., Severe, J. B., Swanson, J. M., Wells, K. C., Wigal, T., & Vitiello, B. (2001). ADHD comorbidity findings from the MTA study: Comparing comorbid subgroups. *Journal of the American Academy of Child & Adolescent Psychiatry, 40*(2), 147–158.

Johnson, C. R., Handen, B. L., Lubetsky, M. J., & Sacco, K. A. (1995). Affective disorders in hospitalized children and adolescents with mental retardation: A retrospective study. *Research in Developmental Disabilities, 16*(3), 221–231.

Johnston, C., & Mash, E. J. (2001). Families of children with attention-deficit/hyperactivity disorder: Review and recommendations for future research. *Clinical Child and Family Psychology Review, 4*, 183–207.

Jones, L., Bellis, M. A., Wood, S., Hughes, K., McCoy, E., Eckley, L., Officer, A. (2012). Prevalence and risk of violence against children with disabilities: A systematic review and meta-analysis of observational studies. *The Lancet, 380*(9845), 899–907. doi:10.1016/S0140-6736(12)60692-8.

Jopp, D. A., & Keys, C. B. (2001). Diagnostic overshadowing reviewed and reconsidered. *American Journal on Mental Retardation, 106*(5), 416–433.

Kabat-Zinn, J., & Hanh, T. N. (2009). *Full catastrophe living: Using the wisdom of your body and mind to face stress, pain, and illness.* Delta.

Kessler, R. C., Berglund, P., Demler, O., Jin, R., Merikangas, K. R., & Walters, E. E. (2005). "Lifetime prevalence and age-of-onset distributions of DSM-IV disorders in the national comorbidity survey replication": Erratum. *Archives of General Psychiatry, 62*(7), 768–768.

Kessler, R. C., Adler, L., Barkley, R., Biederman, J., Conners, C. K., Demler, O., et al. (2006). The prevalence and correlates of adult ADHD in the United States: Results from the national comorbidity survey replication. *American Journal of Psychiatry, 163*(4), 716–723.

Koegel, R. L., Koegel, L. K., & Brookman, L. I. (2003). Empirically supported pivotal response interventions for children with autism. In A. E. Kazdin (Ed.), *Evidence-Based Psychotherapies for Children and Adolescents* (pp. 341–357). New York: Guilford Press.

Kurtz, P. F., Chin, M. D., Huete, J. M., Tarbox, R. S., O'Connor, J. T., Paclawskyj, T. R., & Rush, K. S. (2003). Functional analysis and treatment of self-injurious behavior in young children: A summary of 30 cases. *Journal of Applied Behavior Analysis, 36*(2), 205–219. doi:10.1901/jaba.2003.36-205.

Kurtz, P. F., Boelter, E. W., Jarmolowicz, D. P., Chin, M. D., & Hagopian, L. P. (2011). An analysis of functional communication training as an empirically supported treatment for problem behavior displayed by individuals with intellectual disabilities. *Research in Developmental Disabilities, 32*(6), 2935–2942. doi:10.1016/j.ridd.2011.05.009.

Lahey, B. B., & Loeber, R. (1994). Framework for a developmental model of oppositional defiant disorder and conduct disorder. In D. K. Routh (Ed.), *Disruptive behavior disorders in childhood* (pp. 139–180). New York: Plenum Press.

Lavigne, J. V., Cicchetti, C., Gibbons, R. D., Binns, H. J., Larsen, L., & DeVito, C. (2001). Oppositional defiant disorder with onset in preschool years: Longitudinal stability and pathways to other disorders. *Journal of the American Academy of Child & Adolescent Psychiatry, 40*(12), 1393–1400.

Levy, S. E., Giarelli, E., Lee, L.-C., Schieve, L. A., Kirby, R. S., Cunniff, C., Rice, C. E. (2010). Autism spectrum disorder and co-occurring developmental, psychiatric, and medical conditions among children in multiple populations of the United States. *Journal of Developmental & Behavioral Pediatrics, 31*(4), 267–275. doi:10.1097/DBP.0b013e3181d5d03b.

Lewis, A., & Porter, J. (2004). Interviewing children and young people with learning disabilities: Guidelines for researchers and multi-professional practice. *British Journal of Learning Disabilities, 32*(4), 191–197. doi:10.1111/j.1468-3156.2004.00313.x.

Lin, L. P., Kuan, C. Y., Hsu, S. W., Lee, T. N., Lai, C. I., Wu, J. L., & Lin, J. D. (2013). Outpatient visits and expenditures for children and adolescents diagnosed with autism spectrum disorders and co-occurring intellectual disability: An analysis of the national health insurance claims data. *Research in Autism Spectrum Disorders, 7*(12), 1625–1630. doi:http://dx.doi.org/10.1016/j.rasd.2013.09.003.

Linehan, M. M., & Kehrer, C. A. (1993). Borderline personality disorder. In D. H. Barlow, D. H. Barlow (Eds.), *Clinical handbook of psychological disorders: A step-by-step treatment manual* (2nd ed., pp. 396–441). New York: Guilford Press.

LoVullo, S., & Matson, J. L. (2009). Comorbid psychopathology in adults with autism spectrum disorders and intellectual disabilities. *Research In Developmental Disabilities, 30*(6), 1288–1296. doi:10.1016/j.ridd.2009.05.004.

Ludi, E., Ballard, E. D., Greenbaum, R., Bridge, J., Reynolds, W., & Horowitz, L. (2012). Suicide risk in youth with intellectual disability: The challenges of screening. *Journal of Developmental and Behavioral Pediatrics, 33*(5), 431. doi:10.1097/DBP.0b013e3182599295.

MacLean Jr, W. E., Tervo, R. C., Hoch, J., Tervo, M., & Symons, F. J. (2010). Self-injury among a community cohort of young children at risk for intellectual and developmental disabilities. *The Journal of Pediatrics, 157*(6), 979–983. doi:10.1016/j.jpeds.2010.05.052.

Maenner, M. J., Schieve, L. A., Rice, C. E., Cunniff, C., Giarelli, E., Kirby, R. S., Durkin, M. S. (2013). Frequency and pattern of documented diagnostic features and the age of autism identification. *Journal of the American Academy of Child & Adolescent Psychiatry, 52*(4), 401–413. doi:10.1016/j.jaac.2013.01.014.

Maïano, C. (2011). Prevalence and risk factors of overweight and obesity among children and adolescents with intellectual disabilities. *Obesity Reviews, 12*(3), 189–197. doi:10.1111/j.1467-789X.2010.00744.x.

Mannion, A., Leader, G., & Healy, O. (2013). An investigation of comorbid psychological disorders, sleep problems, gastrointestinal symptoms and epilepsy in children and adolescents with autism spectrum disorder. *Research in Autism Spectrum Disorders, 7*(1), 35–42. doi:10.1016/j.rasd.2012.05.002.

Masi, G., Mucci, M., Favilla, L., & Poli, P. (1999). Dysthymic disorder in adolescents with intellectual disability. *Journal of Intellectual Disability Research, 43*(2), 80–87. doi:10.1046/j.1365-2788.1999.00195.x.

Matson, J. L., & Nebel-Schwalm, M. S. (2007). Comorbid psychopathology with autism spectrum disorder in children: An overview. *Research in Developmental Disabilities, 28*(4), 341–352. doi:10.1016/j.ridd.2005.12.004.

Maughan, B., Rowe, R., Messer, J., Goodman, R., & Meltzer, H. (2004). Conduct disorder and oppositional defiant disorder in a national sample: Developmental epidemiology. *Journal of Child Psychology and Psychiatry, 45*(3), 609–621.

McCarthy, J., & Boyd, J. (2002). Mental health services and young people with intellectual disability: is it time to do better? *J Intellect Disabil Res, 46*(Pt 3), 250–256.

McDiarmid, M., & Bagner, D. M. (2005). Parent-child interaction therapy for children with disruptive behavior and developmental disabilities. *Education of Treatment and Children, 28*, 130–141.

McIntyre, L. L. (2008). Parent training for young children with developmental disabilities: randomized controlled trial. *Am J Ment Retard, 113*(5), 356–368. doi: 10.1352/2008.113:356-368.

McIntyre, L. L. (2013). Parent training to reduce challenging behavior in children and adults with developmental disabilities. In R. P. Hastings & J. Rojahn (Eds.), *International review of research in developmental disabilities: Challenging behavior* (pp. 245–280). San Diego: Academic.

McIntyre, L. L., Blacher, J., & Baker, B. L. (2002). Behaviour/mental health problems in young adults with intellectual disability: the impact on families. *J Intellect Disabil Res, 46*(Pt 3), 239–249.

Moree, B. N., & Davis, T. I. (2010). Cognitive-behavioral therapy for anxiety in children diagnosed with autism spectrum disorders: Modification trends. *Research in Autism Spectrum Disorders, 4*(3), 346–354. doi:10.1016/j.rasd.2009.10.015.

Morgan, C. L., Baxter, H., & Kerr, M. P. (2003). Prevalence of epilepsy and associated health service utilization and mortality among patients with intellectual disability. *Journal Information, 108*(5). doi:10.1352/0895–8017(2003)108 %3C293:POEAAH%3E2.0.CO;2.

Neece C. L., Baker, B. L., Crnic, K., & Blacher, J. (2011). ADHD among children with and without delays: An examination across time. *Journal of Intellectual Disability Research, 55*(7), 623–635.

Neece, C. L., Green, S. A., & Baker, B. L. (2012) Parenting stress and child behavior problems: A transactional relationship across time. *American Journal on Intellectual and Developmental Disabilities, 117*(1), 48–66.

Neece, C. L., Baker, B. L., & Lee, S. S. (2013). ADHD among adolescents with intellectual disabilities: Pre-pathway influences. *Research in developmental disabilities, 34*(7), 2268–2279.

Neece, C. L. (2014). Mindfulness-Based Stress Reduction for Parents of Young Children with Developmental Delays: Implications for Parental Mental Health and Child Behavior Problems. *Journal of Applied Research in Intellectual Disabilities, 27*(2), 174–186.

Nielsen, L. S., Skov, L., & Jensen, H. (2007a). Visual dysfunctions and ocular disorders in children with developmental delay. I. Prevalence, diagnoses and aetiology of visual impairment. *Acta Ophthalmologica Scandinavica, 85*(2), 149–156. doi:10.1111/j.1600-0420.2006.00867.x.

Nielsen, L. S., Skov, L., & Jensen, H. (2007b). Visual dysfunctions and ocular disorders in children with developmental delay. II. Aspects of refractive errors, strabismus and contrast sensitivity. *Acta Ophthalmologica Scandinavica, 85*(4), 419–426. doi:10.1111/j.1600-0420.2007.00881.x.

Nock, M. K., Kazdin, A. E., Hiripi, E., & Kessler, R. C. (2007). Lifetime prevalence, correlates, and persistence of oppositional defiant disorder: Results from the national comorbidity survey replication. *Journal of Child Psychology and Psychiatry, 48*(7), 703–713.

Oguni, H. (2013). Epilepsy and intellectual and developmental disabilities. *Journal of Policy and Practice in Intellectual Disabilities, 10*(2), 89–92. doi:10.1111/jppi.12035.

Oliver, C., Petty, J., Ruddick, L., & Bacarese-Hamilton, M. (2012). The association between repetitive, self-injurious and aggressive behavior in children with severe intellectual disability. *Journal of Autism and Developmental Disorders, 42*(6), 910–919. doi:10.1007/s10803-011-1320-z.

O'Reilly, M., Rispoli, M., Davis, T., Machalicek, W., Lang, R., Sigafoos, J., Didden, R. (2010). Functional analysis of challenging behavior in children with autism spectrum disorders: A summary of 10 cases. *Research in Autism Spectrum Disorders, 4*(1), 1–10. doi:10.1016/j.rasd.2009.07.001.

Orsmond, G. I., Seltzer, M. M., Krauss, M. W., & Hong, J. (2003). Behavior problems in adults with mental retardation and maternal well-being: Examination of the direction of effects. *American Journal on Mental Retardation, 108*(4), 257–271.

Peacock, G., Amendah, D., Ouyang, L., & Grosse, S. D. (2012). Autism spectrum disorders and health care expenditures: the effects of co-occurring conditions. *Journal of Developmental & Behavioral Pediatrics, 33*(1), 2–8.

Pearson, D. A., Lachar, D., Loveland, K. A., Santos, C. W., Faria, L. P., Azzam, P. N., et al. (2000). Patterns of behavioral adjustment and maladjustment in mental retardation: Comparison of children with and without ADHD. *American Journal on Mental Retardation, 105*(4), 236–251.

Pelham, W. E., & Lang, A. R. (1993). Parental alcohol consumption and deviant child behavior: Laboratory studies of reciprocal effects. *Clinical Psychology Review Special Issue: Disinhibition Disorders in Childhood, 13*(8), 763–784.

Pert, C., Jahoda, A., Stenfert Kroese, B., Trower, P., Dagnan, D., & Selkirk, M. (2013). Cognitive behavioural therapy from the perspective of clients with mild intellectual disabilities: A qualitative investigation of process issues. *Journal of Intellectual Disability Research, 57*(4), 359–369. http://doi.org/10.1111/j.1365-2788.2012.01546.x.

Peters-Scheffer, N., Didden, R., Mulders, M., & Korzilius, H. (2010). Low intensity behavioral treatment supplementing preschool services for young children with autism spectrum disorders and severe to mild intellectual disability. *Research in Developmental Disabilities, 31*(6), 1678–1684. doi:10.1016/j.ridd.2010.04.008.

Peters-Scheffer, N., Didden, R., Mulders, M., & Korzilius, H. (2013). Effectiveness of low intensity behavioral treatment for children with autism spectrum disorder and intellectual disability. *Research in Autism Spectrum Disorders, 7*(9), 1012–1025. doi:10.1016/j.rasd.2013.05.001.

Petterson, B., Bourke, J., Leonard, H., Jacoby, P., & Bower, C. (2007). Co-occurrence of birth defects and intellectual disability. *Paediatric and Perinatal Epidemiology, 21*(1), 65–75. doi:10.1111/j.1365-3016.2007.00774.x.

Reichow, B., & Wolery, M. (2009). Comprehensive synthesis of early intensive behavioral interventions for young children with autism based on the UCLA young autism project model. *Journal of Autism and Developmental Disorders, 39*(1), 23–41. doi:10.1007/s10803-008-0596-0.

Reiss, S., Levitan, G. W., & Szyszko, J. (1982). Emotional disturbance and mental retardation: Diagnostic overshadowing. *American Journal of Mental Deficiency, 86*(6), 567–574.

Reiss, S., & Szyszko, J. (1983). Diagnostic overshadowing and professional experience with mentally retarded persons. *American Journal Of Mental Deficiency, 87*(4), 396–402.

Reiter, S., Bryen, D. N., & Shachar, I. (2007). Adolescents with intellectual disabilities as victims of abuse. *Journal of Intellectual Disabilities, 11*(4), 371–387. doi:10.1177/1744629507084602.

Rezaei, M., Rashedi, V., Gharib, M., & Lotfi, G. (2011). Prevalence of feeding problems in children with intellectual disability. *Iranian Rehabilitation Journal, 9*, 56–59.

Rimmer, J., Yamaki, K., Lowry, B., Wang, E., & Vogel, L. (2010). Obesity and obesity-related secondary conditions in adolescents with intellectual/developmental disabilities. *Journal of Intellectual Disability Research, 54*(9), 787–794. doi:10.1111/j.1365-2788.2010.01305.x.

Roberts, R. E., Roberts, C. R., & Xing, Y. (2007). Rates of DSM-IV psychiatric disorders among adolescents in a large metropolitan area. *Journal of Psychiatric Research, 41*(11), 959–967. http://doi.org/10.1016/j.jpsychires.2006.09.006.

Robins, E., & Guze, S. B. (1970). Establishment of diagnostic validity in psychiatric illness: Its application to schizophrenia. *American Journal of Psychiatry, 126*(7), 983–986.

Romaniuk, C., & Miltenberger, R. G. (2001). The influence of preference and choice of activity on problem behavior. *Journal of Positive Behavior Interventions, 3*(3), 152–159.

Ruble, L. A., McGrew, J., Dalrymple, N., & Jung, L. A. (2010). Examining the quality of IEPS for young children with autism. *Journal of Autism and Developmental Disorders, 40*(12), 1459–1470. doi:10.1007/s10803-010-1003-1.

Schreibman, L. (2000). Intensive behavioral/psychoeducational treatments for autism: Research needs and future directions. *Journal of Autism and Developmental Disorders, 30*(5), 373–378. doi:10.1023/A:1005535120023.

Schrojenstein Lantman-de Valk, H. v., Akker, M. v. d., Maaskant, M., Haveman, M., Urlings, H., Kessels, A., & Crebolder, H. (1997). Prevalence and incidence of health problems in people with intellectual disability. *Journal of Intellectual Disability Research, 41*(1), 42–51. doi:10.1111/j.1365-2788.1997.tb00675.x.

Seltzer, M. M., & Krauss, M. W. (2001). Quality of life of adults with mental retardation/developmental disabilities who live with family. *Ment Retard Dev Disabil Res Rev, 7*(2), 105–114. doi: 10.1002/mrdd.1015.

Serra-Pinheiro, M. A., Mattos, P., & Regalla, M. A. (2008). Inattention, hyperactivity, and oppositional–defiant symptoms in Brazilian adolescents: Gender prevalence and agreement between teachers and parents in a non-English speaking population. *Journal of Attention Disorders, 12*(2), 135–140.

Shattuck, P. T., Durkin, M., Maenner, M., Newschaffer, C., Mandell, D. S., Wiggins, L., Cuniff, C. (2009). Timing of identification among children with an autism spectrum disorder: Findings from a population-based surveillance study. *Journal of the American Academy of Child & Adolescent Psychiatry, 48*(5), 474–483. doi: 10.1097/CHI.0b013e31819b3848

Simonoff, E., Pickles, A., Chadwick, O., Gringras, P., Wood, N., Higgins, S., et al. (2006). The croydon assessment of learning study: Prevalence and educational identification of mild mental retardation. *Journal of Child Psychology and Psychiatry, 47*(8), 828–839.

Singh, N. N., Lancioni, G. E., Winton, A. S. W., Singh, J., Curtis, W. J., Wahler, R. G., & McAleavey, K. M. (2007). Mindful parenting decreases aggression and increases social behavior in children with developmental disabilities. *Behav Modif, 31*, 749–771.

Slevin, E., Truesdale-Kennedy, M., McConkey, R., Livingstone, B., & Fleming, P. (2014). Obesity and overweight in intellectual and non-intellectually disabled children. *Journal of Intellectual Disability Research, 58*(3), 211–220. doi:10.1111/j.1365-2788.2012.01615.x.

Smith, T., Eikeseth, S., Klevstrand, M., & Lovaas, O. I. (1997). Intensive behavioral treatment for preschoolers with severe mental retardation and pervasive developmental disorder. *American Journal on Mental Retardation, 102*(3), 238–249.

Soylu, N., Alpaslan, A. H., Ayaz, M., Esenyel, S., & Oruç, M. (2013). Psychiatric disorders and characteristics of abuse in sexually abused children and adolescents with and without intellectual disabilities. *Research in Developmental Disabilities, 34*(12), 4334–4342. doi:10.1016/j.ridd.2013.09.010.

Sparrow, S. S., Balla, D. A., Cicchetti, D. V., Harrison, P. L., & Doll, E. A. (1984). *Vineland adaptive behavior scales* (interview edition). Circle Pines, MN: American Guidance Service.

Speltz, M. L., McClellan, J., DeKlyen, M., & Jones, K. (1999). Preschool boys with oppositional defiant disorder: Clinical presentation and diagnostic change. *Journal of the American Academy of Child & Adolescent Psychiatry, 38*(7), 838–845.

Stahl, B., & Goldstein, E. (2010). *A mindfulness-based stress reduction workbook.* New Harbinger Publications.

Stein, M. A., Szumowski, E., Blondis, T. A., & Roizen, N. J. (1995). Adaptive skills dysfunction in ADD and ADHD children. *Journal of Child Psychology and Psychiatry, 36*(4), 663–670.

Strømme, P., & Diseth, T. H. (2000). Prevalence of psychiatric diagnoses in children with mental retardation: data from a population-based study. *Developmental Medicine & Child Neurology, 42*(4), 266–270. doi:10.1111/j.1469-8749.2000.tb00083.x.

Sturmey, P., Ward-Horner, J., Marroquin, M., & Doran, E. (2007). Structural and functional approaches to psychopathology and case formulation. In P. Sturmey (Ed.), *Functional analysis in clinical treatment* (pp. 1–21). San Diego: Elsevier Academic Press.

Sverd, J. (2003). Psychiatric disorders in individuals with pervasive developmental disorder. *Journal of Psychiatric Practice, 9*(2), 111–127.

Sverd, J., Sheth, R., Fuss, J., & Levine, J. (1995). Prevalence of pervasive developmental disorder in a sample of psychiatrically hospitalized children and adolescents. *Child Psychiatry and Human Development, 25*(4), 221–240.

Szatmari, P., Offord, D. R., & Boyle, M. H. (1989). Correlates, associated impairments and patterns of service utilization of children with attention deficit disorder: Findings from the Ontario child health study. *Journal of Child Psychology and Psychiatry, 30*(2), 205–217.

Taylor, E., Sandber, S., Thorley, G., & Giles, S. (1991). *The epidemiology of childhood hyperactivity.* Oxford: Oxford University Press.

Tonge, B., & Einfeld, S. (2000). The trajectory of psychiatric disorders in young people with intellectual disabilities. *Australian and New Zealand Journal of Psychiatry, 34*(1), 80–84. doi:10.1046/j.1440-1614.2000.00695.x.

von Stauffenberg, C., & Campbell, S. B. (2007). Predicting the early developmental course of symptoms of attention deficit hyperactivity disorder. *Journal of Applied Developmental Psychology, 28*(5-6), 536-552.

Waschbusch, D. A., King, S., & Gregus, A. (2007). Age of onset of ADHD in a sample of elementary school students. *Journal of Psychopathology and Behavioral Assessment, 29*(1), 9–16.

Whitaker, S., & Read, S. (2006). The prevalence of psychiatric disorders among people with intellectual disabilities: An analysis of the literature. *Journal of Applied Research in Intellectual Disabilities, 19*(4), 330–345.

Willoughby, M. T. (2003). Developmental course of ADHD symptomatology during the transition from childhood to adolescence: A review with recommendations. *Journal of Child Psychology and Psychiatry, 44*(1), 88–106.

Wing, L., & Gould, J. (1979). Severe impairments of social interaction and associated abnormalities in children: Epidemiology and classification. *Journal of Autism and Developmental Disorders, 9*(1), 11–29.

Wozniak, J., Biederman, J., Faraone, S. V., Frazier, J., Kim, J., Millstein, R., Snyder, J. B. (1997). Mania in children with pervasive developmental disorder revisited. *Journal of the American Academy of Child and Adolescent Psychiatry, 36*(11), 1552–1559. doi:10.1016/S0890-8567(09)66564-3. (discussion 1559–1560.)

Xenitidis, K., Paliokosta, E., Rose, E., Maltezos, S., & Bramham, J. (2010). ADHD symptom presentation and trajectory in adults with borderline and mild intellectual disability. *Journal of Intellectual Disability Research, 54*(7), 668–677.

Zhang, X., & Ji, C. (2005). Autism and mental retardation of young children in China. *Biomedical and Environmental Sciences, 18*(5), 334.

Chapter 4
Psychopathology: Anxiety, Depression and Schizophrenia

Sarah Helps

Introduction

People with intellectual disabilities (ID) experience higher rates of psychological and psychiatric difficulties compared to their non-disabled counterparts, and experience a similar range of psychological and psychiatric difficulties, although these may appear or be expressed in different ways. The evidence base for psychotherapeutic interventions for people with ID who experience psychological or psychiatric difficulties is growing. There is encouraging evidence that a variety of psychotherapeutic approaches can be effectively adapted to meet the needs of people with ID, and consequently can help improve their well-being and quality of life.

While people with ID still experience some marginalisation in accessing services, there is a push towards the provision of generic, inclusive services delivered by staff who have the training and skills to meet their needs, as well as access to more specialised services for people with more complex needs. People with ID still experience some marginalisation on the research agenda, and more research of a variety of types is still required to inform our practice across the lifespan.

In this chapter I will focus on difficulties of anxiety, depression and severe mental illness in this population, and I will focus on the 'talking therapies'. I will rely on evidence-based practice, small-scale studies, case studies and practice-based evidence.

Mental Health, Psychological Well-being and ID

Identification of the number of people across the lifespan with ID and mental health difficulties is not straightforward due to issues of recognition, classification, service structure and provision and reporting, but it is widely accepted that this population

S. Helps (✉)
London, UK
e-mail: SHelps@tavi-port.nhs.uk

J. L. Matson, M. L. Matson (eds.), *Comorbid Conditions in Individuals with Intellectual Disabilities,* Autism and Child Psychopathology Series,
DOI 10.1007/978-3-319-15437-4_4

has a four- or fivefold increase in mental health difficulties compared to a non-disabled population, with population-based studies reporting rates of between 30 and 41 % (Lund 1985; Cooper et al. 2007; Smiley et al. 2005; Enfield and Emerson 2008; Emerson and Hatton 2007). People with ID are living much longer than in past times and, from the limited available data, the cost of meeting the mental health needs of older people with ID is significant (Strydom et al. 2010).

Nevertheless it remains unclear why people with ID experience higher rates of psychological and psychiatric distress. People with ID are not certainly immune to the stresses and strains of everyday life, and experience the same range of negative life events as people without ID (Hulbert-Williams et al. 2014). However, they may lack the range of adaptive psychological coping strategies and supports to cope with such life events (Bicknell 1983; Taylor et al. 2008). People with ID are also at greater risk than their non-disabled counterparts of experiences of abuse and trauma (Peckham et al. 2007; Robinson 2013) and such experiences are likely to be implicative in the development of a range of psychological and psychiatric disorders, including contributing to the development of disability or secondary handicap (Sinason 1992; Frankish 2013). While there is little evidence to show changes in the prevalence of psychological and psychiatric disorders at particular points over the life course, the clinical view is that, just as for people without ID, people with ID are particularly at risk for the development of difficulties at points of transition or crisis, such as changing school, moving from school to college, moving from living within a family unit to living in a more independent setting, changing jobs and being bereaved.

Service transitions between child and adult services are usually based on chronological age and do not take account of the person's developmental readiness to make the transition, which can lead to young people who are unready and poorly equipped to negotiate adult services falling through the service net. In the UK, recent government legislation on meeting the needs of children and young people with special educational needs and disabilities (2014) has extended the role of educational provision up until the age of 25, which is likely to be very helpful in reducing some of these transitional difficulties.

In exploring the possible causes and links to poor mental health, Cooper et al. (2007) found that poor mental health was associated with experiencing more life events, being of female gender, was linked to type of support received, being of lower ability, having more professional consultations, to smoking, to incontinence, to not having severe physical difficulties and to being mobile. They found no association with living in an area of deprivation, occupation, communication impairment, epilepsy, hearing impairment or previous institutional residence.

It is interesting to consider this alongside the work of researchers such as Emerson (e.g. 2007, 2012) who have highlighted the complex and important links between indices of deprivation, ethnicity and ID for both children and adults with ID. There is not scope in this chapter to explore social and political factors that affect diagnostic classification and rates but it is important to note that social, cultural and political factors may well affect the recognition of psychological difficulties in an ID population and the resources available to meet the needs of the population.

Little is written about the issues facing the growing population of older people with ID. It is clear that they may not share some of the experiences of people who are facing retirement after a lifetime in employment, but are just as likely to experience other life events, such as moving to different places to live or bereavement.

Tools Used to Make a Diagnosis of Mental Health Difficulties in an ID Population

The way in which people with IDs have been viewed by non-disabled counterparts has changed dramatically over the past century. The way in which the needs of people with IDs are assessed and diagnosed has therefore also undergone significant changes. People with ID do not present to services in the same way as their peers and, especially for people with moderate, severe and profound ID, it is incumbent on the clinicians to closely observe aspects of behaviour and emotion that help elucidate the person's difficulties.

The rates of diagnoses are greatly influenced by tools used with people with ID. For example, Cooper et al. (2007) compared different classificatory criteria and found a point prevalence of 40.9% for clinically made diagnoses (i.e. those made by clinicians), 35.2% for diagnoses made using the DC-LD, 16.6% for diagnoses made using the ICD-10-DCR and 15.7% using the DSM-IV-TR. They suggest therefore that using diagnostic classificatory systems that are not specifically tailored to the needs and presentations of people with ID can lead to an undercounting of their difficulties. Perez-Achiaga et al. (2009) undertook a systematic review of the ways in which affective disorders were diagnosed in people with ID. They concluded that further research was required with people with ID to ensure that both cognitive and behavioural symptoms could be both assessed and monitored during therapeutic interventions.

In exploring the utility of ID-specific screening tools, Rojahn et al. (2012) have tested the psychometric properties of the Behavior Problems Inventory-01 (BPI-01), an informant-based behaviour rating instrument for ID with 49 items and three subscales: self-injurious behaviour, stereotyped behaviour and aggressive/destructive behaviour, as well as the Behavior Problems Inventory-Short Form (BPI-S). They report that both BPI versions were found to be equally sound psychometrically and can be endorsed for future use and suggest that the BPI-S is a useful alternative to the BPI-01, especially for research and evaluation purposes involving groups of individuals (Rojahn et al. 2012). They conclude that further research is required to further test the utility of the measures.

In exploring concordance between multi-trait measures of mental health, Beail et al. (2013) administered one measure to informants—the Mini-Psychiatric Assessment Schedule for Adults who have developmental disabilities, and one self-report measure, the Brief Symptom Inventory. Results indicated good concordance between the measures but, as with other multi-trait measures, they did not demonstrate appropriate specificity for particular disorders.

People with severe or profound ID cannot report their own mood and feelings and so staff have to rely on careful observation to assess these. Vos et al. (2013) used an observational scale developed by Petry and Moes (2006). They found that it was possible to distinguish between mood and emotion, and that each aspect could give specific information about a person's affect. Although their findings have some limitations, it is suggested that their finding of diminished emotional reactions towards positive stimuli could potentially identify decreased mood and a potential depressive episode.

There are few measures which have been specifically developed to assess the psychological needs of people with ID following significant life events. One measure in the early stages of development is the Bereavement Needs Assessment Tool (BNAT; Blackman 2008), a nine-domain tool designed to ensure that all aspects of responses to bereavement, both pre- and post-bereavement, can be considered. The tool covers the following domains: emotional responses, cognitive understanding, social responses, social impact, physical lifestyle, continuing relationship with the deceased, changes in functioning, spiritual and changes in identity and comprises a list of questions that accompany each domain. Further work is needed on this and other measures to ensure that clinicians have robust tools to help them assess people with ID who experience significant life events and losses.

Overall, issues such as the diagnostic tools that are used together with the ways in which services for people with IDs are often separated off from general psychological and psychiatric services, serve to make identification and recording of difficulties very complicated. This may be more so for people with mild ID, whose needs might more often be met within generic services. This is likely to be less so for people with moderate and severe ID who are usually known to local child or adult ID services across the lifespan.

Affective Disorders

Depression is the most common disorder of mood and is an episodic disorder characterised by low mood, loss of interest in usual activities and most of the following symptoms: psychomotor retardation or agitation, fatigue, low self-esteem, pessimism, inappropriate excessive guilt, suicidal ideation, impaired concentration and sleep and appetite disturbance (American Psychiatric Association 2000; WHO 1992). Dysthymia does not have the episodic quality that is seen in depression and is a persistent disorder characterised by low mood and at least two of the other symptoms of major depression.

Bipolar affective disorder is diagnosed when a patient experiences two or more episodes of significant disturbance of mood or activity levels, sometimes an elevation or increase in mood and at other times a lowering of these. Mania is considered when there is an elevation of mood and/or activity levels without a related lowering of those levels. Bi-polar affective disorder is considered to be a highly heritable condition, and is often reported to be the most heritable of the psychiatric conditions (Cradock and Sklar 2013).

The prevalence of affective disorders in people with ID is higher than in the general population. The point prevalence of a major depressive illness in people with ID is between 2 and 7 %, which means that depression can be twice as common in this group as in the general population (Prasher 1999; Cooper et al. 2007; Bhaumik 2011).

In their study of those recruited to the 1946 British cohort study, Richards et al. (1997) reported that having an ID was associated with a fourfold increase in risk of affective disorder, which was not accounted for by social and material disadvantage or by medical disorder. They concluded that having an ID was strongly associated with risk of affective disorder, persisting well into midlife. This contrasts with later findings by Colishaw et al. (2004), who found that social disadvantage, and to a lesser extent physical health problems, contributed strongly to the increased risk for depressed mood at age 43 years in a cohort of people with ID.

There is some evidence that people with ID are at greater risk for mania than people without ID, and Deb et al. (2001) found a prevalence of 2.2 % of mania or hypomania in their ID population. In exploring issues of diagnosis of mania in people with severe or profound ID, Matson et al. (2007) found that problems of sleep and psychomotor agitation should alert clinicians that further assessment of bipolar symptomatology is warranted. They suggest that focusing on observable behaviours based on Diagnostic and Statistical Manual of Mental Disorder-IV criteria can be useful in formulating a diagnosis of bipolar disorder in persons with ID.

There has been some concern that symptoms of affective disorders have not been sufficiently recognised in people with ID. Tsiouris et al. (2013) reported an increase over time in the use of antidepressant medication with people with ID, compared with previous reports of use, which they thought might positively indicate the increased recognition and diagnosis of depression in people with ID over the past decades.

There have been reports of episodic mood changes in people with ID over many decades. Because reports of symptoms frequently do not meet the full diagnostic criteria for a diagnosis of bi-polar affective disorder, yet look similar, these patients are often referred to as having unstable mood disorder (Verhoeven and Tuinier 2001). Case reports highlight how carefully patients with rapid cycling mood, and presenting with challenging behaviour, need to be observed (Olubokun and Menon 2004), and how treatment with antipsychotic medication can give rise to obsessive–compulsive symptoms (Ulhaq and Abba-Aji 2012) and dysphagia (Vohra and Patterson 2011) in people with severe ID.

Anxiety Disorders

Anxiety disorders include generalised anxiety, panic disorders, simple phobias, social phobias, obsessive–compulsive disorder and post-traumatic stress disorder (DSM-IV-TR, American Psychiatric Association 2000; World Health Organisation 1992). Anxiety disorders are the most prevalent type of psychiatric disorders in general populations, with studies reporting prevalence between 4 and 8 %, and may be even more common among people with ID. For example Deb et al. (2001) reported that up to 7.8% of their sample showed an anxiety disorder. A recent UK population-based study by Reid et al. (2011) explored the point prevalence of anxiety in a group of over 1,000 adults with ID and found 3.8% of the cohort to have an anxiety disorder, with generalised anxiety being the most common (1.7%) followed by agoraphobia (0.7%). The presence of recent life events and a lack of employment were independently associated with having an anxiety disorder. History of being a long-term hospital resident was independently associated with not having an anxiety disorder.

Phobias

A phobia is an irrational or excessive fear of an object or a situation. There is general acceptance that simple phobias may be more prevalent in an ID population than in the general population, but little solid prevalence data are available (see Jennett and Hagopian 2008).

Post-traumatic Stress Disorder

Post-traumatic stress disorder is a common outcome for people who have experienced highly stressful or life-threatening events or abuse, with a prevalence rate of 5–10% in the general population. It comprises symptoms of re-experiencing the traumatic incident in the form of recurrent and distressing recollections of the event including intrusive images, nightmares and flashbacks, symptoms of avoidance and of arousal.

There appears to be a link between being of lower cognitive ability and the development of PTSD (McNally et al. 1995; Macklin et al. 1998), but clinical experience suggests that there may in fact be a variety of resiliency factors such as coping skills and patterns of support for the person who has experienced the trauma rather than level of cognitive ability that is the determining factor.

Mevissen et al. (2010) highlight the difficulties in getting prevalence data, given that there are no reliable and valid instruments for assessing PTSD in this population. They note the need for further work in this area. Bakken et al. (2014) presented a series of five case studies in which they described their patients with ID who had experienced highly traumatic events and who met the criteria for PTSD.

In one of the few studies to elucidate the psychological consequences of abuse for people with severe ID, Rowsell et al. (2013) used a repeated measures design to interview carers of people with severe ID about their psychological response to experiences of abuse. They found marked increases in the frequency and severity of a range of emotional, physiological and behavioural symptoms of psychological distress in men and women with severe intellectual disabilities following alleged abuse. Over time, there was some alleviation in the victims' difficulties, but up to 2 years after the abuse (at the end point of the study) their psychological functioning remained severely compromised.

Obsessive–Compulsive Disorder

Obsessive–compulsive disorder is characterised by intrusive thoughts, images or ideas, and the engagement in repetitive, apparently nonfunctional overt and covert behaviour to neutralise the obsessions, or in response to rigid rules (DSM-IV-TF, American Psychiatric Association 2000). Given this range of symptomatology, it is often difficult for people with ID to describe their symptoms or indeed those assessing them to elucidate the range of symptoms, hence a definitive diagnosis can be hard to make. Clinically, therefore, people are often described as having obsessive–compulsive behaviours that require intervention.

Severe Mental Illness

People with ID are at three to five times greater risk for the development of a psychotic illness than the general population (Cooper et al. 2007; Morgan et al. 2008), with reported prevalence rates of schizophrenia between 2.6 and 6.5 %, respectively (Corbett 1979; Lund 1985). Most of the existing literature on psychosis focuses on people with mild ID, due to the complexity of making a confident diagnosis in people with moderate or severe ID (Varghese and Banerjee 2011). As Morgan et al. (2008) point out, accurate assessments of the rates of comorbidity are negatively affected by frequent disconnection of services for people with mental illness and those for people with ID.

The aetiology of severe mental illness is unclear, but evidence increasingly suggests a common, perhaps neurodevelopmental pathogenesis (Morgan et al. 2008). From their Australian population-based research, Morgan et al. (2008) found that depending on birth cohort, 37–52 % of those with intellectual disability had co-occurring schizophrenia.

These results contrast with those obtained by Bhaumik et al. (2008) in a UK-based study of people using ID services, in which they reported that 2.2 % were diagnosed with schizophrenia and 1.8 % with other psychotic disorders. They noted a gender difference, in that men were more likely to have a diagnosis of autistic spectrum disorder, behaviour disorder or other psychiatric disorders, and women were more likely to have a diagnosis of schizophrenia, depression or organic disorder. They hypothesise that this may reflect service use patterns, rather than any 'real' difference in the rates of the conditions between men and women.

There has been a long-standing concern that even though the rates of severe mental illness are higher for people with ID than in the general population there has been an overuse of antipsychotic medication, essentially to address behavioural rather than psychiatric issues. In a recent paper by Tsiouris et al. (2013), medication prescription for over 4,000 adults with ID was assessed. They found that 58 % of those in the study were receiving one or more antipsychotropic medications, and 45 % were receiving antipsychotic medications. While the authors noted that prescription of medication was still too high, given the likely rates of psychosis and schizophrenia within the sample, they noted that there had been a reduction in the prescription of antipsychotic medications relative to other studies, and seemingly better evidence-based prescribing on the basis of the treatment of diagnosable psychiatric disorders. They conclude that practitioners now seem to be using psychotropics primarily to treat diagnosed psychiatric disorders and not just to control aggressive behaviour, so indicating that an evidence-based practice of psychiatry is playing an increasing role in the ID population.

In a UK-based case-note audit of the records of 910 people with ID known to local ID services, 28 % were found to have a dual diagnosis of psychosis and ID, with 40 % of these showing moderately severe psychotic symptoms (Varghese and Banerjee 2011). Of those receiving treatment, 25 % were described as treatment-resistant. The authors note that in view of the diagnostic difficulties often encountered in patients with ID and psychosis, the use of symptom rating and drug-related side effect checklists can be a useful supplement to clinical assessments, given the difficulties that people with ID may have in describing or effectively communicating their psychological distress, and given that communications can easily be misunderstood as challenging behaviour.

While in the UK there are guidelines for the treatment of psychosis and schizophrenia (NICE 2014), these do not specifically address the needs of people with ID, and further work is needed to describe the ways in which psychotic illnesses present, including the atypical ways, for people with ID.

Psychotherapeutic Interventions for People with ID

Despite policy stating that people with ID are entitled to receive the same services as people without ID (Valuing People 2001, Valuing People Now 2009), psychological interventions for people with ID are still not widely available. However, the 'therapeutic disdain' that has influenced the lack of provision of psychotherapeutic interventions for people with ID across geography and time (see Taylor et al. 2008) is reducing, and there are pockets of good practice and good research in support of psychotherapeutic services for people with ID.

Clinical Considerations

For young people and adults with ID, it is rarely the person with ID who makes an active decision to seek out psychotherapeutic support. It is therefore important to assess both the referred patient's understanding of the referral together with the understandings and meaning of the referral to those in the referring system.

Most often, meeting with the network of concern prior to meeting with the referred person (assuming that consent has been gained to share information) can be most useful in understanding the context of the referral, including the questions of why now and why here.

It is also important to have a clear and regularly reviewed understanding of the capacity of the referred person to play a part in making decisions about the care they receive. In line with outcome-oriented practices, clarification of goals and desired outcomes between referrer and treatment provider is important. A patient's ability to engage with a therapeutic intervention is complex and based on many factors—this applies just as much to an ID population as to a non-ID population. Bhaumik (2011) notes that there is little available evidence regarding how to motivate people to engage in psychotherapeutic interventions.

Behavioural interventions have been used over many years to help people with ID manage symptoms of distress or behaviour that is challenging. Sturmey and Dibben (2014) provide a thorough review of the evidence-based literature, i.e. studies that meet Chambless and Hollon's (1998) criteria for evidence-based practice. They highlight that there is much to be done in developing the evidence base for psychotherapeutic interventions for people with ID for many symptoms of psychological distress. A broader view of practice-based evidence and evidence-based practice has been selected in reviewing the literature described below.

Cognitive Behavioural Interventions for Symptoms of Anxiety, Depression and PTSD

Cognitive-behavioural therapy (CBT) includes approaches that fall within the realm of learning theory. The treatment method assumes that psychological problems are learned and maintained by cognitive and behavioural social learning processes. The goal of CBT is to resolve the presenting problem. A strong and collaborative therapeutic relationship is required for effective treatment.

CBT has received a great deal of research attention and has a strong evidence base. It is currently seen as the treatment of choice for people who experience symptoms of anxiety and depression. The CBT model underpins IAPT services that are increasingly provided in the UK (NICE 2014). Evidence of the benefits of CBT with an ID population is gradually accumulating, and a number of studies have focussed on how CBT interventions can be adapted to meet the needs of an ID population (e.g. Hassiotis et al. 2011).

A number of case studies have been published that show that CBT can be effective in treating symptoms of anxiety and depression. A number of these studies have been completed with forensic populations in secure units (Sturmey et al. 2004; Taylor et al. 2010), but there are also studies that have been completed with a community population (Willner et al. 2002).

Lindsay et al. (1997) reported on a small trial of 12 patients who received a modified CBT intervention, compared to a wait list control group. Following intervention, the CBT group was reported to be significantly improved when compared with the control group on the global severity index scale of the Brief Symptom Inventory, and these gains were found to be maintained at follow-up.

CBT and Anger

Many people with ID find it very difficult to control their anger, often as a result of trying to manage complicated negative feelings as a result of experiences of abuse, frustration or anxiety. In their systematic review and meta-analysis (2013) Nicoll et al. reviewed 12 studies published since 1999 and reported large uncontrolled effect sizes for treatment of anger in people with ID, but urged caution due to low sample sizes, and noted the need for further high-quality research in the area.

Willner (2005) reviewed eight studies evaluating psychotherapeutic interventions to people with ID. All of these studies showed significant improvements on outcome measures for those in treatment, conditions that were maintained at 3 to 12-month follow-up. With the exception of one controlled study of CBT for depression that yielded very positive outcomes (McCabe et al. 2006), anger research has provided the strongest evidence that CBT can be effective with people with intellectual disabilities.

A CBT group intervention programme designed to reduce inappropriately expressed anger in people with ID was not only successful in significantly reducing levels of anger, but also levels of depression (Rose et al. 2000). In this study the use of CBT techniques applied within a problem-solving framework was found to encourage a sense of self-regulation among the participants.

Lindsay et al. (2014) developed a trans-diagnostic manual for use with people with ID and in testing this with 12 participants, compared to wait-list control data, found that the CBT group made significant improvements compared with the control group on the GSI scale of the BSI, and showed significant improvements on all scales except the depression scale of the BSI from pre- to posttreatment. They suggest that it is therefore possible to treat a range of symptoms and psychiatric diagnoses with a general trans-diagnostic CBT manual.

Although there is very little published literature, clinical practice suggests that the use of a CBT approach to treat simple phobias can be very effective. In one published case study, Newman and Adams (2004) describe the use of systematic desensitisation with relaxation and modelling to help a teenage boy with a moderate ID address his fear of dogs. They report that after 28 sessions the boy was able to manage both his behaviour and anxiety level when in contact with loose, unfamiliar dogs.

Group CBT Interventions

McCabe et al. (2006) conducted a group intervention with 34 people with ID who showed clinical depression or who seemed at risk for the development of symptoms of clinical depression. The group programme was designed to enhance social skills, promote participation in social activities, identify and change negative cognitions and somatic complaints. A group format was deemed to be beneficial as participants were able to practise skills with peers and operate within a social environment where trust and respect for others could be experienced. They found that participation in the intervention programme had a significant impact on depressive symptoms and other psychosocial variables. The results indicated that the treatment group had significantly lower depression scores after completing the intervention programme. The treatment group also experienced an increase in social comparison scores when compared to the control group which did not complete the programme. At 3-month follow-up, there were no significant changes from the assessment scores at posttest, which would indicate that these positive changes were sustained over time.

Marwood and Hewitt (2013) describe a six-session group CBT programme for people with ID who struggled with anxiety. Using a mixed-methods approach, they reported that the group intervention was effective in treating anxiety in the eight group participants, and also improved quality of life for the participants. They highlight some of the complex issues in running a group for people with ID, some of which are similar to groups for people without ID (for example participants not liking each other, age difference between group members) and some of which were specific to this participant group (for example the wide range of cognitive ability of the participants).

Peckham et al. (2007) ran a group for women with ID who had experienced sexual abuse. The group lasted for 20 sessions and involved three stages, establishing relationships and the therapeutic alliance, psychoeducation and helping reprocess the trauma. The group was reported to lead to a reduction in symptoms of depression, self-harm and trauma as well as increased awareness of sexual abuse, and helped both the women and their carers move on with their lives.

Staff Views on CBT Interventions

Linking to the issue of therapeutic disdain, Stenfert et al. (2013) explored staff expectations and views of CBT for people with ID. In their qualitative study, thematic analysis of interviews with a small group ($n=11$) of staff suggested that prior to the intervention, staff did not perceive CBT as a long-term solution for psychological problems, had little knowledge of CBT and did not feel included in the process. These views shifted over the course of the intervention and, following the intervention, staff reported improved psychological well-being for their service user and a wish for longer term involvement of the therapist. Stenfert et al. highlight the importance of working with the wider professional system around the client and negotiating issues of confidentiality and the sharing of information in a way that supports the service users' well-being.

Willner et al. (2013) reported on a group-based 12-week CBT intervention delivered by care staff in day services for people with ID. A total of 179 participants took part. The intervention was found to have only a small, nonsignificant effect on participants' own reports of anger, but keyworker ratings were significantly lower, as were participant ratings on other measures. Both participants and keyworkers reported greater usage of anger coping skills, and professionals reported lower levels of challenging behaviour.

EMDR and PTSD

Eye movement desensitization and reprocessing (EMDR) (Shapiro 1995) is a treatment designed to alleviate symptoms of trauma. In this intervention, patients are asked to bring to mind an image of the distressing or disturbing image, thought or feeling associated with their memory of the trauma while tracking the clinician's moving finger with their eyes, or while the clinician taps on each side of the body. EMDR is a well-researched intervention and many studies highlight its utility for symptoms of both single and multiple traumas (Shaprio 2012).

Mevissen et al. (2010) note that a range of commonly used treatments for PTSD has been described with people with ID (CBT, EMDR and psychodynamic-based treatments) and that these case studies suggest positive treatment effects. They highlight the importance of developing good diagnostic instruments to support further research and treatment. In an effort to add to the very small body of literature, 2011 Mevissen et al. published a case study series in which they described the treatment of four people with ID using EMDR. They reported positive gains from the treatment that was maintained at follow-up. They described how the EMDR intervention could be individually adapted to meet the particular needs of people with ID, often using paradigms designed for use with children.

Clinical experience suggests that people with ID struggle more with the cognitive aspects of EMDR, such as selecting specific negative and positive cognitions, but that they can easily access the affective component of the intervention. A modified storytelling approach, such that reported for use in younger children (see Lovett 1999), has been found to be particularly helpful in working with young adults with ID who have experienced single trauma.

Systemic Interventions

Family therapy, also known as systemic psychotherapy, works to help families develop an understanding of the challenges they face in a relational context and aims to develop alternative ways of thinking, feeling and acting in relation to difficulties faced. Including a person with an ID in a meaningful way often involves working at a slower pace, and can involve active monitoring of language and close attention to the fit between the language used by the therapist, and indeed other family members, with the ways of understanding of the person with ID. It can also involve working at the level of examples, using drawings, photos or videos and providing more sessions than might usually be offered in an episode of care (see Baum and Lynggaard 2006).

The joy and burden of caring for a person with ID most often falls to close family members. This can place a great strain on family members, as they are required to provide information on the well-being of their relative in a way that is not expected for people without ID (Varghese and Banerjee 2011), and the burden of care can be particularly stressful for parents as they get older (Cairns et al. 2013), as they start to think about their own end-of-life issues, and worry about who will meet the needs of their child when they no longer can.

Over the past 15 years, an increasing amount of attention has been paid to the benefits of using family therapy and a systems perspective to address the relational issues associated with living with or caring for a person with ID, and a number of reviews and case studies have been published (e.g. Lynggaard and Scior (2002) Purdy 2012; Baum and Lynngaard 2006; Hill-Weld 2011). Despite this, there have to date been few formal research studies assessing efficacy. Case-study research has shown that a systemic approach can be effective for people with ID not only in working with them and their families, but also with them and their paid supporters (Haydon-Laurelut and Nunkoosing 2010).

Mindfulness

There is a wealth of recent evidence supporting the use of mindfulness to alleviate symptoms of anxiety and depression. There is a small amount of published evidence to suggest that people with ID can derive benefit from attending a mindfulness-based stress reduction group (Charman and Mitchell 2013). In this small study, the authors found that the mindfulness approach was experienced as helpful by their six participants and that participants valued the opportunity to talk to other people about their experiences.

In a study using mindfulness-based cognitive therapy, Idusohan-Moizer et al. (2013) reported an improvement in participants' experiences of anxiety, depression, self-compassion and compassion for others following participation in the group. They reported that gains were maintained at 6-week follow-up.

As therapeutic techniques evolve, it is vital to include people with ID in studies of all aspects of the psychotherapeutic process, to explore what is similar and what is different about the intervention, the way in which it needs to be delivered and the ways in which outcomes and progress can most usefully be monitored.

Psychodynamic Interventions

Psychodynamic psychotherapy refers to a range of treatments based on psychoanalytic concepts and methods (Shedler 2010). Blagys and Hilsenroth (2000) suggested that psychodynamic psychotherapies most usually involve: a focus on affect and expression of emotion; exploration of attempts to avoid distressing thoughts and feelings; identification of recurring themes and patterns; discussion of past experience; a focus on interpersonal relations; a focus on the therapeutic relationship; and an exploration of fantasy life (see Shedler 2010).

Practice-based evidence and case-study research has shown benefits of psychodynamic psychotherapy for adults across the ability spectrum in improving reducing psychological symptoms and improving a variety of aspects of emotional and psychological functioning, including self-esteem and emotional intelligence (Sinason 1992; Beail et al. 1996; MacDonald et al. 2003; Simpson and Miller 2005; Salvadori and Jackson 2009; Alim 2010). However, few well-validated research studies have been conducted. This leads writers such as Flynn (2012) to argue that these approaches continue to be offered on the basis of opinion rather than evidence.

Jackson and Beail (2013) thoroughly reviewed the literature regarding psychodynamic psychotherapeutic interventions with people with ID over the past 30 years. They noted a paucity of descriptive practice in the literature, particularly in relation to how practitioners formulated the information gathered from the patient into an interpretation.

In exploring the effectiveness of psychodynamic psychotherapy, Beail et al. (2007) explored the dose– effect relationships in adults receiving psychodynamic psychotherapy. They reported that the greatest impact was achieved within the first eight sessions, comparable to findings with non-disabled patients.

In a further study, Newman and Beail (2010) explored defence mechanisms used by patients with ID, and found that patients used a wide range of defences. In contrast to their previous findings, they did not find that patients experienced significant change within the first eight sessions, and did not find that patients' defence mechanisms shifted over the course of the sessions. As well as raising some methodological issues, they argued that further work was needed to examine the relationship between anxiety, defence and the hidden content as formulated in psychodynamic interventions and the impact of therapists' interventions.

Common Factors Approach to the Evaluations of Therapeutic Interventions

The work on common factors within psychotherapeutic research highlights the importance of non-modality specific factors on the outcome of interventions (Duncan et al. 2010; Laska et al. 2013). While little common factors analysis has been undertaken with an ID population, it seems highly likely that there will be parallels with other psychotherapy research, where qualities of the therapeutic relationship are as important as are specific aspects of intervention. Further research is therefore needed both on the process of psychotherapy with people with ID as well as the contribution of specific elements of particular modalities. Issues such as staff confidence and competence in delivering services to an ID population are likely to be particularly important variables.

Conclusions

An increasing evidence base shows that people with ID can and do make use of psychotherapeutic interventions to address emotional and mental health difficulties (Beail et al. 2005; Nicoll et al. 2013; Willner et al. 2006). In any form of psychotherapeutic intervention, the 'fit' or relationship between therapist and patient is the key to progress. When working with people with ID an important part of the therapeutic relationship rests on the ability to the therapist to 'meet' the patient in a way that enables the patient to access the therapists' ideas and questions.

Therefore, all forms of psychotherapeutic intervention need to be modified according to the specific needs and profile of the patient. This is particularly important given that there is no clear evidence of a straightforward relationship between aspects of intellectual functioning, or indeed overall IQ and treatment efficacy.

Within UK health services, there is a movement for people with ID to receive the same access to services and indeed to access the same services as people without ID. People with mild ID or intellectual abilities falling above 50 may well be able to make effective use of psychotherapeutic interventions, as delivered in the mainstream or the specialist setting, and further evaluation of the strengths and difficulties of services being delivered in each setting would be helpful in future service planning and delivery and indeed regarding staff training. Much more work is needed to explore whether and indeed how psychotherapeutic interventions can be of benefit to people with moderate or severe ID (Bhaumik et al. 2011).

Access to psychotherapeutic interventions for people with ID remains more limited than for people without ID, which limits the size of the evidence base on clinically effective interventions and treatment approaches (Brown et al. 2011). As evidence for CBT interventions, both individual and group-wise, grows, it is also important to investigate whether and how other interventions that have a good deal of practice-based evidence to recommend them, such as cognitive analytic therapy (Lloyd and Clayton 2013) and dialectical behaviour therapy (Lew 2011; Sakdalan et al. 2010), can be of use.

Further, it will be important to expand the research knowledge regarding the utility of psychotherapeutic interventions for people with ID with a range of other difficulties. For example, given the wealth of research highlighting the benefit of a CBT approach to people who experience chronic pain, McManus et al. (2014) report a pilot study using CBT with five patients with ID who experienced chronic pain. They reported that the patients made good progress in some areas, but that the gains made were not maintained at follow-up. They concluded that further work with larger populations was needed to elucidate how to achieve lasting gains using a CBT approach to pain management with people with mild ID.

There is an increasing evidence base for the open dialogue approach in intervening with people who have severe psychiatric difficulties. This approach is a language-based, community and family-based approach to severe psychiatric crises and conditions developed in Western Lapland to treat people with first-time psychosis. Little work has to date been published involving people with ID who have been treated using the open dialogue approach (Seikkula and Alakare 2014). Given the importance of the network of care and support around a person with an ID it is likely that the open dialogue approach has much to offer people with ID with severe mental health problems.

People with ID are diagnosed as having personality disorders (see for example Alexander et al. 2012; Taylor and Novaco 2013; Turygin et al. 2014) and further research needs to be conducted on how efficacious interventions for people of average cognitive ability might need to be modified for people with mild or even moderate ID. Issues of how to facilitate the development of mentalisation-based skills seem particularly relevant.

What kinds of Research Are Needed: Evidence-Based Practice and Practice-Based Evidence

Good quality research of all kinds will be invaluable in maintaining existing services and in developing effective, efficient and indeed cost-effective services for people with ID (Bhaumik 2011). Much of the existing research on psychotherapeutic interventions for people with ID does not meet the rigorous standards of the randomised-controlled trial. The presence of ID has often been used as exclusion criteria for entry to large-scale research trials (Royal College of Psychiatrists 2004), and this has contributed to the paucity of research produced.

More research using a variety of quantitative and qualitative paradigms is therefore needed. While traditional, quantitative and modernist research paradigms can be very useful, and indeed can provide persuasive evidence for commissioners of services, there is a strong move towards more emancipatory paradigms, which acknowledge the politics of research, involving people with disabilities at all stages of the planning and doing process, addressing the power imbalance inherent in the research endeavour, and focussing on contextual factors and strengths and coping skills of people with disabilities. Such research data are gaining increasing currency with policymakers, and can be just as useful as quantitative data in influencing the shape of clinical practice and services. The transformative paradigm, which focuses on exploring dimensions of diversity, respectfully working in partnership between researcher and participant, exploring resilience and strengths as well as challenges, and explicitly attempting to acknowledge oppressive structures (Mertens 2011), is a particularly helpful paradigm to use with people with ID.

It is also important that service users are asked to give feedback about how they have found the services offered to them (Valuing People Now, Department of Health 2009). McMahon et al. (2014) have recently completed a qualitative study to explore the views of service users with ID following attendance at a CBT group programme to address difficulties with anger. Service users were reported to be able to give valuable feedback on how they had enjoyed the group and found it effective. Further themes of the interviews included 'the importance of relationships', 'a new me', 'new and improved relationships', 'presenting myself in a positive light' and 'what the group didn't change'.

Using a similar methodology, Anslow(2014)) interviewed people with ID who had taken part in family therapy sessions with family members. They used a variety of strategies to support the participants to give feedback on their experiences, including DVD-assisted recall of the family therapy session, and also held a focus group for staff. They reported themes of 'therapists'focus on strengths and difficulties', 'differences in metacognition', 'finding a voice in therapy', 'frustration with the outcome of therapy' and 'managing an unusual experience', and concluded that the study had illuminated useful practice tips for the conduct of family therapy with people with ID.

In their study of the experiences of patients with ID who had received long-term psychodynamic psychotherapy, Merriman and Beail (2009) found that service users reported feeling positive towards their therapist and therapy in general. Positive changes were felt to have been made in both behaviour and emotions. This work was then extended in a further study by Khan and Beail (2013), who explored the views of service users who had received a variety of types of therapeutic intervention. They reported that, overall, service users were highly satisfied with the psychological therapy offered, and felt benefit from attending. They further reported that the qualitative responses in the study highlighted how appropriate adaptation of therapy especially in terms of communication contributes to satisfaction or dissatisfaction with therapy. Overall, there is a good deal of evidence to suggest that people with ID who use psychotherapeutic services are well able to give feedback on their experiences. This can make a valuable contribution to service development and indeed can inform staff training.

Clinical Implications for Providing Therapeutic Interventions for People with ID

A treatment approach informed by the current evidence base in the context of a careful formulation of the needs of the individual is most helpful, where services addressing the biological, social, psychological and developmental aspects of a person's presentation are coordinated and integrated, with the overall aim not on symptoms reduction and quick solutions, but on restoring a person's well-being in the long term (Dosen 2007; Tsiouris 2010; Stenfert Kroze et al. 2014) and improving their felt sense of quality of life.

As well as continuing to develop the increasing evidence for and availability of psychotherapeutic interventions, prevention of mental health problems and the promotion of positive psychological well-being should be a key focus for all involved in caring for and in providing services to people with intellectual disability.

Furthermore, individual, family and systems-based interventions for people with ID need to be seen in the context of broader cultural and social progress to value people with as interwoven layers of intervention that can prevent mental health difficulties and promote positive well-being.

References

Alexander, R. T., Chester, V., Gray, N. S., & Snowden, R. J. (2012). Patients with personality disorders and intellectual disability-closer to personality disorders or intellectual disability? A three-way comparison. *Journal of Forensic Psychiatry & Psychology, 23*(4), 435–451.

Alford, J. D., & Locke, B. J. (1984). Clinical responses to psychopathology of mentally retarded persons. *American Journal of Mental Deficiency, 89,* 195–197.

Alim, N. (2010). Therapeutic progressions of client and therapist throughout a course of psychodynamic therapy with a man with mild learning disabilities and anger problems. *Advances in Mental Health and Learning Disabilities, 4*(1), 42–49.

Anslow (née Atkins Furniss), K. (2014). Systemic family therapy using the reflecting team: The experiences of adults with learning disabilities. *British Journal of Learning Disabilities, 42*(3), 236–243.

American Psychiatric Association (2000) Diagnostic and statistical manual of mental disorders (4th edn, revised) (DSM IV TR). APA.

Azam, K. K., Serfaty, M. M., King, M. M., Martin, S. S., Strydom, A. A., Parkes, C. C., & Hassiotis, A. A. (2012). The development of manualised cognitive behaviour treatment for adults with mild intellectual disability and common mental disorders. *Psychiatriki, 23*(2), 109–116.

Bakken, T., Kildahl, A., Gjersøe, V., Matre, E., Kristiansen, T., Ro, A., & Tveter, A. L., Høidal, S. H. (2014). Identification of PTSD in adults with intellectual disabilities in five patients in a specialised psychiatric inpatient unit. *Advances in Mental Health and Intellectual Disabilities, 8*(2), 91–102.

Baum, S., & Lynggaard, H. (2006). *Intellectual disabilities: A systemic approach.* London: Karnac Books.

Beail, N., Warden, S., Morsley, K., & New man, D. (2005). Naturalistic evaluation of the effectiveness of psychodynamic psychotherapy with adults with intellectual disabilities. *Journal of Applied Research in Intellectual Disabilities, 18*(3), 245–251.

Beail, N., Kellett, S., Newman, D. W., & Warden, S. (2007). The dose-effect relationship in psychodynamic psychotherapy with people with intellectual disabilities. *Journal of Applied Research in Intellectual Disabilities, 20*(5), 448–454.

Beail, N. N., Mitchell, K. K., Vlissides, N. N., & Jackson, T. T. (2013). Concordance of the mini-psychiatric assessment schedule for adults who have developmental disabilities (pasadd) and the brief symptom inventory. *Journal of Intellectual Disability Research, 59*(2), 170–175

Bhaumik, S., Tyrer, F. C., McGrother, C., & Ganghadaran, S. K. (2008). Psychiatric service use and psychiatric disorders in adults with intellectual disability. *Journal of Intellectual Disability Research, 52*(11), 986–995.

Bhaumik, S., Gangadharan, S., Hiremath, A., Russell, P. S. (2011) Psychological treatments in intellectual disability: The challenges of building a good evidence base. *The British Journal of Psychiatry, 198,* 428–430.

Bicknell, J. (1983). The psychopathology of handicap. *British Journal of Medical Psychology, 56,* 167–178.

Blackman, N. (2008). The development of an assessment tool for the bereavement needs of people with learning disabilities. *British Journal of Learning Disabilities, 36*(3), 165–170.

Blagys, M. D., & Hilsenroth, M. J. (2000). Distinctive feature of short-term psychodynamic-interpersonal psychotherapy: A review of the comparative psychotherapy process literature. *Clinical Psychology: Science and Practice, 7*(2), 167–188.

Cairns, D., Tolson, D., Brown, J., & Darbyshire, C. (2013). The need for future alternatives: An investigation of the experiences and future of older parents caring for offspring with learning disabilities over a prolonged period of time. *British Journal of Learning Disabilities, 41,* 73–82.

Chambless, D. L., Hollon, S. D. (1998). Defining empirically supported therapies. *Journal of Consulting and Clinical Psychology, 66*(1), 7–18.

Chapman, M. J., & Mitchell, D. (2013). Mindfully valuing people now: An evaluation of introduction to mindfulness workshops for people with intellectual disabilities. *Mindfulness, 4*(2), 168–178.

Chapman, M. J., Hare, D. J., Caton, S., Donalds, D., McInnis, E., & Mitchell, D. (2013). The use of mindfulness with people with intellectual disabilities: A systematic review and narrative analysis. *Mindfulness, 4*(2), 179–189.

Collishaw, S., Maughan, B., & Pickles, A. (2004). Affective problems in adults with mild learning disability: The roles of social disadvantage and ill health. *British Journal of Psychiatry, 185,* 350 -351.

Cooper, S. A., Smiley, E., Morrison, J., Williamson, A., & Allan, L. (2007). Mental ill-health in adults with intellectual disabilities: Prevalence and associated factors. *British Journal of Psychiatry, 190,* 27–35.

Corbett, J. (1979) Psychiatric morbidity and mental retardation. In F.E. James & R.P. Snaith (Eds.), *Psychiatric Illness and mental handicap* (pp. 11–25). London: Gaskell Press.

Craddock, N., & Sklar, P. (2013). Genetics of bipolar disorder. *Lancet, 381*(9878), 1654–1662.

Dagnan, D., Masson, J., Cavagin, A., Thwaites, R., & Hatton, C. (2014). The development of a measure of confidence in delivering therapy to people with intellectual disabilities. *Clinical Psychology & Psychotherapy*. doi:10.1002/cpp.1898

Deb, S., Thomas, M., & Bright, C. (2001). Mental disorder in adults with intellectual disability. I: prevalence of functional psychiatric illness among a community-based population aged between 16 and 64 years. *Journal of Intellectual Disability Research, 45,* 495–505.

Department of Health. (2001). *Valuing people. A new strategy for learning disability for the 21st Century. Cm 5086.* London: Stationery Office. (http://www.archive.official-documents.co.uk/document/cm50/5086/5086.htm).

Department of Health, Depression in adults: The treatment and management of depression in adults.(2009). http://www.nice.org.uk/guidance/cg90

Dosen, A. A. (2007). Integrative treatment in persons with intellectual disability and mental health problems. *Journal of Intellectual Disability Research, 51*(1), 66–74.

Emerson, E. (2007). Poverty and people with intellectual disabilities. *Mental Retardation and Developmental Disabilities Research Reviews, 13,* 107–113.

Emerson, E. (2012). Deprivation, ethnicity and the prevalence of intellectual and developmental disabilities. *Journal of Epidemiology and Community Health, 66*(3), 218–224

Flynn, A. G. (2012). Fact or faith?: On the evidence for psychotherapy for adults with intellectual disability and mental health needs. *Current Opinion in Psychiatry, 25*(5), 342–347.

Frankish, P. (2013). Thirty years of disability psychotherapy, a paradigm shift? *Advances in Mental Health and Intellectual Disabilities, 7*(5), 257–262.

Hassiotis, A., et al. (2011). Cognitive behaviour therapy (CBT) for anxiety and depression in adults with mild intellectual disabilities (ID): A pilot randomised controlled trial. *Trials, 12,* 95.

Hatton, C. (2002). Psychosocial interventions for adults with intellectual disabilities and mental health problems: A review. *Journal of Mental Health, 11,* 357–373.

Haydon-Laurelut, M., & Nunkoosing, K. (2010). 'I want to be listened to': Systemic psychotherapy with a man with intellectual disabilities and his paid supporters. *Journal of Family Therapy, 32,* 73–86.

Hulbert-Williams, L. L., Hastings, R. R., Owen, D. M., Burns, L. L., Day, J. J., Mulligan, J. J., & Noone, S. J. (2014). Exposure to life events as a risk factor for psychological problems in adults with intellectual disabilities: A longitudinal design. *Journal of Intellectual Disability Research, 58*(1), 48–60. doi:10.1111/jir.12050.

Idusohan-Moizer, H., Sawicka, A., Dendle, J., & Albany, M. (2013). Mindfulness-based cognitive therapy for adults with intellectual disabilities: An evaluation of the effectiveness of mindfulness in reducing symptoms of depression and anxiety. *Journal of Intellectual Disability Research: JIDR, 59,* 93–104

Jackson, T., & Beail, N. (2013). The practice of individual psychodynamic psychotherapy with people who have intellectual disabilities. *Psychoanalytic Psychotherapy, 27*(2), 108–123. doi: 10.1080/02668734.2013.798680.

Jennett, H. K., & Hagopian, L. P. (2008). Identifying empirically supported treatments for phobic avoidance in individuals with intellectual disabilities. *Behavior Therapy, 39*(2), 151–161. doi:10.1016/j.beth.2007.06.003.

Khan, M. M., & Beail, N. (2013) Service user satisfaction with individual psychotherapy for people with intellectual disabilities. *Advances in Mental Health and Intellectual Disabilities, 7*(5), 277–283.

Kroese, B., Jahoda, A., Pert, C., Trower, P., Dagnan, D., & Selkirk, M. (2014). Staff expectations and views of cognitive behaviour therapy (CBT) for adults with intellectual disabilities. *Journal of Applied Research in Intellectual Disabilities, 27*(2), 145–153.

Laska, K. M., Gurman, A. S., & Wampold, B. E. (2013). Expanding the lens of evidence-based practice in psychotherapy: A common factors perspective. *Psychotherapy*. doi:10.1037/a0034332.

Lew, M. (2011). Dialectical behavioral therapy for adults who have intellectual disability. In R. J. Fletcher (Ed.), *Psychotherapy for individuals with intellectual disability* (pp. 37-65). Kingston: NADD Press.

Lindsay, W. R., Neilson, C., & Lawrenson, H. (1997). Cognitive behaviour therapy for anxiety in people with learning disabilities. In B. S. Kroese, D. Dagnan & K. Loumidis (Eds.), *Cognitive behaviour therapy for people with learning disabilities*. (pp. 124–140). London: Routledge.

Lindsay, W. R., Tinsley, S. S., Beail, N. N., Hastings, R. P., Jahoda, A. A., Taylor, J. L., & Hatton, C. C. (2014). A preliminary controlled trial of a trans-diagnostic programme for cognitive behaviour therapy with adults with intellectual disability. *Journal of Intellectual Disability Research*. doi:10.1111/jir.12145

Lloyd, J., & Clayton, P. (2013). *Cognitive analytic therapy for people with intellectual disabilities and their carers*. London: Jessica Kingsley Publishers.

Lovett, J. (1999). *Small wonders: Healing childhood trauma with EMDR*. New York: Free Press.

Lund, J. (1985). The prevalence of psychiatric morbidity in mentally retarded adults. *Acta Psychiatrica Scandinavica, 72,* 563–570.

Lynggaard, H., & Scior, K. (2002) Narrative therapy and people with learning

Marshall, K., & Ferris, J. (2012). Utilising behavioural family therapy (BFT) to help support the system around a person with intellectual disability and complex mental health needs: A case study. *Journal of Intellectual Disabilities, 16*(2), 109–118. doi:10.1177/1744629512443619.

Marwood, H., & Hewitt, O. (2013). Evaluating an anxiety group for people with learning disabilities using a mixed methodology. *British Journal of Learning Disabilities, 41*(2), 150–158. doi:10.1111/j.1468-3156.2012.00749.x.

Matson, J. L., González, M. L., Terlonge, C. C., Thorson, R. T., & Laud, R. B. (2007). What symptoms predict the diagnosis of mania in persons with severe/profound intellectual disability in clinical practice? *Journal of Intellectual Disability Research, 51*(1), 25–31. doi:10.1111/j.1365-2788.2006.00897.x.

McCabe, M. P., McGillivray, J. A., & Newton, D. C. (2006). Effectiveness of treatment programmes for depression among adults with mild/moderate intellectual disability. *Journal of Intellectual Disability Research, 50,* 239–247. doi: 10.1111/j.1365-2788.2005.00772.x.

McMahon, P., Stenfert Kroese, B., Jahoda, A., Stimpson, A., Rose, N., Rose, J., & Willner, P. (2014). 'It's made all of us bond since that course…'—A qualitative study of service users' experiences of a CBT anger management group intervention. *Journal of Intellectual Disability Research: JIDR*. doi:10.1111/jir.12144.

McManus, S., Treacy, M., & McGuire, B. (2014). Cognitive behavioural therapy for chronic pain in people with an intellectual disability: A case series using components of the feeling better programme. *Journal of Intellectual Disability Research: JIDR, 58*(3), 296–306. doi:10.1111/jir.12018

Merriman, C., & Beail, N. (2009). Service user views of long-term individual psychodynamic psychotherapy. *Advances in Mental Health and Intellectual Disabilities, 3*(2), 42–47.

Mertens, D. M. (2011). Mixed methods as tools for social change. *Journal of Mixed Methods Research, 5*(3), 195–197.

Mevissen, L. L., & de Jongh, A. A. (2010). PTSD and its treatment in people with intellectual disabilities: A review of the literature. *Clinical Psychology Review, 30*(3), 308–316. doi:10.1016/j.cpr.2009.12.005.

Mevissen, L. L., Lievegoed, R. R., & de Jongh, A. (2011). EMDR treatment in people with mild ID and PTSD: 4 cases. *Psychiatric Quarterly, 82,* 43–57.

Mevissen, L. L., Lievegoed, R. R., Seubert, A. A., & De Jongh, A. A. (2012). Treatment of PTSD in people with severe intellectual disabilities: A case series. *Developmental Neurorehabilitation, 15*(3), 223–232. doi:10.3109/17518423.2011.654283.

Morgan, V. A., Leonard, H., Bourke, J., & Jablensky, A. (2008). Intellectual disability co-occurring with schizophrenia and other psychiatric illness: Population-based study. *British Journal of Psychiatry, 193*(5), 364–372.

Newman, C., & Adams, K. (2004). Dog gone good: Managing dog phobia in a teenage boy with a learning disability. *British Journal of Learning Disabilities, 32*(1), 35–38. doi:10.1111/j.1468-3156.2004.00259.x.

Newman, D. W., & Beail, N. (2005). Assimilation of problematic experiences during psychotherapy with people who have mental retardation. *American Journal on Mental Retardation, 110,* 359–365.

Newman, D. W., & Beail, N. (2010). An exploratory study of the defence mechanisms used in psychotherapy by adults who have intellectual disabilities. *Journal of Intellectual Disability Research, 54*(7), 579–583.

NICE (2014) Psychosis and schizophrenia in adults: Treatment and management

Nicoll, M., Beail, N., & Saxon, D. (2013). Cognitive behavioural treatment for anger in adults with intellectual disabilities: A systematic review and meta-analysis. *Journal of Applied Research in Intellectual Disabilities, 26*(1), 47–62.

Olubokun, J., & Menon, K. (2004). Rapid cycling affective disorder presenting as challenging behaviour in a service user with mild learning disability: A case report. *British Journal of Developmental Disabilities, 50*(99,Pt2), 99–108. doi:10.1179/096979504799103895

Peckham, N., Corbett, A., Howlett, S., McKee, A., & Pattison, S. (2007). The delivery of a survivors' group for learning disabled women with significant learning disabilities who have been sexually abused. *British Journal of Learning Disabilities, 35*(4), 236–244. doi:10.1111/j.1468-4187.2006.00426.x.

Perez-Achiaga, N. N., Nelson, S. S., & Hassiotis, A. A. (2009). Instruments for the detection of depressive symptoms in people with intellectual disabilities: A systematic review. *Journal of Intellectual Disabilities, 13*(1), 55–76. doi:10.1177/1744629509104487.

Petry, K., & Maes, B. (2006). Identifying expressions of pleasure and displeasure by persons with profound and multiple disabilities. *Journal of Intellectual and Developmental Disability, 31*(1), 28–38. doi:10.1080/13668250500488678.

Prasher, V. (1999). Presentation and management of depression in people with learning disability. *Advances in Psychiatric Treatment, 5,* 447–454.

Prout, H. T., & Nowak-Drabik, K. M. (2003). Psychotherapy with persons who have mental retardation: An evaluation of effectiveness. *American Journal on Mental Retardation, 108,* 82–93.

Purdy, L. (2012). How to fail as a family therapist working with adults with learning disabilities: A paradoxical literature review. *Journal of Family Therapy, 34,* 419–430.

Reid, K. A., Smiley, E., & Cooper, S. A. (2011). Prevalence and associations of anxiety disorders in adults with intellectual disabilities. *Journal of Intellectual Disability Research: JIDR, 55*(2), 172–181. doi:10.1111/j.1365-2788.2010.01360.x. (Epub 2011 Jan 4).

Robinson, S. (2013) *Preventing the emotional abuse and neglect of people with intellectual disability.* London: Jessica Kingsley. (ISBN: 9781849052306).

Rojahn, J. M. (2012). The behavior problems inventory-short form for individuals with intellectual disabilities: Part II: reliability and validity. Journal Of Intellectual Disability

Rojahn, J. J., Rowe, E. W., Sharber, A. C., Hastings, R. R., Matson, J. L., Didden, R. R., & Dumont, E. M. (2012). The behavior problems inventory-short form for individuals with intellectual disabilities: Part I: Development and provisional clinical reference data. *Journal of Intellectual Disability Research, 56*(5), 527–545. doi:10.1111/j.1365-2788.2011.01507.x.

Rose, J. (2010). Carer reports of the efficacy of cognitive behavioral interventions for anger. *Research in Developmental Disabilities, 31*(6), 1502–1508. doi:10.1016/j.ridd.2010.06.007. (Epub 2010 Jul 2).

Rowsell, A. C., Clare, I. H., & Murphy, G. H. (2013). The psychological impact of abuse on men and women with severe intellectual disabilities. *Journal of Applied Research in Intellectual Disabilities, 26*(4), 257–270. doi:10.1111/jar.12016.

Royal College of Psychiatrists. (2004). Psychotherapy and learning disability. Council, Report CR116. London: Royal College of Psychiatrists. Journal of Intellectual Disability Research. doi: 10.1111/j.1365-2788.2005.00772.x.

Sakdalan, J. A., Shaw, J. J., & Collier, V. V. (2010). Staying in the here-and-now: A pilot study on the use of dialectical behaviour therapy group skills training for forensic clients with intellectual disability. *Journal of Intellectual Disability Research, 54*(6), 568–572. doi:10.1111/j.1365-2788.2010.01274.x.

Salvadori, A., & Jackson, T. (2009). A structured account of short-term psychodynamic psychotherapy with a man with learning disabilities. *Advances in Mental Health and Learning Disabilities, 3*(4), 31–35.

Seikkula, J., & Alakare, B. (2014). In a severe mental health crisis, it should be normal psychiatric. *Creative Positions in Adult Mental Health: Outside In-Inside Out*, 131.

Shapiro, F. (1995). *Eye movement desensitization and reprocessing: Basic principles, protocols, and procedures*. New York: Guilford Press.

Shapiro, F. (2012). EMDR therapy: An overview of current and future research. *Revue Européenne de Psychologie Appliquée/European Review of Applied Psychology, 62*(4), 193–195.

Shedler, J. (2010). The efficacy of psychodynamic psychotherapy. *American Psychologist, 65*(2), 98–109. doi:10.1037/a0018378.

Sinason, V. (1992). *Mental handicap and the human condition: New approaches from the tavistock*. London: Free Association Books.

Simpson, D., Miller, L. (2005). *Unexpected gains: Psychotherapy with people with learning disabilities*. London: Karnac Publications.

Smiley, E. (2005). Epidemiology of mental health problems in adults with learning disability: An update. *Advances in Psychiatric Treatment, 11*, 214–222.

Stimpson, A., Kroese, B., MacMahon, P., Rose, N., Townson, J., Felce, D., & Willner, P. (2013). The experiences of staff taking on the role of lay therapist in a group-based cognitive behavioural therapy anger management intervention for people with intellectual disabilities. *Journal of Applied Research in Intellectual Disabilities, 26*(1), 63–70. doi:10.1111/jar.12006.

Strydom, A., Romeo, R., Perez-Achiaga, N., Livingston, G., King, M., Knapp, M., & Hassiotis, A. (2010). Service use and cost of mental disorder in older adults with intellectual disability. *The British Journal of Psychiatry, 196*(2), 133–138. doi:10.1192/bjp.bp.108.060939.

Sturmey, P. (2004). Cognitive therapy with people with intellectual disabilities: A selective review and critique. *Clinical Psychology & Psychotherapy, 11*, 222–232.

Sturmey, P., & Didden, R. (Eds.) (2014) Evidence-based practice and intellectual disabilities. Chichester: Wiley Blackwell

Taylor, J. L., & Novaco, R. W. (2013). A brief screening instrument for emotionally unstable and dissocial personality disorder in male offenders with intellectual disabilities. *Research in Developmental Disabilities, 34*(1), 546–553. doi:10.1016/j.ridd.2012.09.018.

Taylor, J., Lindsay, W., & Willner, P. (2008). CBT for people with intellectual disabilities: Emerging evidence, cognitive ability and IQ effects. *Behavioural and Cognitive Psychotherapy, 36*(6), 723-733. (ISSN 1352–4658).

Tsiouris, J. A. (2010). Pharmacotherapy for aggressive behaviours in persons with intellectual disabilities: Treatment or mistreatment? *Journal of Intellectual Disability Research, 54*(1), 1–16. doi:10.1111/j.1365-2788.2009.01232.x.

Tsiouris, J. A., Kim, S. Y., Brown, W. T., Pettinger, J., & Cohen, I. L. (2013). Prevalence of psychotropic drug use in adults with intellectual disability: Positive and negative findings from a large scale study. *Journal of autism and developmental disorders, 43*(3), 719–731. doi:10.1007/s10803-012-1617-6.

Turygin, N., Matson, J. L., & Adams, H. (2014). Prevalence of co-occurring disorders in a sample of adults with mild and moderate intellectual disabilities who reside in a residential treatment setting. *Research in Developmental Disabilities, 35*(7), 1802–1808. doi:10.1016/j.ridd.2014.01.027.

Ulhaq, I., & Abba-Aji, A. (2012). Haloperidol induced obsessive compulsive symptom (OCS) in a patient with learning disability and bipolar affective disorder. BMJ Case Reports, 2012doi:10.1136/bcr.11.2011.5161

Varghese, S., & Banerjee, S. (2011). Psychotic disorders in learning disabilities-Outcome of an audit across community teams. *British Journal of Learning Disabilities, 39*(2), 148–153. doi:10.1111/j.1468-3156.2010.00641.x.

Verhoeven, W. A., & Tuinier, S. (2001). Cyclothymia or unstable mood disorder? A systematic treatment evaluation with valproic acid. *Journal of Applied Research in Intellectual Disabilities, 14*(2), 147–154. doi:10.1046/j.1468-3148.2001.00063.x.

Vohra, A., & Patterson, J. (2011). Quetiapine-induced dysphagia in a developmentally disabled woman with bipolar affective disorder. *German Journal of Psychiatry, 14*(2), 95–97.

Vos, P. P., De Cock, P. P., Petry, K. K., Van Den Noortgate, W. W., & Maes, B. B. (2013). Investigating the relationship between observed mood and emotions in people with severe and profound intellectual disabilities. *Journal of Intellectual Disability Research, 57*(5), 440–451. doi:10.1111/jir.12021.

Willner, P. (2005). The effectiveness of psychotherapeutic interventions for people with learning disabilities: A critical overview. *Journal of Intellectual Disability Research, 49,* 73–85.

Willner, P., Jones, J., Tams, R., & Green, G. (2002). A randomized controlled trial of the efficacy of a cognitive-behavioural anger management group for clients with learning disabilities. *Journal of Applied Research in Intellectual Disabilities, 15,* 224–235. doi:10.1046/j.1468-3148.2002.00121.x.

Chapter 5
Feeding Disorders

Alison M. Kozlowski, Tessa Taylor, Melissa L. González and Peter A. Girolami

Introduction

Oral consumption of food and drink is often viewed as one of the most basic behaviors in which people engage; it is ideally present immediately following birth and continues throughout the lifespan, with advancements in variety, volume, texture, and independence occurring following a developmental trajectory. However, for many children with intellectual and other developmental disabilities (ID/DD), this natural progression never commences or is disrupted. Some of these derailments are not atypical, such as toddlers and other young children experiencing varying periods of "picky eating" (Mascola et al. 2010). However, there comes a point when these deviations from typical eating patterns are a concern, at which point a pediatric feeding disorder is diagnosed. According to the *Diagnostic and Statistical Manual of Mental Disorders, Fifth Edition* (American Psychiatric Association 2013), a pediatric feeding disorder, now referred to as avoidant/restrictive food intake disorder, is diagnosed when an individual fails to consistently orally consume an adequate number of calories and amount of nutrients, which is associated with weight loss or lack of appropriate weight gain, nutritional deficiencies, dependence on enteral feedings or oral nutritional supplements, and/or interference with psychosocial functioning. Though this leaves some room for interpretation, this diagnosis may ultimately be given for a variety of feeding concerns, including when an individual has a weight for height or body mass index below normal limits or that would be below normal limits without supplemental feedings (de Moor et al. 2007;

A. M. Kozlowski (✉)
Kennedy Krieger Institute, 21205 Baltimore, MD, USA
e-mail: kozlowski@kennedykrieger.org

T. Taylor
Lizard Centre, Eastwood, South Australia, Australia

M. L. González · P. A. Girolami
Kennedy Krieger Institute/Johns Hopkins University School of Medicine, 21205 Baltimore, MD, USA

J. L. Matson, M. L. Matson (eds.), *Comorbid Conditions in Individuals with Intellectual Disabilities,* Autism and Child Psychopathology Series,
DOI 10.1007/978-3-319-15437-4_5

Farrell et al. 2001), consumes a limited variety of solid foods that do not represent a number of foods from all of the major food groups (Allison et al. 2012), is liquid dependent (Kelley et al. 2003), consumes only solids of a modified texture (Shore et al. 1998), and/or does not engage in developmentally appropriate self-feeding (Vaz et al. 2011). Additionally, these individuals often engage in refusal whenever nonpreferred foods/drinks are presented (Borrero et al. 2010; LaRue et al. 2011; Piazza et al. 2003a; Rivas et al. 2010; Wilder et al. 2005).

Although eating and drinking are often viewed as simple behaviors, each response actually contains multiple steps with which difficulties can arise. From a behavioral perspective, refusal can occur at many steps along this chain. Among the most commonly discussed groups of behaviors identified as refusal, inappropriate mealtime behavior (IMB), also referred to as disruptions and/or simply as refusal, involves the child preventing the deposit of food or drink by pushing the food/drink or the feeding hand away, turning one's head from the bite/drink presentation, and/or covering one's mouth (Allison et al. 2012; Piazza et al. 2003a). However, other forms of refusal also exist.

Nonacceptance, which is defined as not allowing the bite or drink to be deposited, may occur with or without IMB. For example, a child may "passively refuse," "hold out," or "wait out" the bite/drink by holding his/her mouth closed while not exhibiting IMB until the bite/drink is ultimately removed due to time constraints (Kadey et al. 2013b; Rubio et al. in press). Once the food or drink is deposited, refusal may take the form of expels or packs. An expel occurs when any food or drink, typically of at least a minimum size (e.g., larger than the size of a pea), is present outside of the mouth following acceptance of a bite or drink that has not been observed to be previously swallowed (Sevin et al. 2002). A pack occurs after accepting a bite or drink when any food or drink, once again, typically of at least a minimum size (e.g., larger than the size of a pea), remains inside the mouth following a specified period of time (e.g., 30 s) (Gulotta et al. 2005; Sevin et al. 2002). Although these forms of refusal are not always given as much attention as IMB, they too can significantly interfere with a child's feeding.

Prevalence of Feeding Difficulties in Individuals with Intellectual Disabilities

Estimates of the prevalence of feeding problems vary as a function of having no universally accepted definition of what constitutes a feeding problem or an agreed upon classification system (Benjasuwantep et al. 2013). A wide variety of different disorders, diagnoses, skill deficits, and problematic behaviors fall under the term "feeding problems" and include categories such as: (a) self-feeding deficits (e.g., acquisition and maintenance of independent self-feeding skills) (Luiselli 1991); (b) limited food intake (e.g., eating small quantities or being highly selective); (c) texture selectivity (e.g., consuming only smooth or puree textures); (d) coughing, gagging, and choking; (e) improper pacing (i.e., self-feeding, but at a very fast or slow rate); (f) food refusal; and (g) vomiting and rumination (i.e., voluntary regurgitation of stomach contents) (Sisson and Van Hasselt 1989). Further complicating the determination of prevalence, the etiology, severity, and clinical presentation of feeding problems varies across children of various ages, developmental trajectories, and medical histories (Williams et al. 2010).

The general consensus is that feeding problems in children are common, affecting typically developing children, as well as children and adolescents with ID/DD, and medical conditions. Prevalence rates for typically developing children exhibiting feeding problem ranges from 18 to 50% (Beautrais et al. 1982; Bentovim 1970; Carruth et al. 2004; Forsyth et al. 1985; Palmer and Horn 1978; Palmer et al. 1975). In individuals with ID/DD, estimates of prevalence increase from anywhere between 33 to almost 100% (Gal et al. 2011; Matson and Kuhn 2001; Palmer and Horn 1978; Palmer et al. 1975; Reilly et al. 1996; Rezaei et al. 2011; Sullivan et al. 2000; Williams et al. 2010). In their review of the literature, Williams et al. (2010) found that 139 of 178 (78%) children described in the treatment literature for food refusal were reported to have developmental disabilities. This finding is similar to previous estimates of developmental delay in this population (Budd et al. 1992; Burklow et al. 1998; Field et al. 2003). Further, Gal et al. (2011) found that among a sample of 91 children (ages 4–9 years) with a diagnosis of ID, over 95% had at least one problem related to eating/feeding, with a high percentage of feeding problems represented across mild, moderate, and severe levels of ID. Finally, Rezaei et al. (2011) examined the prevalence of feeding problems in 144 individuals with ID referred to speech and language pathology clinic. Results demonstrated that all participants exhibited some type of feeding problem.

Feeding problems are also common in children diagnosed with an autism spectrum disorder (ASD). Ledford and Gast (2006) reported in their review that 46–89% of children with ASD have feeding problems, most commonly in the form of food and texture selectivity. Previous studies have found that children with autism have lower nutritional variety relative to the other children, even when the social environment (i.e., adult models and food offered) is held constant (Berlin et al. 2011; Nadon et al. 2011). Specifically, Nadon et al. (2011) found that 52% of children with ASD were reported to have feeding problems that were considered to be moderate to severe by their caregivers. Moreover, these children had significantly more problems during the transition from puree to textured foods as infants, remained texture-selective for longer periods, and exhibited more behaviors including drooling, coughing, gagging, vomiting, and out-of-seat behavior during mealtimes. In addition, it has been suggested that children with ASD may be more susceptible to feeding problems of this nature (i.e., food selectivity) than children with other developmental disabilities.

Feeding issues are also very common in individuals diagnosed within the subgroup of cerebral palsy with rates of up to 90% experiencing some form of oral–motor or feeding problem (Reilly et al. 1996; Sullivan et al. 2000). Sullivan et al. (2000) reported finding that the greater the severity of motor impairment, the longer the meal duration. Significant concerns with swallowing function, including aspiration, have also been identified with individuals with cerebral palsy (Schwarz et al. 2001).

Some feeding problems may occur more frequently than others. Using the Screening Tool for Feeding Problems (STEP) (Matson and Kuhn 2001) to examine feeding problems exhibited by individuals with ID, Matson et al. (2008) reported the most common feeding related issue was problems with feeding skills (e.g., lack of independent eating, need of special equipment, and positioning modifications were all deemed significant variables). Similar findings were reported in recent studies (Reilly et al. 1996; Williams et al. 2010), including by Gal et al. (2011) and Rezaei et al. (2011) where feeding skills were significant problems for over 75% of their respective samples. Gender and level of ID severity also appear to be relevant factors in feeding problems. When comparing feeding problems in males and females across mild, moderate, and severe levels of ID, males demonstrated more significant feeding issues while the severity of feeding problems was greatest for those with severe and profound ID compared to the mild and moderate levels of ID (Matson et al. 2008; Rezaei et al. 2011). Food refusal and selective eating are also commonly identified feeding issues with individuals with ID (Williams et al. 2010) with some studies demonstrating rates as high as 60–70% (Gal et al. 2011; Rezaei et al. 2011; Williams and Seiverling 2010).

The high rate of occurrence of feeding problems in individuals with ID reported in the literature underscores a need for early assessment and preemptive measures to prevent serious physical impairment or quality of life issues. Although there are similarities across studies in regard to prevalence and type of feeding problem, each individual will compromise his or her own constellation of feeding issues based on their physical and developmental status, learning history, and environment. Thus, individual assessment to detect the presence of current or emerging feeding problems will help ensure the individuals safety and ability to reach their eating potential.

Comorbid Difficulties in Children with Feeding Disorders/Food Refusal

The higher frequency of food refusal in children with ID/DD, relative to typically developing children, may be due to the increased frequency of medical conditions and other complications that frequently co-occur with developmental delays (Sullivan 2008). Given the complex nature and multitude of factors that may be associated with the development of feeding difficulties, it is not surprising that children who present with food refusal frequently have a history of (or ongoing) medical complications, structural/physical abnormalities, and/or developmental concerns (Nicholls and Bryant-Waugh 2009). Moreover, it is common for these children to present with multiple conditions associated with food refusal (e.g., developmental disabilities and gastroesophageal reflux) (Burklow et al. 1998). Berlin et al. (2011) conducted a review of 286 children seen in a feeding clinic, and they reported the mean number of co-occurring medical and developmental conditions to be 3.74 per patient.

Co-occurring Medical Complications

Williams and Seiverling (2010), in their review of 38 intervention studies for pediatric food refusal, reported 212 out of 218 (97%) participants had some form of medical complication. Of 144 children dependent upon gastrostomy/nasogastric tube feedings seen in a hospital-based intensive feeding program from 2003 to 2008, 96% were found to have a history of or current gastroesophageal reflux (Gulotta 2012). In a separate sample of 121 children (including those with tube dependency, liquid dependency, and food selectivity) seen in the same hospital-based intensive program from February 2012 to September 2013, 39% were found to have a history of gastroesophageal reflux (original data collected by current authors). These findings match previous studies with a relatively higher percentage of children with total food refusal (i.e., insufficient consumption of daily caloric needs; nasogastric or gastrostomy tube dependence) having history of reflux as compared to those with problems of selectivity (Field et al. 2003; Ledford and Gast 2006; Rommel et al. 2003; Williams et al. 2010). Other associated problems related to the gastrointestinal tract include food allergies, delayed gastric emptying, constipation, and other types of motility difficulties (Field et al. 2003; Schwarz et al. 2001; Williams et al. 2010; Zangen et al. 2003). In many cases, these comorbid difficulties when unidentified and/or untreated play a role in the development or maintenance of the feeding problem due to the discomfort experienced during or immediately following meals.

Medical problems (not related to the gastrointestinal tract) noted to co-occur with feeding problems include chronic kidney disease, congenital cardiac disease, and esophageal atresia (Ramsay and Birnbaum 2013; Sables-Baus et al. 2011; Samaan and Secker 2014). Thirty-seven to 40% of infants and children assessed for feeding and swallowing difficulties were born premature and are at increased risk for cardiac, respiratory, neurologic (e.g., cerebral palsy), and developmental difficulties (Budd et al. 1992; Burklow et al. 1998; Lefton-Greif 2008; Schädler et al. 2007). In such cases, repeated exposure to invasive medical interventions such as intubation, mechanical ventilation, oral gastric or nasogastric tube feeding, frequent oral suctioning, or other devices in and around the child's throat may have caused ongoing distress or gagging establishing a learning history in which the child associates activities involving the child's mouth or swallowing with pain or discomfort. Thus, the child may remain resistant or otherwise hypersensitive to stimuli presented to his or her mouth (Hawdon et al. 2000; Schuberth et al. 2010). For children who are premature, they may not have the neurologic or digestive maturation necessary for successful oral feedings. With many of these cases, enteral feedings by nasogastric and gastrostomy tubes are necessary to ensure proper nutrition (Mason et al. 2005). However, prolonged tube feedings have been found to disrupt the development of age-appropriate oral motor skills and are often associated with increases in refusal when oral feeds are presented (Berlin et al. 2011). The lack of early eating experiences for these children either because of acute illness or maturation-related difficulties may be related to later difficulties with feedings.

Structural and Physical Abnormalities

Structural and/or anatomical abnormalities such as cleft palate, tracheoesophageal fistula, and microgastria may also contribute to difficulties with feeding and subsequent food refusal (de Moor et al. 2007). Oral-motor dysphagia, which typically results from a lack of experience in managing oral feeds, may maintain food refusal over time because the child has not developed the specific skills needed to advance oral-motor development (Schuberth et al. 2010).

Behavioral Difficulties

Environmental variables are often involved in the development and maintenance of food refusal. The child may learn that specific behaviors (i.e., turning head, crying, blocking mouth) during mealtime (or otherwise) are associated with different responses from caregivers such as a variation in the amount or quality of caregiver attention provided (i.e., coaxing or comforting) or the demands that are placed (i.e., amount or type of food presented or duration of the meal) (Babbitt et al. 1994; Palmer et al. 1975; Piazza et al. 2003a). Given the learning experiences that take place in the meal context, it should not be surprising that behavioral difficulties outside of meals are also common. Johnson et al. (2014) conducted a study involving 256 children with ASD with the aim of describing the relationship between core and associated behaviors of ASD and feeding/mealtime difficulties. Regression analyses indicated strong relationships between higher rates of repetitive behavior, sensory differences, and both externalizing and internalizing behavioral, and increasingly problematic feeding/mealtime behavior regardless of functioning level. These data suggest that children who display disruptive behavior outside of meals also engage in the same behavior at mealtimes.

Given the complex, bio-psychosocial nature of feeding problems, co-occurring medical, structural, and/or developmental disabilities are the rule rather than the exception. It is important that providers consider potential comorbidities that may be contributing to the maintenance of the feeding problem. Multiple disciplines are often required to properly assess and intervene in order to successfully treat/manage the feeding and comorbid difficulties.

Assessment

Interdisciplinary Assessment

As discussed previously, feeding disorders often have multiple comorbidities and etiologies, and thus may require assessment by a team of professionals from multiple disciplines so a comprehensive evaluation can be completed. Interdisciplinary assessment may take place in an interdisciplinary clinic setting format which involves record review, caregiver interview and questionnaires, and a direct meal observation. First and foremost, if necessary, potential medical issues should be assessed prior to beginning intensive therapy. Referrals to medical specialists such as allergists, gastroenterologists, and otolaryngologists may be warranted. A dietitian evaluates growth and nutritional deficiencies and recommendations regarding specific conditions (e.g., glycogen storage disease, diabetes). Speech-language pathologists and/or occupational therapists may conduct swallow studies to evaluate safety and aspiration risk, assess oral motor and self-feeding skills, and evaluate necessity of adaptive equipment for seating arrangements during mealtimes and/or utensils. Behavioral psychologists or behavior analysts conduct data-based assessments (e.g., functional assessments) and treatment evaluations, and conduct caregiver training and assess integrity once a mealtime protocol is established. This area will be the focus of this chapter and discussed in detail.

Behavioral Assessment

A variety of direct assessments may be conducted to inform treatment. Direct toy preference assessments and food/liquid preference assessments (Babbitt et al. 1994; e.g., paired-choice similar to Fisher et al. 1992; Levin and Carr 2001) may be administered to inform functional analysis (FA) design, identify potential reinforcers, and assess/manipulate edible demand level in treatment evaluations. Various antecedent assessments examining mealtime behavior in relation to variables such as food variety, texture, bolus, or presentation method may also be utilized to inform treatment (e.g., Kadey et al. 2013a; Munk and Repp 1994; Patel et al. 2002b; Sharp et al. 2010a).

With respect to behavioral assessments to assist in determining function-based components of treatment, researchers have adapted FA methodology for severe problem behavior (Iwata et al. 1982/1994) to evaluate IMB (e.g., Bachmeyer et al. 2009; Girolami and Scotti 2001; Najdowski et al. 2003; Najdowski et al. 2008; Piazza et al. 2003a). Girolami and Scotti (2001) conducted an FA of IMB in a home setting with six conditions (attention, demand, tangible toy, tangible food, alone, and control) and demonstrated concurrent validity with interview, questionnaire, and direct observations. Lower rates of refusal in the alone and control conditions were observed for all three children. Piazza et al. (2003a) conducted an FA of IMB in 15 children with four conditions: baseline (toy), attention, escape, and tangible. Out of those with differentiated responding, the majority ($n = 6$) had both escape and attention functions, and for the other children, functions included escape; attention; escape and tangible; and escape, attention, and tangible. Najdowski et al. (2003) and Najdowski et al. (2008) evaluated parent-conducted FAs of IMB in natural settings, and escape functions were found for all seven children. González et al. (2014) also found that during FA conditions for the majority of participants, IMB was lower when noncontingent access (NCA) to preferred tangibles was provided; however, for one out of nine participants, IMB was higher during the attention test condition with NCA to tangibles included. Multiple sources of control were found for all participants ($n = 9$); more specifically, nine (all) with escape, seven with attention, and six with tangible. In summary, FAs for IMB identify escape as a maintaining function in most cases, and IMB is often multiply maintained.

Descriptive analyses have also been employed to evaluate variables associated with IMB. Based on observation data from caregiver-fed meals, Piazza et al. (Piazza et al. 2003a) found that caregivers provided escape and attention following IMB for all six children assessed, and for half ($n = 3$), tangible delivery was also observed. Casey and colleagues (Casey et al. 2006; Casey et al. 2009) used descriptive assessment to evaluate and manipulate reinforcement schedules, demonstrating utility of this method to inform treatment. The researchers found that IMB was on a rich schedule of negative reinforcement for all three children. Positive reinforcement for bite acceptance was on a lean schedule for one child and a rich schedule for two children. Borrero et al. (2010) evaluated conditional and unconditional probabilities of delivery of escape, attention, and tangibles following refusal and acceptance in 25 children. Responses that were most likely to follow refusal were meal termination, spoon/cup removal, and coaxing. Responses varied depending on the topography of refusal (e.g., attention in the form of concern/comfort following emesis; switching to a previously accepted food following expulsion; meal termination following disruption). Extending this work, Woods et al. (2010) used lag sequential analyses to specifically evaluate the temporal impact of various forms of attention on mealtime behavior. Reprimands and statements of comfort/concern were followed by an immediate temporary decrease in IMB, while coaxing was followed by an immediate temporary increase in acceptance.

Thus, a wide variety of behavioral assessment technologies have been established. Assessments can be utilized to gather information about tangible and edible preferences, antecedent variables impacting specific mealtime behavior(s), and maintaining environmental variables for IMB. The benefit of these assessments is that they provide objective, measurable data to directly inform treatment. Various antecedent- and consequence-based procedures utilized in the treatment of pediatric feeding disorders will be described in the following section.

Behavioral Treatment

Antecedent-based Procedures

Various antecedent-based strategies have been examined (both with and without other components such as escape extinction and positive reinforcement, which are strategies that will be discussed in detail later in this chapter) to target mealtime behavior. Such strategies have included stimulus and demand fading, simultaneous presentation, and the high-probability (high-p) instructional sequence. In addition, various strategies have been utilized to teach mealtime skills.

Stimulus fading involves gradually changing properties of the mealtime stimulus (e.g., food/drink, utensil) from a response within the child's repertoire to a novel or target response. Stimulus fading, in combination with escape extinction (EE) and/or differential reinforcement of alternative behavior (DRA)/noncontingent reinforcement (NCR), has been used to gradually transition from liquids in a bottle to purees on a spoon (Johnson and Babbitt 1993), spoon to cup drinking via taping the spoon at varying distances to the cup (Groff et al. 2011), thickened liquids on spoon to cup (Babbitt et al. 2001), lower to higher food textures (Shore et al. 1998), liquid to baby food (Bachmeyer et al. 2013), water to a nutritional caloric drink (milk with Carnation Instant Breakfast™) via blending (Patel et al. 2001), chocolate to plain milk (Tiger and Hanley 2006), and preferred to nonpreferred foods via blending (Mueller et al. 2004). Rivas et al. (2010) evaluated fading of spoon distance from the child's lips, and found that IMB was lower at a distance compared to at the lips. Spoon distance fading alone did not increase acceptance, and acceptance increased more rapidly with EE alone compared to EE with spoon distance fading.

Demand fading involves increasing mealtime response requirements. In the absence of EE, demand fading has been used to increase food portion sizes with paced prompting and DRA (Knox et al. 2012) and increase bite number with cueing and DRA (Luiselli 2000). In conjunction with EE and/or DRA, demand fading has been employed to increase food portion size and variety (Freeman and Piazza 1998; Riordan et al. 1980), number of bites/sips (Najdowski et al. 2003; Riordan et al. 1980), food bolus on the spoon (Kerwin et al. 1995), and liquid bolus of cup drinking in conjunction with backward chaining (Hagopian et al. 1996).

Simultaneous presentation involves placing a preferred food item on or behind a nonpreferred food and presenting them together. Piazza et al. (2002) found that simultaneous presentation increased consumption without EE for two out of three participants. Without EE, simultaneous presentation has been shown to reduce packing (Buckley and Newchok 2005), increase solid variety via condiments such as ketchup (Ahearn 2003), and increase milk consumption via chocolate syrup which was later eliminated via stimulus fading (Tiger and Hanley 2006). This procedure has also been utilized in conjunction with EE to increase variety (Kern and Marder 1996; Riordan et al. 1984; VanDalen and Penrod 2010).

Researchers have applied the high-probability (high-p) instructional sequence used to target noncompliance (e.g., Mace et al. 1988) to mealtime behavior with mixed results. The high-p instructional sequence involves delivering a sequence of demands which have a high probability of compliance (e.g., accepting an empty spoon, pushing a button) prior to delivering a demand with a low probability of compliance (e.g., accepting a food bite). Researchers have utilized both topographically similar (mealtime-related) and dissimilar (unrelated to mealtime) high-p demands to increase consumption of nonpreferred foods. McComas et al. (2000) evaluated topographically dissimilar high-p instructions in conjunction with a treatment package consisting of choice, EE, DRA, and NCR to target bite acceptance for one child. Initially, compliance was higher when the high-p component was in place, but this effect was transient (compliance increased and maintained without high-p component). Dawson et al. (2003) also used topographically dissimilar high-p instructions and found that this procedure was ineffective alone, and it also did not enhance the effectiveness of EE when in conjunction with treatment packages. Using mealtime-related high-p instructions, Patel et al. (2006) found mixed results. When added to EE, the high-p instructional sequence increased acceptance for one participant, and increased acceptance and decreased IMB for another participant. For the third participant, the high-p instructional sequence alone was ineffective and did not enhance acceptance in conjunction with EE; however, with EE, the addition of the high-p instructional sequence resulted in lower and more stable IMB. Finally, Patel et al. (2007) found the high-p instructional sequence alone (using empty spoon presentations) increased acceptance for one participant.

Many antecedent-based (as well as some consequence-based) procedures are frequently employed in clinical practice to specifically target skill development in relation to pediatric feeding disorders (e.g., opening mouth, closing lips on spoon/cup, chewing, self-feeding/drinking). Such strategies include shaping, modeling, prompting, chaining, reinforcement, and physical guidance. However, aside from chewing (see chewing section of this chapter) and chaining and physical guidance targeting independence (e.g., Luiselli 1993; Piazza et al. 1993), there is a dearth of literature on application of these strategies to teach skills in this area. In addition, in clinical practice it is found that with continued practice/exposure many of these skills (as well as other responses such as gagging/coughing and expulsion) may improve over time without specific treatment changes (e.g., over time during a texture assessment, Shore et al. 1998).

Reinforcement and Punishment Procedures

Reinforcement Procedures In line with implementing the least restrictive treatments necessary to increase consumption, positive reinforcement, NCR/access, and negative reinforcement in various combinations have all been evaluated in regard to their impact on the treatment of food refusal.

Several researchers have documented success with providing positive reinforcement for appropriate behaviors (e.g., acceptance, mouth cleans) to increase the consumption of nonpreferred foods and drinks in children with pediatric feeding disorders without the use of EE (Casey et al. 2006; Koegel et al. 2012; Riordan et al. 1980). For example, Riordan et al. (1980) successfully increased the consumption of a variety of solids in two girls with ID who were previously maintained on limited diets. The treatment involved providing access to preferred foods and verbal praise contingent on bite acceptance, and later swallowing due to the emergence of packing and expelling, nonpreferred foods. Similarly, Casey et al. (2006) increased the volume of solids consumed by a 20-month-old typically developing girl who had been diagnosed with failure to thrive by providing verbal praise and attention contingent on bite acceptance while still providing escape from bites contingent on refusal.

However, other researchers have found that positive reinforcement alone is not always effective in treating pediatric feeding disorders such that it is necessary to implement other treatment components, such as EE, in conjunction (Hoch et al. 1994; Najdowski et al. 2003; Patel et al. 2002a; Piazza et al. 2003b; Seiverling et al. 2012). Seiverling et al. (2012) attempted to increase consumption of solids in a 3-year-old boy who consumed several foods, though most of them were starches. In the initial stages of treatment, access to a preferred food was provided contingent on consuming a bite of a nonpreferred food. With refusal continuing to result in escape from the nonpreferred food, the child's consumption of nonpreferred foods did not increase. However, once EE was added to the treatment, consumption of nonpreferred foods increased. Although EE was necessary for initial treatment gains in addition to the DRA procedure, the authors were able to remove the EE element and return to providing access to preferred foods contingent on consuming nonpreferred foods during maintenance. The authors, therefore, concluded that although EE was necessary for introducing nonpreferred foods, only the DRA procedure was necessary for maintenance, thereby decreasing the intrusiveness of treatment overall.

Patel et al. (2002a) compared DRA for acceptance to DRA for mouth cleans in three children with gastrostomy tube dependence. EE was not implemented initially, such that refusal resulted in escape from the bite/drink. Neither DRA treatment in the absence of EE resulted in increases in consumption. However, a comparison of the same procedures with the addition of EE in the form of nonremoval resulted in equal increases in acceptance and mouth cleans as well as equally low rates of IMB and expels.

NCR, also commonly referred to as NCA, has also been evaluated with respect to its impact on treating pediatric feeding disorders. Although NCR does not reinforce specific behaviors, it is believed that it may decrease the aversive properties of the mealtime context, thereby increasing consumption (Reed et al. 2004). Similar to the support for positive reinforcement to treat pediatric feeding disorders, NCR has also been found to be effective for some children (Wilder et al. 2005) and ineffective for others (Reed et al. 2004; Sharp et al. 2010b) when used without other treatment components. Wilder et al. (2005) evaluated the use of NCR in the context of escape in a 40-month-old girl who consumed puree/baby foods, but engaged in self-injurious behavior as a means of food refusal and did not consume a wide variety of foods. During treatment, the girl was provided NCA to a preferred video and removal of the spoon remained contingent on self-injurious behavior. Treatment resulted in an increase in acceptance and a decrease in self-injurious behavior.

However, when Reed et al. (2004) evaluated the effect of NCR in the context of escape in four children ages 15 months to 4 years who engaged in severe food refusal but did consume some foods/drinks orally, they found NCR in the context of escape to be ineffective. EE was necessary in order to significantly increase consumption and decrease IMB. Nevertheless, a comparison of EE alone and EE in conjunction with NCR showed that NCR was beneficial for some participants during EE treatments because it resulted in lower rates of IMB and less negative vocalizations.

Although some researchers have found that positive reinforcement and NCR may be effective in treating pediatric feeding disorders, whether in conjunction with EE or not, a comparison of the two reinforcement-based procedures for food refusal has received little attention. Allison et al. (2012) compared DRA for acceptance and NCR, both with highly preferred tangibles and attention, in the context of EE in a 3-year-old boy with ASD who ate several foods, but had limited variety. The interventions were equally effective in increasing acceptance and decreasing IMB and negative vocalizations. However, the NCR procedure was ultimately chosen for treatment by the caregiver, primarily because of ease of implementation compared to the DRA procedure.

Despite food refusal being commonly maintained by negative reinforcement in the form of escape from the bite or drink (Borrero et al. 2010; Girolami and Scotti 2001; Piazza et al. 2003a), thereby supporting the use of negative reinforcement as part of a function-based treatment, there is a paucity of research on the use of negative reinforcement in the form of breaks to treat food refusal. LaRue et al. (2011) evaluated the use of breaks for mouth cleans (i.e., swallowing bites/drinks within 30 s of acceptance) as a form of negative reinforcement in the treatment of food refusal in five children in an intensive feeding program after verifying through an FA that escape at least partially maintained each child's refusal. In the context of escape for IMB (i.e., the child continued to receive escape from each bite/drink contingent on IMB), mouth cleans never occurred so that no child ever came into contact with the contingencies for negative reinforcement, although they continued to receive breaks due to IMB. In a comparison of a treatment consisting only of nonremoval of the spoon/cup and one consisting of nonremoval of the spoon/cup and a 30-s break for each mouth clean (i.e., the next bite/drink was not delivered for an additional 30 s after the mouth clean as opposed to immediately following the mouth clean), the authors concluded that the treatments were equally effective. Therefore, it was concluded that negative reinforcement in the form of a break was not a necessary component of treatment. Further research is needed to evaluate the effectiveness of negative reinforcement in the form of breaks in treating food refusal, although it may be hypothesized that its effectiveness is likely similar to that of positive reinforcement and NCR.

Overall, although some researchers have provided support for reinforcement-based procedures used alone, many others have found these procedures to be ineffective when not used in conjunction with EE procedures. The rationale for this difference in outcomes may be attributed to a difference in participants; reinforcement-based procedures may be more effective by themselves when the participants currently consume some foods orally, consume foods from more than just one food group, and/or have only recently begun eliminating foods.

Punishment Procedures When reinforcement procedures alone are ineffective in treating pediatric feeding disorders, or it is hypothesized their solitary use will be ineffective, a punishment procedure may be incorporated. While some punishment procedures may include feeding-specific techniques, to be reviewed later in this chapter, response cost is also sometimes utilized. Kahng et al. (2001) implemented response cost in the context of escape with a 5-year-old boy with ID who exhibited problem behavior during meals. Preferred tangibles were provided at the commencement of each meal and removed following any instance of problem behavior (response cost), and also for not accepting a bite within 30 s (negative reinforcement). Within this treatment, positive reinforcement was provided contingent on subsequent acceptance. With treatment in place, acceptance increased and IMB decreased. This method was replicated and expanded upon by Buckley and Newchok (2005), who compared response cost procedures with NCR and with DRA. During these comparisons, access to tangibles was provided at the beginning of each meal and removed contingent on IMB or for not accepting a bite within 30 s, and then returned either 30 s after the removal regardless of behavior (NCR) or after swallowing a subsequent bite (differential reinforcement). Both procedures resulted in an increase in mouth cleans and a decrease in IMB and expels, but the procedure with NCR resulted in greater initial treatment gains such that overall mouth clean percentages were higher and overall IMB and expels were lower compared to the response cost procedure with differential reinforcement.

Specific Procedural/Behavioral Interventions for Acceptance

Acceptance, or allowing a bolus of food/drink to be deposited in the mouth, is generally one of the first behaviors targeted during treatment alongside a reduction in IMB so that acceptance is possible. Although numerous topographies of food refusal exist, many of these behaviors can only occur once acceptance has already occurred. While reinforcement procedures may be effective in treating pediatric feeding disorders, this is commonly felt to only be the case when the child is presently orally consuming some foods or drinks, thereby increasing the probability of him/her coming into contact with the reinforcement contingencies. However, in more severe pediatric feeding disorder cases where the child is consuming little if anything orally, more intensive procedures are often necessary, as reinforcement procedures alone generally tend to be ineffective.

Because food/drink refusal is often maintained by negative reinforcement in the form of escape from nonpreferred foods and drinks (Borrero et al. 2010; Girolami and Scotti 2001; Piazza et al. 2003a), elimination of this form of reinforcement through EE is frequently incorporated into treatments. EE involves not allowing the problem behavior, in this case one or more forms of refusal, to result in escape from the demand, in this case eating and/or drinking (Piazza et al. 2003a). In children with pediatric feeding disorders, implementing EE in its truest form would result in the child consuming the food or drink presented; with eating and drinking, this is a multistep demand and first requires the child to accept the bite or drink by mouth. Various feeding-specific procedures have been developed to ensure that EE occurs at least for acceptance of the bite/drink into the mouth, including nonremoval of the spoon, jaw prompts, finger prompts, and side deposits.

Nonremoval Presentation One of the most commonly cited methods of EE, a nonremoval presentation involves holding the spoon, cup, or other utensil to the child's mouth until the bite or drink is accepted regardless of the child's behavior (Allison et al. 2012; Kozlowski et al. 2011; LaRue et al. 2011). Attempts by the child to move the presentation away (e.g., pushing the spoon away) and to move oneself away from the presentation (e.g., turning head, covering mouth) are prevented by blocking and following the child's mouth with the utensil. Across the literature, there have been variations in precisely where the utensil is held, with recommendations to hold it to the upper lip (Rubio et al. in press), lower lip (Ahearn 2002; Kerwin et al. 1995), or at the midline (Kadey et al. 2013b; LaRue et al. 2011). Some researchers have not specified precisely where the utensil should be held. Once the mouth is open wide enough, the food/drink is deposited by inserting the utensil across the plane of the lips. Although specific rules regarding depositing the food/drink may vary depending on treatment providers, it is usually deposited unless the child is coughing, gagging, or having emesis. That is, if the child's mouth is open due to screaming or crying, the utensil is still inserted into the mouth.

The effectiveness of nonremoval presentations has been demonstrated by many researchers both in isolation and in conjunction with other procedures (Allison et al. 2012; Bui et al. 2013; Kozlowski et al. 2011; LaRue et al. 2011; Patel et al. 2002a; Patel et al. 2006; Piazza et al. 2003b; Reed et al. 2004; Rivas et al. 2010; Sharp et al. 2010b). For example, following a comparison of differential reinforcement for acceptance and for mouth cleans without the use of EE procedures (i.e., the presentation was still removed contingent on refusal), which did not increase consumption in three children with gastrostomy-tube dependence, Patel et al. (2002a) compared both reinforcement procedures with the addition of a nonremoval presentation. Both treatments were equally successful in increasing acceptance and mouth cleans and decreasing IMB and expels. When the nonremoval component was removed, similar performance continued for some children, but eventually decreased. An occasional maintenance of improvement sometimes occurs when the nonremoval component is removed, which is hypothesized to be the result of the child never coming into contact with the contingency for escape (i.e., not engaging in IMB).

Another example of support for nonremoval presentations was provided by Piazza et al. (2003b), who also evaluated the effectiveness of EE in the form of a nonremoval presentation following ineffective results when differential reinforcement alone was implemented for two children with total food refusal. They found that nonremoval presentations were effective in treating severe food refusal regardless of whether or not differential reinforcement was also implemented. However, nonremoval presentations with differential reinforcement occasionally resulted in a reduction in extinction bursts, less IMB, and less negative vocalizations.

Although nonremoval presentations have proven effective in increasing acceptance of nonpreferred foods and drinks, some negative consequences of implementing the procedure have been documented. Due to a history of IMB (e.g., pushing the bite/drink away, turning one's head) often being negatively reinforced (i.e., escape is provided contingent on these behaviors), an extinction burst often immediately follows implementation of nonremoval presentations since escape from the presentation is no longer provided, such that these behaviors increase temporarily in frequency and/or intensity before improving. The extinction burst may also be accompanied by increases in negative vocalizations (e.g., screaming, crying) (Piazza et al. 2003b). Although these bursts many times only last for up to a few meals, caregivers may be resistant to the implementation of such procedures due to these immediate consequences. In an effort to decrease the initial negative consequences associated with nonremoval presentations, reinforcement procedures be used in conjunction with nonremoval presentations.

In addition to the initial negative consequences of implementing nonremoval presentations, in some cases nonremoval presentations may prove ineffective because the child will learn to simply hold his/her mouth closed so that the food or drink cannot be deposited (Borrero et al. 2013; Kadey et al. 2013b; Rubio et al. in press). In these cases, the child will "passively refuse," "hold out," or "wait out" the presentation until the time cap is reached and the meal is terminated, thereby ultimately resulting in escape from the bite/drink. When this occurs, additional procedural interventions may be required in conjunction with a nonremoval presentation.

Alternative Deposit Methods In some cases, a child may open his/her mouth to allow a bite to be deposited, but then not close his/her lips around the spoon to complete the deposit. Behavioral strategies may then be used to increase the likelihood of the child closing his/her lips around the spoon (e.g., prompts, reinforcement-based procedures). Additionally, alternate deposit methods, such as sliding the spoon against the upper teeth/lip, flipped spoon deposits, and NUK® deposits, have also been used to target this behavior, as well as others (e.g., expels), during treatment, though research has not been published with respect to its effect on acceptance. With an upright spoon presentation, the bite may be deposited by sliding the upright spoon against the upper teeth/lip when removing the spoon from the mouth so that the bolus is scraped off into the mouth (Sharp et al. 2010a; Sharp et al. 2012). A flipped spoon deposit involves inserting the spoon upright into the mouth above the midline of the tongue and then rotating it 180 degrees so that the top of the spoon faces the tongue (Sharp et al. 2010a; Sharp et al. 2012). The spoon is then gently pressed down against the tongue while pulling the spoon out of the mouth, which results in the bolus being deposited directly onto the tongue. Lastly, an NUK® deposit involves transferring a lower texture food (e.g., puree) from the spoon to an NUK® brush, inserting the brush into the mouth over the midline of the tongue while holding the brush horizontally, and then depositing the bolus by gently pressing the brush down against the midline of the tongue while rotating the brush forward and concurrently pulling the brush out of the mouth (Sharp et al. 2010a).

Physical Guidance Procedures To date, several physical guidance procedures have been developed and evaluated in the context of food/drink refusal, including jaw prompts, finger prompts, NUK prompts, and side deposits. Perhaps the first documented form of physical guidance, often simply referred to as "physical guidance," a jaw prompt involves applying slight pressure at the mandibular junction of the jaw with the nonfeeding hand's thumb on one side of the mandibular joint and the forefinger on the other until the mouth opens so that the bite/drink can be deposited (Ahearn et al. 1996; Borrero et al. 2013). To date, the effectiveness of jaw prompts has been demonstrated repeatedly (Ahearn et al. 1996; Borrero et al. 2013; Kerwin et al. 1995; Piazza et al. 2003b), especially when positive reinforcement-based strategies or nonremoval presentations have been ineffective or less preferred by caregivers.

Kerwin et al. (1995) initially evaluated a jaw prompt procedure for two children with ID and total food refusal for which positive reinforcement procedures alone were ineffective in significantly increasing solid consumption. After introducing a jaw prompt in conjunction with a positive reinforcement procedure, consumption increased. However, with these children, nonremoval of the spoon had not been attempted, thereby not allowing for a comparison of the two procedures. When Ahearn et al. (1996) compared a jaw prompt procedure to nonremoval of the spoon in three children who exhibited severe food refusal and limited acceptance of solids, the authors found that while both treatments ultimately produced comparable results, the jaw prompt procedure resulted in a quicker reduction in "corollary behaviors" (i.e., IMB, negative vocalizations, and self-injury) and was also more preferred by caregivers.

Although many researchers have found jaw prompts, generally in conjunction with other behavioral interventions (e.g., positive reinforcement), to be effective in increasing acceptance of nonpreferred foods, there are some concerns regarding the procedure. First, the slight or gentle pressure to be used during this procedure is subjective (Kadey et al. 2013b). Because there is not a standard level of pressure described, other than the terms "slight" or "gentle," individuals may apply too much or too little pressure, each carrying its own consequences. If too little pressure is applied, the procedure may be unsuccessful in physically guiding the mouth open. On the other hand, if too much pressure is applied, there is a risk of harm to the child. Furthermore, with the application of only slight or gentle pressure, children are capable of continuing to hold their mouth closed. Due to these potential difficulties with jaw prompts, other forms of physical guidance have also been evaluated.

Another form of physical guidance that can be implemented when a child will not open his/her mouth entails the feeder inserting his/her index finger at the corner of the child's mouth and holding it along the child's upper gum line between the gums and cheek until the child opens his/her mouth wide enough for the food/drink to be deposited. Although this method is used quite frequently with high effectiveness in some feeding programs, published research to date has been scant. Borrero et al. (2013) evaluated the effectiveness of the finger prompt in comparison to the jaw prompt in four children with severe food refusal in the context of comprehensive treatment packages which included nonremoval along with other function-based treatment components (e.g., NCA). The finger prompt and jaw prompt in conjunction with other identical treatment components were equally effective in increasing consumption, decreasing latency to accept, and decreasing IMB. However, caregivers of all participants indicated a preference for the finger prompt over jaw prompt. Borrero et al. (2013) note that, while the finger prompt is also an intrusive procedure, it provides less ambiguity in comparison to the jaw prompt due to the absence of the application of pressure being involved. Additionally, although the child attempting to bite the feeder is an added risk when using a finger prompt procedure, no child attempted to bite the feeder during the study. In cases in which children do attempt to bite the feeders, protective equipment may be used to alleviate this risk and/or the jaw prompt procedure may be judged more appropriate.

An NUK® brush has also been evaluated more recently as a physical guidance procedure. Kadey et al. (2013b) described a procedure in which, if the child passively refused with nonremoval and other reinforcement-based procedures, an NUK® brush was maneuvered between the child's lips, slid between the cheek and teeth past the last molar, and held against the gums while turning it approximately 10°. Once this resulted in the child's mouth opening at least 1 cm, the food or drink was deposited with a spoon or cup. The authors stated that, therefore, the child could not escape the bite or drink being deposited; however, it was not explicitly stated where the food was deposited if the child opened his/her lips but continued to clench his/her teeth. They evaluated this treatment for two children, ages 3 and 9 years, with intellectual and/or developmental disabilities following either a lack of success in increasing consumption with a nonremoval presentation and NCR or an inability to appropriately implement a nonremoval presentation due to the child's size. For both children, the NUK® brush prompt was effective in increasing acceptance/consumption, decreasing meal duration, and decreasing IMB. Therefore, the NUK® prompt procedure may be a viable option when other EE procedures and reinforcement-based procedures are either ineffective or not appropriate options due to the child's size or high rate of IMB and/or physical aggression.

Despite multiple physical guidance procedures having been developed to assist the child in opening his/her mouth during passive refusal, the fact remains that many children may be able to continue avoiding bite/drink presentations even with the implementation of these procedures by forcefully holding their lips closed or clenching their teeth. Therefore, if a child continues to passively refuse when nonremoval and other physical guidance procedures have been implemented, the side deposit method may be used to place the food in the child's mouth (Rubio et al. in press). Following implementation of the finger prompt, as described by Borrero et al. (2013), the feeder gently moves his/her index finger away from the gum line toward the inside of the cheek and continues this horizontal movement until a space is created to deposit food/drink. Even in cases in which the child clenches his/her teeth, a space will still be available for the deposit of food/drink in the side of the mouth. With lower texture food, the food is transferred to an NUK® brush, which is then inserted in the space at the corner of the mouth to deposit the food by rolling the brush downward against the inside of the cheek. The index finger is then removed from the child's mouth immediately once the food/drink has been deposited. If the child opens his/her mouth prior to the deposit, the food may be deposited on the midline of the tongue using the previously mentioned NUK® brush deposit method. With regular texture food, the feeder may place the bite along the inside of the cheek using a pincer grasp with the feeding hand. Rubio et al. (in press) demonstrated the effectiveness of a side deposit procedure with lower texture food with two children for whom treatment packages consisting of nonremoval of the spoon and physical guidance (jaw prompt and finger prompt) were ineffective in increasing and maintaining high levels of consumption due to passive refusal. With the addition of the side deposit procedure, both children consistently consumed their entire meal volume. Additionally, rates of IMB remained low and comparable to prior treatment packages.

Specific Procedural/Behavioral Interventions for Expulsion and Packing

While nonremoval of the spoon/cup targets acceptance, expulsion and packing may emerge as topographies of refusal following acceptance to escape consumption of the food/liquid and/or due to oral motor skill deficits. For example, Sevin et al. (2002) demonstrated that sequentially introducing treatment targeting acceptance increased expulsion, and treatment targeting expulsion increased packing. Multiple methods of treatment for expulsion and packing have been investigated. In addition to preventing escape, hypothesized behavioral mechanisms for expulsion and packing treatments have included increased response effort to expel and decreased response effort to swallow, reduction of the aversive properties of swallowing, triggering a swallow response, or negative reinforcement in the form of avoidance of the treatment procedures.

Expulsion Expulsion can vary in form, such as actively spitting out the food/liquid using the mouth, using an implement (e.g., sleeve, napkin, finger) to wipe away/pull the food/liquid out of the mouth, or passively allowing the food/liquid to dribble or fall out of the mouth. Treatment for expulsion typically involves re-presentation (Ahearn et al. 1996; Coe et al. 1997; Patel et al. 2002a), but additional methods may also be necessary. Re-presentation involves collecting the expelled food/liquid (or a fresh, equivalent amount of food/liquid) and continuing to present the bite/drink until consumption occurs. Variations in the utensils used during the initial presentation and the re-presentation method have been examined. Girolami et al. (2007) found that compared to using a spoon to re-present the expelled bite, an NUK® brush re-presentation reduced expulsion, and utilizing an NUK® brush for both the initial presentation and subsequent re-presentations even further reduced expulsion. In addition to the NUK® brush, using a flipped spoon for initial presentations and re-presentations has also been shown to reduce expulsion (Sharp et al. 2010a; Sharp et al. 2012). To decrease expulsion due to absence of mouth closure (e.g., passive refusal), Wilkins et al. (2011) utilized a chin prompt (applying gentle upward pressure to the upper lip using the thumb and to the chin using the forefinger). Antecedent manipulations such as decreasing texture have also been shown to reduce expulsion (Patel et al. 2002a).

Packing Various treatment methods have been evaluated to target packing and increase swallowing. Redistribution involves collecting packed food from the mouth and placing it on the tongue until consumption occurs. Redistribution has been implemented with an NUK® brush (Gulotta et al. 2005; Sevin et al. 2002) and a flipped spoon (Volkert et al. 2011). Flipped spoon presentations and re-presentations have been demonstrated to increase mouth cleans (Rivas et al. 2011; Sharp et al. 2010a; Sharp et al. 2012). Swallow facilitation (or induction) has also been utilized to target packing, and involves placing food on the posterior of the child's tongue (e.g., Hoch et al. 1995). Dempsey et al. (2011) found that adding a chin prompt to a flipped spoon presentation and re-presentation increased mouth cleans for honey consistency liquids, although a chin support alone did not. Vaz et al. (2012) demonstrated the effectiveness of utilizing a chaser (presenting, either immediately or 15 s post acceptance, a solid or liquid that the child consistently accepted and swallowed) to reduce packing.

Antecedent manipulations such as decreasing texture, blending, and simultaneous presentation have also been used for packing to increase swallowing. Patel et al. (2005) demonstrated that reducing texture reduced packing, and increased gram consumption and weight. Kadey et al. (2013a) also found that mouth cleans were higher for lower textures, and that for specific foods (e.g., chicken nuggets, green beans, asparagus, grilled chicken, and broccoli and cheese), mouth cleans were lower compared to other specific foods at the same pureed texture. Mueller et al. (2004) gradually blended nonpreferred foods into preferred foods to increase mouth cleans. Buckley and Newchok (2005) found that simultaneous presentation (placing a highly preferred ground chocolate cookie on the spoon behind the target food) decreased packing.

Specific Procedural/Behavioral Interventions for Chewing

Developmentally typical chewing patterns do not emerge naturally for children with feeding difficulties (Kadey et al. 2013a; Patel et al. 2005; Patel et al. 2002b; Sheppard 2008). Unlike typical eaters, these children do not chew when presented with food; instead, they often expel (i.e., spit out the bite), pocket, or pack the food in their cheek, swallow the bite prematurely, mash the food on their palate, or demonstrate an immature munching pattern that is not conducive to functional chewing. In order for chewing to be functional, the individual must not only be able to chew the food, but also chew the food sufficiently so that it can be safely swallowed. Some of these issues may be the result of inexperience or insufficient practice with regular textured foods, or a preference for lower texture foods over higher textures. And for others, difficulty chewing may be the result of structural or anatomical differences such as tongue thrusting, which is often observed in children with Down syndrome (Frazier and Friedman 1996; Gisel et al. 1984). Prevalence estimates of chewing difficulties are relatively high among children with feeding problems. Krom et al. (2013) described a sample of 33 children seen in an outpatient feeding program in which 50% of the children had inadequate chewing skills. Likewise, Field et al. (2003), in a sample of 350 children referred to their feeding program, reported that

26% consumed inappropriate food textures (i.e., only lower textured food) and many did not exhibit any chewing.

Overall, there is limited empirical evidence in the literature for treatments to advance texture and chewing in the developmentally delayed population (Sheppard 2008). This is likely due to a number of difficulties related to this type of research. One challenge is that there is no agreed upon operational definition for chewing. Previous studies have either failed to define or used inconsistent definitions; thus, it is difficult to draw any conclusions from the current literature base (Volkert et al. 2013). A second obstacle in this type of research is obtaining a product measure of functional chewing. A recent study has incorporated a measure of *mastication,* which was defined as food with pieces no larger than 0.2 x 0.2 cm in a liquid medium after chewing (Volkert et al. 2013). Further, obtaining adequate interobserver agreement with the use of observational (duration or frequency) measures of chewing/mastication may be a challenge when patients present with atypical/idiosyncratic chewing patterns, a closed-mouth chew, or swallow bites prior to checks for mastication. Despite the aforementioned challenges, there are some treatment studies to guide future improvements in the literature. Existing treatment studies that focus on advancing texture and/or chewing in those with feeding difficulties can be divided into two main strategic approaches: texture fading and chewing skills training.

Texture Fading Luiselli and Gleason (1987) and Shore et al. (1998) used stimulus fading in which food acceptance remained high as the food texture was gradually increased to the point of age-appropriate textures. Shore et al. (1998) advanced four children with food refusal/selectivity to the target texture (identified by an occupational therapist) with a treatment package involving texture fading, reinforcement contingent upon acceptance and swallowing, and EE for IMB and expulsion. The authors posited that an advantage of this approach is that higher amounts of gagging and an increased risk of aspiration during the meals may have been avoided compared to an approach where the target texture would be presented from the outset. These authors acknowledged that studies are needed to determine when or if chewing skill training is needed to advance textures.

Sheppard (2008) reported a case in which the child was trained to bite off small pieces of a crisp, soft-to-munch, moist cracker (e.g., graham cracker), which was placed on his preferred side for chewing. Subsequently, the foods presented progressed from soft pieces (e.g., banana, soft fish, soft meats, cooked carrots), mixed textures, and finally, firm and fibrous foods (e.g., raisins, pretzel rods, and firm meats). While other studies have since demonstrated the effectiveness of manipulating texture gradually (Eckman et al. 2007), clinically there are times when professionals question this approach. While this technique may be effective in increasing acceptance of higher textured foods (compliance), it may not actually teach chewing. For those whom chewing skills do not emerge through experience with the progressively higher textures, this may result in some children swallowing foods whole without sufficient mastication, putting them at an increased risk for choking or aspiration.

Chewing Skills Training Of the few treatment studies available related to teaching chewing, the majority do not show a clear demonstration of experimental control to determine what treatment components are responsible for the increase in chewing. In addition, many of the studies available are conducted with children who have demonstrated some chewing skills prior to the intervention (Shore et al. 1999; Volkert et al. 2013). The following techniques have been combined in treatment packages for chewing skills training.

Modeling and Reinforcement Butterfield and Parson (1973) described a treatment to increase chewing for a moderately delayed individual with no prior evidence of chewing which involved removal of attention following the absence of chewing, repeated modeling and reinforcement (e.g., a caregiver demonstrated chewing a cracker resulting in an audible "crunch," following the "crunch" he/she was provided a preferred food of the participant), and praise and preferred edible following successful approximation of chewing (i.e., shaping). This treatment was effective in teaching the child to chew saltine crackers, OREO® cookies, graham crackers, cake, eggs, and meat.

Descriptive Prompting and Differential Reinforcement Shore et al. (1999) developed a treatment to increase safe eating in a 14-year-old who had developmental delays, reflux, and esophageal stricture (i.e., a narrowing of the esophagus). A treatment package including prompting, response blocking (of large bites and bite rate >30 s), and reinforcement of a 30 s bite rate, small bite size, and a prespecified number of chews per bite was found to be effective in increasing his safety during self-feeding of chopped and regular texture food. Similarly, Volkert et al. (2013) systematically demonstrated that descriptive verbal prompts and praise were responsible for increases in chewing and mastication for a 14-year-old male with developmental delays who had some evidence of chewing prior to treatment.

Negative Reinforcement Kadey et al. (2013c) increased a 6-year-old boy's compliance with chewing and swallowing. The child reportedly possessed the necessary oral motor skills to chew, sufficiently masticate, and safely swallow table foods, but refused to do so. The initial treatment involved differential reinforcement in the form of delivery of a preferred edible and activity for chewing and swallowing bites. Following low levels of compliance under the initial condition, a rule was added that following noncompliance, a physical prompt to chew would be provided. This resulted in increased compliance with chewing; however, swallowing did not occur. Thus, a rule was added that following noncompliance to swallow a physical prompt to swallow would be implemented. This prompt involved moving an NUK® brush along the midline of the tongue. The implementation of the rule resulted in increased swallowing and further increases in chewing. These components were subsequently removed from the treatment while high levels of chewing and swallowing maintained. It was speculated that the physical prompts to chew and swallow functioned as aversive stimuli (i.e., negative reinforcement).

Molar Placement, Lip Closure, and Tongue Lateralization Prior research by Gisel (1994), Gisel and Alphonce (1995), and Gisel et al. (1996) noted increases in chewing following teaching the skills of tongue lateralization (e.g., moving tongue side-to-side), lip control (i.e., lip closure around a straw/cup), and vigor of chewing (achieved with a molar placement). With these findings, Eckman et al. (2007) increased chewing in two children with delays and no previous chewing skills utilizing a multicomponent treatment package involving a molar placement, reinforcement in the form of praise and a preferred tangible for biting/chewing and swallowing, and EE (in the form of nonremoval of the bite). Concurrently, other sessions in which larger volumes of lower textured foods were presented, these children also practiced tongue lateralization and lip control. Thus, it is not clear which components were necessary to increase chewing skills in these children.

Overall, there is much work to be done to better isolate the treatment variables that are necessary for advancing texture and chewing skills in children with feeding difficulties. It remains unclear what approach, texture fading, or chewing skills training, is most effective and for whom. Further work in this area would improve the efficiency and effectiveness of treatments to achieve more developmentally and age-appropriate eating.

Caregiver Training

A key test to any behavioral intervention is the extent to which behavior change generalizes beyond the hospital/clinic setting with the treating therapist to the natural environment with the caregivers (Mueller et al. 2003; Stokes and Baer 1977; Werle et al. 1993). To accomplish this goal, it is necessary to program for generalization by training those caregivers who will maintain the progress in the home/community setting over time. McCartney et al. (2005) noted that for this programming to occur, it is necessary to evaluate the efficacy of such training programs, the degree to which caregivers are able to adhere to the intervention (i.e., treatment integrity), and also the extent to which caregivers report satisfaction and a willingness to use the intervention (i.e., social validity).

Individual Caregiver Training

Werle et al. (1993) examined the effectiveness of a treatment involving basic nutrition education, contingent attention, rewards, and planned ignoring (for two participants a brief time-out was also used) that was implemented by caregivers in the home environment. Treatment sessions incorporated a period of 20–30 min to discuss the techniques with the caregiver, a meal observation, and then a brief discussion regarding the caregiver's implementation and the child's response to the treatment. Specific training methods included instruction, discussion, handouts, role-play, behavioral rehearsal during mealtimes, verbal feedback, and periodic videotape review. The results demonstrated that home-based behavioral training resulted in systematic changes in caregiver and child responding during meals. Anderson and McMillan (2001) also provided in-home training to caregivers of a child with feeding problems. Caregiver training methods included verbal and written instructions, modeling, videotape review, and performance feedback during and after feeding sessions. Following several sessions and a gradual introduction of nonpreferred foods, the caregivers fed with high levels of integrity. McCartney et al. (2005) evaluated a systematic procedure in training caregivers to implement a commonly used treatment component, EE in the form of nonremoval of the spoon (Hoch et al. 1994). Caregivers watched videos of therapist-fed meals, participated in video review, and observed meals through a one-way mirror and within the feeding room. Initial caregiver-fed meals consisted of one bite. The number of bites was increased systematically as latency to accept bites and refusal remained low. Levels of integrity during treatment implementation were high for caregivers feeding in the clinic, home setting, and at follow-up.

Najdowski et al. (2010) evaluated the effectiveness of training parents to implement a treatment for food selectivity within the home setting. Investigators were present in the home only twice per week and caregivers video recorded one meal per week (for evaluating procedural integrity and accuracy of data collection). Similar to McCartney et al. (2005), the number of nonpreferred bites presented was increased gradually across meals. Caregivers were involved with data collection, implementation of the procedures, and conducting generalization probes with nonpreferred foods that were not previously exposed to the treatment. Training components involved data collection procedures (demonstrating high levels of IOA with therapists), written and verbal instructions, modeling, role-play, and in-vivo coaching while the caregivers implemented the treatment with the child in the home setting. The results indicated that the caregivers' implementation of the treatment was effective in increasing their child's consumption of nonpreferred foods and decreasing IMB in the home setting with relatively little time spent in training and with supervision.

Caregiver training for individual feeding interventions has been demonstrated to be effective in both clinic and home settings (Anderson and McMillan 2001; Najdowski et al. 2010; Werle et al. 1999), with varying levels of supervision and durations of training (Najdowski et al. 2010) and to have high social validity and high levels of caregiver acceptability (Binnendyk and Lucyshyn 2009; McCartney et al. 2005; Najdowski et al. 2010; Pangborn et al. 2013). However, as these previous studies utilized multicomponent training packages, it is not clear what component(s) of the training package were responsible for the change in the caregiver responses during meals.

In order to examine and increase the efficiency of training packages for feeding interventions, Mueller et al. (2003) examined the effectiveness of a training package involving verbal instructions, role-modeling, and rehearsal (written instructions were provided under baseline conditions). Following the implementation of this training package, two caregivers demonstrated consistently high levels of treatment integrity. For the third caregiver, post-session feedback was required prior to achieving high levels of treatment integrity. In a second study, these authors examined the components separately (i.e., verbal instruction + modeling, verbal instruction + rehearsal, and verbal instruction only) to determine the necessary training components. Consistently low levels of treatment integrity were observed when caregivers were provided written instructions only (i.e., baseline condition). Verbal instructions + modeling and verbal instructions + rehearsal were sufficient to lead to high levels of treatment integrity. Verbal instruction, when delivered only once, was insufficient. However, when verbal instruction was delivered a second time, caregivers implemented the treatment with high levels of integrity (above 90 %). Based on these results, the authors suggested all training components are not necessary; however, reiteration of the information may be an important factor during the training process.

To extend the work of Mueller et al. (2003), Pangborn et al. (2013) applied a multicomponent training package in a sequential manner to evaluate levels of caregivers' correct implementation of a feeding protocol following each step of training. Training phases included observation, written and verbal protocol review (including a brief quiz), video review, structured observation (i.e., in-room observation of therapist-fed meal with caregiver data collection), modeling, role-play, and immediate feedback. Following the completion of each training component, caregiver-fed probe meals were conducted in which caregivers were asked to feed a meal using the training procedures reviewed immediately prior to the session. If the caregivers' implementation during the probe meal did not meet training criteria (i.e., less than 80 % integrity, less than 95 % total consumption, or IMB > 0.5 rpm), verbal feedback was provided that was consistent with the appropriate training step, and a second probe meal was conducted. If during the second probe meal performance failed to meet training criteria, the next training phase was conducted. Results demonstrated that caregivers could be taught to successfully implement feeding interventions by training successive components and thus, training steps could be individualized to meet the needs of the individual caregiver. None of the caregivers required all seven phases, yet there were individual differences regarding the number of phases that were required to meet training criteria. The authors suggest sequential application of the training phases may be a more time-and resource-efficient training delivery method.

Caregiver Group Interventions

Caregiver group interventions have been shown to have some beneficial effects with nonclinical feeding difficulties (e.g., picky eating, fussy eaters, mealtime behavioral difficulties) in typically developing, healthy children (Adamson et al. 2013; Morawska et al. 2014). Similar caregiver group-based approaches to intervention have been investigated with children with clinically significant feeding difficulties (Jones and Bryant-Waugh 2012) and those with autism and food selectivity (Sharp et al. 2013a). Jones and Bryant-Waugh (2012) conducted a preliminary evaluation of a skills-and-support group intervention for mothers of children with feeding problems whose children were receiving services in the Feeding and Eating Disorder Service in a tertiary referral hospital. The content of the group covered seven themes including "food preparation and provision," "mealtime interactions," "identity, parental expectations and support," "impact on the general parent-child relationship," "concerns about the future," "stress," and "need for control." Overall, results of the study showed little change on measures of caregivers' mood and stress; however, there were some changes in caregiver ratings of the severity and number of child feeding problems.

Similarly, with an effort to develop an economical alternative with the potential for replication and rapid treatment dissemination, Sharp et al. (2013a) conducted a preliminary examination of a group-based caregiver training targeted for caregivers of children with ASD and food selectivity. The Autism MEAL Plan is a curriculum specifically developed to assist caregivers to Manage Eating Aversions and Low intake among children with ASD. The intervention consisted of eight, 1-h, didactic caregiver training sessions covering general behavior management strategies applied during meals (e.g., routine and consistency, positive attending), specific interventions for feeding problems associated with ASD (e.g., extinction and stimulus fading), and strategies for promoting self-feeding (e.g., graduated prompting and backward chaining). Other concepts emphasized throughout the sessions were the gradual process of behavior change, importance of monitoring behavior (e.g., antecedent-behavior-consequence charts and data sheets), the use of operational definitions, using the child's behavior to guide the course of treatment through the use of decision rules, and the possibilities for an increase in problem behavior following the introduction of treatment (i.e., an extinction burst). Caregivers were encouraged to individualize the recommendations during homework assignments following each session. Questions and feedback regarding the assignments were reviewed at the start of the next session. The training did not include direct observation of the feeding sessions of caregiver–child dyads. Overall, following completion of the group, caregivers reported a significant reduction in caregiver stress as measured by the *Parenting-Stress Index-Short Form* (Abidin 1995) and reported overall high levels of satisfaction with the program. However, no significant change was observed in feeding behaviors as captured by the *Brief Autism Mealtime Behavior Inventory* (Lukens and Linscheid 2008) or dietary variety as measured by the *Food Preference Inventory* (Sharp et al. 2013b) selectivity score. The authors suggested that future variations of the treatment will likely include live observations of meals that will allow for coaching, modeling, and role plays that have been found to be effective in other individualized training programs (Kaminski et al. 2008; Mueller et al. 2003), and incorporation of measures of procedural fidelity (Najdowski et al. 2010).

Caregiver Training Conclusions

The number of systematic investigations of feeding interventions has increased in the past decade (Sharp et al. 2010c). With the increased evaluations of feeding interventions, there has also been an increased focus on determining best practices for training caregivers who will implement these interventions in the home/community setting. To date, several individualized and a few preliminary group training programs have been evaluated for children with severe feeding difficulties. Overall, many of the individual training methods have been found to be effective in changing caregiver responses during meals and demonstrated high levels of treatment fidelity, which in turn has resulted in increased appropriate mealtime behavior in the patient. High levels of treatment fidelity have been associated with lower levels of IMB (Pangborn et al. 2013; Wilder et al. 2006). However, Mueller et al. (2003) noted that high levels of treatment integrity may not be necessary for child responding to persist in some cases. Relatively high levels of appropriate eating maintained even when treatment implementation failures occurred. Additional investigation is warranted to determine under what conditions will appropriate eating maintain when treatment fidelity is less than optimal. With the end goal of developmentally appropriate eating, caregivers and clinicians alike typically intend to gradually normalize the child's mealtime routine and discontinue the use of treatment components when they are no longer necessary. Determining when this fading of components could successfully occur and what methods could be trained so that caregivers understand how and when to do so with minimal assistance is an area for future study. The majority of studies reviewed reported high levels of caregiver satisfaction and many also noted corresponding decreases in caregiver stress and increased caregiver confidence (Adamson et al. 2013; Binnendyk and Lucyshyn 2009; McCartney et al. 2005; Najdowski et al. 2010; Pangborn et al. 2013; Sharp et al. 2013a). These findings are important given the impact that caregiver stress/confidence may have on parent–child interactions and the caregiver's ability to follow through with recommendations in the home setting (Garro et al. 2005).

General Conclusions

Pediatric feeding disorders, though not specific to children with ID/DD, are highly comorbid with such diagnoses. Children with feeding disorders may present with a variety of one or more difficulties, including problems with variety, volume, texture, proportionality of solids/liquids, self-feeding, and others. The etiology of this class of disorders often varies from child to child and may be multifaceted, with medical, developmental, and/or oral-motor concerns playing a role in the development, maintenance, and exacerbation of feeding difficulties, in addition to behavioral variables. Therefore, an interdisciplinary approach to assessment and treatment is often advised in order to provide comprehensive care. From a behavioral perspective, which was the focus of this chapter, refusal is often a primary target of assessment and treatment. Function-based treatments following a functional behavioral assessment have proven to be most effective in the treatment of refusal, with escape being identified as a maintaining variable in the majority of cases. Over the past 10 years, research on the behavioral components related to feeding disorders has significantly expanded, which has resulted in an increase in available assessments and treatments to effectively alleviate feeding difficulties in children with ID/DD, as well as in children with feeding difficulties without these diagnoses. Caregiver training has also been highlighted more in the literature, which is a key component to the success of any behavioral treatment targeting feeding problems. Overall, significant advancements have been made within the field and are expected to continue as the field continues to grow.

References

Abidin, R. R. (1995). *Parenting Stress Index (PSI) Professional Manual* (Third ed.). Lutz: Psychological Assessment Resources, Inc.

Adamson, M., Morawska, A., & Sanders, M. R. (2013). Childhood feeding difficulties: A randomized controlled trial of a group-based parenting intervention. *Journal of Developmental and Behavioral Pediatrics, 34*(5), 293–302. doi:10.1097/DBP.0b013e3182961a38.

Ahearn, W. H. (2002). Effect of two methods of introducing foods during feeding treatment on acceptance of previously rejected items. *Behavioral Interventions, 17*(3), 111–127. doi:10.1002/Bin.112.

Ahearn, W. H. (2003). Using simultaneous presentation to increase vegetable consumption in a mildly selective child with autism. *Journal of Applied Behavior Analysis, 36*(3), 361–365. doi:10.1901/jaba.2003.36-361.

Ahearn, W. H., Kerwin, M. E., Eicher, P. S., Shantz, J., & Swearingin, W. (1996). An alternating treatments comparison of two intensive interventions for food refusal. *Journal of Applied Behavior Analysis, 29*(3), 321–332. doi:10.1901/jaba.1996.29-321.

Allison, J., Wilder, D. A., Chong, I., Lugo, A., Pike, J., & Rudy, N. (2012). A comparison of differential reinforcement and noncontingent reinforcement to treat food selectivity in a child with autism. *Journal of Applied Behavior Analysis, 45*(3), 613–617. doi:10.1901/jaba.2012.45-613.

American Psychiatric Association (Ed.). (2013). *Diagnostic and statistical manual of mental disorders* (5th ed.). Arlington: American Psychiatric Publishing.

Anderson, C. M., & McMillan, K. (2001). Parental use of escape extinction and differential reinforcement to treat food selectivity. *Journal of Applied Behavior Analysis, 34*(4), 511–515. doi:10.1901/jaba.2001.34-511.

Babbitt, R. L., Hoch, T. A., Coe, D. A., Cataldo, M. F., Kelly, K. J., Stackhouse, C., & Perman, J. A. (1994). Behavioral assessment and treatment of pediatric feeding disorders. *Journal of Developmental and Behavioral Pediatrics, 15*(4), 278–291. doi:10.1097/00004703-199408000-00011.

Babbitt, R. L., Shore, B. A., Smith, M., Williams, K. E., & Coe, D. A. (2001). Stimulus fading in the treatment of adipsia. *Behavioral Interventions, 16*(3), 197–207. doi:10.1002/Bin.94.

Bachmeyer, M. H., Piazza, C. C., Fredrick, L. D., Reed, G. K., Rivas, K. D., & Kadey, H. J. (2009). Functional analysis and treatment of multiply controlled inappropriate mealtime behavior. *Journal of Applied Behavior Analysis, 42*(3), 641. doi:10.1901/jaba.2009.42-641.

Bachmeyer, M. H., Gulotta, C. S., & Piazza, C. C. (2013). Liquid to baby food fading in the treatment of food refusal. *Behavioral Interventions, 28*(4), 281–298. doi:10.1002/bin.1367.

Beautrais, A. L., Fergusson, D. M., & Shannon, F. T. (1982). Family life events and behavioral problems in preschool-aged children. *Pediatrics, 70*(5), 774–779.

Benjasuwantep, B., Chaithirayanon, S., & Eiamudomkan, M. (2013). Feeding problems in healthy young children: Prevalence, related factors and feeding practices. *Pediatric Reports, 5*(2), 38–42.

Bentovim, A. (1970). The clinical approach to feeding disorders of childhood. *Journal of Psychosomatic Research*. doi:http://dx.doi.org/10.1016/0022-3999(70)90053-X.

Berlin, K. S., Lobato, D. J., Pinkos, B., Cerezo, C. S., & LeLeiko, N. S. (2011). Patterns of medical and developmental comorbidities among children presenting with feeding problems: A latent class analysis. *Journal of Developmental and Behavioral Pediatrics, 32*(1), 41–47. doi:10.1097/DBP.0b013e318203e06d.

Binnendyk, L., & Lucyshyn, J. M. (2009). A family-centered positive behavior support approach to the amelioration of food refusal behavior an empirical case study. *Journal of Positive Behavior Interventions, 11*(1), 47–62. doi:10.1177/1098300708318965.

Borrero, C. S. W., Woods, J. N., Borrero, J. C., Masler, E. A., & Lesser, A. D. (2010). Descriptive analyses of pediatric food refusal and acceptance. *Journal of Applied Behavior Analysis, 43*(1), 71–88. doi:10.1901/jaba.2010.43-71.

Borrero, C. S. W., Schlereth, G. J., Rubio, E. K., & Taylor, T. (2013). A comparison of two physical guidance procedures in the treatment of pediatric food refusal. *Behavioral Interventions, 28*(4), 261–280. doi:10.1002/bin.1373.

Buckley, S. D., & Newchok, D. K. (2005). An evaluation of simultaneous presentation and differential reinforcement with response cost to reduce packing. *Journal of Applied Behavior Analysis, 38*(3), 405–409. doi:10.1901/jaba.2005.71-04.

Budd, K. S., McGraw, T. E., Farbisz, R., Murphy, T. B., Hawkins, D., Heilman, N., & Werle, M. (1992). Psychosocial concomitants of children's feeding disorders. *Journal of Pediatric Psychology, 17*(1), 81–94. doi:10.1093/jpepsy/17.1.81.

Bui, L. T. D., Moore, D. W., & Anderson, A. (2013). Using escape extinction and reinforcement to increase eating in a young child with autism. *Behaviour Change, 30*(1), 48–55. doi:10.1017/Bec.2013.5.

Burklow, K. A., Phelps, A. N., Schultz, J. R., McConnell, K., & Rudolph, C. (1998). Classifying complex pediatric feeding disorders. *Journal of Pediatric Gastroenterology and Nutrition, 27*(2), 143–147. doi:10.1097/00005176-199808000-00003.

Butterfield, W. H., & Parson, R. (1973). Modeling and shaping by parents to develop chewing behavior in their retarded child. *Journal of Behavior Therapy and Experimental Psychiatry, 4*(3), 285–287. doi:10.1016/0005-7916(73)90090-6.

Carruth, B. R., Ziegler, P. J., Gordon, A., & Barr, S. I. (2004). Prevalence of picky eaters among infants and toddlers and their caregivers' decisions about offering a new food. *Journal of the American Dietetic Association, 104* (Supplement 1), 57–64. doi:http://dx.doi.org/10.1016/j.jada.2003.10.024

Casey, S. D., Cooper-Brown, L. J., Wacker, D. P., & Rankin, B. E. (2006). The use of descriptive analysis to identify and manipulate schedules of reinforcement in the treatment of food refusal. *Journal of Behavioral Education, 15*(1), 39–50. doi:10.1007/s10864-005-9001-7.

Casey, S. D., Perrin, C. J., Lesser, A. D., Perrin, S. H., Casey, C. L., & Reed, G. K. (2009). Using descriptive assessment in the treatment of bite acceptance and food refusal. *Behavior Modification, 33*(5), 537–558. doi:10.1177/0145445509341457.

Coe, D. A., Babbitt, R. L., Williams, K. E., Hajimihalis, C., Snyder, A. M., Ballard, C., & Efron, L. A. (1997). Use of extinction and reinforcement to increase food consumption and reduce expulsion. *Journal of Applied Behavior Analysis, 30*(3), 581–583. doi:10.1901/jaba.1997.30-581.

Dawson, J. E., Piazza, C. C., Sevin, B. M., Gulotta, C. S., Lerman, D., & Kelley, M. L. (2003). Use of the high-probability instructional sequence and escape extinction in a child with food refusal. *Journal of Applied Behavior Analysis, 36*(1), 105–108. doi:10.1901/jaba.2003.36-105.

de Moor, J., Didden, R., & Korzilius, H. (2007). Behavioural treatment of severe food refusal in five toddlers with developmental disabilities. *Child: Care, Health and Development, 33*(6), 670–676. doi:10.1111/j.1365-2214.2007.00734.x.

Dempsey, J., Piazza, C. C., Groff, R. A., & Kozisek, J. M. (2011). A flipped spoon and chin prompt to increase mouth clean. *Journal of Applied Behavior Analysis, 44*(4), 961–965. doi:10.1901/jaba.2011.44-961.

Eckman, N., Williams, K. E., Riegel, K., & Paul, C. (2007). Teaching chewing: A structured approach. *The American Journal of Occupational Therapy: Official Publication of the American Occupational Therapy Association, 62*(5), 514–521. doi:10.5014/ajot.62.5.514.

Farrell, D. A., Hagopian, L. P., & Kurtz, P. F. (2001). A hospital-and home-based behavioral intervention for a child with chronic food refusal and gastrostomy tube dependence. *Journal of Developmental and Physical Disabilities, 13*(4), 407–418. doi:10.1023/A:1012241630667.

Field, D., Garland, M., & Williams, K. (2003). Correlates of specific childhood feeding problems. *Journal of Paediatrics and Child Health, 39*(4), 299–304. doi:10.1046/j.1440-1754.2003.00151.x.

Fisher, W., Piazza, C. C., Bowman, L. G., Hagopian, L., Owens, J., & Slevin, I. (1992). A comparison of two approaches for identifying reinforcers for persons with severe and profound disabilities. *Journal of Applied Behavior Analysis, 25*(2), 491. doi:10.1901/jaba.1992.25-491.

Forsyth, B. C., Leventhal, J. M., & McCarthy, P. L. (1985). Mothers' perceptions of problems of feeding and crying behaviors: A prospective study. *American Journal of Diseases of Children, 139*(3), 269–272. doi:10.1001/archpedi.1985.02140050063023.

Frazier, J. B., & Friedman, B. (1996). Swallow function in children with Down syndrome: A retrospective study. *Developmental Medicine and Child Neurology, 38*(8), 695–703. doi:10.1111/j.1469-8749.1996.tb12139.x.

Freeman, K. A., & Piazza, C. C. (1998). Combining stimulus fading, reinforcement, and extinction to treat food refusal. *Journal of Applied Behavior Analysis, 31*(4), 691–694. doi:10.1901/jaba.1998.31-691.

Gal, E., Hardal-Nasser, R., & Engel-Yeger, B. (2011). The relationship between the severity of eating problems and intellectual developmental deficit level. *Research in Developmental Disabilities, 32*(5), 1464–1469. doi:10.1016/j.ridd.2010.12.003.

Garro, A., Thurman, S. K., Kerwin, M. E., & Ducette, J. P. (2005). Parent/caregiver stress during pediatric hospitalization for chronic feeding problems. *Journal of Pediatric Nursing, 20*(4), 268–275. doi:10.1016/j.pedn.2005.02.015.

Girolami, P. A., & Scotti, J. R. (2001). Use of analog functional analysis in assessing the function of mealtime behavior problems. *Education and Training in Mental Retardation and Developmental Disabilities, 36*(2), 207–223.

Girolami, P. A., Boscoe, J. H., & Roscoe, N. (2007). Decreasing expulsions by a child with a feeding disorder: Using a brush to present and re-present food. *Journal of Applied Behavior Analysis, 40*(4), 749–753. doi:10.1901/jaba.2007.749.

Gisel, E. G. (1994). Oral-motor skills following sensorimotor intervention in the moderately eating-impaired child with cerebral palsy. *Dysphagia, 9*(3), 180–192. doi:10.1007/BF00341263.

Gisel, E. G., & Alphonce, E. (1995). Classification of eating impairments based on eating efficiency in children with cerebral palsy. *Dysphagia, 10*(4), 268–274. doi:10.1007/BF00431421.

Gisel, E. G., Lange, L. J., & Niman, C. W. (1984). Chewing cycles in 4-and 5-year-old Down's syndrome children: A comparison of eating efficacy with normals. *The American Journal of Occupational Therapy, 38*(10), 666–670. doi:10.5014/ajot.38.10.666.

Gisel, E. G., Applegate-Ferrante, T., Benson, J., & Bosma, J. F. (1996). Oral-motor skills following sensorimotor therapy in two groups of moderately dysphagic children with cerebral palsy: Aspiration vs nonaspiration. *Dysphagia, 11*(1), 59–71. doi:10.1007/BF00385801.

González, M. L., Rubio, E. K., & Taylor, T. (2014). Inappropriate mealtime behavior: The effects of noncontingent access to preferred tangibles on responding in functional analyses. *Research in Developmental Disabilities, 35*(12), 3655–3664. doi:10.1016/j.ridd.2014.08.016

Groff, R. A., Piazza, C. C., Zeleny, J. R., & Dempsey, J. R. (2011). Spoon-to-cup fading as treatment for cup drinking in a child with intestinal failure. *Journal of Applied Behavior Analysis, 44*(4), 949–954. doi:10.1901/jaba.2011.44-949.

Gulotta, C. S. (2012). Pediatric tube dependency: Outcomes of an intensive interdisciplinary feeding program. Unpublished manuscript.

Gulotta, C. S., Piazza, C. C., Patel, M. R., & Layer, S. A. (2005). Using food redistribution to reduce packing in children with severe food refusal. *Journal of Applied Behavior Analysis, 38*(1), 39–50. doi:10.1901/jaba.2005.168-03.

Hagopian, L. P., Farrell, D. A., & Amari, A. (1996). Treating total liquid refusal with backward chaining and fading. *Journal of Applied Behavior Analysis, 29*(4), 573–575. doi:10.1901/jaba.1996.29-573.

Hawdon, J., Beauregard, N., Slattery, J., & Kennedy, G. (2000). Identification of neonates at risk of developing feeding problems in infancy. *Developmental Medicine and Child Neurology, 42*(4), 235–239. doi:10.1111/j.1469-8749.2000.tb00078.x.

Hoch, T. A., Babbitt, R. L., Coe, D. A., Krell, D. M., & Hackbert, L. (1994). Contingency contacting: Combining positive reinforcement and escape extinction procedures to treat persistent food refusal. *Behavior Modification, 18*(1), 106–128.

Hoch, T. A., Babbitt, R. L., Coe, D. A., Ducan, A., & Trusty, E. M. (1995). A swallow induction avoidance procedure to establish eating. *Journal of Behavior Therapy and Experimental Psychiatry, 26*(1), 41–50. doi:10.1016/0005-7916(94)00067-V.

Iwata, B. A., Dorsey, M. F., Slifer, K. J., Bauman, K. E., & Richman, G. S. (1982/1994). Toward a functional analysis of self-injury. *Journal of Applied Behavior Analysis, 27*(2), 197–209. doi:10.1901/jaba.1994.27-197.

Johnson, C. R., & Babbitt, R. L. (1993). Antecedent manipulation in the treatment of primary solid food refusal. *Behavior Modification, 17*(4), 510–521. doi:10.1177/01454455930174006.

Johnson, C. R., Turner, K., Stewart, P. A., Schmidt, B., Shui, A., Macklin, E., Reynolds, A., James, J., Johnson, S. L., Courtney, P. M., & Hyman, S. L. (2014). Relationships between feeding problems, behavioral characteristics and nutritional quality in children with ASD. *Journal of Autism and Developmental Disorders,* 1–10. doi:10.1007/s10803-014-2095-9

Jones, C., & Bryant-Waugh, R. (2012). Development and pilot of a group skills-and-support intervention for mothers of children with feeding problems. *Appetite, 58*(2), 450–456. doi:10.1016/j.appet.2011.12.017.

Kadey, H. J., Piazza, C. C., Rivas, K. M., & Zeleny, J. (2013a). An evaluation of texture manipulations to increase swallowing. *Journal of Applied Behavior Analysis, 46*(2), 539–543. doi:10.1002/jaba.33.

Kadey, H. J., Roane, H. S., Diaz, J. C., & McCarthy, C. M. (2013b). Using a Nuk® brush to increase acceptance of solids and liquids for two children diagnosed with autism. *Research in Autism Spectrum Disorders, 7*(11), 1461–1480. doi:10.1016/j.rasd.2013.07.017.

Kadey, H. J., Roane, H. S., Diaz, J. C., & Merrow, J. M. (2013c). An evaluation of chewing and swallowing for a child diagnosed with autism. *Journal of Developmental and Physical Disabilities, 25*(3), 343–354. doi:10.1007/s10882-012-9313-1.

Kahng, S., Tarbox, J., & Wilke, A. E. (2001). Use of a multicomponent treatment for food refusal. *Journal of Applied Behavior Analysis, 34*(1), 93–96. doi:10.1901/jaba.2001.34-93.

Kaminski, J. W., Valle, L. A., Filene, J. H., & Boyle, C. L. (2008). A meta-analytic review of components associated with parent training program effectiveness. *Journal of Abnormal Child Psychology, 36*(4), 567–589. doi:10.1007/s10802-007-9201-9.

Kelley, M. E., Piazza, C. C., Fisher, W. W., & Oberdorff, A. J. (2003). Acquisition of cup drinking using previously refused foods as positive and negative reinforcement. *Journal of Applied Behavior Analysis, 36*(1), 89–93. doi:10.1901/jaba.2003.36-89.

Kern, L., & Marder, T. J. (1996). A comparison of simultaneous and delayed reinforcement as treatments for food selectivity. *Journal of Applied Behavior Analysis, 29*(2), 243–246. doi:10.1901/jaba.1996.29-243.

Kerwin, M. E., Ahearn, W. H., Eicher, P. S., & Burd, D. M. (1995). The costs of eating: A behavioral economic analysis of food refusal. *Journal of Applied Behavior Analysis, 28*(3), 245–260. doi:10.1901/jaba.1995.28-245.

Knox, M., Rue, H. C., Wildenger, L., Lamb, K., & Luiselli, J. K. (2012). Intervention for food selectivity in a specialized school setting: Teacher implemented prompting, reinforcement, and demand fading for an adolescent student with autism. *Education & Treatment of Children, 35*(3), 407–417.

Koegel, R. L., Bharoocha, A. A., Ribnick, C. B., Ribnick, R. C., Bucio, M. O., Fredeen, R. M., & Koegel, L. K. (2012). Using individualized reinforcers and hierarchical exposure to increase food flexibility in children with autism spectrum disorders. *Journal of Autism and Developmental Disorders, 42*(8), 1574–1581. doi:10.1007/s10803-011-1392-9.

Kozlowski, A. M., Matson, J. L., Fodstad, J. C., & Moree, B. N. (2011). Feeding therapy in a child with autistic disorder: Sequential food presentation. *Clinical Case Studies, 10*(3), 236–246. doi:10.1177/1534650111405189.

Krom, H., Otten, M.-A. G., van der Sluijs Veer, L., van Zundert, S. M., Khawaja, F. K., Benninga, M. A., & Kindermann, A. (2013). Multidisciplinary approach in young children with severe

feeding disorders. *Tijdschrift Voor Kindergeneeskunde, 81*(1), 72–72. doi:10.1007/s12456-013-0070-6.
LaRue, R. H., Stewart, V., Piazza, C. C., Volkert, V. M., Patel, M. R., & Zeleny, J. (2011). Escape as reinforcement and escape extinction in the treatment of feeding problems. *Journal of Applied Behavior Analysis, 44*(4), 719–735. doi:10.1901/jaba.2011.44-719.
Ledford, J. R., & Gast, D. L. (2006). Feeding problems in children with autism spectrum disorders a review. *Focus on Autism and Other Developmental Disabilities, 21*(3), 153–166. doi:10.1177/10883576060210030401.
Lefton-Greif, M. A. (2008). Pediatric dysphagia. *Physical Medicine and Rehabilitation Clinics of North America, 19*(4), 837–851. doi:10.1016/j.pmr.2008.05.007.
Levin, L., & Carr, E. G. (2001). Food selectivity and problem behavior in children with developmental disabilities analysis and intervention. *Behavior Modification, 25*(3), 443–470. doi:10.1177/0145445501253004.
Luiselli, J. K. (1991). Acquisition of self-feeding in a child with Lowe's syndrome. *Journal of Developmental and Physical Disabilities, 3*(2), 181–189. doi:10.1007/bf01045932.
Luiselli, J. K. (1993). Training self-feeding skills in children who are deaf and blind. *Behavior Modification, 17*(4), 457–473. doi:10.1177/01454455002430003.
Luiselli, J. K. (2000). Cueing, demand fading, and positive reinforcement to establish self-feeding and oral consumption in a child with chronic food refusal. *Behavior Modification, 24*(3), 348–358. doi:10.1177/0145445500243003.
Luiselli, J. K., & Gleason, D. J. (1987). Combining sensory reinforcement and texture fading procedures to overcome chronic food refusal. *Journal of Behavior Therapy and Experimental Psychiatry, 18*(2), 149–155. doi:10.1016/0005-7916(87)90029-2.
Lukens, C. T., & Linscheid, T. R. (2008). Development and validation of an inventory to assess mealtime behavior problems in children with autism. *Journal of Autism and Developmental Disorders, 38*(2), 342–352. doi:10.1007/s10803-007-0401-5.
Mace, F. C., Hock, M. L., Lalli, J. S., West, B. J., Belfiore, P., Pinter, E., & Brown, D. K. (1988). Behavioral momentum in the treatment of noncompliance. *Journal of Applied Behavior Analysis, 21*(2), 123–141. doi:10.1901/jaba.1988.21-123.
Mascola, A. J., Bryson, S. W., & Agras, W. S. (2010). Picky eating during childhood: A longitudinal study to age 11 years. *Eating Behaviors, 11*(4), 253–257. doi:10.1016/j.eatbeh.2010.05.006.
Mason, S. J., Harris, G., & Blissett, J. (2005). Tube feeding in infancy: Implications for the development of normal eating and drinking skills. *Dysphagia, 20*(1), 46–61. doi:10.1007/s00455-004-0025-2.
Matson, J. L., & Kuhn, D. E. (2001). Identifying feeding problems in mentally retarded persons: Development and reliability of the Screening Tool of Feeding Problems (STEP). *Research in Developmental Disabilities*. doi:http://dx.doi.org/10.1016/S0891-4222(01)00065-8.
Matson, J. L., Fodstad, J. C., & Boisjoli, J. A. (2008). Cutoff scores, norms and patterns of feeding problems for the Screening Tool of Feeding Problems (STEP) for adults with intellectual disabilities. *Research in Developmental Disabilities, 29*(4), 363–372. doi:10.1016/j.ridd.2007.06.001.
McCartney, E. J., Anderson, C. M., English, C. L., & Horner, R. H. (2005). Effect of brief clinic-based training on the ability of caregivers to implement escape extinction. *Journal of Positive Behavior Interventions, 7*(1), 18–32. doi:10.1177/10983007050070010301.
McComas, J. J., Wacker, D. P., Cooper, L. J., Peck, S., Golonka, Z., Millard, T., & Richman, D. (2000). Effects of the high-probability request procedure: Patterns of responding to low-probability requests. *Journal of Developmental and Physical Disabilities, 12*(2), 157–171. doi:10.1023/A:1009411706876.
Morawska, A., Adamson, M., Hinchliffe, K., & Adams, T. (2014). Hassle Free Mealtimes Triple P: A randomised controlled trial of a brief parenting group for childhood mealtime difficulties *Behaviour Research and Therapy, 53*, 1–9. doi:10.1016/j.brat.2013.11.007.
Mueller, M. M., Piazza, C. C., Moore, J. W., Kelley, M. E., Bethke, S. A., Pruett, A. E., Oberdorff, A. J. & Layer, S. A. (2003). Training parents to implement pediatric feeding protocols. *Journal of Applied Behavior Analysis, 36*(4), 545–562. doi:10.1901/jaba.2003.36-545.

Mueller, M. M., Piazza, C. C., Patel, M. R., Kelley, M. E., & Pruett, A. (2004). Increasing variety of foods consumed by blending nonpreferred foods into preferred foods. *Journal of Applied Behavior Analysis, 37*(2), 159–170. doi:10.1901/jaba.2004.37-159.

Munk, D. D., & Repp, A. C. (1994). Behavioral assessment of feeding problems of individuals with severe disabilities. *Journal of Applied Behavior Analysis, 27*(2), 241–250. doi:10.1901/jaba.1994.27-241.

Nadon, G., Feldman, D. E., Dunn, W., & Gisel, E. (2011). Mealtime problems in children with autism spectrum disorder and their typically developing siblings: A comparison study. *Autism: The International Journal of Research and Practice, 15*(1), 98–113. doi:10.1177/1362361309348943.

Najdowski, A. C., Wallace, M. D., Doney, J. K., & Ghezzi, P. M. (2003). Parental assessment and treatment of food selectivity in natural settings. *Journal of Applied Behavior Analysis, 36*(3), 383–386. doi:10.1901/jaba.2003.36-383.

Najdowski, A. C., Wallace, M. D., Penrod, B., Tarbox, J., Reagon, K., & Higbee, T. S. (2008). Caregiver-conducted experimental functional analyses of inappropriate mealtime behavior. *Journal of Applied Behavior Analysis, 41*(3), 459–465. doi:10.1901/jaba.2008.41-459.

Najdowski, A. C., Wallace, M. D., Reagon, K., Penrod, B., Higbee, T. S., & Tarbox, J. (2010). Utilizing a home-based parent training approach in the treatment of food selectivity. *Behavioral Interventions, 25*(2), 89–107. doi:10.1002/bin.298.

Nicholls, D., & Bryant-Waugh, R. (2009). Eating disorders of infancy and childhood: Definition, symptomatology, epidemiology, and comorbidity. *Child and Adolescent Psychiatric Clinics of North America, 18*(1), 17–30. doi:10.1016/j.chc.2008.07.008.

Palmer, S., & Horn, S. (1978). Feeding problems in children. In S. Palmer & S. Ekvall (Eds.), *Pediatric nutrition in developmental disorders* (6th ed., pp. 107-129). Springfield: Charles C. Thomas.

Palmer, S., Thompson, R. J. Jr., & Linscheid, T. R. (1975). Applied behavior analysis in the treatment of childhood feeding problems. *Developmental Medicine and Child Neurology, 17*(3), 333–339. doi:10.1111/j.1469-8749.1975.tb04671.x.

Pangborn, M. M., Borrero, C. S., & Borrero, J. C. (2013). Sequential application of caregiver training to implement pediatric feeding protocols. *Behavioral Interventions, 28*(2), 107–130. doi:10.1002/bin.1356.

Patel, M. R., Piazza, C. C., Kelly, M. L., Ochsner, C. A., & Santana, C. M. (2001). Using a fading procedure to increase fluid consumption in a child with feeding problems. *Journal of Applied Behavior Analysis, 34*(3), 357–360. doi:10.1901/jaba.2001.34-357.

Patel, M. R., Piazza, C. C., Martinez, C. J., Volkert, V. M., & Santana, C. M. (2002a). An evaluation of two differential reinforcement procedures with escape extinction to treat food refusal. *Journal of Applied Behavior Analysis, 35*(4), 363–374. doi:10.1901/jaba.2002.35-363.

Patel, M. R., Piazza, C. C., Santana, C. M., & Volkert, V. M. (2002b). An evaluation of food type and texture in the treatment of a feeding problem. *Journal of Applied Behavior Analysis, 35*(2), 183–186. doi:10.1901/jaba.2002.35-183.

Patel, M. R., Piazza, C. C., Layer, S. A., Coleman, R., & Swartzwelder, D. M. (2005). A systematic evaluation of food textures to decrease packing and increase oral intake in children with pediatric feeding disorders. *Journal of Applied Behavior Analysis, 38*(1), 89–100. doi:10.1901/jaba.2005.161-02.

Patel, M. R., Reed, G. K., Piazza, C. C., Bachmeyer, M. H., Layer, S. A., & Pabico, R. S. (2006). An evaluation of a high-probability instructional sequence to increase acceptance of food and decrease inappropriate behavior in children with pediatric feeding disorders. *Research in Developmental Disabilities, 27*(4), 430–442. doi:10.1016/j.ridd.2005.05.005.

Patel, M. R., Reed, G. K., Piazza, C. C., Mueller, M. M., Bachmeyer, M. H., & Layer, S. A. (2007). Use of a high-probability instructional sequence to increase compliance to feeding demands in the absence of escape extinction. *Behavioral Interventions, 22*(4), 305–310. doi:10.1002/Bin.251.

Piazza, C. C., Anderson, C., & Fisher, W. (1993). Teaching self-feeding skills to patients with Rett syndrome. *Developmental Medicine and Child Neurology, 35*(11), 991–996. doi:10.1111/j.1469-8749.1993.tb11581.x.

Piazza, C. C., Patel, M. R., Santana, C. M., Goh, H. L., Delia, M. D., & Lancaster, B. M. (2002). An evaluation of simultaneous and sequential presentation of preferred and nonpreferred food to treat food selectivity. *Journal of Applied Behavior Analysis, 35*(3), 259–270. doi:10.1901/jaba.2002.35-259.

Piazza, C. C., Fisher, W. W., Brown, K. A., Shore, B. A., Patel, M. R., Katz, R. M., Blakely-Smith, A. (2003a). Functional analysis of inappropriate mealtime behaviors. *Journal of Applied Behavior Analysis, 36*(2), 187–204. doi:10.1901/jaba.2003.36-187.

Piazza, C. C., Patel, M. R., Gulotta, C. S., Sevin, B. M., & Layer, S. A. (2003b). On the relative contributions of positive reinforcement and escape extinction in the treatment of food refusal. *Journal of Applied Behavior Analysis, 36*(3), 309–324. doi:10.1901/jaba.2003.36-309.

Ramsay, M., & Birnbaum, R. (2013). Feeding difficulties in children with esophageal atresia: Treatment by a multidisciplinary team. *Diseases of the Esophagus, 26*(4), 410–412. doi:10.1111/dote.12062.

Reed, G. K., Piazza, C. C., Patel, M. R., Layer, S. A., Bachmeyer, M. H., Bethke, S. D., & Gutshall, K. A. (2004). On the relative contributions of noncontingent reinforcement and escape extinction in the treatment of food refusal. *Journal of Applied Behavior Analysis, 37*(1), 27–42. doi:10.1901/jaba.2004.37-27.

Reilly, S., Skuse, D., & Poblete, X. (1996). Prevalence of feeding problems and oral motor dysfunction in children with cerebral palsy: A community survey. *The Journal of Pediatrics, 129*(6), 877–882.

Rezaei, M., Rashedi, V., Gharib, M., & Lotfi, G. (2011). Prevalence of feeding problems in children with intellectual disability. *Iranian Rehabilitation Journal, 11*(14), 56–59.

Riordan, M. M., Iwata, B. A., Wohl, M. K., & Finney, J. W. (1980). Behavioral treatment of food refusal and selectivity in developmentally disabled children. *Applied Research in Mental Retardation, 1*(1), 95–112. doi:10.1016/0270-3092(80)90019-3.

Riordan, M. M., Iwata, B. A., Finney, J. W., Wohl, M. K., & Stanley, A. E. (1984). Behavioral assessment and treatment of chronic food refusal in handicapped children. *Journal of Applied Behavior Analysis, 17*(3), 327–341. doi:10.1901/jaba.1984.17-327.

Rivas, K. D., Piazza, C. C., Patel, M. R., & Bachmeyer, M. H. (2010). Spoon distance fading with and without escape extinction as treatment for food refusal. *Journal of Applied Behavior Analysis, 43*(4), 673–683. doi:10.1901/jaba.2010.43-673.

Rivas, K. D., Piazza, C. C., Kadey, H. J., Volkert, V. M., & Stewart, V. (2011). Sequential treatment of a feeding problem using a pacifier and flipped spoon. *Journal of Applied Behavior Analysis, 44*(2), 387–391. doi:10.1901/jaba.2011.44-387.

Rommel, N., De Meyer, A.-M., Feenstra, L., & Veereman-Wauters, G. (2003). The complexity of feeding problems in 700 infants and young children presenting to a tertiary care institution. *Journal of Pediatric Gastroenterology and Nutrition, 37*(1), 75–84. doi:10.1097/00005176-200307000-00014.

Rubio, E. K., Borrero, C. S. W., & Taylor, T. (in press). Use of a side deposit to increase consumption in children with food refusal. *Behavioral Interventions.*

Sables-Baus, S., Kaufman, J., Cook, P., & da Cruz, E. M. (2011). Oral feeding outcomes in neonates with congenital cardiac disease undergoing cardiac surgery. *Cardiology in the Young, 22*(1), 42. doi:10.1017/S1047951111000850.

Samaan, S., & Secker, D. (2014). Oral feeding challenges in infants with chronic kidney disease assessment and intervention. *ICAN: Infant, Child, & Adolescent Nutrition*, 1941406414524273. doi:10.1177/1941406414524273

Schädler, G., Süss-Burghart, H., Toschke, A. M., Von Voss, H., & Von Kries, R. (2007). Feeding disorders in ex-prematures: Causes-response to therapy-long term outcome. *European Journal of Pediatrics, 166*(8), 803–808. doi:10.1007/s00431-006-0322-x.

Schuberth, L. M., Amirault, L. M., & Case-Smith, J. (2010). Feeding intervention. In J. Case-Smith & J. O'Brien (Eds.), *Occupational therapy for children* (6th edn., pp. 446–473). St. Louis: Mosby/Elsevier.

Schwarz, S. M., Corredor, J., Fisher-Medina, J., Cohen, J., & Rabinowitz, S. (2001). Diagnosis and treatment of feeding disorders in children with developmental disabilities. *Pediatrics, 108*(3), 671–676. doi:10.1542/peds.108.3.671.

Seiverling, L., Kokitus, A., & Williams, K. (2012). A clinical demonstration of a treatment package for food selectivity. *The Behavior Analyst Today, 13*(2), 11–16.

Sevin, B. M., Gulotta, C. S., Sierp, B. J., Rosica, L. A., & Miller, L. J. (2002). Analysis of response covariation among multiple topographies of food refusal. *Journal of Applied Behavior Analysis, 35*(1), 65–68. doi:10.1901/jaba.2002.35-65.

Sharp, W. G., Harker, S., & Jaquess, D. L. (2010a). Comparison of bite-presentation methods in the treatment of food refusal. *Journal of Applied Behavior Analysis, 43*(4), 739–743. doi:10.1901/jaba.2010.43-739.

Sharp, W. G., Jaquess, D. L., Bogard, J. D., & Morton, J. F. (2010b). Additive, multi-component treatment of emerging refusal topographies in a pediatric feeding disorder. *Child & Family Behavior Therapy, 32*(1), 51–69. doi:10.1080/07317100903539931.

Sharp, W. G., Jaquess, D. L., Morton, J. F., & Herzinger, C. V. (2010c). Pediatric feeding disorders: A quantitative synthesis of treatment outcomes. *Clinical Child and Family Psychology Review, 13*(4), 348–365. doi:10.1007/s10567-010-0079-7.

Sharp, W. G., Odom, A., & Jaquess, D. L. (2012). Comparison of upright and flipped spoon presentations to guide treatment of food refusal. *Journal of Applied Behavior Analysis, 45*(1), 83–96. doi:10.1901/jaba.2012.45-83.

Sharp, W. G., Burrell, T. L., & Jaquess, D. L. (2013a). The Autism MEAL Plan: A parent-training curriculum to manage eating aversions and low intake among children with autism. *Autism: The International Journal of Research and Practice*. doi:10.1177/1362361313489190.

Sharp, W. G., Jaquess, D. L., & Lukens, C. T. (2013b). Multi-method assessment of feeding problems among children with autism spectrum disorders. *Research in Autism Spectrum Disorders, 7*(1), 56–65. doi:10.1016/j.rasd.2012.07.001.

Sheppard, J. J. (2008). Using motor learning approaches for treating swallowing and feeding disorders: A review. *Language, speech, and hearing services in schools, 39*(2), 227–236. doi:10.1044/sasd20.3.82.

Shore, B. A., Babbitt, R. L., Williams, K. E., Coe, D. A., & Snyder, A. (1998). Use of texture fading in the treatment of food selectivity. *Journal of Applied Behavior Analysis, 31*(4), 621–633. doi:10.1901/jaba.1998.31-621.

Shore, B. A., LeBlanc, D., & Simmons, J. (1999). Reduction of unsafe eating in a patient with esophageal stricture. *Journal of Applied Behavior Analysis, 32*(2), 225–228. doi:10.1901/jaba.1999.32-225.

Sisson, L., & Van Hasselt, V. (1989). Feeding disorders. In J. Luiselli (Ed.), *Behavioral medicine and developmental disabilities* (pp. 45-73). New York: Springer.

Stokes, T. F., & Baer, D. M. (1977). An implicit technology of generalization. *Journal of Applied Behavior Analysis, 10*(2), 349–367. doi:10.1901/jaba.1977.10-349.

Sullivan, P. B. (2008). Gastrointestinal disorders in children with neurodevelopmental disabilities. *Developmental Disabilities Research Reviews, 14*(2), 128–136. doi:10.1002/ddrr.18.

Sullivan, P. B., Lambert, B., Rose, M., Ford-Adams, M., Johnson, A., & Griffiths, P. (2000). Prevalence and severity of feeding and nutritional problems in children with neurological impairment: Oxford Feeding Study. *Developmental Medicine and Child Neurology, 42*(10), 674–680. doi:10.1111/j.1469-8749.2000.tb00678.x.

Tiger, J. H., & Hanley, G. P. (2006). Using reinforcer pairing and fading to increase the milk consumption of a preschool child. *Journal of Applied Behavior Analysis, 39*(3), 399–403. doi:10.1901/jaba.2006.6-06.

VanDalen, K. H., & Penrod, B. (2010). A comparison of simultaneous versus sequential presentation of novel foods in the treatment of food selectivity. *Behavioral Interventions, 25*(3), 191–206. doi:10.1002/bin.310.

Vaz, P. C. M., Volkert, V. M., & Piazza, C. C. (2011). Using negative reinforcement to increase self-feeding in a child with food selectivity. *Journal of Applied Behavior Analysis, 44*(4), 915–920. doi:10.1901/jaba.2011.44-915.

Vaz, P. C. M., Piazza, C. C., Stewart, V., Volkert, V. M., Groff, R. A., & Patel, M. R. (2012). Using a chaser to decrease packing in children with feeding disorders. *Journal of Applied Behavior Analysis, 45*(1), 97–105. doi:10.1901/jaba.2012.45-97.

Volkert, V. M., Vaz, P. C., Piazza, C. C., Frese, J., & Barnett, L. (2011). Using a flipped spoon to decrease packing in children with feeding disorders. *Journal of Applied Behavior Analysis, 44*(3), 617–621. doi:10.1901/jaba.2011.44-617.

Volkert, V. M., Piazza, C. C., Vaz, P. C. M., & Frese, J. (2013). A pilot study to increase chewing in children with feeding disorders. *Behavior Modification, 37*(3), 391–408. doi:10.1177/0145445512474295.

Werle, M. A., Murphy, T. B., & Budd, K. S. (1993). Treating chronic food refusal in young children: Home-based parent training. *Journal of Applied Behavior Analysis, 26*(4), 421–433. doi:10.1901/jaba.1993.26-421.

Werle, M. A., Murphy, T. B., & Budd, K. S. (1999). Broadening the parameters of investigation in treating young children's chronic food refusal. *Behavior therapy, 29*(1), 87–104. doi:10.1016/S0005-7894(98)80033-6.

Wilder, D. A., Normand, M., & Atwell, J. (2005). Noncontingent reinforcement as treatment for food refusal and associated self-injury. *Journal of Applied Behavior Analysis, 38*(4), 549–553. doi:10.1901/jaba.2005.132-04.

Wilder, D. A., Atwell, J., & Wine, B. (2006). The effects of varying levels of treatment integrity on child compliance during treatment with a three-step prompting procedure. *Journal of Applied Behavior Analysis, 39*(3), 369–373. doi:10.1901/jaba.2006.144-05.

Wilkins, J. W., Piazza, C. C., Groff, R. A., & Vaz, P. C. (2011). Chin prompt plus re-presentation as treatment for expulsion in children with feeding disorders. *Journal of Applied Behavior Analysis, 44*(3), 513–522. doi:10.1901/jaba.2011.44-513.

Williams, K. E., & Seiverling, L. (2010). Eating problems in children with autism spectrum disorders. *Topics in Clinical Nutrition, 25*(1), 27–37. doi:10.1097/TIN.0b013e3181d10958.

Williams, K. E., Field, D. G., & Seiverling, L. (2010). Food refusal in children: A review of the literature. *Research in Developmental Disabilities, 31*(3), 625–633.

Woods, J. N., Borrero, J. C., Laud, R. B., & Borrero, C. S. W. (2010). Descriptive analyses of pediatric food refusal: The structure of parental attention. *Behavior Modification, 34*(1), 35–56. doi:10.1177/0145445509355646.

Zangen, T., Ciarla, C., Zangen, S., Di Lorenzo, C., Flores, A. F., Cocjin, J., Reddy, S. N., Rowhani, A., Schwankovsky, L., & … Hyman, P. E. (2003). Gastrointestinal motility and sensory abnormalities may contribute to food refusal in medically fragile toddlers. *Journal of Pediatric Gastroenterology and Nutrition, 37*(3), 287–293. doi:10.1097/00005176-200309000-00016.

Chapter 6
Sleep Problems

Lynn M. Breau

Introduction

Sleep problems are very common for those with intellectual disabilities (IDs). There is evidence that they experience serious difficulties with many aspects of sleep and show bedtime behaviour problems. There is also evidence that sleep problems lead to troubles with behaviour and function for many. The majority of research has targeted children, rather than adults, and the greatest number of studies has included either heterogeneous samples of individuals, with ID due to a broad range of aetiologies, or those with an autism spectrum disorder (ASD). Most studies have been questionnaire based, utilizing the report of parents or caregivers, whereas only a few have used direct observation. Only a handful of studies have examined sleep problems longitudinally. Thus, although the literature clearly points to sleep problems being a common, chronic and distressing issue for those with ID and their families or caregivers, our knowledge is not cohesive or comprehensive, and a great deal of work remains to be done.

Sleep problems are commonly grouped into two categories. Dyssomnias include primary sleep disorders that can be due to internal factors, such as circadian rhythm abnormalities or external factors, such as inappropriate sleep-related routines. Examples include problems with sleep initiation or onset, night waking or early morning waking. Parasomnias refer to abnormal events that disrupt sleep. The parasomnias most of us have experienced at some point in time are nightmares, but teeth grinding, enuresis, sleep walking and sleep talking also fall into this category. In addition to sleep disorders, many children may display resistance to going to sleep. This often manifests as noncompliance, tantrums or oppositional behaviour. These are sometimes referred to as "settling problems". For the most part, research focused on individuals with ID has targeted these three concerns. Sleeping with a parent, also called "co-sleeping" can also be a problem. Although this may actually

L. M. Breau (✉)
Psychology Services, Glenrose Rehabilitation Hospital, Edmonton, Alberta, Canada
e-mail: lynnbreau@gmail.com

J. L. Matson, M. L. Matson (eds.), *Comorbid Conditions in Individuals with Intellectual Disabilities,* Autism and Child Psychopathology Series,
DOI 10.1007/978-3-319-15437-4_6

improve sleep onset and reduce night wakings for children, it can be disruptive for families. Sleep-related breathing disorders, such as sleep apnoea, are also common in this population and included in some research. However, because they are a complex phenomenon with various physiological aetiologies that require medical intervention, they will not be covered in detail in this chapter.

Although, much less is known about the sleep disorders of children and adults with ID than their peers in the general population, early studies with children with severe ID indicated rates of sleep problems as high as 80 % (Bartlett et al. 1985). More recent studies suggest rates from 46 % (Krakowiak et al. 2008) to close to 100 % (Wiggs and Stores 1996a; Didden et al. 2002b) in heterogeneous groups with ID. The sleep problems of those with ID are particularly problematic, in part because of their persistence (Wiggs 2001). In one longitudinal study of 200 children ages 1–18 years 'with severe ID, follow up...' 3 years later indicated that close to half still experienced problems. Thus, these sleep problems are not time-limited but appear to be protracted. They have also been linked to behaviour problems in both children (Didden et al. 2002) and adults (Matson et al. 2008). Despite this, many do not get treatment (Kronk et al. 2009; Maas et al. 2010) with one author suggesting this may be because professionals lack experience with these problems and because parents may perceive the sleep problems as unsolvable (Wiggs 2001).

This chapter will provide an overview of the literature regarding sleep problems in children and adults with ID. Research regarding heterogeneous groups will be discussed first, followed by a review of studies that have looked at groups with ID due to specific aetiologies. The factors that have been shown to relate to sleep problems will then be examined, followed by a description of the potential consequences of sleep problems in this group. The chapter will end with a review of possible treatments for sleep problems in children and adults.

Rates of Sleep Problems

Heterogeneous Groups of Children

Over 20 years of research exists that details the sleep problems of children with ID. Most studies have been based on parent report via questionnaires, although some have included direct observation or actigraphy.

Quine investigated the sleep problems of 200 children with severe ID and followed up with 166 of them 3 years later (Quine 1991). A large proportion of this group had sleep problems when first assessed, based on the semi-structured interview that was used. Although the overall prevalence of any type of sleep problem in their sample is not reported, 41 % of children had problems with settling and 45 % with night waking, whereas 1–33 % experienced at least one form of parasomnia. Only night waking and sleeping in a parent's bed decreased with age. As would be expected, both settling and night waking problems were more common in children 5 years of age and younger. An interesting finding was that 48 % of those with settling problems at Time 1 continued to have these at Time 2, and 64 % of those with night waking problems at Time 1 continued to have these at Time 2, suggesting the problems were persistent.

Shortly after, Piazza et al. used observational methods to examine the sleep problems of 51 children and adolescents age 3–21 years who had been admitted to an inpatient centre for severe behaviour problems (Piazza et al. 1996). All had a diagnosis of ID, including 2 with mild ID, 7 with moderate, 8 with severe and 34 with profound ID. Using a time-sampling procedure over an average of 22 days for each patient, observers recorded every 30 min whether the individual was awake or asleep, in bed or out of bed. The authors report that the children displayed night wakings an average of 2.6 times per week and early morning waking was shown on 30 % of days. In all, 88.2 % of the sample showed either delayed sleep onset, night waking or early waking on at least 43 % of the nights observed.

The same year, Wiggs and Stores also investigated sleep problems in children with severe ID (Wiggs and Stores 1996a). For their study, parents of 209 children attending special schools completed questionnaires. They found that all children had at least one sleep problem either most nights or every night, with 44 % indicating it was severe. In addition, 27 % of those without a current sleep problem or with an infrequent sleep problem had also had a sleep problem in the past. The authors note that the average duration of a sleep problem was 7.13 years (SD = 4.04) indicating these problems were longstanding for most of the children. Younger children in their study were more likely to have sleep problems.

In a smaller sample of 52 children, 11 with mild ID, 25 with moderate, 13 with severe and 2 with profound, Richdale et al. found that 58 % had a current sleep problem (Richdale et al. 2000). Of these children, aged 2–17 years, 59 % had had a sleep problem for 2 or more years. Among the group, 69 % had frequent night waking, and this had been a problem for 2 or more years for 53 % of these.

Didden's group studied 286 children aged 1–19 years who lived at home in the Netherlands (Didden et al. 2002b). The children were recruited through daycare centres and special schools in the Netherlands to complete questionnaires regarding their child's sleep and sleep problems. The children ranged from 1 to 19 years of age and had mild (17.4 %), moderate (40.3 %), severe (33.8 %) and profound (8.5 %) ID. Using the same questionnaire as Wiggs and Stores (Wiggs and Stores 1996a), Didden et al. found that 38.8 % of parents reported their child had settling problems and 69 % reported their child woke at night at least once per week. Overall, they found almost the identical overall rate of difficulties to Wiggs and Stores' earlier study; 99.4 % of parents reported their child had at least one problem related to going to bed or sleep.

In the most recent study located regarding children with ID, Krakowiak et al. included 63 children age 2–5 years with a developmental delay (Krakowiak et al. 2008). Overall, 46 % of parents reported their child had a sleep problem. In this group, sleep onset and settling problems were most prevalent, followed by night waking and parasomnias.

Overall, this literature is small. However, the results are sufficient to develop a preliminary sense of the pattern of problems in this population. Based on the rates reported, night waking appears to be the most common difficulty parents face. Settling and sleep onset problems follow close behind in frequency. Parasomnias and early morning waking are relatively less common. Although not an overwhelming trend, some authors have found that problems appear to be more severe in younger children. However, unlike typically developing (TD) children, sleep problems in children with ID appear to be chronic; they do not appear to "grow out" of them. Because no studies have followed children into adulthood, we do not know whether these problems continue into adulthood or remit and resurface later. However, a look at the studies that have included adults with ID suggests that, for many, they remain static.

Heterogeneous Groups of Adults

Much less research exists regarding sleep problems in adults with ID. In a 1998 study, Brylewski and Wiggs surveyed the caregivers of 205 people with ID aged 21–83, who were living in community housing (Brylewski and Wiggs 1998). They found that 26.8 % had problems preparing for sleep, such as resistance, 34.1 % were "light sleepers" and 14 % had parasomnias. Overall, fewer than 32 % of these individuals had no sleep problems, with over 38 % having 2–5 problems. The authors also report that there were few factors found that affected differences in sleep problems. However, women did have more problems preparing for bed, older residents were more likely to snore, and residents with Down syndrome were less likely to wake at night, whereas those with less ability to communicate were more likely. Enuresis was also more common in those who had a seizure disorder, were taking an antiepileptic medication or had less ability to communicate.

Harvey et al. conducted a telephone survey with the 67 caregivers of 237 adults with mild to profound ID living in group homes (Harvey et al. 2003). These individuals were 18–70 years of age. Their results indicated many had night wakings, with 36 % being awake more than 1 h each night. There was also a high rate of sleep onset problems, with 60 % being awake more than 30 min after retiring.

As part of their study comparing the sleep of adults with ID and adults with ASD and ID, Matson et al. report on 166 adults aged 27–88 years from developmental centres in the southeastern USA (Matson et al. 2008). Their results indicated that 13.7 % had at least one sleep problem listed on the sleep disorders scale of the Diagnostic Assessment of the Severely Handicapped-II (Matson 1995), an observational scale that was administered to direct care workers.

In a more recent study, Boyle et al. recruited individuals with ID within a health district in Scotland (Boyle et al. 2010). This group used a subset of items from a larger questionnaire to assess psychiatric problems. The 1023 individuals were age 16 years or older (52 % < 45 years) and had mild (39 %), moderate (24 %), severe (19 %) or profound ID (18 %). Among them, 18 % had Down syndrome and 7.5 % had been diagnosed with ASD. They report that 8.5 % of the group had initial insomnia, 9.9 % experienced early morning waking and 12 % had broken sleep.

Overall, the rates of sleep problems in adults with ID do appear somewhat lower than for children. Rates also appear to vary depending on the manner information was collected. When subsets of items from more general behavioural or psychiatric measures are used, rates are less than 15 %. In contrast, when more detailed information is collected using questionnaires that are sleep-specific, rates are as high as 68 %. This variation may be due to two things. First, sleep problems may be less easily recognized in adults with ID. They may be less likely to seek comfort or attention or to act out when having difficulties sleeping or when waking. Thus, caregivers may be less cognizant of their problems, making very detailed questioning necessary to uncover them. Second, adults with ID are more likely to live outside of a family home than children. This means caregivers may change frequently. The result may be that staff is less aware of the continuity of sleep problems because they are not dealing with a specific resident on an ongoing basis. This may lead them to believe problems are transitory, and therefore, to under-report them. Nonetheless, the data do suggest that sleep problems are a lingering problem for adults with ID, no less deserving of attention than for children.

Differences in Sleep Problems Between Groups With ID and Peers From the General Population

Although studies suggest sleep problems are common for those with ID, the question has been asked as to whether these differ substantially from individuals without ID. This is especially relevant in the case of children, for whom sleep problems are not uncommon in the general population.

Several studies have included both children with ID and typically developing (TD) peers in their samples. In Quine's 2001 study, parents of children aged 4–12 years who attended 12 primary and special schools in the UK were recruited. They compared the report of parents of the 182 children at special schools to those of the parents of the 576 primary school pupils. A larger proportion of children at the special schools experienced settling problems (41 versus 27 %), night waking problems (45 versus 13 %), early waking (14 versus 5 %), restlessness during sleep (53 versus 26 %), snoring (27 versus 14 %), apnoeic episodes (3 versus 1 %), gagging or choking during sleep (3 versus 1 %), head banging (4 versus 2 %) and bedwetting (33 versus 5 %). A larger number of children from the special schools also slept in their parents' bed (17 versus 11 %). Children from the special schools did not have more night-time fears, sleep talking, sleep walking, tooth grinding, nightmares or sleep terrors. Of note, several dyssomnias decreased with age in the mainstream school group, including settling, night waking and early waking, as well as sleeping in a parent's bed. In contrast, only night waking and sleeping in a parent's bed decreased with age for the children from the special schools. Neither group showed changes with age in sleep apnoea problems or parasomnias.

Goodlin-Jones et al. used parent report with the Children's Sleep Habits Questionnaire (CSHQ) as well as actigraphy to compare 57 children with a developmental disability to 69 TD children age 2–6.5 years (Goodlin-Jones et al. 2009). The CSHQ is the most commonly used tool to assess sleep problems in children with ID (Owens et al. 2000). It includes subscales that assess the frequency and severity of several aspects of sleep, including bedtime resistance, sleep onset delay, sleep duration, sleep anxiety, night wakings, parasomnias, sleep-disordered breathing and daytime sleepiness. Cut-off scores were developed by the authors to determine when sleep problems reach levels that would be considered a sleep disorder. Because data have been published with both TD children in the community and TD children diagnosed with a sleep disorder, the difficulties of children with ID can be viewed relative to these groups.

In Goodlin-Jones et al.'s study, children with a developmental disability (DD) were 3.3 times more likely to have a score above 60 on the CSHQ (OR=3.3, 95% CI=1.1–10.0) and less likely to have actigraphy readings that were indicative of a sleep onset insomnia (OR=0.3, 95% CI=0.1 to 0.8). However, they did not differ from TD children in terms of parent report of a sleep problem (OR=1.5, 95% CI=0.9–2.7) or actigraphy recordings indicative of night waking insomnia (OR=1.4, 95% CI=0.7–2.8).

Because children were followed up 3 and 6 months later, Goodlin-Jones et al. were able to examine the stability of problems for comparison across groups. More children with DD had scores above 60 on the CSHQ (10%) at all three time points than TD children (2%). In addition, children with a DD had more persistent reports by parents of a sleep problem (OR=2.1, 95% CI=1.0–4.4) and less persistent sleep-onset type insomnia based on actigraphy reading (OR=0.3, 95% CI=0.1–0.8). However, they did not differ from TD children in relation to the persistence of problems as measured by the CSHQ or persistence of actigraphy scores indicative of night waking insomnia. The authors suggest that the decrease in insomnia may have been due to maturation, although only 6 months had passed. However, it may have also been due to the focus on sleep in the families during the study. In other words, parents may have paid more attention to sleep routines and inadvertently helped improve their child's sleep over the course of the study. The authors also suggest the possibility that the discrepancy between the measures of sleep problems, CSHQ and actigraphy, may reflect the fact that parents of children with a DD may have heightened general stress, which may alter their experience of their child's sleep behaviours independent of their severity.

Krakowiak et al. also compared preschool children with developmental delays to a TD group, both of whom ranged from 2 to 5 years of age (Krakowiak et al. 2008). They solicited information as part of a larger study by using 39 questions regarding sleep, sleep behaviour and sleep problems. Parents of the 63 children with a DD did not report more problems with sleep than the parents of the 163 TD children. This lack of difference could be due to the fact that data were not collected using a standardized and validated questionnaire. The lack of difference may also be due to the fact that there is a higher prevalence of sleep problems in younger TD children, which tends to decrease with age (van Litsenburg et al. 2010).

Another study also reports no difference due to having a DD. Buckley et al. compared the sleep patterns of 15 TD children and 13 with DD who were 2–7 years old (Buckley et al. 2010). They completed an overnight polysomnogram. The DD group did not show a shorter total sleep time, longer time to sleep onset or more minutes awake after sleep onset. The authors caution that some differences in the data from data obtained for children at sleep labs suggest that the fact they were collected during admission to a regular paediatric unit may have negatively impacted children's sleep. It is possible that this attenuated differences between the groups.

In summary, Quine's study of school age children generally found more sleep problems in children attending a special school than a mainstream school (Quine 2001). The exception was parasomnias. In contrast, studies with younger children (Goodlin-Jones et al. 2009; Krakowiak et al. 2008) do not find differences between children with ID and TD peers. Although this may simply reflect differences in methodology, it is also possible that the underlying factor is age. Probably because sleep problems are more prevalent in younger TD children, but decrease with age, only children with ID that are school age or older show more sleep problems than their peers. Quine's data suggesting that dyssomnias decreased with age in that study for TD children, but not children with ID, support this possibility. No studies could be found comparing adolescents or adults with ID to a TD group, making it difficult to know whether these differences stabilize. However, given the high rates of reported sleep problems in adults with ID, and their nature, such as bedtime resistance and parasomnias (Brylewski and Wiggs 1998) it is likely that a direct comparison would yield significant differences.

Sleep Problems in Groups With ID due to Specific Aetiologies

In addition to studies using heterogeneous groups of children or adults with ID, many authors have examined sleep problems in groups with specific disorders or have included analyses of subgroups with specific disorders within their report. This can add to our knowledge. Because each disorder carries with it specific attributes, neurological, physiological and behavioural, investigations such as these may lead to a better understanding of factors that contribute to poor sleep or to better sleep within the ID population as a whole. This section describes the studies that could be found that focus on subgroups with ID. As with most work in this area, unfortunately, the preponderance of studies do focus on children. However, in some cases both children and adults are included in the same study. Although this is uncommon in the research literature, it did allow for the researchers to recruit sample sizes that were sufficiently large to examine problems in some detail.

Angelman Syndrome

Only one study has included data specific to individuals with Angelman syndrome (Didden et al. 2004b). They included 109 individuals aged 3–44 years, 33% of whom lived in residential centres and 67% of whom lived in a family home. Within that group, 29% experienced early waking, 37% night waking and 10% settling problems. Overall, 40% had severe sleep problem and for 90% of these the sleep problems had lasted for at least a year, with a mean duration of 9.7 years (SD = 8.0). The authors report that 33 % had received advice or help for either their current or past sleep problems (6 % psychological, 11 % education, 23 % medication and 3 % surgery). Of those receiving help, the greatest percentage believed psychological was effective (43 %), rather than education (33 %) or medication (24 %). The authors also report there was no impact of age on the sleep problems reported.

Autism Spectrum Disorder

More studies have been published regarding sleep problems in individuals with ASD than any other specific group of individuals with ID. Generally, parents of children with ASD report more sleep problems than TD peers (Goodlin-Jones et al. 2009; Krakowiak et al. 2008; Cotton and Richdale 2010; Couturier et al. 2005). This may be one reason for the focus on this group.

A number of studies have used the CSHQ (Owens et al. 2000) to investigate the sleep problems of children with ASD (Table 6.1). In 2002, Honomichl et al. used the CSHQ, along with diaries, to examine sleep problems in 100 children age 2–11 years with pervasive developmental disorders (PDDs). Among these, 65 had ASD, 8 had Asperger's syndrome (AS) and 23 had pervasive developmental disorder-not otherwise specified (PDD-NOS) (Honomichl et al. 2002). Parents completed the CSHQ at study entry, followed by a daily sleep diary for 4 weeks and completion of the CSHQ again. Six weeks later, they completed the CSHQ a second time, followed by completing the daily sleep diary for 2 additional weeks, and a final completion of the CSHQ.

CSHQ and sleep diary values were stable over the two time periods, suggesting steady problems. Children typically took 30 min to fall asleep at night, woke at night more than twice per week and were awake approximately 60 min at each time they woke. Children slept an average of 9.5 h per night. The authors report that at entry to the study, 54 parents reported their child had a sleep problem. This group had significantly higher scores on the CSHQ for bedtime resistance, sleep onset delay, sleep duration, sleep anxiety, night waking and parasomnia scales than those whose parents did not report a sleep problem. They found no differences in scores when children aged 2–5 years were compared to children 6–11 years, suggesting sleep problems did not decrease with age.

Three studies have used the CSHQ to compare the sleep problems of children with ASD and TD children (Couturier et al. 2005; Hoffman et al. 2006; Souders et al. 2009) and provide subscale scores for the children with ASD in their study (Table 6.1). Couturier et al. report that children with ASD and normal intelligence in their study had more frequent and more severe sleep problems than the TD children in the study. Of those with ASD, 78 % had a score above the cut-off on the CSHQ, indicating a sleep problem, compared to only 26 % of the TD group, and the difference was still significant when children taking stimulants were excluded from the analyses (79 versus 21 %). Children with ASD also had higher scores on the CSHQ

Table 6.1 Studies with children using the Children's Sleep Habits Questionnaire

Study	Group (age years; n)	Bedtime resistance	Sleep onset delay	Sleep duration	Sleep anxiety	Night wakings	Parasomnias	Sleep disordered breathing	Daytime sleepiness
Owen et al. 2000	TD community (M = 7.6, SD = 1.5; 469)	7.06 (1.89)	1.25 (0.53)	3.41 (0.93)	4.89 (1.45)	3.51 (0.89)	8.11 (1.25)	3.24 (0.63)	9.64 (2.80)
Owen et al. 2000	TD Sleep Clinic (M = 6.6, SD = 1.6; 154)	9.43 (3.49)	1.80 (0.88)	4.94 (1.98)	7.09 (2.44)	5.69 (1.60)	11.22 (2.53)	4.71 (2.54)	11.99 (3.39)
Breau and Camfield 2011	ID: no pain (3–21; 86)	7.3 (2.2)	1.6 (0.8)	4.1 (1.5)	5.1 (1.5)	4.3 (1.3)	9.0 (1.8)	3.8 (1.3)	14.5 (2.6)
Couturier et al. 2005	ASD (5–12; 23)	8.3 (2.8)	1.8 (0.8)	4.7 (1.5)	6.4 (1.8)	4.3 (1.5)	10.3 (2.7)	4.0 (1.3)	11.5 (2.9)
Souders et al. 2009	ASD (4–10; 59)	8.15 (2.16)	1.61 (0.77)	4.67 (1.83)	5.81 (1.98)	4.74 (1.64)	9.59 (1.85)	3.32 (0.57)	12.3 (3.22)
Hoffman et al. 2006	ASD (4–16; 106)	9.49 (2.66)	1.92 (0.78)	5.00 (1.92)	6.62 (2.10)	4.82 (1.74)	9.63 (2.09)	3.92 (1.33)	10.59 (2.93)
Tudor et al. 2014	ASD (3–18; 62)	9.33 (3.20)	2.03 (0.81)	5.62 (1.95)	6.64 (2.13)	5.06 (1.78)	10.72 (2.57)	3.99 (1.22)	13.82 (3.30)
Carter et al. 2009	Down syndrome (4–12; 24)	9.75 (1.5)	1.67 (0.9)	3.88 (1.6)	5.92 (1.7)	5.75 (1.9)	11.46 (2.3)	5.75 (2.0)	15.2 (4.2)
Carter et al. 2009	Down syndrome (13–17;1 6)	9.13 (1.6)	1.63 (0.8)	4.25 (1.8)	5.69 (2.0)	4.44 (1.8)	10.0 (1.7)	5.38 (2.0)	15.2 (3.4)
Ashworth et al. 2013	Down syndrome (6-12; n = 22)	8.55 (2.48)	1.55 (0.76)	4.85 (1.81)	6.25 (1.33)	6.35 (1.73)	10.40 (2.30)	5.45 (1.64)	12.45 (2.83)
Annaz et al. 2011	William syndrome (6–12; 64)	8.87 (2.7)	2.03 (0.9)	4.25 (1.9)	5.5 (2.1)	4.94 (2.1)	8.86 (2.9)	3.50 (1.5)	10.8 (3.3)

Table 6.1 (Continued)

Study	Group (age years; n)	Bedtime resistance	Sleep onset delay	Sleep duration	Sleep anxiety	Night wakings	Parasomnias	Sleep disordered breathing	Daytime sleepiness
Ashworth et al. 2013	William syndrome (6-12; n = 24)	7.21 (1.44)	1.83 (0.76)	4.71 (1.73)	5.08 (1.98)	5.25 (1.59)	9.29 (1.55)	3.63 (1.10)	11.75 (2.98)
Breau and Camfield 2011	ID: treated pain (3–21; n = 21)	7.3 (2.1)	1.7 (0.9)	5.0 (2.2)	5.5 (1.6)	5.2 (1.6)	9.2 (1.9)	4.8 (1.5)	13.7 (1.78)
Breau and Camfield 2011	ID: untreated pain (3–21; n = 16)	7.1 (2.3)	1.8 (0.8)	4.0 (1.6)	5.5 (1.9)	4.5 (1.5)	10.8 (2.8)	4.1 (1.3)	13.9 (3.08)

M mean, *SD* standard deviation, *TD* typically developing, *ID* intellectual disability, *ASD* autism spectrum disorder

subscales of sleep onset delay, sleep duration, sleep anxiety and parasomnias. There was also a trend for those with ASD to have higher scores for bedtime resistance and night wakings subscales.

In their study, Souders et al. compared 59 children with PDDs (26 ASD, 21 PDD-NOS, 12 AS) who were age 4–10 years with 40 TD children. Parents of 57.6% of the children with PDDS reported concerns with sleep compared to 12.5% of parents of TD children. Significantly more children with PDDS were also taking medication to help sleep (37.3%) than TD children (0%). Interestingly, the CSHQ scores of the children taking medication for sleep were higher than those who were not, suggesting the effects of the medication were limited. Actigraphy recordings also did not differ due to taking sleep medication.

In another study, Hoffman et al. compared their group of 106 children with ASD age 4–16 to a comparison group of TD children age 4–15 years (Hoffman et al. 2006). In this case, children with ASD scored higher on all CSHQ subscales except daytime sleepiness (Table 6.1).

Finally, in addition to a TD comparison group, Goodlin-Jones et al. used parent report with the CSHQ as well as actigraphy to compare the 68 children in their study with ASD to 57 with a DD in addition to 69 TD children (Goodlin-Jones et al. 2009). The children in the study were preschoolers, ranging from 2 to 6.5 years. Children with ASD (42%) were more than twice as likely to have their parents report a generic sleep problem than TD children (14%), but not children with DD (48%). In contrast, based on actigraphy, children with ASD were less likely to have sleep onset problems or night waking insomnia than TD children. Over the three time periods used in the study, covering a 6-month period, the same proportion of children had a problem at all three time periods as TD children according to CSHQ scores. However, 16% of the ASD group, compared to 5% of the TD group had a problem at all three time points based on parent report. As the authors discuss, these discrepancies raise the question as to whether children with ASD actually have more sleep problems than TD children, or, whether their parents of experience their children's sleep behaviour and sleep patterns as more stressful due to other factors associated with having a child with ASD.

One study used the Behavior Evaluation of Disorders of Sleep (BEDS) to investigate sleep problems in children with ASD/PDD. The BEDS includes 28 items that fall into five domains: expressive sleep disturbances, sensitivity to the environment, sleep facilitators, disoriented awakenings and apnoea/bruxism. Shreck and Mulick (Schreck and Mulick 2000) included 55 children age 5–12 years with ASD or PDD in their study, comparing them to 22 children with ID and 49 with borderline ID and 43 TD children. Parents of children with ASD/PDD were more likely to indicate their child had a sleep problem. Based on the BEDS, they determined that children with ASD/PDD had more dyssomnias and parasomnias than the other groups.

Polimeni et al. (Polimeni et al. 2005) also used the BEDS in addition to a survey developed for their study. They included 53 children with ASD, 52 with Asperger's disorder (AD) and 66 TD children in their study. They ranged from 2 to 17 years. A total of 50% of the TD group reported sleep problems, whereas 73% each of ASD and AD groups did. Parents reported 1.2 problems on average, but they found no difference between groups in the severity of sleep problems. Parents reported mild problems in 22% of the ASD group, 25% of the AD group and 23% of the TD group, moderate problems in 57% of the ASD group, 39.5% of the AD group and 42% of the TD group and severe problems in 17% of the ASD group, 33% of the AD group and 30% of the TD group. Despite this, the AD group had significantly higher BEDS total scores than the ASD or TD groups, but there were no differences in BEDS subscale scores, with the exception of being disoriented upon waking being more common for AD children than TD children.

Krakowiak included 303 children in their study with ASD and compared them to 63 DD children and 163 TD children (Krakowiak et al. 2008). Children with ASD tended to get less sleep than TD children (11 h versus 12 h). Parents of 53% of children with ASD reported at least one "frequent" or "always" sleep problem, compared to 46% of those in the DD group and 32% of those in the TD group. Further, more children in the ASD group (13%) than in the DD (9.5%) or TD groups (3.7%) had elevated scores for sleep onset problems and night waking (11 versus 6.3 versus 4.3%). However, the differences between the ASD and DD groups were no longer significant after controlling for medical and demographic characteristics (gender; age; use of allergy, CNS or respiratory medications; and frequent gastrointestinal symptoms, birth order). Of note, cognitive and adaptive delays were not associated with sleep problems in the ASD group, although they were across the larger sample.

Mayes and Calhoun used 10 items of the Pediatric Behaviour Scale, developed by the authors, to investigate sleep problems in 477 children with ASD age 1–15 years. Data were collected from charts of a psychiatry diagnostic clinic (Mayes and Calhoun 2009). They report that "sometimes" to "very often" 35% of children walked or talked in their sleep, 36% wet their bed, 39% had nightmares, 45% woke too early, 50% woke often during the night, 56% were restless during sleep and 60% had difficulty falling asleep. No problems were associated with age, except waking during the night, which decreased with age, and nightmares, which increased with age. Overall, sleep problems were not correlated with IQ.

Williams et al. asked 210 parents of children with ASD (127 with ID also) to complete a survey regarding their child's sleep (Williams et al. 2004). Parents reported that "frequently" or "almost always" 53% had difficulty falling asleep, 40% had restless sleep, 33.8% had frequent wakings, 39.5% insisted on co-bedding, 27.7% had enuresis, 21% each had bruxism and snoring, 10.5% vocalized in their sleep, 5.2% woke up screaming, 3.8% had nightmares and 1% experienced sleep walking. No difference in the frequency of problems between the groups with and without ID was found except for night wakings, which were more frequent in the group with ASD and ID than the group with ASD alone (63.8 versus 45.3%). Only enuresis was related to age. It was more common in younger children (<6 years versus 6–11 versus 11+).

Matson's group conducted the only study that could be located to specifically examine sleep problems in adults with ASD (Matson et al. 2008). In their study, 168 adults with ASD and ID (age 16–78) were compared to 166 with ID alone. They report that 44.7% of those with ASD and ID had sleep problems, compared to 13.7% of those with ID only. Those with ASD and ID also had higher DASH-II scores reflecting difficulty staying awake, waking up frequently at night, difficulty getting to sleep and waking up screaming. There was no difference between groups for sleepwalking.

In summary, the data regarding individuals with an ASD are mixed. Some studies find no difference in sleep problems between those with ASD relative to those with ID (Krakowiak et al. 2008; Goodlin-Jones et al. 2009; Williams et al. 2004). In addition, the highest rates in two studies were for children with AS (Couturier et al. 2005; Krakowiak et al. 2008). Finally, one study found that, although parents of children with ASD reported more problems, the data did not support this (Goodlin-Jones et al. 2009). This raises the question regarding whether parents of children with ASD perceive their child's sleep differently. This may be due to parents of children with ASD having high levels of stress related to parenting that make them more sensitive to issues related to sleep, as suggested by Goodlin-Jones et al. (Goodlin-Jones et al. 2009). It may also be due to the methodologies used. However, there is no way to know if the results reported apply to adults with ASD as only one study exists at this time. What is clear is that parents are experiencing frequent and serious difficulties with getting their child with ASD to go to sleep and stay asleep. More studies with objective measures are needed with this group to back up these findings based primarily on parent-completed questionnaires. More studies are also needed with adults with ASD.

Cri du chat Syndrome

Only two reports by the same group have included those with cri du chat syndrome (Maas et al. 2009; Maas et al. 2012). In their first study, Maas et al. compared the sleep of 30 individuals with cri du chat syndrome who were 2–47 years old to that of 30 with Down syndrome and 30 with ID due to mixed aetiologies. Although more individuals with cri du chat had sleep problems (30 %) than with those with Down syndrome (10 %) or ID (23 %), the difference was not significant. Night waking was the most common problem in the cri du chat group, being a severe problem for 20 %. Severe early waking was a problem for 3 % and none had a severe settling problem. Otherwise, there was no increased prevalence of sleep problems for those with cri du chat relative to other groups. In a subsequent study, 25 individuals who took part in the 2009 study were compared to a group with Jacobsen syndrome. No differences in sleep problems between groups emerged. These two studies suggest that having cri du chat syndrome is unlikely to increase the likelihood of having a sleep problem relative to people with Down syndrome, Jacobsen syndrome or ID due to a variety of aetiologies.

Cornelia de Lange

Only one study could be found that specifically examined sleep problems in individuals with Cornelia de Lange syndrome (Hall et al. 2008). A total of 55 % of the 54 youth (mean age = 13.9 years, SD = 8.6) had sleep problems. This did not differ from the proportion of a comparison group of 46 individuals with ID of mixed aetiologies in terms of overall sleep problems, going to bed problems or waking at night. These results tentatively suggest that having Cornelia de Lange syndrome does not increase risk of sleep problems relative to individuals with ID of other aetiologies.

Down Syndrome

A group from the UK studied 58 children with Down syndrome ranging from less than 1 to 17 years of age (Carter et al. 2009). They report that, using the CSHQ, 33 % of the children under age 4 had restless sleep, although the scale was not designed for that age group. They also found that children aged 4–12 had elevated scores on all scales except sleep duration relative to the US same-age norms provided by Owens et al. (Owens et al. 2000). In their group 13 years and older with Down syndrome, the children showed significantly elevated scores for bedtime resistance, parasomnias, sleep-disordered breathing and daytime sleepiness. The most noted problems were resisting going to bed (25 %), sleeping in another's bed (33 %), restlessness during sleep (58 %), waking more than once per night (40 %) and waking at least twice per night (28 %). Parasomnias that were reported included bruxism at least 2 nights per week (45 %) and sleep talking (45 %). Only 5 % each reported sleep walking or night terrors.

Two years later, Breslin et al. used the CSHQ to investigate the sleep problems of a group of 35 children age 7–18 years (Breslin et al. 2011). Their data indicated 85 % had scores above the cut-off for a clinical problem. The children exhibited a variety of problems. Compared to norms generated with a community sample of TD children by Owens et al. (2000), this group had significantly elevated scores for bedtime resistance, sleep anxiety, night wakings, parasomnias, sleep-disordered breathing and daytime sleepiness. There was a trend to have higher scores for the sleep onset delay subscale, but there was no difference on the sleep duration subscale.

Very recently Stores and Stores enrolled 78 parents of children with Down syndrome age 4–19 years (Stores and Stores 2013). They report that 20 % had problems with settling, 26 % were reluctant to go to bed and 9 % insisted on sleeping with someone else. They also found that 12 % had apnoeic episodes. Parasomnias that were reported included sleep talking (19 %), teeth grinding (17 %) and bed wetting (16 %). Fewer children banged their head (7 %) or walked in their sleep (3 %). None reported nightmares or night terrors.

The same year, Ashworth et al. compared 22 children 6–12 years of age with Down syndrome to a group of 24 with Williams syndrome and 52 TD children (Ashworth et al. 2013). They used both parent report, with the CSHQ, and actigraphy which was collected for a minimum of four nights. Children with Down syndrome had higher scores on all subscales of the CSHQ, relative to both the Williams syndrome and the TD group, except for the sleep onset delay and daytime sleepiness subscales. Analyses of specific items of the CSHQ indicated that, relative to TD children, those with Down syndrome had more restless sleep, were more likely to move to another bed, snore loudly, wake early and seem sleepy during the day on 2 or more nights per week. Actigraphy recordings also indicated that children with Down syndrome had the most disrupted sleep.

Maas et al. also compared sleep problems of children with Down syndrome to other groups (Maas et al. 2012). In their case-control study of children with Down syndrome, cri du chat syndrome, Jacobsen syndrome and nonspecific ID, they found no difference in the number of children with a severe sleep problem among groups. However, children with Jacobsen syndrome showed significantly more sleep complaints than Down syndrome.

Taken together, these studies suggest that having Down syndrome does increase the risk of sleep problems relative to TD children. One exception may be children's sleep duration; two studies did not report a difference in this aspect (Carter et al. 2009; Breslin et al. 2011). This suggests that those with Down syndrome sleep the same number of hours, but have more disrupted sleep. There is less evidence that Down syndrome increases risk for sleep problems relative to other children with ID of different aetiologies. In one study, they showed more of some problems than children with Williams syndrome, but in another study they showed no more than children with Jacobsen syndrome. Thus, although the data suggest that these children do have more sleep problems than TD children, more research is needed before a strong argument can be made that they show more problems than other groups with a DD or ID alone.

Fragile X Syndrome

Only two studies could be located that examined the sleep problems of children with fragile X syndrome. The first included 13 children aged 3–19 years (Richdale 2003). Parents completed a questionnaire asking about various aspects of sleep. Seven parents reported a past sleep problem that had begun when their child was 3 years old or younger. Four reported a current problem, with three of these indicating it had begun more than 2 years ago. Parents of eight children reported settling problems, three for more than 2 years, and five reported frequent night waking for more than 2 years.

In the second study, Kronk et al. used the CSHQ (Owens et al. 2000) with 90 children with fragile X syndrome aged 3–17 years (Kronk et al. 2009). They report that 47 % of their sample had total scores at or above the cut-off score of 41, indicating a clinically significant problem, whereas another 38 % had scores between 38 and 40 indicating a subclinical problem. They also found no difference in CSHQ scores due to age, gender or whether the child was taking medication for sleep. They report that 21 % struggled at bedtime, 41 % showed a sleep onset delay, 54 % had insufficient sleep, 52 % woke once per night and 27 % more than once, 21 % moved to another`s bed at night, 38 % experienced bedwetting, 20 % talked during sleep, 33 % ground their teeth during sleep, 57 % had restless sleep and 34 % snored loudly.

Clearly, rates are higher than for TD children. However, studies comparing this population to other groups are needed to confirm that there is an added risk for sleep problems when a child has ID due to fragile X syndrome specifically.

Jacobsen Syndrome

Only one group has published research regarding sleep problems in children and young adults with Jacobsen syndrome (Maas et al. 2008; Maas et al. 2012). Data from the same sample were used in both reports. In their 2008 study, data regarding sleep were collected for 43 individuals. Of these, 23 % had a sleep problem, including settling problems (94 %), frequent night waking (16 %) and early waking (6 %). Of the 43, 54 % also had a history of sleep problems. They found no associations between the presence of a sleep problem and age, or level of ID. In their 2012 study, more details were provided regarding the 25 who had reported a sleep problem in the first study. Of the 25, 19 were classed as having a severe sleep problem and this did not differ from comparison groups with cri du chat syndrome, Down syndrome or nonspecific ID. The group of individuals with Jacobsen syndrome showed more sleep complaints than those with Down syndrome but not the other groups. Until more research is conducted with additional samples, these studies provide a brief overview of sleep problems in one sample of individuals with Jacobsen syndrome. However, there is insufficient data at this time to develop hypotheses regarding the relative rate or quality of sleep problems for people with Jacobsen syndrome relative to individuals with ID due to other aetiologies.

Prader-Willi Syndrome

Maas' group also produced the only study that could be located looking at sleep problems in individuals with Prader-Willi syndrome (Maas et al. 2010). The 79 participants in this study were adults, ranging from 18 to 65 years of age. Only one was reported to have a settling problem, 13 % had a night waking problem and 4 % had an early waking problem. A total of 15 % had some type of current sleep problem. Three participants met criteria for sleep apnoea. Relative to reported rates for those with ID of other aetiologies, there are not sufficient data to determine whether this group differs in terms of risk of sleep problems.

Rett Syndrome

In an early study, Piazza et al. examined sleep problems in 20 girls and women age 1–32 years with Rett syndrome and severe to profound ID (Piazza et al. 1990).

Parents recorded sleep and wake information for 30 min periods during the day until the participant was put to bed and fell asleep and then at 02:00 and 04:00. This was collected for 3–18 days. The authors report that night wakings occurred on 21 % of nights, delayed sleep onset on 68 % of nights and early wakings on 25 %. There was no relation between these three sleep problems.

In a subsequent study, Piazza et al. compared the data collected in their first study to a group of 51 youth aged 3–21 years with ID and severe behaviour problems (Piazza et al. 1996). They report that the group with Rett syndrome slept significantly more at all ages and did not show the age-related decrease in night sleep displayed by children and youth with ID only. In addition, the individuals with Rett syndrome had more daytime sleep than those with ID and showed an increase in daytime sleep with age. Thus, they had more hours sleep per day as they aged when night-time and daytime sleep were combined.

More recently, Young and her group conducted a study on 237 individuals with Rett syndrome age 2–29 years in Australia, using information collected as part of the Australian Rett Syndrome Database (Young et al. 2007). Of these, 131 had information for three time points separated by 2 years each. Depending on the time point, 79–85 % reported any sleep problem. At the last time point, reports from 202 indicated that, at least "weekly or more often", 18 % displayed night laughing, 13 % displayed night screaming, 11 % had night seizures, 33 % teeth grinding, 9 % of those who were mobile showed sleep walking, 6 % talked in their sleep and 4 % had night terrors. Only night laughing decreased significantly with age, whereas night seizures increased, peaking in the age 13–17 group and then showing a small decrease in those over age 18.

Several results are intriguing within this small literature. First, children with Rett syndrome were found to increase their daily amount of sleep with age over childhood. Second, they experienced increased night seizures in adolescence in another study. Finally, the report of laughing during sleep is unique. It is possible that this is another form of parasomnia.

Sanfillipo Syndrome

In the only study that could be found to investigate individuals with Sanfillipo syndrome, Colville et al. surveyed the parents of 80 people age 4–25 years in the UK (Colville et al. 1996). Parents reported 78 % had a sleep problem, and 29 of those whose family member had a sleep problem said it was severe. The authors report that, surprisingly, given the age of the sample, 19 were sleeping in their parents' room. The problems reported included settling (56 %), night waking (59 %), early morning waking (28 %), moving to parents' bed (30 %) and sleep talking (23 %). Some parents also described their child singing ($n=9$) or laughing ($n=3$) during sleep. Although there was a high rate of past sleep problems (92 %), there was no association between age and amount of sleep, night waking or overall sleep problems.

Williams Syndrome

Annaz et al. studied the sleep of 64 children with Williams syndrome aged 6–12 years and a comparison group of 92 age-matched healthy children (Annaz et al. 2011). Children with Williams syndrome received higher scores than the control group for the bedtime resistance, sleep onset delay, sleep anxiety, night waking and daytime sleepiness subscales of the CSHQ. Analyses also revealed that sleep problems decreased in children with Williams syndrome with age at a significantly slower rate than in the control group, suggesting, as with children with ID due to mixed aetiologies (Quine 2001) and ASD (Honomichl et al. 2002), that problems do not disappear with age. Asthma and allergies were a predictor of sleep onset delay, and cardiac problems had a significant effect on sleep duration. However, there was no effect on sleep of ear infections, constipation, tonsillitis or epilepsy. In terms of specific problems, 45 % resisted going to bed, 40 % moved to someone else's bed in the night, 15 % sleep talked, 97 % had two or more wakings per night, 60 % experienced restless during sleep, 51 % had enuresis and 36 % snored. These problems were reported to occur "sometimes" or "often".

As described earlier, Ashworth et al. compared 22 children age 6–12 years with Down syndrome ($n=22$) to 24 children with Williams syndrome and 52 TD children (Ashworth et al. 2013). They used both parent report based on the CSHQ, and actigraphy which was collected for a minimum of four nights. Children with Williams syndrome had higher scores on sleep onset delay, sleep duration and night waking subscales of the CSHQ than the TD children, but lower scores on all subscales than the Down syndrome group except for the sleep onset delay and daytime sleepiness subscales. Actigraphy showed that children with Williams syndrome had the longest sleep latency, with the average being 48 min to fall asleep, 23–25 min longer than the other two groups.

At this time, there are insufficient data to determine that those with Williams syndrome have more sleep problems or a specific pattern of sleep problems than children with ID due to other aetiologies. However, there is some indication that health problems may play a role for some.

In summary, studies of individuals with specific aetiologies of ID reveal that problems occur across groups. The number of studies is small, and the methods used are varied. Thus, the findings are difficult to compare. In some cases, authors have reported unique behaviours, such as laughing at night. However, without more studies using equivalent measures, it is hard to say whether these behaviours do not occur with other groups, or whether parents were just not provided with the opportunity to report them.

It could be helpful to know if having ID due to a specific aetiology leads to differences in sleep problems. In many cases, specific medical conditions are associated with specific diagnoses and these may contribute to sleep problems or exacerbate sleep problems that are more related to having an ID. It is also possible that having a sleep problem is related to the level of ID, which may also vary due to aetiology, along with behavioural problems. Finally, it is also possible that parents react differently to sleep and sleep problems in different groups. As noted by

Goodlin-Jones et al. (Goodlin-Jones et al. 2009), some groups of parents may have more stress related to their child. It is also possible that others may have different expectations, such as when ID is typically less severe for those with that specific syndrome, leading to greater frustration when sleep problems persist into middle childhood. Finally, ID aetiologies that are associated with serious medical conditions may make it more difficult for parents to maintain a consistent approach to sleep and sleep problems because of their worry over the child's health problems. Large studies, with multiple groups of different aetiologies, are needed to address these questions.

Risk Factors for Sleep Problems

Few studies have focused solely on potential contributors to sleep problems for those with ID. However, many studies that have looked at the prevalence or have compared sleep problems among groups within the ID population have included some examination of factors that are related to sleep problems. The sections below describe those studies that have provided some information.

Age

For the most part, in children with ID, sleep problems have not been found to be related to age (Didden et al. 2002). This is in contrast to the typical pattern in most children, where sleep problems generally decrease over childhood (Meltzer and Mindell 2006). Honomichl et al. studied 100 children age 2–11 years with PDDs and found no difference in CSHQ scores for sleep problems when they compared a 2–5-year-old group to a 6–11-year-old group (Honomichl et al. 2002). Kronk et al. also reported no age differences in CSHQ scores within their sample of 90 children with fragile X syndrome (Kronk et al. 2009).

Some studies, however, have reported differences. When Annaz et al. examined the data for 64 children with Williams syndrome aged 6–12 years and a comparison group of 92 age-matched healthy children (Annaz et al. 2011), they found that sleep problems decreased in children with Williams syndrome with age, but at a significantly slower rate than in the control group. Others have found that some types of sleep problems decrease. Two studies have described decreases in night waking with age. In their study of 477 children age 1–15 years with ASD seen at a psychiatry diagnostic clinic, Mayes and Calhoun found that only waking during the night decreased with age in their group (Mayes and Calhoun 2009). Night waking also decreased with age in the 4–12-year-olds with ID studied by Quine (Quine 2001). Quine also found that sleeping with a parent decreased with age. Williams et al. report that only enuresis decreased with age in their study. They investigated sleep problems of 210 children with ASD and found this difference when they compared <6 versus 6–11 versus 11+year groups. Finally, the study to report the greatest effect of age was conducted with children age 3–18 years with Down syndrome

(Breslin et al. 2011). Bresin et al. investigated the sleep of 35 children based on parent report of sleep problems using the CSHQ. Although there was no difference due to age on total CSHQ score, younger children received higher scores for sleep anxiety, bed resistance, parasomnias and lower scores sleep onset delay than older children in the study.

In studies including both children and adults, differences are also not generally reported. Didden et al. found no effect of age in a sample of 109 individuals with Angelman syndrome age 2–44 years (Didden et al. 2004b). Similarly, no effect of age was found in a study of 43 children and young adults with Jacobsen syndrome (Maas et al. 2008) or in Colville et al.'s study of 80 people age 4–25 years with Sanfillipo syndrome (Colville et al. 1996). Thus, it would appear that problems do not always decrease in adulthood.

In the only study to follow individuals over time, few changes were also found. Young and her group conducted a study of 237 individuals with Rett syndrome aged 2–29 years in Australia, using information collected as part of the Australian Rett syndrome database (Young et al. 2007). Of these, 131 had information for three time points separated by 2 years each. Only night laughing decreased significantly with age, whereas night seizures increased, peaking in the age 13–17 group and then showing a small decrease in those over age 18.

Overall, these studies report inconsistent relations between sleep problems and age in individuals with ID. Change with increasing age has been reported for night waking, sleeping with a parent and enuresis, but not in all studies that have investigated these aspects. Decreased night laughing and increased night seizures, peaking in adolescence, were also reported in one longitudinal study. Perhaps the most striking pattern that emerges across studies is the lack of change over childhood, which is in contrast to the pattern most studies suggest for typical children (Meltzer and Mindell 2006).

This lack of improvement suggests that, just as with other aspects of their functioning, those with ID are not following typical developmental patterns. This may also be a reason that differences between those with ID and TD children appear to be less significant in preschool groups. Clearly, TD children have a tendency to "outgrow" many sleep problems that are common in this age group, whereas children with ID do not. Little is known about sleep problems over the lifespan of adults with ID. This area is important because changes in sleep and the development of sleep problems are common in the elderly in the general population. There is no reason to believe a similar pattern does not exist for those with ID and there is a possibility that the changes may be more complex or present in different ways or at different ages. Given the increasing lifespan of those with ID over the past few decades, this area is vitally in need of further study.

Level of ID

Most studies have not found differences in sleep problems in relation to intellectual level, whether studying children (Mayes and Calhoun 2009; Richdale et al. 2000) or children and adults (Didden et al. 2004). Interestingly, although they found no difference in reported problems in relation to level of ID, Richdale et al. did find that parents of children with severe/profound ID were more stressed by their child's waking than parents of children with mild or moderate ID.

One study with children did find a difference. Didden et al. report that in their sample having a more severe ID was significantly related to having a severe sleep problem and more children had a sleep problem as the level of ID became more severe. They fund that fewer children in the mild group had a sleep problem (8.6%), whereas 14.8% of the moderate group, 27.9% of the severe group and 35.3% of the profound group were experiencing sleep problemsproblems. (Didden et al. 2002b).

Similarly, in their sample of adults age 18–70, Harvey et al. found that the frequency of multiple sleep problems was greater in those with more significant ID (Harvey et al. 2003). While only 19% of those with mild ID had multiple problems, 30% of those with moderate ID, 38% of those with severe ID and 53% of those with profound ID had multiple sleep problems. They also found those with more significant ID were more likely to have nocturnal enuresis. In their group, 15% of those with mild ID, 23% of those with moderate, 66% of those with severe and 77% of those with profound ID experienced bed wetting.

Clearly, more work needs to be done in this area. The mixed results do not provide a good evidence base to suggest that sleep problems are related to an individual's level of ID. Nonetheless, the two reports that have examined level of ID appear to suggest that some sleep problems may increase with level of impairment. Because it is possible that concomitant factors may account for this, such as the increased rate of physical disabilities and medical conditions in those with more severe ID, it is essential that future studies account for these confounding factors when they investigate the impact of the level of ID on sleep problems.

Medical Conditions

Only one study has specifically evaluated the role of general medical conditions on sleep problems in children with ID. Ghanizadeh and Faghih used the CSHQ to assess sleep problems in children with ID with ($n=58$) and without ($n=75$) a medical condition in the previous month (Ghanizadeh and Faghih 2009). The most common medical condition was abdominal pain (23.1%), followed by allergies (9.5%), ear infections (3.9%), seizures (1.8%) and surgery (0.6%). Comparisons were made on factor scores of the CSHQ derived from the full sample that also included 83 TD children and 121 siblings of the children with ID. Children with ID who had medical conditions had higher scores on three factors: parasomnias, daytime sleepiness and "other" problems (falls asleep with rocking, sleepwalks, awakes more than once during the night, seems tired). Their factor scores were not higher for problems with bedtime resistance/sleep duration or sleep anxiety behaviours. After excluding children with a medical condition from all subgroups, children with ID did not differ in sleep problems from TD children or the siblings of the children with ID. Because of this, the authors suggest that it may be that medical conditions, more frequent in children with ID, lead to more sleep problems in this population, and, that managing those medical conditions may reduce sleep problems.

Breau et al. also studied the effect of medical conditions on sleep in a sample of 37 children with ID who ranged from 3 to 21 years (Breau and Camfield 2011). In this case, the purpose was to examine the effect of pain on sleep. Children with pain had higher total CSHQ scores and higher scores on night waking, parasomnias and sleep-disordered breathing subscales. Sleep medications did not affect sleep. Children taking medications to manage pain did not experience fewer sleep problems than those with untreated pain. Those with medicated pain slept fewer hours than those with no pain as well as had more night wakings than children without pain. Children with untreated pain had more parasomnias. The authors speculate that the intensity of pain may be related to whether it was being treated and that treatments may not have been sufficient to relieve pain. Thus, it may be that treated pain was more severe and woke the child, whereas untreated pain was less intense and lead to disrupted sleep in the form of parasomnias.

In a similar investigation, Tudor et al. had parents of 62 children aged 3–18 years with ASD complete the CHSQ (Tudor et al. 2014). Pain predicted overall sleep disturbance and three CSHQ subscale scores: sleep duration, parasomnias and sleep-disordered breathing. Interestingly, they report that children who scored higher on the social subscale of the pain measure used the Non-communicating Children's Pain Checklist - Revised (Breau et al. 2002) were more likely to have sleep duration problems. Because that subscale includes behaviours that may reflect attempts to communicate pain, such as seeking comfort, the authors speculate that it is possible that the children's attempts to communicate their pain are what interfered with sleep.

Others have examined specific medical problems as part of larger studies regarding sleep problems. In their 2002 study, Didden et al. studied 286 children age 1–19 with mild to profound ID (Didden et al. 2002b). Having a diagnosis of cerebral palsy was significantly related to having a severe sleep problem. Of children with cerebral palsy, 33.3 % had a sleep problem, whereas only 15.8 % of those without cerebral palsy had a sleep problem. In contrast, the same group reports that in their group of 109 children and adults with Angelman syndrome, having epilepsy had no relation to sleep problems (Didden et al. 2004b). Finally, Krakowiak et al.'s study involved a large sample of 529 children with ASD (303), DD (63) and TD children (163) (Krakowiak et al. 2008). They found that having gastrointestinal problems was associated with more problems with sleep onset.

In all, there is very little research focused specifically on medical factors that may affect sleep problems in those with ID. No study examining the role of neurological conditions, such as ADHD, in sleep problems for those with ID could be found. With the exception of three studies specifically addressing the impact of medical conditions on sleep problems, two of which examined pain specifically, most research addressing the role of medical conditions on sleep have included those with specific medical conditions (Batista and Nunes 2007) or physical disabilities (Hemmingsson et al. 2009) who do not necessarily have intellectual limitations.

However, the existing studies point to discomfort or pain having an impact, often due to gastrointestinal conditions or orthopaedic conditions, which are both more common in those with ID than in the general population. As this population ages, it is also likely that rates of conditions that may cause discomfort, such as arthritis, will also be common in this group, as in those without ID who are aging. Other conditions may also have an impact, and it is fair to assume this should be similar in magnitude to that reported for the general population. In the interim, it is appropriate to consider medical conditions that cause pain or discomfort when attempting to manage sleep problems for an individual with ID.

Medication

Many individuals with ID take medication on a regular basis to manage health problems. Psychotropic medications are also not uncommon, frequently given to manage behaviour or anxiety. Anecdotally, many parents of children with ID report that they believe some medications their child has used did affect sleep. For some, the effect is sufficient that the medication is discontinued.

Some studies have examined whether taking medication is a risk factor for having sleep problems. In their study with children in the community, Didden et al. found that children whose parents reported they were taking medication were more likely to have a sleep problem (Didden et al. 2002b). Almost 28 % of those taking medication had a sleep problem compared to 10.6 % of those who were not. Unfortunately, the types of medications used were not examined in detail. Krakowiak also found that those in their large study of 529 children with ASD who taking CNS medications had more problems with sleep onset (Krakowiak et al. 2008).

In contrast, in a similar sample of children with ASD or AS, Polimeni's group found that taking medication was not related to report of sleep problems (Polimeni et al. 2005). No differences were found in the sample of children and adults with Angelman syndrome in Didden at al.'s study (Didden et al. 2004b).

In a somewhat different study, focused on sleep patterns, Luiselli et al. did report a difference (Luiselli et al. 2005). They asked staff in 16 suburban group homes in the northeastern USA to observe 59 participants aged 23–71 years with mild to profound ID from 19:00 to 07:00 over a 1-month period. Staff made recordings every 30 min to document whether the residents were awake, awake and disruptive or asleep. They found that only taking medication impacted sleep; those taking selective serotonin reuptake inhibitors (SSRIs) slept less. This is not surprising because, although sleepiness has been associated with SSRIs in the short term, long-term effects include sleep disturbance.

Another unusual result was reported by Valdovinos et al. based on their chart review of 30 people age 31–75 with ID (mild, 23 %; moderate, 10 %; severe, 23 %; and profound, 43 %) over a 2-year period. The goal of their study was to investigate the side effects of psychotropic medications. Of their sample, 67 % had sleep problems and they report a significant relation between the number or medication *changes* over the two years ($r = .50$) and sleep problems (Vladovinos et al. 2005). Over the 2 years, there were 69 changes for 21 of the participants; most often increases in dose (47 % of participants) or addition of another medication (43 % of participants). Because the analysis is correlational, this raises the question of whether ongoing sleep problems were judged as a side effect requiring a medication change, or whether medication changes contributed to sleep problems. This is an important issue worth further study because management of psychotropic medications can be difficult in those with ID, often necessitating changes to best manage psychological or behavioural problems.

At this time, the evidence regarding the role of medications in sleep problems for those with ID is mixed. Some have found effects, whereas others have not. Given that many medications are specifically associated with sleep problems, it is logical to assume that these will impact sleep for individuals with ID just as they do in the general population. However, it is also possible that those caring for individuals with ID are more likely to stop use of medications that are causing sleep problems if their family member of client already has pre-existing sleep problems that are worsened by the medication.

Consequences of Sleep Problems

Sleep problems are unpleasant for those who have them, and for their family members or caregivers. They also disrupt and attenuate sleep, leading to daytime tiredness. Those with ID are not immune to these effects. A growing literature points to several aspects of functioning that are impacted by sleep problems in those with ID. These include both increased maladaptive behaviour, as well as reduced performance in other areas of function.

Behaviour Problems

One major concern regarding the sleep problems of those with ID, above and beyond their inconvenience and disruption within a family or other home, is that there is growing research indicating that sleep problems can lead to significant behaviour problems in both children and adults.

Studies of Children

Quine indicates that, of the 200 children with severe ID in that study (Quine 1991), those who had settling problems were significantly more likely to show daytime behaviour problems. This included behaviour management problems, hyperactivity, concentration problems, attention seeking, a lack of social awareness and inappropriate behaviour with strangers, interrupting others' activities, being destructive, scattering objects, pica, swearing, embarrassing behaviours and being disruptive at school. In addition to being linked to these, night-time waking was also significantly associated with encopresis, tantrums, mood problems, problems with peers, sucking objects, making noises, repetitive activities and delayed echolalia.

Wiggs and Stores examined behaviour problems and their relation to sleep problems in 209 children with ID (Wiggs and Stores 1996a). The 92 children with reported sleep problems showed significantly more irritability, lethargy, stereotypies and hyperactivity than those without sleep problems on the aberrant behaviour checklist (Aman and Singh 1986).

Richdale et al. (2000) also reports that children in their study that had sleep problems also had more behaviour problems. Within the group with ID, having a sleep problem was associated with disruptive behaviour and self-absorbed behaviour as measured by the Developmental Behaviour Checklist (Einfeld and Tonge 1994). Interestingly, sleep problems were not significantly associated with anxiety in the group with ID, although they were in the group of TD children.

Didden et al. (2002b) reported that, in a group of children who lived at home they found significantly more aggression, screaming, temper tantrums, noncompliance and impulsivity based on the Aberrant behavior Checklist (Aman and Singh 1986) in children with severe sleep problems. In that study, a sleep problem was designated as severe if it involved three or more nights per week with at least one problem out of settling, night-time waking and early waking. Sleep problems were not related to self-injury.

Overall, these studies of children with ID of mixed aetiology suggest more problem behaviour with sleep problems. The specific type of problem behaviour appears to differ between studies. This may reflect the differences in the samples or in the tools used to assess problem behaviour.

Several groups have investigated behaviour problems in relation to sleep problems in groups of children with ASD. Rzepecka et al. studied 167 children with ID and/or ASD age 5–18 who attended a health service in the UK (Rzepecka et al. 2011). For this study, they used the CSHQ to assess sleep problems and the Aberrant behavior Checklist to assess behaviour. In a hierarchical multiple regression, they found that, after accounting for the effect of medication, CSHQ scores added significantly to predicting problem behaviour.

In a large group of 1193 children aged 4–10 years with ASD, Sikora et al. used the Aberrant behavior Checklist to elicit parent report of problem behaviours in relation to sleep problems assessed with the CSHQ. (Sikora et al. 2012). They found that those with no sleep problems received a lower score than those with mild sleep problems (CSHQ 41–55) or moderate to severe sleep problems (CSHQ > 55) for both internalizing and externalizing behaviours composites.

In an intriguing investigation of the effect of sleep on autism symptoms, Schreck et al. looked at parent reports of sleep problems in 55 children aged 5–12 years diagnosed with ASD (Schreck et al. 2004). They found that increased communication problems were predicted by a combination of increased sensitivity to stimuli in the sleeping environment and periods of screaming during the night. Screaming during the night together with fewer hours slept per night also predicted increased stereotypic behaviour. Finally, fewer hours of sleep per night alone predicted more difficulties with social interactions and overall ASD symptoms as measured by the GARS (Gilliam Autism Rating Scale) (Gilliam 1995), a parent report questionnaire that provides scores on four subscales and an overall autism quotient (AQ).

Hoffman et al. report a similar finding. They enrolled 80 children ranging from 4 to 15 years of age in their study focused on examining the relations between ASD characteristics and sleep problems (Hoffman et al. 2005). ASD characteristics were assessed using the GARS (Gilliam 1995). They report that sleep-disordered breathing scores of the CSHQ predicted GARS scores for stereotyped behaviour and social interaction, a combination of the parasomnias and sleep duration scores predicted developmental disturbances, and a combination of sleep-disordered breathing and parasomnia scores predicted AQ. The authors speculate that sleep-disordered breathing and parasomnias would both affect sleep duration, suggesting that sleep deprivation may be a factor in the relation between poor sleep and increased ASD behaviour.

In a study using the same methodology, Tudor et al. examined the relation between sleep problems on the CSHQ and autistic characteristics assessed via the GARS with 80 children who had ASD but no comorbid developmental disabilities (Tudor et al. 2014). In this sample, stereotyped behaviour scores on the GARS were predicted by sleep onset delay scores, social interaction scores were predicted by a combination of sleep onset delay and night waking scores, communication scores were predicted by sleep anxiety and parasomnia scores, and AQ WAS predicted by sleep onset delay scores alone. This group also proposes that these results support the theory that lack of sleep is the underlying factor in the relation between sleep problems and severity of autistic behaviour.

These findings are significant because they suggest that, not only do sleep problems increase general problem behaviour, they may also increase autism-specific behaviours that are problematic. This possibility definitely deserves further study. From a clinical perspective, this small group of studies suggests it may be worthwhile considering sleep problems when trying to uncover the reason for increased behaviour problems or autistic behaviour. From the opposite perspective, decreases in these behaviors may be a sign that interventions aimed at improving sleep are working. This may be particularly helpful when the sleep problem in question (e.g. parasomnias, night waking) may not be easy to monitor to determine efficacy of the intervention.

Studies of Adults

As in other areas of sleep problem research, fewer studies have examined the impact of sleep problems on adults with ID. An early study in a UK health district investigated the relation between sleep problems and challenging behaviour in 205 individuals living in community housing (Brylewski and Wiggs 1999). They ranged from 21 to 83 years of age. Using the Aberrant behavior Checklist, the authors determined that residents who had sleep problems were more likely to show aggression, self-injury and screaming and they showed more severe forms of these behaviours. They were not more likely to be noncompliant. They also scored higher on the Aberrant behavior Checklist factor scores for irritability, stereotypies and hyperactivity but not lethargy or inappropriate speech.

Over 10 years later, Matson et al. investigated this in 168 adults with ASD and ID using the DASH-II to assess sleep problems, which incorporates both frequency, duration and severity of behaviours (Matson et al. 2008). They found a relationship between the degree of sleep problems and number of problem behaviours. Those with a mild sleep problem had an average of eight problem behaviours whereas those with a moderate sleep problem had a mean of 15 problem behaviours. There were multiple significant relationships between sleep problems and problem behaviour, regardless of whether the sleep problems were mild, moderate or severe. For example, those with mild difficulties getting to sleep showed more unusual play with objects, inappropriate sexual behaviour, throwing objects at others and yelling or shouting at others, whereas those with moderate or severe problems with waking up, screaming or crying showed more kicking objects, banging objects with their hands, leaving supervisions or caregiver without permission and yelling or shouting at others.

Shortly afterwards, Lenjavi et al. studied 20 women with developmental disabilities residing in an institution (Lenjavi et al. 2010). Maladaptive behaviour was recorded daily for 4 months along with nightly sleep/wake logs. For each, specific maladaptive behaviours were monitored. These included head banging, hitting, kicking, scratching, biting or grabbing others; throwing objects, screaming, other forms of self-injury. They report that reduced sleep efficiency was related to maladaptive behaviour up to 8 days following a specific night observed. Conversely, maladaptive behaviour up to 8 days prior to a specific night of sleep decreased sleep efficiency. The authors suggest that this means there is a chronic relationship between the two.

Only one study could be found that reports no relation between sleep problems and problem behaviour. It included 79 adults aged 18–65 with Prader-Willi syndrome. Maas et al. found no relation between sleep problems and behaviour problems (Maas et al. 2010). However, it is possible that this is due, in part, to methodological differences. They assessed settling problems, sleep apnoea and daytime sleepiness only, whereas other studies have also examined night waking, parasomnias and early morning waking.

This small group of studies provides some evidence that sleep problems lead to problem behaviours for adults with ID as much as they do for children. One difference appears to be that the behaviours observed in adults with sleep problems appear to have more of an aggressive nature to them. This may reflect the fact that the adults studied tended to not reside in family homes, suggesting they may have more severe ID or more pre-existing behavioural problems. However, longitudinal research would provide a better indication of whether this is the case, or whether there is a developmental pattern in the relation between sleep and problems behaviour.

Studies of Self-Injurious Behaviour

Several studies have examined the relation between sleep problems and self-injurious behaviour. Two of these included children. Didden et al. did not report a relation between having a severe sleep problem and scores for self-injury on the aberrant behaviour checklist among the 286 children age 1–19 years with mild to profound ID in their study (Didden et al. 2002b). In another study that included 54 children with Cornelia de Lange syndrome, Hall et al. also report that the presence of self-injury was not related to having sleep problems and the severity of sleep problems was not related to severity of sleep problems (Hall et al. 2008). They assessed sleep problems with an adapted version of the Infant Sleep Questionnaire that includes 10 items to assess sleep problems over the past month and self-injury was determined through a standardized interview. Thus, the available information at this time does not suggest that sleep problems are related to increased self-injury in children.

One study has examined this question with adults. Symons et al. studied 30 individuals with profound ID who displayed chronic severe self-injury and 30 matched controls with profound ID who did not (Symons et al. 2000). They ranged in age from 25 to 69 and resided in a large residential centre in the midwest USA. Participants' behaviour related to sleep was recorded every 30 min from 23:00 to 07:00 nightly for 60–330 nights. Those who self-injured slept almost 30 min less per night than their counterparts who did not self-injure. Age, and whether individuals were taking medication, were not related to time sleeping. Perhaps most interesting, the authors report that the variability in sleep patterns was significantly larger for those who self-injured. Although no data were collected detailing why the individuals with SIB had less sleep and more variability in their sleep pattern, these results do suggest that poor sleep may be a contributor to self-injury in adults with ID.

In addition to the fact that this sample was adult, it is possible that the fact that Symon et al.'s study was based on direct observation, rather than questionnaires, lead to the different results. More comprehensive studies such as this may be needed to definitively determine whether sleep problems lead to self-injury or increased frequency, intensity or quality of self-injury.

Executive Function

Although parents and caregivers anecdotally report that their child or client with ID does not perform as well cognitively when they have sleep problems, there have been few studies examining this. Two studies that examined the relation between sleep problems and intelligence test scores (IQ) did not find a significant relationship in children with ID (Richdale et al. 2000) and ASD (Taylor et al. 2012). However, one study has reported relations. In their very well-designed study, Chen et al. enrolled 29 adolescents and young adults with Down syndrome living at home with their parents (Chen et al. 2013). Having more problems with sleep initiation and maintenance, based on responses to the sleep questionnaire (Simonds and Parraga 1982), was associated with having poorer verbal fluency and having obstructive sleep apnoea was associated with several executive functioning tasks the participants completed, including verbal fluency and inhibition. The authors speculate that their results raise the possibility that obstructive sleep apnoea may impact prefrontal cortex development in individuals with Down syndrome.

Because so few studies exist, no conclusions can be drawn at this time regarding the effect of sleep problems on executive function in those with ID specifically. However, based on the literature with the general population, there are likely to be some impacts. These may be attenuated in this population because their abilities are more limited, leading to floor effects. Conversely, the tenuousness of their cognitive function may also make them more susceptible to negative impacts due to sleep problems.

Development and Adaptive Function

Only two studies could be found that have investigated the relation between sleep problems and adaptive functioning in those with ID, both involving children with ASD. With their large group of 1193 children aged 4–10 years with ASD, Sikora et al. used the Vineland Adaptive Behavior Scales, Second Edition (VABS-II) (Sparrow et al. 2005) to elicit parent report of adaptive function in relation to sleep problems assessed with the CSHQ (Sikora et al. 2012). They grouped children into two groups; preschoolers (age 4–5 years) and school-age children (6–10 years). They then grouped the children as being good sleepers (CSHQ total score of 40 or less), having mild sleep problems (CSHQ total score of 41–55) or having moderate to severe sleep problems (CSHQ total score greater than 55). Using multivariate analyses of variance, they investigated the effects of sleep group, across the sample and by age group, on VABS-II composite scores, reflecting overall adaptive function, as well as on the functional domains of communication, daily living skills and socialization. Their results indicated that good sleepers had higher VABS-II composite scores than both mild and moderate/severe sleep problem groups. This was also the case for daily living skills. However, in relation to communication and socialization, good sleepers differed from the moderate/severe problem group, but the mild group did not differ from moderate/severe group.

Looking at age groups, Sikora et al. also found that, within the preschool group, there were differences among the three groups on communication (Sikora et al. 2012). However, only the good sleeper group and moderate/severe groups differed in socialization, not the good sleeper and mild groups. For school-age children, the good sleepers differed from the moderate/severe group on communication and socialization, but not daily living skills. There were no differences between mild and moderate/severe problem groups on the domain scores within the age groups, suggesting that the severity of sleep problems was not as important within the age groups. For the sample as a whole, poorer communication and socialization was found with a sleep problem, regardless of its severity.

In a second study published the same year, Taylor et al. also examined this question in children with ASD by collecting data from a diagnostic database at a paediatric disability assessment clinic (Taylor et al. 2012). Parents of the 335 children (219 with ASD, 116 with PDD-NOS) had completed questionnaires regarding sleep, as well as standardized measures of adaptive function. Their results indicated that more hours slept predicted better daily living skills and more hours slept combined with fewer night wakings predicted better communication skills.

These early results do suggest that sleep problems may impact functioning. Although there are only two studies, both included large samples and used well-validated measures of adaptive behaviour. Perhaps the most important limitation of the two investigations is that they both included children with ASD. Because this group within the ID population have specific patterns of adaptive functioning strengths and weaknesses, it is possible that these results do not apply to children with ID due to other aetiologies. The lack of adult studies is also important. Although most adults in the general population have developed adult-level skills, those with ID may continue to develop skills well into adulthood. It would be important to know whether they too have that development attenuated by sleep problems. Similarly, it would be helpful to know if the loss of skills that happens in older adults is affected by their sleep problems.

In summary, studies have found that sleep problems are associated with problems in behaviour for those with ID across the lifespan. The exact relation, however, is not yet known. We also do not know whether specific sleep problems lead to behaviour problems or whether sleep problems are a surrogate for sleep deprivation. It is also not clear which aspects of behaviour are most affected by sleep problems. We know less about the impact of sleep on cognitive, executive and adaptive functioning. This lack of research in this area is very relevant. Those with ID experience high rates of sleep problems. They also have deficits in functioning that reduce their quality of life and can increase the burden of families and caregivers. A better understanding of the relation between sleep problems and function could be vital to improving their daily function, and, ultimately their development. Until then, it is prudent to assume that the impacts are likely to be the same as, or greater than, that reported for the general population and to take action appropriately.

Treatment

Wiggs has suggested that one reason that children with ID are not routinely treated for sleep problems is that professionals lack training (Wiggs 2001). However, she also posits that parents may view these problems as longstanding and unsolvable because they are a part of the child's underlying condition. Both views have some support in the small literature that exists. Studies have shown that parents have been given inappropriate advice, that parents have not all sought help, and that parents may feel some approaches to managing sleep problems are unacceptable to them. They also feel that they need information and treatment that is specific to their child. For example, Adkins et al. (Adkins et al. 2012) enrolled 36 children aged 2–10 years with ASD in a study where parents were randomly assigned to receive an educational pamphlet or no intervention. Follow-up revealed no differences between groups, and parents who had been given the pamphlet indicated they would prefer a more individualized approach. In contrast, Colville reports on five children provided an individualized behavioural intervention for sleep problems by a psychologist over a 6-week period. It included both home visits and telephone contact. Reducing night wakings was the most common goal. All but one showed clinically significant improvement during treatment. In the three cases that were followed up, some gains were maintained (Colville et al. 1996). These results suggest that treatment for sleep problems in those with ID most likely requires an individualized approach that includes several modalities and is matched to each individual's unique limitations and abilities, as well as the goals and situation of their family or caregivers.

Studies Examining Treatment Rates and Parent Reported Effectiveness

Several studies have examined the efforts of parents to manage sleep problems in their child with ID and their perceptions of the treatments' effectiveness and acceptability. As these studies describe, parents' views are mixed. Wiggs and Stores (Wiggs and Stores 1996b) found that only 47 % of 124 parents of children with ID due to mixed aetiologies had received advice or treatment for their child's sleep problems. Of these, 36 % had been offered medication, 27 % behavioural techniques and 24 % both. More parents reported that the behavioural advice had been helpful (79 %) than medication (58 %) or medication and behavioural advice combined (15.5 %). Of the 92 with a current sleep problem, only 55 % said they wanted help in addressing it. Interestingly, parents' reasons for the failure of behavioural interventions fell into several broad categories: (1) parents had tried the intervention as instructed but felt it did not work; (2) parents felt that the programme was not appropriate for the child (e.g. did not accommodate for medical conditions); (3) parents were actually given incorrect advice; or (4) parents felt the advice was unacceptable because it conflicted with their approach to parenting. These categories of views provide some indication of why so few parents indicated they would like help for their child's current sleep problem, because they suggest a frequent mismatch between child and treatment, poor advice or a treatment that was difficult for parents to maintain sufficiently long to see progress. This may, in turn, make them less likely to repeat attempts to manage sleep problems.

Keenan et al. looked at the issue of parental acceptance of sleep problem interventions in an even more detailed way. They explored this in a study of 58 parents of children age 1–19 years of age who had developmental disabilities and were experiencing a sleep problem (Keenan et al. 2007). They assessed parents' beliefs about their child's sleep problem as well as their perception of psychological/behavioural treatment or taking melatonin for sleep. They report that 60 % of parents had sought help for sleep problems in the past, with 27.6 % having had psychological/behavioural help, 17.2 % melatonin and 13.8 % other medications. Of those who had tried treatment, 60 % thought it had been helpful. Most parents indicated they believed their child's sleep problem was chronic, to have severe consequences and to be curable or controllable. Parents' acceptability ratings of psychological/

behavioural treatment and melatonin did not differ significantly. However, they did indicate they believed melatonin would be more effective in the short term, but that it would have more side effects. Further, parents who had rated their child's sleep problem as more severe tended to rate melatonin acceptability higher. Parents' past experiences with either treatment type were not related to their preferences for current treatment. This latter result suggests a lack of overwhelming belief in the efficacy of their child's past treatment approach, because they did not have strong feelings that they would return to that modality.

Williams et al. also studied parent perceptions of sleep problem treatment (Williams et al. 2006), but focused on parents of children with ASD. Their sample included 127 parents of children with ASD and ID and 75 whose child had ASD only. Parents were first asked about the type of behavioural treatments they had tried in the past. The most common were a regular bedtime (92 %), a regular waking time (78 %), a darkened room (76 %), reading a story (76 %), taking toys to bed (71 %), using a night-light (68 %), restricting caffeine (66 %) and a quiet time before bed (65 %). Fewer parents reported having tried medication; 35 % of parents had tried diphenhydramine, 23 % clonidine, 16 % melatonin and 7 % chloral hydrate. Twenty-one percent had tried other medications.

The authors report that parents rated a regular bedtime as most effective of the behavioural interventions (78 %), followed by sleeping in the parents' bed (72 %) and wrapping the child in a blanket (61 %). There were few differences in the ratings of effectiveness between the groups of children with and without ID. However, using a night-light and reading a story were viewed as less effective for children with ID, whereas playing music was more often effective for children with ID. No significant differences were found in the reported effectiveness of medications based on whether the child had ID or not. In the full sample, 63 % found clonidine helpful, 57 % chloral hydrate and 38 % melatonin. Williams et al. point to the interesting finding that some of the interventions that were used relatively less, such as wrapping the child in a blanket, were perceived as more effective by parents. It is also important to note that taking the child into a parent's bed was deemed relatively effective, although this action is most often viewed as a type of sleep problem by health professionals. One can assume that parents' goal is for their child to sleep, and they are prepared to offer this option to make that happen. It is also interesting to note that a regular bedtime was rated so highly. This leads to questions regarding whether irregular bedtimes may be more common when a child has ID. It may be that bedtime resistance and other behaviours lead parents to be less consistent in this aspect of sleep than parents of TD children.

Unfortunately, no studies have examined concerns of caregivers or family members of adults with ID in relation to treatment approaches and efficacy for sleep problems. It would be helpful to know the views of caregivers who work with adults in community homes or residential settings. These caregivers often work with their clients over many years and can gain perspective on the strategies that are most helpful and those that are most easily implemented. Managing sleep problems in an adult with ID who is living at a residential home provides some advantages, because staff in these settings may have more access to professionals to advise them.

However, it may also be more challenging because of the involvement of multiple caregivers in some situations, which may make implementation of behavioural approaches that require consistency more difficult. Nonetheless, these three studies raise some important issues regarding treatment for sleep problems in children with ID. Although behavioural approaches appear to have been tried more frequently, parents are not necessarily averse to medication and do not feel that behavioural approaches have always been effective. A brief overview of the behavioural and pharmacological approaches that have been investigated in studies of people with ID follows below. It is important to note that this is not an exhaustive review and not all available treatments have been researched in this population.

Behavioural Interventions for Sleep Problems

Most research investigating the effects of behavioural strategies for sleep problems have involved children and describe case series. Behavioural approaches to sleep problems require that parents make changes to the events leading up to their child going to bed, to their reaction when their child does not sleep or to their reaction when their child wakes at night or too early in the morning. Because of this, parents carry the burden of implementing treatment and their belief in the strategies used is essential to success. This is particularly important because many interventions do not lead to positive, sustained results unless the strategies are used consistently and for some time, typically several weeks. Thus, parents are faced with making changes that may not provide immediate results, and, in some cases, may lead to a short-term exacerbation of problems.

Sleep Hygiene

At the most basic level, sleep hygiene should be considered and addressed before other changes are made. This can often be quite simple, most often involving changes to routines and the environment to facilitate better sleep onset and maintenance. Jan et al. provide an excellent review of sleep hygiene for children with neurodevelopmental disabilities (Jan et al. 2008). Common sleep hygiene practices include taking actions to provide a good sleep environment. For example, sleeping position and bedding can be very important for individuals with ID. Jan et al. note that the high rate of medical and physical conditions in this group mean that positioning may have a serious impact on comfort. For example, individuals with ID may be immobile, requiring turning by a parent. They may also have other motor disorders, such as cerebral palsy, that may make it difficult for the child to turn voluntarily or may make finding a comfortable position difficult. Other medical problems that are common for children with ID that may make positioning important include gastroesophegeal reflux, seizures, respiratory disorders and pressure sores.

Jan et al. also propose that the sleeping environment may also have a significant impact on sleep and sleep problems. Those with ID who are mobile may wander at night. This may necessitate a bed designed to contain them to prevent injury. Although these may be purchased, they can be expensive for many families. This can lead them to improvise, to keep their child's door locked or to allow their child to sleep in the parent's bed so that they are aware when the child wakes and moves. Lighting is another relevant environmental factor. Many children with ID can be anxious and prefer to sleep with lights turned on or with a night-light. This can cause problems for melatonin levels and disrupt circadian-mediated sleep onset. Similarly, the common practice of providing sensory objects for young children, such as music boxes and mobiles, may not be appropriate for those with ID who may be more easily overstimulated. The presence of televisions and computers in older children's rooms may also cause problems with overstimulation at bedtime, or when children awake and use these during the night, just as in the general population. Jan et al. suggest that white noise machines, although not researched with this population, are often reported to be helpful, especially for children who tend to easily become overstimulated.

Sleep hygiene can be a good first step for most children or adults with ID when sleep problems occur. Although the strategies may appear simple, they can eliminate possible factors that are creating or exacerbating sleep problems. Parents and caregivers can generally use sleep hygiene approaches recommended for children and adults in the general population, as most require changing the environment, not the individual's behaviour. Thus, there should generally be no constraint on their effectiveness due to the individual's intellectual level or physical functioning. It is also advised that these approaches be attempted under the supervision of a clinician who can help parents or caregivers to implement them in a staged fashion, while monitoring impact, so that it will be apparent which strategies lead to improvement and whether they are additive.

Functional Assessment as a Foundation for Treatment Selection and Implementation

Once basic environmental factors have been dealt with, it is important to understand the aetiology and function of sleep problems prior to developing a behavioural treatment. As mentioned by some parents in Wiggs and Stores' study (Wiggs and Stores 1996b), some strategies may not be appropriate for a specific child due to medical conditions. Approaches may also have to account for the individual's cognitive limitations. Other factors, such as sensory processing disorders, may make some treatments ineffective or intolerable for some people. Because of that, and the multiple potential contributors to sleep problems, a functional analysis is a good way to start (Didden et al. 2002a). This can involve a detailed interview with parents. Use of a standardized tool, such as the CSHQ can also help fully capture all possible sleep problems, as typically more than one exists.

Didden et al. conducted a functional assessment for four individuals with ID age 1–25 years living with their family (Didden et al. 2002a). Three had problems with night waking and two with settling. However, it became apparent that the onset of the settling problems for two children may have been related to an early childhood illness and insistence at that time on having a parent with them at bedtime. Extinction was used for all four. This is a procedure whereby parental attention when the individual is not settling or is awake is minimized. In these cases, parents were instructed to not re-enter their family member's room after putting them to bed until morning. If the individual did not show problems over the night, they were told so in the morning and that they had earned positive attention. Importantly, in one case, medication was also deemed appropriate in addition to extinction. This demonstrates how individuals may have multiple factors contributing to sleep problems. In one case, night waking increased in the short term, known as a "burst", before decreasing. This highlights the fact that response can also vary from individual to individual. In this study, extinction was applied fully from the onset, without gradual implementation. Didden et al. report that parents found this stressful, worrying that they may traumatize their family member. This is an important consideration when one decides to use extinction. Parent acceptance will impact their ability to stay with the treatment and to implement it correctly. In some cases, graduated extinction, withdrawing the positive reinforcement of a behaviour, which in this study and in many cases of sleep problems is parent attention, in a stepped fashion.

Behavioural Approaches That Have Been Studied in Children

Extinction was also used with a larger group of five children with ASD, one with Asperger's syndrome and seven with Fragile X syndrome in a study by Weiskop et al. (Weiskop et al. 2005). They also determined that child behaviours were being reinforced by parent response, either attention or co-sleeping. Parents were provided with three training sessions that covered learning theory principles, including the role of antecedents and consequences on behaviour. Parents were also helped to improve sleep hygiene and taught how to use modelling to teach their child about the new bedtime routines. Finally, they were taught how to utilize rewards to positively reinforce desirable behaviour at bedtime. Given a choice of graduated extinction or standard extinction, all parents chose standard extinction.

The authors provide results for 10 participants who completed the training and data collection. Seven children displayed an extinction burst, an increase in sleep problems with initiation of treatment. However, all participants showed improvement over the treatment period in the goals that were set by their parents. This was maintained at 3 month follow-up for seven of the children and at 12 month follow-up for all four who provided data. Weiskop et al. note that extinction was not effective for early morning waking. They posit that this is because it was not maintained by parent attention prior to the treatment.

Another study, including five children with Angelman syndrome, combined sleep hygiene changes, extinction and sleep scheduling in combination (Allen et al.

2013). All children showed disruptive bedtime behaviour and/or sleep onset problems. None were going to sleep independently. Sleep hygiene changes included ensuring that there was low or no light and auditory stimulation (television, music) and ensuring temperature was appropriate in the child's room. Extinction included ignoring the child once he or she was in bed. In this case, extinction was less stringent. Parents were permitted to check on their child if the child was calm and quiet, thereby reinforcing sleep compatible behaviours. Finally, sleep scheduling was used to alter bedtimes. Sleep scheduling typically refers to making changes in the time an individual is put in bed, or leaves bed, so that minimal time is spent in bed awake. For example if a child usually is awake 60 min after they are put in bed, their bedtime is moved to a later time closer to their actual sleep onset time. Most often, this results in a shorter sleep onset latency. Once that is established, the bedtime can be moved earlier in small increments, typically 30 min. In this study, parents were asked to put their child to bed 30 min after they typically were asleep. The authors report that all children were sleeping independently at the end of the treatment, had CSHQ scores that had moved from the "problem sleeper" to "nonproblem sleeper" range, and had markedly reduced disruptive behaviour during the day. Although the design of the study makes it impossible to know which of the three components of the treatment had the greatest impact, this combination of sleep hygiene changes, sleep scheduling and extinction is one that is often employed clinically.

Christodulu and Durand followed a similar procedure with four children with developmental disabilities 2–5 years of age (Christodulu and Durand 2004). All showed disruptive behaviour at bedtime, irregular sleep schedules and night wakings. In this study, changes were made to bedtime routines first. Once these were established, sleep restriction was implemented. This refers to reducing the amount of time a person is allowed in bed to a portion of their typical sleep time, often 90 %. For example if a child falls asleep inconsistently between 8:00 and 11:00, but typically sleeps 8 h, they could be put on a sleep restriction schedule where they are put in bed at 11:30 and woken at 7:00 every morning. It is expected that this will increase their drive to sleep. Once the person is falling asleep well, the bedtime can be moved in a stepwise manner to a time more preferred by parents. This type of approach is commonly used when sleep onset and night waking problems are reported.

All children showed less disruptive behaviour at bedtime after treatment. All also showed a reduction in the frequency and duration of night wakings. Thus, the combination of good sleep hygiene and restricting the time that children spent awake in bed was successful in reducing sleep problems. As with Allen et al.'s study (Allen et al. 2013), this study does not allow for determination of which component of the treatment was most effective. However, visual data presented in the report suggest that there was an additive effect.

Interestingly, the results also indicated that three children were sleeping 30–90 min less after the treatment. This could reflect the fact, as posited by the authors, that their sleep quality was now improved. They were also awake less during the night, so that almost all time in bed was time asleep. The authors indicate no child appeared to be having problems due to the reduced sleep, although it was also below a level that was developmentally typical.

In a clinical setting, it may be important as part of assessment to determine why parents have selected a specific bedtime for their child. In some cases, parents may be following cultural norms, accommodating parent work schedules (e.g. some parents who work into the evening want their child to be awake when they get home), or following guidelines from family members, healthcare providers or other sources. In some cases, however, parents of children with ID may be inclined to put their child to bed at a time that is not typical for the child's chronological age. In some cases, parents have not changed the bedtime as the child has aged, perhaps because they are basing bedtime on the child's developmental age. In other cases, clinicians may sense that putting the child to bed provides respite from the stresses of parenting a very high-needs child. It is important that, in these cases, a discussion be held with the parents regarding the benefits and costs of a later bedtime that goes smoothly, versus an earlier bedtime that is wrought with conflict.

Other case reports also reveal success using behavioural techniques, including sleep scheduling for night waking (Durand and Christodulu 2004; DeLeon et al. 2004), and self-injury upon waking (DeLeon et al. 2004), extinction for disruptive bedtime behaviour, sleep onset problems and night waking (Curfs et al. 1999; Didden et al. 2004) and even use of social stories for one young boy with ASD who had several sleep problems (Moore 2004).

This is a small literature, primarily of case reports and case series. In all, only several dozen children with ID have taken part in research regarding behavioural treatment of sleep problems. This is a serious gap in the literature given the prevalence of the problem in this group. It is also troubling because so many parents have indicated they have used behavioural approaches (Wiggs and Stores 1996b; Keenan et al. 2007; Williams et al. 2006), when so little research exists to guide them or the professionals who are recommending the treatment.

Behavioural Approaches That Have Been Studied in Adults

A group from the Netherlands studied 41 individuals, living in residential centres, who were provided with an individualized treatment (Hylkema and Vlaskamp 2009). In the group, 7 individuals had moderate ID, 17 severe and 17 profound. Ten had a diagnosis of ASD. They ranged in age from 8 to 66 years, with only seven being under age 18, primarily adolescents. The residents took an average 50 min to fall asleep nightly, and spent an average of over 11 h in bed each night, but were asleep only approximately 8 h of that time. Fifteen were provided sleep scheduling, 11 with increased activity during the day, 9 with both sleep scheduling and increased activity during the day, 2 with a different daily routine and the remainder other behavioural approaches. After treatment, which lasted approximately 22 weeks for each individual, 15 individuals were being put in bed at a more age appropriate time, later in all cases. In addition, 80.5 % spent less time in bed awake, and 85.3 %

had a shorter sleep onset latency, with most showing an improvement in both. Of the group, 13 had epilepsy, and the authors report that the treatment was less effective for this subgroup. The authors also note that after treatment the average time spent in bed awake was still 2 h per night, more than is desirable. However, they cite agreements with families, unique individual schedules and workload issues as contributors to this.

In a second study with adults, Gunning and Espie provided nine adults with sleep problems with a 4-week behavioural intervention (Gunning and Espie 2003). They were selected from a pool of 118 individuals attending an adult training centre, based on the presence of a significant sleep problem. They ranged from 20 to 47 years of age. Two had a diagnosis of mild ID, three moderate and four severe. The individuals attended the weekly 60 min treatment sessions with a caregiver. The treatment included information on sleep hygiene, scheduling and relaxation (progressive muscle relaxation) with some cognitive behavioural therapy (CBT) components regarding psychopathological and psychological factors than can interfere with sleep. Six of the individuals had at least one significant change in sleep problems. Of these, two had improved sleep onset latency, two had fewer times getting out of bed before sleep onset, one had less day-time napping, one had less time spent in bedtime rituals and one had less consumption of caffeine during the day. Although this study showed some positive effects, they were not overwhelming. This may be due to the manner in which it was delivered. First, in three cases where individuals had mild/moderate ID, their caregiver was minimally involved in the treatment. Second, only four 60 min sessions were provided, which appears much less than that reported in others studies (Colville et al. 1996; Hylkema and Vlaskamp 2009).

As with children, the literature regarding behavioural approaches to sleep problems in adults with ID is seriously lacking. These two studies suggest some efficacy for changes in sleep scheduling. However, it is also apparent that some sleep problems in adults with ID may be due, in part, to their spending an excessive amount of time in bed. This may require institutional culture to change, rather than individual treatment. It is interesting that increased daily activity was helpful in one study, as this also suggests that the programming offered to those with ID who are not living at home may actually contribute to sleep problems. This also means that institution wide changes, such as more programming involving physical activity, may alleviate some sleep problems in these settings.

Treatment for individuals with ID may also require intensive long-term training, with an adult caregiver or parent taking the lead role, as evidenced by the inconsistent results in Gunning and Espie's study. They provided only four sessions and some individuals with ID took the lead in their education and treatment. Given that those with ID have cognitive limitations that will affect their learning rate and style, more time, simplified information and other adaptations to the material taught and method of instruction may need to be applied to psychological approaches to sleep problems.

Pharmacological Treatment Approaches

There appears to be much more research on use of medication for sleep problems in individuals with ID than use of non-pharmacological approaches. In a recent review regarding pharmacological treatment of sleep problems in children, Hollway and Aman report that they identified 58 studies that included children or adults, which investigated use of medications for dyssomnias or parasomnias that interfere with sleep onset or maintenance (Hollway and Aman 2011). Most (58 %) focused on children. They conclude that melatonin has the most empirical evidence to support its use in children with ID and suggest that it should be considered the first line of treatment when behavioural approaches have not been successful. The authors suggest that other commonly used medications, including diphenhydramine, clonidine, zolpidem and benzodiazepines have either insufficient evidence to support use or have some evidence of negative side effects, including effects on sleep architecture.

Hollway and Aman's conclusions regarding melatonin coincide with the conclusions of Braam et al.'s meta-analysis of melatonin for sleep problems in people with ID conducted 2 years earlier (Braam et al. 2009). In nine studies with 183 participants, they found that melatonin decreased sleep latency by an average of 34 min, increased time asleep by an average of 50 min and significantly reduced the number of wakings per night. It is important to note that only one of the studies included a significant number of adults (Braam et al. 2008). Further, the doses given, time of administration and the aetiology of ID in the studies found differed. Thus, they indicate further research is needed to determine dose and administration recommendations.

Despite the lack of evidence, many studies of sleep problems in children and adults with ID report that a healthy proportion are using, or have used, medications. For example, Kronk et al. report that 19 % of their sample of 90 children with Fragile X were taking medication for sleep, including melatonin ($n=8$), clonidine ($n=3$) and 1 each risperidone, quetiapine, aripiprazole, mirtazapine and buspirone (Kronk et al. 2009). All had clinically significant sleep problems as measured on the CSHQ. Medication had been used by 5 % of those age 3–6 years, 32 % of 7–11-year-olds and 20 % of 12–17-year-olds.

An even larger proportion (37.3 %) of those in another study of 59 children with ASD had used medication (Souders et al. 2009). In that study, 15 had used melatonin, 3 clonidine, 4 risperidone, 2 aripiprazole, 1 hydroxyzine and 1 fluoxetine. Polimeni et al. report that of the 53 children with ASD in their study, 50 % had attempted medication treatment. In that same study, of the 52 children with AD, 43 % had tried medication (Polimeni et al. 2005). In a study of 167 children with ID and/or ASD aged 5–18 who attended a health service in the UK (Rzepecka et al. 2011) only 13.7 % were using melatonin. Williams et al., who asked parents of children with ASD with and without ID about their use of interventions report that 16 % of their sample had tried melatonin (Williams et al. 2004).

In a study including both children and adults, Colville et al. report that 52 of the 80 parents of individuals with Sanfillipo syndrome age 4–26 years had used medication for sleep problems at some point (Colville et al. 1996). However, participants did not appear to feel medication was a long-term solution. Twenty-two parents said it was useful as a last resort, for short periods or for times when problems were severe. Of the 79 adults with Prader-Willi syndrome in another study, only 1 was using melatonin, 3 modafinil, 1 temazepam and 1 venlaflaxine for sleep (Maas et al. 2010).

The success of medication for sleep problems has varied, according to family reports. In Taylor et al.'s study, children with ASD who were taking medication for sleep continued to have more sleep problems than children who were not (Taylor et al. 2012). In the Williams et al. study, only 38% reported melatonin effective (Williams et al. 2004). In Polimeni's study, the average rating of success or medication by parents of children with ASD on a 0–7 scale was 3.95, and for parents of children with AD it was 3.96.

This research suggests that medication is a common approach for parents and caregivers attempting to manage sleep problems in those with ID. The results, however, are mixed. On the positive side, Braam et al.'s meta-analysis of melatonin for sleep indicates there is some efficacy. Why so many parents report that melatonin was not effective is not clear. Because melatonin is an over-the-counter medication in North America, it may be that it is not used optimally. Parents may not have the guidance of a physician in making decisions about dose and timing of administration. Some authors have also noted that the improvements in sleep for children with ID taking melatonin are variable (Appleton et al. 2012). To investigate this, Appleton et al. conducted a randomized controlled trial of melatonin with 110 children age 3–15 years with neurodevelopmental disabilities. Those in the treatment group received an initial dose of .5 mg, which could increase up to 12 mg over the first 3 weeks. They found a 22.4 min improvement in sleep time based on diaries and 13.3 min improvement based on actigraphy for those taking melatonin relative to placebo and accounting for baseline. Although this was statistically significant, it was not clinically significant. Similarly, Gingras et al. report, based on the same trial, that improved sleep onset was accompanied by a mean earlier waking of 29.9 min (Gringras et al. 2012). Thus, it is possible that many parents who have tried melatonin with their children found that the changes were too small to be deemed a success. This may be one reason for discontinuation being common. Very recently, Braam has also proposed that the presence of a single nucleotide polymorphism in those with ASD may be linked to slow metabolism of melatonin, reducing its effectiveness over time (Braam et al. 2013). In summary, although the existing data do suggest that melatonin is effective for those with ID, especially children, the effects may not be clinically significant for many. This does not mean that melatonin should not be considered. However, it may be best used as part of a multi-modal treatment. Parents and caregivers should also be advised that it is not a "magic pill".

The literature regarding treatment for sleep problems in those with ID is in its naissance. There a very small number of studies of psychological or behavioural treatment, and most provide case reports or case series with no quantitative evaluation of the treatment effectiveness. The samples used also vary widely, and the techniques evaluated vary. Nonetheless, parents do report that these approaches can be helpful. In particular, extinction techniques for settling problems and sleep onset problems appear to hold promise. The limitations of behavioural approaches lay in the demands they place on parents and caregivers. This suggests that professional involvement to help parents implement, maintain and adapt these techniques is essential.

The literature regarding medication treatment is somewhat larger. However, most has focused on melatonin. The results point to melatonin having some effectiveness, although the effects may not always be as large as parents hope for or need to feel the treatment was effective. Other medications used for sleep, primarily off-label, have not been investigated with this population. Thus, there is no evidence base upon which to make recommendations regarding their use.

Conclusions

Almost all of us have experienced a sleep problem or cared for an individual with a sleep problem. When these are transient, we typically recover and do not seek help. This is not the case for many individuals with ID and their parents or caregivers. They may have chronic sleep problems that persist for years, disrupting their behaviour and function, and causing significant disruption for those who care for them.

This chapter has provided an overview of the existing literature regarding sleep problems in those with ID. It is admittedly small. Despite this, several basic facts appear to have some evidence to support them. Sleep problems are inarguably more common for children with ID who are school age and older than their TD same age peers. Sleep problems in adults with ID are also prevalent; however, there are no direct comparisons at this time to know whether they differ in frequency from same-age peers. Nonetheless, it is likely that they do differ in quality. Whereas existing reports suggest that adults with ID appear to still experience sleep problems commonly seen in children, such as settling problems and sleeping in a parent's bed, those in the general population rarely display these, but may have more sleep problems related to life stress and lifestyle. Thus, although the rate of sleep problems may not differ between adults with ID and their peers without ID, it is very likely the nature of the problems does differ.

There are a growing number of studies of individuals with ID due to specific aetiologies. In terms of determining whether a given diagnosis increases risk for sleep problems, there are some hints this may be the case, but the evidence is still inconclusive. Until further research is conducted where groups can be compared based on identical methodologies, we should not base assessment or treatment on the handful of studies that have been conducted with a group with a specific diagnosis. Similarly, the literature that has accumulated does not suggest that specific characteristics of these individuals put them at greater risk for sleep problems, with one exception. Health problems, and particularly those that cause pain or discomfort, do appear to be linked to increased sleep problems, although the specific nature of the problems most exacerbated by this is not yet clear. Given this relation between pain and sleep is common in the general population, this is not unexpected.

The research to date does suggest that sleep problems do have consequences for those with ID. The greatest impact appears to be on their problem behaviour. This is not surprising. This information can be useful for management of either sleep or behaviour problems. Sleep problems can be addressed as part of a programme to manage problem behaviour. Likewise, behaviour can be monitored to assess the effectiveness of strategies aimed at improving sleep.

This chapter finished with a brief review of the research regarding treatment for sleep problems in those with ID. It is undeniably sparse. However, two approaches do hold promise. Although the studies of behavioural treatments, extinction and sleep scheduling/restriction in particular, are few, they have been successful with some. Parents also report that many have tried these, suggesting they are open to them. However, as suggested by some authors, individualized treatment may be needed to have success. This may also promote parent or caregiver adherence and long-term results. Thus, a clinician trained in behavioural techniques' should be included in attempts to use these techniques with this population. Melatonin also appears to show some effectiveness, although there is some suggestion that this may wear off in time for some. Unfortunately, there is not good information regarding dose and timing of administration. Thus, a physician should guide and monitor use of this approach with individuals with ID to ensure that these are optimal. This may be especially important because parents and caregivers may be quick to deem this approach as ineffective without knowing whether use was optimal.

Good sleep is a pleasure and a need. Poor sleep is unpleasant and a burden. Because those with ID have increased risk for sleep problems from very early childhood, they may not be aware of the contrast between these two, which means they may not seek help. Instead, their behaviour most often alerts us once sleep problems are entrenched and significant. It would be useful to include education about sleep and sleep problems as part of routine clinical visits to help alert parents to the potential signs of problems early, to provide them with information regarding typical sleep patterns for children and to encourage good basic sleep habits such as good sleep hygiene and parenting strategies that minimize positive attention for sleep problems. This type of education and coaching may provide the ounce of prevention that is worth more than extraordinary "cures" once problems are deep-rooted.

References

Adkins, K. W., Molloy, C., Weiss, S. K., Reynolds, A., Goldman, S. E., Burnette, C., et al. (2012). Effects of a standardized pamphlet on insomnia in children with autism spectrum disorders. *Pediatrics, 130*(Suppl 2), 139–S144.

Allen, K. D., Kuhn, B. R., DeHaai, K. A., & Wallace, D. P. (2013). Evaluation of a behavioral treatment package to reduce sleep problems in children with Angelman Syndrome. *Research in Developmental Disabilities, 34,* 676–686.

Aman, M. G., & Singh, N. N. (1986). *Manual for the Aberrant Behavior Checklist.* East Aurora: Slosson Educational Publications, Inc.

Annaz, D., Hill, C. M., Ashworth, A., Holley, S., & Karmiloff-Smith, A. (2011). Characterisation of sleep problems in children with Williams syndrome. *Research in Developmental Disabilities, 32,* 164–169.

Appleton, R. E., Jones, A. P., Gamble, C., Williamson, P. R., Wiggs, L., Montgomery, P., et al. (2012). The use of Melatonin in children with neurodevelopmental disorders and impaired sleep: A randomised, double-blind, placebo-controlled, parallel study (MENDS). *Health Technology Assessment, 16,* i–239.

Ashworth, A., Hill, C. M., Karmiloff-Smith, A., & Dimitriou, D. (2013). Cross syndrome comparison of sleep problems in children with Down syndrome and Williams syndrome. *Research in Developmental Disabilities, 34,* 1572–1580.

Bartlett, L. B., Rooney, V., & Spedding, S. (1985). Nocturnal difficulties in a population of mentally handicapped children. *British Journal of Mental Subnormality, 31,* 54–59.

Batista, B. H., & Nunes, M. L. (2007). Evaluation of sleep habits in children with epilepsy. *Epilepsy & Behavior, 11,* 60–64.

Boyle, A., Melville, C. A., Morrison, J., Allan, L., Smiley, E., Espie, C. A., et al. (2010). A cohort study of the prevalence of sleep problems in adults with intellectual disabilities. *Journal of Sleep Research, 19,* 42–53.

Braam, W., Didden, R., Smits, M., & Curfs, L. (2008). Melatonin treatment in individuals with intellectual disability and chronic insomnia: A randomized placebo-controlled study. *Journal of Intellectual Disability Research, 52,* 256–264.

Braam, W., Smits, M. G., Didden, R., Korzilius, H., Van Geijlswijk, I. M., & Curfs, L. M. (2009). Exogenous melatonin for sleep problems in individuals with intellectual disability: A meta-analysis. *Developmental Medicine & Child Neurology, 51,* 340–349.

Braam, W., Keijzer, H., Struijker, B. H., Didden, R., Smits, M., & Curfs, L. (2013). CYP1A2 polymorphisms in slow melatonin metabolisers: A possible relationship with autism spectrum disorder? *Journal of Intellectual Disability Research, 57,* 993–1000.

Breau, L. M., & Camfield, C. S. (2011). Pain disrupts sleep in children and youth with intellectual and developmental disabilities. *Research in Developmental Disabilities, 32*(6), 2829–2840.

Breau, L. M., McGrath, P. J., Camfield, C. S., & Finley, G. A. (2002). Psychometric properties of the non-communicating children's pain checklist-revised. *Pain, 99,* 349–357.

Breslin, J. H., Edgin, J. O., Bootzin, R. R., Goodwin, J. L., & Nadel, L. (2011). Parental report of sleep problems in Down syndrome. *Journal of Intellectual Disability Research, 55,* 1086–1091.

Brylewski, J. E., & Wiggs, L. (1998). A questionnaire survey of sleep and night-time behaviour in a community-based sample of adults with intellectual disability. *Journal of Intellectual Disability Research, 42*(Pt 2), 154–162.

Brylewski, J. E., & Wiggs, L. (1999). Sleep problems and daytime challenging behaviour in a community-based sample of adults with intellectual disability. *Journal of Intellectual Disability Research, 43,* 504–512.

Buckley, A. W., Rodriguez, A. J., Jennison, K., Buckley, J., Thurm, A., Sato, S., et al. (2010). Rapid eye movement sleep percentage in children with autism compared with children with developmental delay and typical development. *Archives of Pediatrics & Adolescent Medicine, 164,* 1032–1037.

Carter, M., McCaughey, E., Annaz, D., & Hill, C. M. (2009). Sleep problems in a Down syndrome population. *Archives of Disease in Childhood, 94,* 308–310.

Chen, C. C., Spano, G., & Edgin, J. O. (2013). The impact of sleep disruption on executive function in Down syndrome. *Research in Developmental Disabilities, 34,* 2033–2039.

Christodulu, D. V., & Durand, V. M. (2004). Reducing bedtime disturbance and night waking using positive bedtime routines and sleep restriction. *Focus on Autism and Other Developmental Disabilities, 19,* 130–139.

Colville, G. A., Watters, J. P., Yule, W., & Dax, M. (1996). Sleep problems in children with Sanfilippo syndrome. *Developmental Medicine & Child Neurology, 38,* 538–544.

Cotton, S. M., & Richdale, A. L. (2010). Sleep patterns and behavior in typically developing children and children with autism, Down syndrome, Prader-Willi syndrome and intellectual disability. *Research in Autism Spectrum Disorders, 4,* 490–500.

Couturier, J. L., Speechley, K. N., Steele, M., Norman, R., Stringer, B., & Nicolson, R. (2005). Parental perception of sleep problems in children of normal intelligence with pervasive developmental disorders: Prevalence, severity, and pattern. *Journal of the American Academy of Child & Adolescent Psychiatry, 44,* 815–822.

Curfs, L. M., Didden, R., Sikkema, S. P., & De Die-Smulders, C. E. (1999). Management of sleeping problems in Wolf-Hirschhorn syndrome: A case study. *Genetic Counseling, 10,* 345–350.

DeLeon, I. G., Fisher, W. W., & Marhefka, J. M. (2004). Decreasing self-injurious behavior associated with awakening in a child with autism and developmental delays. *Behavioral Interventions, 19,* 111–119.

Didden, R., Curfs, L. M., van, D. S., & de Moor, J. M. (2002a). Sleep problems in children and young adults with developmental disabilities: Home-based functional assessment and treatment. *Journal of Behavior Therapy and Experimental Psychiatry, 33,* 49–58.

Didden, R., Korzilius, H., van Aperlo, B., van Overloop, C., & de Vries, M. (2002b). Sleep problems and daytime problem behaviours in children with intellectual disability. *Journal of Intellectual Disability Research, 46,* 537–547.

Didden, R., de Moor, J. M., & Curfs, L. M. G. (2004a). Behavioral treatment of sleep problems in three children with developmental disabilities. *British Journal of Developmental Disabilities, 50(1),* 13–19.

Didden, R., Korzilius, H., Smits, M. G., & Curfs, L. M. (2004b). Sleep problems in individuals with Angelman syndrome. *American Journal on Mental Retardation, 109,* 275–284.

Durand, V. M., & Christodulu, D. V. (2004). Description of a sleep-restriction program to reduce bedtime disturbances and night wakening. *Journal of Positive Behavior Interventions, 6,* 83–91.

Einfeld, S. L., Tonge, B. J., & Florio, T. (1994). Behavioural and emotional disturbance in fragile X syndrome. *American Journal of Medical Genetics, 51*(4), 386–391.

Ghanizadeh, A., & Faghih, M. (2009). The impact of general medical condition on sleep in children with mental retardation. *Sleep and Breathing, 15,* 57–62.

Gilliam, J. E. (1995). *Gilliam Autism Rating Scale: Examiners Manual.* Austin, TX: Pro-Ed Publishers.

Goodlin-Jones, B., Schwichtenberg, A. J., Iosif, A. M., Tang, K., Liu, J., & Anders, T. F. (2009). Six-month persistence of sleep problems in young children with autism, developmental delay, and typical development. *Journal of the American Academy of Child & Adolescent Psychiatry, 48,* 847–854.

Gringras, P., Gamble, C., Jones, A. P., Wiggs, L., Williamson, P. R., Sutcliffe, A., et al. (2012). Melatonin for sleep problems in children with neurodevelopmental disorders: Randomised double masked placebo controlled trial. *British Medical Journal, 345,* e6664.

Gunning, M. J., & Espie, C. A. (2003). Psychological treatment of reported sleep disorder in adults with intellectual disability using a multiple baseline design. *Journal of Intellectual Disability Research, 47,* 191–202.

Hall, S. S., Arron, K., Sloneem, J., & Oliver, C. (2008). Health and sleep problems in Cornelia de Lange Syndrome: A case control study. *Journal of Intellectual Disability Research, 52,* 458–468.

Harvey, M. T., Baker, D. J., Horner, R. H., & Blackford, J. U. (2003). A brief report on the prevalence of sleep problems in individuals with mental retardation living in the community. *Journal of Positive Behavior Interventions, 5,* 195–200.

Hemmingsson, H., Stenhammar, A. M., & Paulsson, K. (2009). Sleep problems and the need for parental night-time attention in children with physical disabilities. *Child: Care, Health and Development, 35,* 89–95.

Hoffman, C. D., Sweeney, D. P., Gilliam, J. E., Apodaca, D. D., Lopez-Wagner, M. C., & Castillo, M. M. (2005). Sleep problems and symptomology in children with autism. *Focus on Autism and Other Developmental Disabilities, 20,* 194–200.

Hoffman, C. D., Sweeney, D. P., Gilliam, J. E., & Lopez-Wagner, M. C. (2006). Sleep problems in children with autism and in typically developing children. *Focus on Autism and Other Developmental Disabilities, 21,* 146–152.

Hollway, J. A., & Aman, M. G. (2011). Pharmacological treatment of sleep disturbance in developmental disabilities: A review of the literature. *Research in Developmental Disabilities, 32,* 939–962.

Honomichl, R. D., Goodlin-Jones, B. L., Burnham, M., Gaylor, E., & Anders, T. F. (2002). Sleep patterns of children with pervasive developmental disorders. *Journal of Autism and Developmental Disorders, 32,* 553–561.

Hylkema, T., & Vlaskamp, C. (2009). Significant improvement in sleep in people with intellectual disabilities living in residential settings by non-pharmaceutical interventions. *Journal of Intellectual Disability Research, 53,* 695–703.

Jan, J. E., Owens, J. A., Weiss, M. D., Johnson, K. P., Wasdell, M. B., Freeman, R. D., et al. (2008). Sleep hygiene for children with neurodevelopmental disabilities. *Pediatrics, 122,* 1343–1350.

Keenan, R. A., Wild, M. R., McArthur, I., & Espie, C. A. (2007). Children with developmental disabilities and sleep problems: Parental beliefs and treatment acceptability. *Journal of Applied Research in Intellectual Disabilities, 20,* 455–465.

Krakowiak, P., Goodlin-Jones, B., Hertz-Picciotto, I., Croen, L. A., & Hansen, R. L. (2008). Sleep problems in children with autism spectrum disorders, developmental delays, and typical development: A population-based study. *Journal of Sleep Research, 17,* 197–206.

Kronk, R., Dahl, R., & Noll, R. (2009). Caregiver reports of sleep problems on a convenience sample of children with fragile X syndrome. *American Journal on Intellectual and Developmental Disabilities, 114,* 383–392.

Lenjavi, M. R., Ahuja, M. A., Touchette, P. E., & Sandman, C. A. (2010). Maladaptive behaviors are linked with inefficient sleep in individuals with developmental disabilities. *Journal of Neurodevelopmental Disorders, 2,* 174–180.

Luiselli, J. K., Magee, C., Sperry, J. M., & Parker, S. (2005). Descriptive assessment of sleep patterns among community-living adults with mental retardation. *Mental Retardation, 43*(6), 416–420.

Maas, A. P., Grossfeld, P. D., Didden, R., Korzilius, H., Braam, W. J., Smits, M. G., et al. (2008). Sleep problems in individuals with 11q terminal deletion disorder (Jacobsen syndrome). *Genetic Counseling, 19,* 225–235.

Maas, A. P., Didden, R., Korzilius, H., Braam, W., Smits, M. G., & Curfs, L. M. (2009). Sleep in individuals with cri du chat syndrome: A comparative study. *Journal of Intellectual Disability Research, 53,* 704–715.

Maas, A. P., Sinnema, M., Didden, R., Maaskant, M. A., Smits, M. G., Schrander-Stumpel, C. T., et al. (2010). Sleep disturbances and behavioural problems in adults with Prader-Willi syndrome. *Journal of Intellectual Disability Research, 54,* 906–917.

Maas, A. P., Didden, R., Korzilius, H., & Curfs, L. M. (2012). Exploration of differences in types of sleep disturbance and severity of sleep problems between individuals with cri du chat syndrome, Down's syndrome, and Jacobsen syndrome: A case control study. *Research in Developmental Disabilities, 33,* 1773–1779.

Matson, J. L. (1995). *Diagnostic Assessment for the Severely Handicapped -II.* Baton Rouge: Scientific Publishers.

Matson, J. L., Ancona, M. N., & Wikins, J. (2008). Sleep disturbances in adults with autism spectrum disorders and severe intellectual disabilities. *Journal of Mental Health Research in Intellectual Disabilities, 1,* 129–139.

Mayes, S. D., & Calhoun, S. L. (2009). Variables related to sleep problems in children with autism. *Research in Autism Spectrum Disorders, 3,* 931–941.

Meltzer, L. J., & Mindell, J. A. (2006). Sleep and sleep disorders in children and adolescents. *Psychiatric Clinics of North America, 29,* 1059–1076.

Moore, P. S. (2004). The use of social stories in a psychology services for children with learning disabilities. A case study of a sleep problem. *British Journal of Learning Disabilities, 32,* 133–138.

Owens, J. A., Spirito, A., & McGuinn, M. (2000). The Children's Sleep Habits Questionnaire (CSHQ): Psychometric properties of a survey instrument for school-aged children. *Sleep, 23,* 1043–1051.

Piazza, C. C., Fisher, W., Kiesewetter, K., Bowman, L., & Moser, H. (1990). Aberrant sleep patterns in children with the Rett syndrome. *Brain & Development, 12*(5), 488–493.

Piazza, C. C., Fisher, W. W., & Kahng, S. W. (1996). Sleep patterns in children and young adults with mental retardation and severe behavior disorders. *Developmental Medicine & Child Neurology, 38,* 335–344.

Polimeni, M. A., Richdale, A. L., & Francis, A. J. (2005). A survey of sleep problems in autism, Asperger's disorder and typically developing children. *Journal of Intellectual Disability Research, 49,* 260–268.

Quine, L. (1991). Sleep problems in children with mental handicap. *Journal of Mental Deficiency Research, 35*(Pt 4), 269–290.

Quine, L. (2001). Sleep problems in primary school children: Comparison between mainstream and special school children. *Child: Care, Health and Development, 27,* 201–221.

Richdale, A. L. (2003). A descriptive analysis of sleep behavior in children with Fragie X. *Journal of Intellectual & Developmental Disability, 28,* 135–144.

Richdale, A., Francis, A., Gavidia-Payne, S., & Cotton, S. (2000). Stress, behaviour, and sleep problems in children with an intellectual disability. *Journal of Intellectual & Developmental Disability, 25,* 147–161.

Rzepecka, H., McKenzie, K., McClure, I., & Murphy, S. (2011). Sleep, anxiety and challenging behaviour in children with intellectual disability and/or autism spectrum disorder. *Research in Developmental Disabilities, 32,* 2758–2766.

Schreck, K. A., & Mulick, J. A. (2000). Parental report of sleep problems in children with autism. *Journal of Autism and Developmental Disorders, 30,* 127–135.

Schreck, K. A., Mulick, J. A., & Smith, A. F. (2004). Sleep problems as possible predictors of intensified symptoms of autism. *Research in Developmental Disabilities, 25,* 57–66.

Sikora, D. M., Johnson, K., Clemons, T., & Katz, T. (2012). The relationship between sleep problems and daytime behavior in children of different ages with autism spectrum disorders. *Pediatrics, 130*(Suppl 2), 83–S90.

Simonds, J. F., & Parraga, H. (1982). Prevalence of sleep disorders and sleep behaviors in children and adolescents. *Journal of the American Academy of Child Psychiatry, 21*(4), 383–388.

Souders, M. C., Mason, T. B., Valladares, O., Bucan, M., Levy, S. E., Mandell, D. S., et al. (2009). Sleep behaviors and sleep quality in children with autism spectrum disorders. *Sleep, 32,* 1566–1578.

Sparrow, S. S., Cicchetti, D. V., & Balla, D. A. (2005). *Vineland-II Adaptive Behavior Scales.* Circle Pines: American Guidance Service.

Stores, G., & Stores, R. (2013). Sleep disorders and their clinical significance in children with Down syndrome. *Developmental Medicine & Child Neurology, 55,* 126–130.

Symons, F. J., Davis, M. L., & Thompson, T. (2000). Self-injurious behavior and sleep disturbance in adults with developmental disabilities. *Research in Developmental Disabilities, 21,* 115–123.

Taylor, M. A., Schreck, K. A., & Mulick, J. A. (2012). Sleep disruption as a correlate to cognitive and adaptive behavior problems in autism spectrum disorders. *Research in Developmental Disabilities, 33,* 1408–1417.

Tudor, M. E., Walsh, C. E., Mulder, E. C., & Lerner, M. D. (2014). Pain as a predictor of sleep problems in youth with autism spectrum disorders. *Autism: The International Journal of Research and Practice.*

van Litsenburg, R. R., Waumans, R. C., van den, B. G., & Gemke, R. J. (2010). Sleep habits and sleep disturbances in Dutch children: A population-based study. *European Journal of Pediatrics, 169, 1009–1015.*

Vladovinos, M. G., Caruso, M., Roberts, C., Kim, G., & Kennedy, C. H. (2005). Medical and behavioral symptoms as potential side effects in adults with developmental disabilities. *American Journal on Mental Retardation, 110,* 164–170.

Weiskop, S., Richdale, A., & Matthews, J. (2005). Behavioural treatment to reduce sleep problems in children with autism or fragile X syndrome. *Developmental Medicine & Child Neurology, 47,* 94–104.

Wiggs, L. (2001). Sleep problems in children with developmental disorders. *Journal of the Royal Society of Medicine, 94*, 177–179.

Wiggs, L., & Stores, G. (1996a). Severe sleep disturbance and daytime challenging behaviour in children with severe learning disabilities. *Journal of Intellectual Disability Research, 40*(Pt 6), 518–528.

Wiggs, L., & Stores, G. (1996b). Sleep problems in children with severe intellectual disabilities: What help is being provided? *Journal of Applied Research in Intellectual Disabilities, 9*, 160–165.

Williams, P. G., Sears, L. L., & Allard, A. (2004). Sleep problems in children with autism. *Journal of Sleep Research, 13*, 265–268.

Williams, G., Sears, L. L., & Allard, A. (2006). Parent perceptions of efficacy for strategies used to facilitate sleep in children with autism. *Journal of Developmental and Physical Disabilities, 18*, 25–33.

Young, D., Nagarajan, L., de Klerk, N., Jacoby, P., Ellaway, C., & Leonard, H. (2007). Sleep problems in Rett syndrome. *Brain & Development, 29*, 609–616.

Part III
Medical Disorders

Chapter 7
Epilepsy

Megan A. Hattier, Lauryn M. Toby and Lindsey W. Williams

Introduction

Epilepsy is currently the most common serious neurological condition, affecting nearly 70 million people in the world. In high-income countries, approximately 6 per 1000 people will develop epilepsy during their lifetime, and 45 people per 100,000 will develop new-onset epilepsy each year. These figures are nearly twice as high in low- and middle-income countries (Brodie et al. 2012). Epilepsy is also the most common serious neurological disorder affecting people with intellectual disabilities (ID), with prevalence rates reaching up to 30 times higher than the general population rate (Espie et al. 2003). Epilepsy in people with ID is more difficult to manage, and several studies have reported increased risk of epilepsy with increased severity of ID (Bowley and Kerr 2000; Corbett 1993; Kerr et al. 1996). As such, when considering individuals with ID, it is important to acknowledge the potential for the occurrence of comorbid epileptic seizures and the complex array of factors that may accompany such a dual diagnosis.

Therefore, the following review outlines the current types and classifications of epileptic seizures, provides information regarding the prevalence and etiology of epilepsy in the ID population, reviews assessment methods and diagnostic considerations, and presents current treatment options from relevant literature. These options may include psychopharmacological methods, surgical procedures as well as various alternative treatments (i.e., dietary and neurobehavioral). Furthermore, the potential for additional psychopathology commonly associated with the

M. A. Hattier (✉)
Department of Psychology, Johns Hopkins School of Medicine, Baltimore, MD, USA
e-mail: megan.h.binder@gmail.com

L. M. Toby
Neurobehavioral Unit—Outpatient Clinic, Department of Behavioral, Psychology Kennedy Krieger Institute, Johns Hopkins University School of Medicine, Baltimore, MD, USA

L. W. Williams
Department of Psychology, Louisiana State University, Baton Rouge, LA, USA

J. L. Matson, M. L. Matson (eds.), *Comorbid Conditions in Individuals with Intellectual Disabilities,* Autism and Child Psychopathology Series,
DOI 10.1007/978-3-319-15437-4_7

co-occurrence of epilepsy and ID is discussed. Finally, the psychosocial impact of the presence of comorbid epilepsy and ID is considered, including individual and familial stressors that may commonly occur.

The International League Against Epilepsy (ILAE) has defined *epilepsy* as a chronic condition of the brain characterized by an enduring propensity to generate epileptic seizures and lead to neurobiological, cognitive, psychological, and/or social consequences due to the condition. In practice, this diagnosis implies two or more spontaneous seizures in a greater than 24-h period. Similarly, the ILAE describes an epileptic *seizure* as "a transient occurrence of signs and/or symptoms due to abnormal excessive and synchronous neuronal activity in the brain" (Fisher et al. 2005, p. 471). An epileptic seizure can consist of impaired higher mental function or altered consciousness, involuntary muscle movements or cessation of movement, sensory or psychic experiences, or autonomic disturbances. Seizures typically occur as a combination of dysfunctions and a progression of signs and symptoms. Furthermore, epileptic seizures occur with a variety of diseases and disorders that alter neuronal functioning and produce epileptogenic activity. The behavioral features of an epileptic seizure typically tend to reflect the functions of the cerebral areas where the abnormal neuronal activity originates and spreads (Engel 2013).

Types of Seizures and Symptom Expression

A simplistic view of brain disturbances is that they consist of either neuronal under-activity, giving rise to negative signs and symptoms such as paralysis and blindness, or over-activity, giving rise to positive signs and symptoms, the most common of which are epileptic seizures (Engel 2013). In general, the nervous system has a limited repertoire of responses to injury or stimuli. During an epileptic seizure, neuronal activity either increases or decreases, leading to symptoms such as paralysis, blindness, rigidity, hemiballismus, spasticity, overall weakness, and coma. The occurrence of an epileptic seizure is generally characterized as either brief, intermittent, spontaneous, or paroxysmal (implying a sudden or severe event). In addition, status epilepticus refers to either a prolonged seizure or repeated epileptic seizures lasting for over 30 min, without intervening recovered consciousness.

Terms commonly associated with the description of epileptic seizures include ictal, postictal, and interictal. An *ictal* event refers to the epileptic seizure itself. *Postictal* phenomena are transient abnormalities in brain function that appear after the ictal event has ended. The time during which postictal symptoms persist (a few seconds to a few days) is called the postictal period. The *interictal* period is the time between the resolution of postictal abnormalities and the beginning of the next ictal event (this term applies only to patients with recurrent epileptic seizures; Engel 2013).

Many specific types of seizures may occur in individuals with epilepsy, often reflecting different pathological mechanisms. The ILAE publishes the International Classification of Epileptic Seizures, first introduced in 1970 and revised in 1981.

This classification scheme is based on distinctive behavioral and electrophysiological features of epileptic ictal events. Table 7.1 lists the current classification of epileptic seizure types.

Epileptic seizures are commonly divided into *focal* (previously known as partial) seizures or *generalized* seizures, the former referring to seizures that originate in a part of only one hemisphere, while the latter describes a seizure originating simultaneously in both hemispheres (Berg et al. 2010). However, this distinction has become problematic over the years due to the fact that focal seizures are almost always due to widespread areas of cerebral dysfunction and are not necessarily localized as the name implies. Many seizures are preceded by something known as an *aura.* An aura is a warning that precedes an epileptic seizure, and can include specific sensations or mood changes that can begin up to several hours before the seizure's onset.

Focal seizures are then commonly further divided into *simple focal* seizures (i.e., without impairment of consciousness) and *complex focal* seizures (i.e., with impairment of consciousness). Most focal-onset seizures arise in the temporal or frontal lobes. Features of temporal lobe seizures include flushing, pupillary dilatation,

Table 7.1 ILAE International Classification of Epileptic Seizures (1981)

1. Partial (focal, local) seizures
a. Simple partial seizures
i. With motor signs
ii. With somatosensory or special sensory symptoms
iii. With autonomic symptoms or signs
iv. With psychic symptoms
b. Complex partial seizures
i. Simple partial onset followed by impairment of consciousness
ii. With impairment of consciousness at onset
c. Partial seizures evolving to secondarily generalized seizures
i. Simple partial seizures evolving to generalized seizures
ii. Complex partial seizures evolving to generalized seizures
iii. Simple partial seizures evolving to complex partial seizures evolving to generalized seizures
2. Generalized seizures (convulsive or nonconvulsive)
a. Absence seizures (formally petit mal)
i. Typical absences
ii. Atypical absences
b. Myoclonic seizures
c. Clonic seizures
d. Tonic seizures
e. Tonic–clonic seizures (formerly grand mal)
F. Atonic seizures (astatic seizures; drop attacks)
3. Unclassified epileptic seizures

apnea, and heart rate changes. Motor phenomena during the seizure may include lip smacking, nose wiping, hand automatisms, and upper limb dystonic posturing. Frontal lobe seizures include a variety of seizure types, and may manifest as limb jerking spreading from the hand to the whole side of the body; others may manifest as forced head and eye turning with arm jerking or elevation.

Generalized seizures are further divided into absence seizures (i.e., brief lapses in consciousness), minor motor events (e.g., myoclonic and atonic), and major motor events (e.g., tonic, clonic, and tonic–clonic). *Absence* seizures are typically characterized by an abrupt loss of consciousness, with momentary loss of contact and cessation of activity. There may be eyelid myoclonus, altered axial tone, and even automatisms. Atypical absence seizures are more prolonged, have less abrupt onset and offset, and are often associated with myoclonus and changes in muscle tone.

Other generalized seizures include *myoclonic* seizures, typically involving brief limb jerks, especially of the arms. *Tonic–clonic* seizures manifest as loss of consciousness followed by a "tonic phase" (i.e., extension and stiffening, sometimes with a cry, cyanosis, and tongue biting) followed by the "clonic phase" (i.e., rhythmical jerking of the limbs). There may be injuries and incontinence. Afterwards, patients are drowsy, and report headache and aching muscles. *Tonic* seizures manifest as a tonic muscle contraction of the limbs and trunk, with altered consciousness and often a fall with potential for injury. Finally, *atonic* seizures are caused by an abrupt loss of muscle tone, and often result in falls or injury.

The 1981 ILAE Classification scheme, although widely used across the world, has been criticized because post hoc etiologic information from observers and EEG data are often required to use it properly, and as noted above the dichotomy of "partial/focal" versus "generalized" is problematic in its anatomic implications. Furthermore, the division of partial/focal seizures into "simple" and "complex" falsely created the impression that impairment of consciousness had certain implications related to limbic system involvement. Research over the past 20 years has yielded detailed investigations of the anatomic substrates of ictal semiology, and results have strongly suggested that the fundamental mechanisms of limbic seizures are different from those of neocortical seizures, but both can be associated with impairment of consciousness or not. Thus, recent attempts at revising the terminology for the classification and organization of seizures and epilepsy were published by Berg et al. in 2010. These revisions can be found in Table 7.2 and have emphasized that impairment of consciousness, a focus of the 1981 classification scheme, is not a useful criterion for classifying epileptic seizure types. Additionally, effort has been made to clarify the relatively blurry distinction between focal seizures and generalized seizures, and as such the current list of recognized seizure types includes primarily types of generalized seizures, while focal seizures no longer include a simple/complex distinction.

Prevalence

As previously noted above, the frequency of epilepsy occurring in people with an ID is much higher than in the general population. Large epidemiological studies suggest

Table 7.2 ILAE classification of epileptic seizures (2010)

Generalized seizures
1. Tonic– clonic (in any combination)
2. Absence
a. Typical
b. Atypical
3. Absence with special features
a. Myoclonic absence
b. Eyelid myoclonia
4. Myoclonic
a. Myoclonic
b. Myoclonic atonic
c. Myoclonic tonic
5. Clonic
6. Tonic
7. Atonic
8. Focal seizures
9. No agreement on how best to characterize or classify
10. Epileptic spasms

that about 30% of people with ID have epilepsy, compared to 2–5% in the general population (Brodie et al. 2012). Additional data on prevalence rates can be further described by the specific disorder or genetic condition for which comorbid epilepsy is common. For example, it is estimated that epilepsy occurs in up to 13% of individuals with Down syndrome, 34–60% of individuals with Cerebral Palsy, 50% of individuals with Rett syndrome, 80% of individuals with Angelman syndrome, 28–46% of those with Prader–Willi syndrome, 80% of those with Tuberous Sclerosis, and 10–50% of individuals with Autism (Prasher and Kerr 2008; Robinson 2012). For individuals with autism spectrum disorder (ASD) and epilepsy, a study of 542 children with epilepsy showed that 5% had ASD; however, this prevalence increased to 13.8% among those who had impaired cognitive levels (Berg and Scheffer 2011).

Similar to the above findings of Berg et al., several additional studies have found that the prevalence of epilepsy is significantly associated with higher levels of cognitive impairment. This association has been found present in both children and adults with ID. This marked increase in the prevalence of epilepsy in those with more severe ID is understandable, as many have overt signs of neurological damage (McGrother et al. 2006). In addition, those conditions in which epilepsy is most commonly found tend to be genetic disorders with higher incidences of ID. For example, epilepsy is typically observed at higher rates in those individuals with Angelman syndrome, Fragile X syndrome, Down syndrome, Tuberous sclerosis, Rett syndrome, and Cerebral Palsy, and is most prevalent in those with diagnosed ID (Bowley and Kerr 2000; Clarke 1996; Matsumoto et al. 1992; Musumeci et al. 1991; Webb et al. 1991).

Etiology

Traditionally, when epileptic seizures occur as the sole manifestation of a genetic disturbance, the epileptic disorder or syndrome is said to be primary or *idiopathic*. This indicates that the condition is a direct result of a known or presumed genetic defect in which seizures are a core symptom. Idiopathic refers to a syndrome that is only epilepsy, with no underlying structural brain lesion or other neurologic signs or symptoms. Seizures that are idiopathic are presumed to be genetic and are usually age dependent. When epileptic seizures occur as symptoms of specific structural or metabolic pathology, the epileptic disorder is said to be secondary or *symptomatic*. Symptomatic refers to a syndrome in which the epileptic seizures are the result of one or more identifiable structural lesions of the brain. However, as many epileptic conditions may involve both genetic and acquired components, recent research has recommended that when an etiological designation is appropriate, the terms genetic and structural/metabolic should be used in place of idiopathic and symptomatic, which recognizes that these concepts are not dichotomous (Berg et al. 2010; Engel 2013). In addition, some types of epileptic seizures can be thought of as natural reactions to physiological stress or transient causes, and as such are typically labeled *provoked* seizures. Provoked seizures do not reflect chronic neurological disturbances, but rather may reflect various documented causes such as sleep deprivation, alcohol withdrawal, acute head trauma, and certain reversible infections.

Due to the aforementioned high prevalence rates of the occurrence of epilepsy in individuals with ID, coupled with the fact that epilepsy in people with ID is more likely to be treatment resistant (McGrother et al. 2006) and is associated with higher rates of mortality (Forsgren et al. 2005), a specific examination into the etiological relationship between epilepsy and ID appears essential. However, when it comes to discussions of etiology in the ID population, it appears as though both epilepsy and ID can be caused by a range of genetic, congenital, traumatic, and other pathological processes. It is generally accepted that epilepsy arises secondarily to brain damage or abnormality, which is typically the presumed cause of ID, but unfortunately the precise relationship between ID and epilepsy is often unclear (McGrother et al. 2006).

Epilepsy in the ID population is presumably caused by a multitude of factors that likely depend on the specific nature of the disorder or disability. Specifically, congenital brain abnormalities, developmental anomalies (e.g., cerebral palsy), or chromosomal abnormalities (e.g., Down syndrome, Fragile-X syndrome, tuberous sclerosis, or Angelman syndrome) all may account for the development of epilepsy in populations with ID. However, although these associations are assumed, exact pathways are variable and the precise mechanisms by which epilepsy may manifest are currently uncertain. For example, some evidence speculates interplay between hyper-excitable ion channels, abnormal dendritic spines, lower synaptic density, and fewer inhibitory neurons in individuals with trisomy 21 that may contribute to the development of seizures. The major question remains, though, as to how these structural and functional abnormalities are generated (Stafstrom 1993). More recent research has made substantial gains in linking the precise mechanisms by which epilepsy tends to manifest in specific genetic syndromes. Specifically, changes in the functioning of the glutamatergic and GABAergic neurotransmitter systems have been found across several ID syndromes (e.g., Rett syndrome, Fragile-X syndrome, and Angelman syndrome) and may be involved in the etiology of epilepsy and ID. The precise mechanisms connecting genetic pathology to neurotransmitter system changes and subsequent phenotypic characteristics have not yet been fully determined, but these advances in molecular biology have nonetheless helped to clarify causal links and potential pathways through which epilepsy may develop (Leung and Ring 2013).

Furthermore, interactions between astrocytes and neurons have also been found to be important in the etiology of both epilepsy and ID. Astrocytes entertain a close relationship with neurons and are critical in the regulation of excitatory synapses and the homeostasis of the internal milieu within neurons. Both of these functions may be implicated in the initiation of neuronal excitability and the maintenance of abnormal synchronized discharge. The establishment and subsequent pruning of synaptic connections within neuronal networks are guided by factors secreted by astrocytes, and defects in these processes have been linked with cognitive impairment (Kaufmann and Moser 2000). Clearly, research has not yet succeeded in fully describing how genetic mutations may have led to the presence of epileptic seizures described in these syndromes. Nonetheless, the aforementioned studies investigating what appears to be relevant pathological processes may actually imply potential therapeutic interventions that in the future may not only help manage epilepsy, but also ameliorate the harmful effects of these processes on intellectual functioning and overall quality of life. An undoubtedly important contribution towards reaching this goal is the use of appropriate and comprehensive assessment procedures that yield an accurate diagnosis and the subsequent selection of effective treatment options.

Assessment

Assessment and diagnosis of epilepsy in individuals with ID poses unique challenges. Receptive and expressive communication deficits may limit self-report, and for those with severe ID it may be impossible to obtain self-report regarding some aspects of seizures, such as auras. Furthermore, it may be difficult to obtain a complete medical history, historical description of seizures, and EEG recordings. Consequently, it is of particular importance to work closely with all primary caregivers to seek relevant information, and to actively solicit information that caregivers may not immediately regard as relevant (e.g., changes in mood and symptoms of absence seizures). The clinician may need to train caregivers in how to systematically collect data important for accurate diagnosis. Various assessment methods for determining the presence of an epilepsy diagnosis are discussed below.

Medical History and Seizure Topography

A thorough medical history of early childhood can help classify both the epileptic syndrome and, in some cases, the cause of ID. Epilepsy syndromes associated with ID include: Ohtahara's syndrome, West syndrome, Lennox–Gastaut syndrome, Dravet syndrome, Doose syndrome, early infantile epileptic encephalopathy or myoclonic encephalopathy, severe myoclonic epilepsy in infancy, epilepsy with myoclonic absences, epilepsy with myoclonic-astatic seizures (Engel 2006), and cerebral palsy (Vargha-Khadem et al. 1992). Children with autism also have an increased risk (estimated at up to 49 %) of experiencing seizures, with greatest risk during early childhood and again at adolescence (Danielsson et al. 2005). For a more inclusive list of cerebral developmental disorders and other syndromes associated with ID and seizures, along with prevalence and incidence rates, see Martin 2008. Behavioral and psychiatric history of the patient and family members should also be recorded at this time.

The medical history should outline the onset and course of epilepsy, including a thorough description of objective and subjective aspects of seizures. The clinician should also assess for changes over time in seizure frequency, changes in pre- or post-ictal events, and topographical expression of reported seizure activity. The clinician should inquire carefully about affect and behavior before and after seizures. The observant caretaker may notice nonverbal individuals giving indication of auras, such as symptoms of fear (e.g., clinging to caregiver, fearful expression, and vocalizations) or changes in consciousness before motor symptoms become apparent. Such symptoms could indicate an aura, in which case the individual or caregivers may be able to help avoid injury or to quickly administer emergency medication to prevent a partial seizure from progressing to a more generalized seizure. Commonly reported prodromal symptoms (i.e., symptoms occurring 30 min or more before seizure onset) include dysphoria, irritability, restlessness or hyperactivity, impaired concentration, dizziness, and headache (Schulze-Bonhage et al. 2006). These symptoms can be difficult to assess in individuals with severe ID or who are nonverbal, especially as caregivers may mistakenly attribute these symptoms to the ID or comorbid psychiatric diagnoses.

Possible precipitating factors should also be assessed and systematically recorded, keeping in mind that factors that precipitate seizures in some patients may decrease seizure activity in others. For example, it is not uncommon for infections or fevers to worsen seizure activity, particularly when occurring in the context of Angelman Syndrome or Dravet Syndrome (Galván-Manso et al. 2005; Genton et al. 2011). Conversely, for others, seizure activity may be tempered in the presence of infections associated with fever (Ernst 2004). Some precipitating factors may be readily apparent to caregivers, such as sensory stimuli (e.g., flashing lights). Other sensory precipitants reported in the literature include changes in temperature, intestinal or stomach distention, certain noises, or even very specific tactile sensations such as brushing ones' teeth (Kasteleijn-Nolst Trenité 2012; Navarro et al. 2006). Sleep deprivation, emotional stress, or conflict at home or work are also commonly self-reported precipitants of seizures in the non-ID population (Malow 2004; Nakken et al. 2005). However, caregivers may not think these factors are related to seizure activity and thus fail to report recent changes in the home, restless sleep, or other potentially stressful environmental events if not specifically asked. The clinician should also consider the possibility that seizures may be self-induced. This is more common in individuals with photosensitivity; epileptiform discharges may induce a pleasant feeling for some individuals and thus become reinforcing (Kasteleijn-Nolst Trenité 2012). In some cases, seizures may be induced relatively quickly; in other cases, repetitive stimulation may be necessary such as repeated rubbing of the skin (Kanemoto et al. 2001). Behaviors which self-induce seizures may look topographically identical to stereotypies common in the ID population (e.g., waving fingers in front of the eyes; Kasteleijn-Nolst Trenité 2012), requiring careful observation and differentiation by the clinician, particularly if the self-induced seizure is a simple partial seizure less likely to be readily noticed by caregivers.

In assessing the frequency and duration of seizures, one must be careful not to overlook seizures occurring during sleep or associated with wakening. In many settings, caregivers are unlikely to witness such events. Because of compromised sleep quality and postictal fatigue, sleep-associated seizures are likely to lead to daytime sleepiness as well as behavioral and cognitive changes. If sleep-associated seizures are suspected, risk of asphyxiation and falling from the bed should be assessed. Video cameras can assist in determining the presence of nighttime seizures, although a sleep study may be warranted if such seizures are suspected.

EEG and Magnetic Resonance Imaging (MRI)

In addition to obtaining a descriptive account of an individual's medical history, EEG is a critical method of assessing actual seizure seismology, though this assessment in individuals with ID may prove challenging and time intensive. By coordinating with the medical facility, caregivers can facilitate a successful procedure. Prior exposure to the environment and aspects of the EEG testing to foster familiarity with the equipment and procedures may help reduce anxiety; the individual may also be provided with comforting items during the procedure such as a favorite object to hold or a favorite playlist of music. The ease of application and time efficiency of EEG electrode caps may provide an advantage over other electrode application techniques for some individuals. Obtaining EEG recordings during sleep significantly increases the sensitivity of the EEG recording, particularly after sleep deprivation (Leach et al. 2006; Mendez and Brenner 2006; Veldhuizen et al. 1983). In some cases, this may be most readily obtained by ambulatory EEG recording under the supervision of familiar caretakers in the home environment. Ambulatory EEG monitoring can allow monitoring for longer periods of time (e.g., all night) and in the individuals' normal environment, perhaps increasing compliance for individuals distressed by medical settings. Ambulatory EEG or video-EEG monitoring can help obtain more information on seismology, discover sleep-related seizures, assess seizure correlates for use in planning surgery, differentiate between epileptic and nonepileptic seizures, and reveal subtle seizures which may have otherwise passed unnoticed.

Many of the disorders that cause both ID and epilepsy are associated with specific EEG tendencies; for example, depressed interictal amplitude is usually found over the affected hemisphere in Sturge–Weber syndrome (Arzimanoglou 1997; for additional detail on EEG characteristics in various disorders, see Martin 2008). EEG assessment is a critical method by which physicians differentiate between epileptic and nonepileptic seizures. Additionally, in individuals with ID, care must be taken to differentiate between seizures and other paroxysmal nonepileptic motor and behavior happenings. This will be discussed in more detail under the differential diagnosis section of this chapter.

MRI and computed tomography (CT) are also useful methods for identifying possible epileptogenic anomalies. MRI has the advantage of greater sensitivity and specificity to detect anomalies; on the other hand, CT scans can be conducted more rapidly due to a faster scan speed and thus can be essential in emergencies. The goal of such scans is to locate underlying epileptogenic lesions, which can help in the diagnosis of particular epileptic syndromes and etiologies. If a confined epileptogenic lesion is identified, surgery may be possible for individuals with otherwise unmanageable epilepsy.

Differential Diagnosis

The diagnostic process should be undertaken with great care; the risks of misdiagnosis of epileptic syndromes should not be underestimated. In all individuals, misdiagnosis can lead to inappropriate medical treatments resulting in deleterious side effects of antiepileptic drugs (AEDs). Side effects can be difficult to recognize in those with ID due to language delays or impairments in communication skills, making it difficult for these individuals to verbally express symptoms. Cognitive side effects are common with AED use (Arif et al. 2009), thus exacerbating the problems associated with unnecessary pharmacological treatment. Therefore, any diagnosis of epilepsy must not rely solely on caretaker report and medical history, but should be well supported with additional evidence.

The clinician must make a distinction between epileptic and nonepileptic seizures, keeping in mind that both epileptic and nonepileptic disorders may co-occur. This distinction is important because the treatments for seizures will differ depending on the underlying cause. Seizures that are truly epileptic in nature are distinctly marked by a hypersynchronous neuronal discharge. Nonepileptic seizures may be caused by a number of factors and are sometimes called anoxic, psychogenic, or pseudoseizures. Zuberi (2008) categorized nonepileptic seizures into six categories: syncope and anoxia, psychological disorders, disordered sleep, paroxysmal movement disorders (PMDs), migraines or related disorders, and other miscellaneous neurological events; familiarity with these categories will aide in differential diagnosis of disorders which may be misdiagnosed as epilepsy in individuals with intellectual disability. These categories will be briefly discussed below.

Syncopal Convulsions The most common nonepileptic seizure is the syncopal convulsion, caused by sudden decrease in perfusion of oxygenated blood throughout the brain (Crompton and Berkovic 2009). Crompton and Berkovic posit that syncopal attacks with associated jerking movements are likely the most common cause for misdiagnosis of epilepsy. Syncope attacks often occur with myoclonic jerks, but unlike the cortically based epileptic seizures, jerky movements during syncope are thought to be caused by brainstem activity (Lempert et al. 1994). Myoclonic jerks generally occur after about 10 s of asystole in adults, but the threshold is lower in children (Hoefnagels et al. 1991). Hoefnagels et al. (1991) outline several features which may help distinguish a syncopal convulsion from an epileptic seizure. For example, epileptic seizures may begin while standing, be cyanotic, last 5 min or more, include postictal confusion, and are more likely to involve tongue biting or incontinence. Syncopal convulsions are usually 2 min or less, begin after falling, cause pale complexion, and post-episode confusion is typically mild or absent although fatigue is common.

Syncope resulting in convulsions can be due to a number of causes. While some causes of syncopal convulsions are relatively benign, other causes may be life threatening (e.g., cardiac arrhythmias), further highlighting the importance of differential diagnosis. In some individuals, syncopal convulsions may be induced by a vasovagal response, in which case the use of a tilt table will assist differential diagnosis. Vasovagal syncope may be induced by long periods of standing motionless, pain, emotional distress, or response to the sight of blood or injury (Wieling et al. 2004). Interestingly, a majority of individuals with this vasovagal response have a close relative affected (Wieling et al. 2004). Syncopal convulsions may also be caused by hyperventilation, orthostasis, prolonged expiratory apnea, reflex anoxic syncope (RAS), or response to Valsalva maneuver. Prolonged expiratory apnea often may occur after periods of prolonged crying, tantrums, or breath holding, but may also include cardiac anomalies (DiMario 2001; Southall et al. 1985). RAS is commonly seen after a bump to the head, particularly in children. The Valsalva maneuver is performed by attempting to exhale against a closed airway; this is a technique often used, for example, to equalize pressure in the ears and sinuses during changes in air pressure. As a medical test to elicit cardiovascular response without forcing air into the Eustachian tube, one may expire against a closed glottis.

The clinician should not rule out the possibility that syncopal convulsions are self-induced, nor that both nonepileptic and epileptic seizures may occur in the same individual. For example, individuals with Rett syndrome are at an increased risk for epilepsy, but the prevalence may be overestimated due to confusion with nonepileptic seizures. In a study of 82 females with Rett syndrome and abnormal EEGs, Glaze et al. (1998) found that some individuals engaged in hyperventilation followed by Valsalva maneuver with a closed glottis, effectively obstructing cerebral circulation and inducing episodes closely resembling epileptic seizures. These episodes may, in turn, lead to an anoxic epileptic seizure, presenting a medical emergency (Horrocks et al. 2005). To further complicate differential diagnosis, individuals with Rett syndrome often engage in complex stereotypies, which may also be mistaken for seizure activity.

Psychological Causes Some behaviors resembling epileptic seizures have a more psychological basis. A variety of terms have been used to describe self-induced, nonepileptic and nonsyncopal seizures, including pseudoseizures, psychogenic nonepileptic seizures, and pseudoepileptic seizures. These episodes may differ widely in expression, and at times may share resemblance to complex motor behaviors exhibited in some frontal lobe seizures (Carreno et al. 2005). However, these types of episodes more often contain a sexual or aggressive element. Long duration, asynchronous movements, pelvic thrusting, rolling from side to side with eyes closed, memory recall, sudden cessation, and lack of postictal confusion are signs that may help distinguish pseudoseizures from epileptic seizures (Avbersek and Sisodiya 2010).

Stereotypic motor movements such as hand flapping, head banging, and body rocking are common in individuals with pervasive developmental delay and other disorders commonly occurring with ID, and these repetitive motor movements may resemble seizure activity in some individuals, making differential diagnosis in these cases important. Stereotypies frequently occur in response to excitement or anxiety, but may also be a form of self-stimulation. Self-stimulatory behavior may also be seen, often occurring with rhythmic extension of the lower limbs, hip flexion, and a distant expression (Nechay et al. 2004; Yang et al. 2005). Daydreams from which it is difficult to distract the individual may be mistaken for absence seizures; epileptic absences are likely to include mild loss of muscle tone and eye flickering, which are not seen in daydream spells. Dissociative states, perceptual disturbances, or panic attacks may also be confused with seizures, particularly since changes in perception are associated with some seizures, and panic attacks are sometimes an indicator of an epileptic seizure (Sazgar et al. 2003).

Sleep Disorders Abnormal paroxysmal episodes during sleep may be either parasomnias or seizures. The difficulty in differentially diagnosing is increased by the fact that paroxysmal, nonepileptic events during sleep are more common both in individuals with epilepsy and individuals with ID (Bisulli et al. 2010; Brylewski and Wiggs 1998). The features of nocturnal frontal lobe epilepsy are especially likely to be confused with epileptic seizures; frontal lobe seizures often occur during sleep and in many cases are entirely restricted to sleep (Derry et al. 2006). A detailed history with the use of video, EEG, or polysomnograph may be useful in differentiating sleep disorders from epilepsy. The Frontal Lobe Epilepsy and Parasomnias (FLEP) scale is an assessment tool for use in differentiating features of nocturnal frontal lobe epilepsy from those of parasomnias (Derry et al. 2006). Features which may help differentiate seizures from paroxysmal sleep disorders include the frequency and duration of events per night, the stage of sleep in which the events arise, presence of stereotypies, characteristics of vocalizations, and what aspects of the event, if any, are later recalled by the individual. Disorders to consider during differential diagnosis include non-Rapid Eye Movement (REM) partial arousal disorders, REM sleep disorders, sleep-wake transition disorders, and narcolepsy.

Movement Disorders PMDs share many characteristics with seizures, and in the past were often mistaken as such. Indeed, the clinical distinctions between PMDs and seizures are not entirely clear (Swoboda et al. 2000). While both epileptic seizures and PMDs are associated with unusual motor movements, epileptic seizures are coupled with abnormal, hypersynchronous cortical discharges, and PMDs are generally not associated with epileptiform discharges. However, the distinction between the two disorders is challenged by reports of interictal EEG abnormalities in persons with PMDs, and the beneficial response to AEDs by persons with PMDs (Berkovic 2000). Epilepsy syndromes and PMDs may co-occur in the same individual, or more frequently, in separate individuals within the same families (Swoboda 2000). Generally, diagnostic distinctions between PMDs and epileptic seizures include the frequency of antecedent triggers and preserved consciousness during paroxysmal dyskinesias and ataxias. As an example, paroxysmal exercise-induced dyskinesia is marked by a clear antecedent (i.e., exercise), followed by dystonia in the exerted muscle after at least 10–15 min of exercise. However, identifying triggers and assessing states of consciousness may be more challenging within the context of ID. Careful data recording by caregivers may help identify antecedent triggers.

Hemiplegic Migraine and Alternating Hemiplegia Familial hemiplegic migraine is a subtype of migraine with aura, in which hemiplegia is a defining characteristic of the aura. Affected individuals may also have episodic or nonepisodic ataxia (Koeppen 2003). This disorder has an autosomal dominant pattern of inheritance.

Alternating hemiplegia is rare disorder that also has an autosomal dominant inheritance. Alternating hemiplegia is characterized by episodes of hemiplegia lasting from a few minutes to several days. Common symptoms include cognitive impairment, gait and balance issues, and excessive sweating. Symptoms are observed before 18 months of age and often co-occur with other paroxysmal disorders including dystonia, nystagmus, and strabismus. A clue to differential diagnosis is that in alternating hemiplegia, symptoms resolve after falling asleep although they may come back 10–20 min after waking during prolonged episodes (Bourgeois et al. 1993). The clinician should bear in mind, however, that alternating hemiplegia often co-occurs with epilepsy and changes in consciousness during episodes are thought to be epileptic in nature (Sweney et al. 2009).

Other Neurologic Events Tics are marked by strong subjective urges to produce the tic movement, although the urges can be suppressed to some degree. In typically developing individuals, the subjective urge and the ability to suppress tics in some instances are key diagnostic features that easily differentiate tics from seizures. In individuals with ID, however, neither the subjective experience of the compulsion nor the ability to suppress the action may be readily apparent. Ideally, an EEG recording would be obtained during a tic, perhaps accompanied by video recording.

Myoclonus is a brief, involuntary twitching of a muscle or group of muscles. Myoclonic jerks are not uncommon; for example, both hiccups and hypnic jerks while falling asleep can be considered brief myoclonic episodes. However, myoclonic jerks can also signify a number of neurological disorders, including epilepsy, multiple sclerosis, Creutzfeldt–Jakob disease, serotonin toxicity, Alzheimer's disease, and Parkinson's disease. Myoclonus is common in situations involving reduced cortical inhibition of brainstem and spinal reflexes, as may be seen in cerebral palsy or microcephaly (Zuberi 2008). EEG recordings can differentiate epileptic from nonepileptic myoclonus.

Cataplexy is a sudden episode of muscle weakness, commonly but not always occurring within the context of narcolepsy. Cataplexy without narcolepsy is rare but may be seen in disorders commonly associated with ID, including Prader–Willi syndrome, Norrie disease, and Niemann–Pick type C. Emotional triggers, such as laughing or emotional shock, usually precede a cataplectic episode. In cataplexy without narcolepsy, conscious awareness is maintained throughout the episode, differentiating cataplexy from epileptic seizures (Krahn et al. 2005). In Coffin–Lowry syndrome, cataplectic episodes are triggered by laughter and the startle response (Crow et al. 1998; Stephenson et al. 2005).

Glut-1 deficiency syndrome is a genetic disorder that has only recently been described and researched. At least three different phenotypes have emerged, all of which are marked by movement disorders that could be mistaken for epileptic seizure activity. The first phenotype is marked by encephalopathy, epileptic seizures, and paroxysmal events such as atonic drop attacks and cyanotic spells (Wang et al. 2005). Interestingly, patients in this first phenotypic group either did not respond to or experienced worsened symptoms when given AEDs including phenobarbital, but responded to a ketogenic diet (Wang et al. 2005). The second phenotype is marked by ID, dysarthria, and sporadic ataxia, but no seizures. The third phenotype described by Wang et al. (2005) is characterized by choreoathetosis, atonia, and developmental delay, but no seizures. In all phenotypes, motor symptoms responded to a ketogenic diet. Glut-1 deficiency syndrome can be identified by genetic testing; the clinician should bear in mind that this disorder may occur either with or without epileptic seizures, and that if epileptic seizures are present, AEDs are less likely to be effective than in other epileptic syndromes.

In sum, accurate diagnosis of seizures and other causes of movement disorders are critical both in implementing effective treatment and in avoiding potentially harmful effects of misguided interventions. The clinician must differentiate seizures from other paroxysmal, nonepileptic behaviors or movements, as well as from stereotypies and other atypical behaviors that are common in individuals with ID. For example, while it is true that individuals with brain injury are at greater risk to experience epileptic seizures than the general population, these individuals also have a higher risk of nonepileptic myocolonus, sleep disturbances, and movement disorders (Castriotta et al. 2009; Jankovic 1994). Furthermore, nonepileptic, self-induced seizures that are rarely seen in the non-ID population may be more common in those with ID; for example, compulsive Valsalvas resulting in anoxic seizures may be seen in children with autism or ID (Gastaut et al. 1981; Stephenson et al. 2004). Finally, to further complicate differential diagnosis, it is possible for epileptic and nonepileptic disorders to co-occur. Unsurprisingly, the diagnosis of epilepsy in individuals with ID is a complex task. Differential diagnosis should be carefully considered to ensure that the individual receives the treatment most appropriate for the problems he or she is experiencing, whether that be epilepsy, some other cause, or a combination of factors.

Treatment

Following a comprehensive assessment, individuals with ID and epilepsy are often treated early on to prevent any further neurological damage that may be caused by ongoing seizures. Research has shown that prolonged seizure activity over time can have many deleterious effects on one's physical health, cognitive ability, psychological well-being, adaptive functioning, and quality of life. While epilepsy is commonly found in individuals with ID (Fitzgerald and Ring 2009; Martin and Brown 2009; Welsh Office 1995; Weston et al. 2008), randomized controlled trials are often difficult to conduct within this specific subsection of the total epilepsy population often due to methodological issues and measurement bias (IASSID Guidelines Group 2001; Lennox et al. 2005; Oguni 2013; Rai et al. 2012). Therefore, the treatment of those with comorbid diagnoses of ID and epilepsy is difficult and often complicated by additional variables, including other diagnoses or additional impairments (e.g., communication impairments, behavioral problems; Alvarez et al. 1998; IASSID Guidelines Group 2001; Kerr et al. 2013; Weston et al. 2008).

To assist practitioners in treating this population, the International Association of the Scientific Study of Intellectual Disability (IASSID) formed a working group to develop specific guidelines for the management of epilepsy in those with ID (IASSID Guidelines Group 2001). This working group consisted of professionals from various disciplines (e.g., clinical psychologists, clinical neurophysiologists, ID nurses, neurologists, pediatric neurologists, neuropsychiatrists, ID psychiatrists, and representatives of caregivers of those with ID). These guidelines provide clinicians with specific recommendations regarding increasing dosages and slowly titrating certain antiepileptic medications.

While AEDs are the most common path of treatment for individuals with ID and epilepsy (Martin and Brown 2009), a number of other forms of treatment have been studied as well. These include: nerve stimulation therapy, surgery, dietary treatments, neurobehavioral approaches, and other alternative therapies. Regardless of the method, the goal of treatment is always to prevent future seizure activity, avoid adverse effects, and allow the individual to lead active lives (Goldenberg 2010). These various methods of managing epilepsy within the ID population will be reviewed.

Antiepileptic Medications

Although AEDs are sometimes used to treat other ancillary psychotic or behavioral problems commonly present in those with ID, these medications are more often than not prescribed for the specific treatment of seizures. Arshad et al. conducted a study in 2011 comparing individuals with ID and epilepsy and individuals with ID without a diagnosis of epilepsy. Anticonvulsant use was found to be significantly higher in those carrying a diagnosis of epilepsy (Arshad et al. 2011). However, as previously stated, due to the dearth of empirical research investigating the efficacy of AEDs for the treatment of epilepsy specifically in the ID population, most clinicians base their pharmacological treatment decisions on extrapolations from research of the general population and on personal clinical experience (Wilcox and Kerr 2008).

While many clinicians and researchers believe that early intervention leads to better prognoses (Goldenberg 2010), others have argued that the timing of the initiation of epilepsy treatment has little effect on the long-term outcomes (Wilcox and Kerr 2008). Nevertheless, practitioners should conduct a comprehensive assessment confirming the presence of a seizure disorder prior to starting any treatment regimen, especially pharmacological treatments. Currently, it is common practice to delay treatment until the individual has experienced at least two unprovoked seizures (Goldenberg 2010; Wilcox and Kerr 2008). However, some support the treatment of those with only a single seizure if that seizure was caused by an identified lesion (e.g., tumor, infection, or trauma) shown to be epileptogenic in nature (Lowenstein 2008).

Researchers have found that approximately 25 % of individuals with epilepsy are unresponsive to medication management, and this estimation is believed to be even greater in the ID population (Kwan and Brodie 2000; Martin et al. 2009). Although specific recommendations regarding dosages and other medication management are beyond the scope of this chapter, two of the primary AEDs used to treat epilepsy will be reviewed.

Lamotrigine (Sodium Valproate) According to the IASSID guidelines referenced above, the recommended first line of treatment consists of monotherapy using lamotrigine (also known as sodium valproate or Lamictal), a common antiepileptic or anticonvulsant medication (IASSID Guidelines Group 2001). Lamitrogine is currently approved for the treatment of epilepsy in individuals above the age of 16; however, it has also been approved for children at least 2 years of age as an adjunctive treatment for Lennox–Gastaut syndrome, primary generalized tonic–clonic seizures, and/or partial seizures (Glaxo Smith Kline 2013).

In 2001, Crawford et al. conducted a randomized open-label study comparing the effects of gabapentin and lamotrigine in 109 adults with epilepsy and a learning disability. Approximately 49 % of participants in the lamotrigine group experienced at least a 50 % reduction in seizure frequency. Based upon caregiver report, the improvement in seizure severity was also significantly greater for those prescribed lamotrigine as compared to the gabapentin group (Crawford et al. 2001).

Topiramate Although few studies have focused specifically on those with ID and epilepsy, topiramate has been proven to be an efficacious AED in treating a range of seizure types in the general population (Goldenberg 2010). The IASSID guidelines also state that if lamotrigine is either unsuccessful or produces adverse side effects, then topiramate is another viable option (IASSID Guidelines Group 2001).

In 2002, an open-label clinical trial was conducted to determine the utility of topiramate in individuals with epilepsy and ID (Singh and White-Scott 2002). Initially, topiramate was administered in addition to each participant's baseline AED regimen. Over approximately 42 weeks, the dosage of topiramate was increased while any other AEDs were slowly titrated and many were discontinued. Following the topiramate therapy, the authors found that the frequency of seizures was reduced by at least 50 % in approximately 70 % of the sample, and two participants were actually seizure free. Seizure activity either remained stable or worsened for five participants. Reductions in seizure duration and/or severity were observed in 44 % of the sample. While 11 of the 16 participants (69 %) had reported improved alertness, many experienced adverse side effects (e.g., behavior problems, decreased alertness, drowsiness, abnormal movements, and disorientation).

That same year, Kelly et al. (2002) published an open-label study exploring the efficacy of topiramate as an adjunctive therapy for individuals with refractory epilepsy and a learning disability. Compared to baseline levels, 25 % of participants had no reported seizures for at least 6 months following the topiramate adjunctive therapy. Forty-five percent experienced a reduction of at least 50 % in seizure frequency. Others showed modest improvements as well. Of the 55 participants who continued to take the drug, no adverse effects on appetite, behavior, alertness, or sleep were reported by caregivers, in fact many reported improvements in these areas.

Kerr et al. (2005) later published the first randomized, placebo-controlled trial studying the effects of topiramate in individuals with epilepsy and ID. Although the study was underpowered due to problems with recruitment, the results suggested that topiramate reduced seizure frequency by more than 30 % from baseline levels without producing a negative impact on behavioral problems. Similar results were found in a study published in Finland (Arvio and Sillanpaa 2005). The authors found that 17 % of participants achieved seizure freedom for at least 6 months following the use of topiramate as an adjunctive treatment to other AEDs. Additionally, 46 % of the sample had at least a 50 % reduction in their seizure frequency. Interestingly, topiramate was found to be significantly more efficacious in participants with localization-specific epilepsy rather than those with generalized epilepsies. For example, 100 % of participants with temporal lobe epilepsy experienced at least a 50 % reduction in seizure frequency. Additionally, adverse effects were only reported in 10 % of the sample.

Since many authors have reported mixed findings of adverse behavioral side effects of AEDs, Martin et al. (2009) investigated the effects of topiramate on seizure activity and other behavioral symptoms in individuals diagnosed with epilepsy and ID. Seizure frequency reduced by half in 52 % of participants; however, 38 % of the sample experienced an increase in seizure activity. For a subset of the sample, caregiver-report measures were administered to track any behavioral changes following the topiramate therapy. Improvements were reported with respect to irritability, lethargy, stereotypic behavior, and inappropriate speech.

Surgery

Although epilepsy surgery has largely excluded patients with ID, this may be an option for treatment of refractory epilepsy within this population only after careful evaluation. Until recently, cognitive impairment was considered a strong contraindication for surgical intervention of epilepsy. Past research linked poor postoperative seizure control with low IQ (Chelune et al. 1998; Duchowny 1989; Lieb et al. 1982; Lieb et al. 1980; Rausch and Crandall 1982); however, more recent studies have not found this to be the case (Khoury et al. 2005; Levisohn 2000). Davies et al. (2009) note that many of these early surgical procedures were conducted prior to the dawn of MRI, which is now used to identify patients with generalized, widespread epileptogenicity prior to surgery for exclusion purposes. Surgical treatment is only considered appropriate in situations of localized seizure foci (Nicolson 2008).

Over the past two decades, epilepsy surgery has evolved from being a last resort option to being a feasible treatment method due to the advent of utilizing MRI as a preoperative candidate selection tool (Reiser et al. 2013). Now, many clinicians offer this as a second treatment option early on when anticonvulsant medications have not been effective, as early surgery has shown to lead to better outcomes (Mathern et al. 1999). Epilepsy surgery consists of a number of various procedures including, temporal lobectomy, focal cortical resection, hemispherectomy, corpus callosotomy, and subpial transection. Each procedure is selected based upon a number of factors, such as patient population, type of seizure, seizure severity, and the location of seizure activity within the brain, among other factors (Nicolson 2008; Shields 2004). Shields (2004) states that "seizure control is much better with cortical resection than with any other treatment option if the patient is an appropriate surgical candidate" (p. 63). Unfortunately, there are very few studies examining outcomes in patients with epilepsy and ID following surgery.

In 1998, the first study to examine postoperative seizure outcomes specifically in adults with epilepsy and ID was conducted (Chelune et al. 1998). The authors found no significant increase in risk for those with ID when no structural lesions were extant other than mesial temporal sclerosis. However, when these other structural lesions were present, participants with ID had nearly a 390 % increase in risk for continued seizure activity following surgery. It is important to note than only 2.3 % (n=24) of the sample had an IQ falling below 70, likely confounding the results of this study.

In 2004, Bjornaes et al. examined the effects of resective surgery in 31 children and adults with epilepsy and ID. Seizure freedom was acquired in 48 % of the sample 2 years following surgery. Duration of epilepsy was also significantly associated with seizure outcome, specifically 80 % those with epilepsy for less than 12 years became seizure free. Therefore, seizure outcome was better in children that in adult patients. Outstandingly, improvements in Full Scale IQ scores were even observed in the adults from the sample who became seizure free. Significant improvements were also reported in regard to vocational adjustment for many adults.

Gleissner et al. (2006) also conducted a study comparing the postoperative outcomes among three groups: individuals with ID, participants with below average intelligence, and participants with average-range intelligence. No significant differences were found between groups with respect to seizure outcome at a 1 year follow-up. Seizure freedom was achieved for all groups as well (67 % for the ID group, 77 % in the below average intelligence group, and 78 % in the average-range intelligence group). Interestingly, the ID group was the only group with significant improvements in their executive functioning following surgery. The authors concluded that "IQ alone does not appear to be a good predictor of seizure outcome" and "early intervention may be imperative for good seizure outcome in patients with low IQ" (Gleissner et al. 2006, p. 412).

A similar study was conducted in 2009 investigating the outcomes following a temporal lobectomy in individuals with epilepsy (Davies et al. 2009). Among all 313 patients who received the surgery, no significant differences were found between those who were seizure free and those who continued to experience seizures postoperatively. Of that sample, a small subset ($n=15$) each had a preoperative verbal IQ of 70 or below. Sixty-six percent of this ID cohort had no reported seizures at 1 year follow-up.

Most recently, Wethe et al. (2013) examined changes in cognitive functioning after epilepsy surgical resection. Participants with ID showed significantly larger gains in intellectual functioning following the surgical procedure as compared to participants of typical development. Taken together, these studies provide support for the use of epilepsy surgery as a treatment option for individuals with epilepsy and cognitive impairment.

There are many advantages to epilepsy surgery in those with ID. For example, many patients who receive resective surgery experience a decrease in seizure frequency and/or severity. Many are also able to reduce or discontinue the use of anticonvulsant medications. Successful surgical outcomes have also been associated with reductions in the burden of care placed on many caregivers (Karakis et al. 2013).

Careful consideration should be paid, however, to the many problems and risks associated with epilepsy surgery. First, clinicians often conduct a comprehensive neuropsychological evaluation with each candidate prior to surgery to determine if surgery is a good fit for treatment. Due to communication problems often associated with cognitive impairment, individuals with ID may not be able to express their seizure symptomatology to their physician. Likewise, many of the assessment tools used during these assessments are not normed on or developed specifically for the ID population. Second, extensive medical testing is usually required prior to surgery (e.g., MRI and invasive EEG recording), and many of these procedures may be difficult to perform in persons with ID without using a general anesthetic.

Although a number of studies examining the effectiveness of epilepsy surgery in persons with ID were reviewed above, research in this area is still needed. Specifically, future studies should include larger sample sizes to improve upon the accuracy and reliability of any findings. Researchers should also consider inspecting the effectiveness of the various types of epilepsy surgeries within the ID population.

Vagus Nerve Stimulation (VNS) Therapy

As previously discussed, treating persons diagnosed with ID and epilepsy with AEDs is particularly challenging due to additional comorbidities and an increased sensitivity to the many adverse side effects of these medications (Buelow and Shore 2010). Approximately 20–30% of individuals are resistant to pharmacological treatments for their epilepsy, despite many clinicians' best efforts to find an effective combination of AEDs (Goldenberg 2010). Furthermore, many individuals with ID and epilepsy experience seizures that cannot be treated surgically either (e.g., multifocal or generalized seizures) and/or possess characteristics that exclude them from being an appropriate candidate for surgery (Davies et al. 2009; Devinsky 2002). Therefore, other innovative options for epilepsy treatment have been studied, one of those being VNS therapy.

VNS therapy was first proposed as a treatment for seizures by Dr. Jacob Zabara in 1985. He suggested that by desynchronizing the brain's electrical activity, seizures could be prevented, since they were essentially uncontrollable and irregular synchronicities in the brain (Zabara 1985). VNS therapy involves implanting a generator, similar to a pace-maker, under the skin in the left chest area which is then attached to a stimulation lead on the left vagus nerve. This nerve controls muscular movements including, swallowing, coughing, and voice production. Usually, the generator is set to stimulate the nerve for 30 s every 3 min; however, the generator can also be manually activated by waving a magnet over the stimulator. In 1997, VNS therapy was approved by the FDA to treat refractory epilepsy as an adjunctive therapy for individuals over 12 years of age (McGoldrick and Wolf 2012). Renfroe and Wheless (2002) advise that individuals should pursue VNS therapy after having two or three AED failures and a duration of epilepsy of less than 2 years. It is suggested that earlier intervention of VNS therapy leads to better seizure control and quality of life, and unlike medications, VNS therapy has been shown to work better over time.

A retrospective study was conducted in 2001 examining the effectiveness of VNS specifically for the ID population (Andriola and Vitale 2001). The charts of 21 patients (age range 3–56 years) were reviewed. A greater than 50% reduction in seizures was reported for 68% of the sample 6 months following the implantation of the VNS. Some reported adverse effects, however, including: hoarseness, unilateral vocal cord paralysis, muscle tightness in the neck, and coughing. One participant had several years of success with VNS therapy. Unfortunately, the stimulator was later removed due to an infection that formed following a battery change.

Interestingly, however, this participant did not experience an increase in seizure activity following the removal of the VNS.

In 2005, Huf et al. followed 40 individuals diagnosed with epilepsy and ID for 2 years. All participants had epilepsies resistant to pharmacological treatments and were, thus, treated with VNS therapy. Eighty-five percent of participants experienced some decrease in the frequency of their seizures, while seizure frequency decreased by at least half for 28 % of the sample. Briefer postictal periods were reported in over 75 % of the sample. Several other quality-of-life factors also significantly improved at both 1 and 2 year follow-up assessments. These factors included: attention span, word usage, clarity of speech, standing balance, ability to wash dishes, and ability to perform other household chores. According to caregivers, great improvement was also observed with regard to alertness, overall mood, and verbal ability. It should be noted, however, that a few of the participants experienced adverse side effects including, increased aggressive behavior and decreased appetite (Huf et al. 2005).

This approach to treatment for epilepsy in those with ID offers a number of advantages: (1) VNS therapy does not have interaction effects with AEDs (Handforth et al. 1998; McGoldrick and Wolf 2012; Prasher et al. 2008); (2) many patients and caregivers report quality-of-life improvements unrelated to a reduction in seizures (Huf et al. 2005); (3) caregivers report less burden due to the automatic nature of VNS therapy; (4) VNS therapy does not cause many of the side effects common with AEDs (e.g., sedation, psychomotor slowing, and weight gain; Prasher et al. 2008); (5) many patients are able to discontinue the use of AEDs with this treatment in place (Tatum et al. 2001); and (6) VNS therapy is comparatively very cost-effective (Boon et al. 1999).

Clinicians, caregivers, and patients should, however, be aware of the common side effects of VNS therapy and adverse effects specific to the ID population prior to pursuing this course of treatment. Common side effects include: hoarseness, pain or tingling in the neck, and coughing. These symptoms, however, typically subside over time and with slight modifications to the stimulator settings (McGoldrick and Wolf 2012; Prasher et al. 2008). One of the less common side effects is wound infection, which occurs in about 3–6 % of patients and rarely requires removal of the device (Handforth et al. 1998). Other less common adverse side effects include: muscle pain, chest pain, headaches, chronic diarrhea, Horner syndrome, psychotic episodes, nausea, vomiting, device failure, and vocal cord paralysis (Charous et al. 2001; Higgins et al. 2010; Kersing et al. 2002; Schaffer et al. 2005; Shaw et al. 2006; Zalvan et al. 2003).

There are many problems that may arise after the initiation of VNS therapy specifically in those with ID. First, individuals with ID may experience difficulties with swallowing and aspiration. This is particularly concerning since many individuals with ID also have a comorbid feeding disorder (Ashworth et al. 2008; Matson et al. 2009; Williams et al. 2009) and so should be closely monitored. The stimulator, however, can be temporarily deactivated during mealtimes by taping a specialized magnet over the VNS. Second, a seizure can be shortened or even prevented in the moment by waving the magnet over the stimulator. Many individuals with ID, however, also have communication impairments, which may impact their ability to alert a caregiver when they feel a seizure may soon occur. Fortunately, the stimulator can be set to automatically activate on a frequent basis. Third, while many VNS patients tend to keep the magnet nearby or even wear it around their wrist, caregivers of individuals with ID should be cautious of this, as many individuals with ID have stereotyped and involuntary motor movements. If worn on the wrist, then involuntarily and repetitively waving one's arm near the chest where the VNS is located may unnecessarily activate the stimulator. Similarly, communication impairments may also impede one's ability to communicate the presence of any of the common side effects mentioned above, which may worsen in some cases if not identified and treated early on. Finally, many individuals with ID undergo frequent medical testing due to the many common comorbid conditions that may be present. However, patients of VNS therapy are not advised to receive MRI testing without specific precautions being taken (e.g., wearing a special head coil and deactivating the stimulator; McGoldrick and Wolf 2012).

Clinicians and caregivers should carefully weigh these advantages and disadvantages of VNS therapy for any potential candidate. However, growing research supports VNS therapy as a viable and beneficial treatment option for those with ID and epilepsy. When other approved mainstream medical treatment options for epilepsy (e.g., AEDs, surgery, dietary treatments) prove to be ineffective, VNS therapy is another innovative treatment consideration for many. Nevertheless, there continues to be a need for randomized controlled clinical trials examining the effectiveness of VNS therapy within the ID population, specifically. Further information is also needed regarding the long-term effects for the ID population. Additionally, given the wide range of functioning and behavioral presentations observed across varying severity levels of ID, it would be informative to the scientific community for researchers to compare the effects of VNS therapy in all forms of ID, ranging from mildly to profoundly impaired. Given that researchers have shown the severity of epilepsy to be correlated with the severity of ID (Huttenlocher and Hapke 1990), this research would aid clinicians in determining predictors of good response in VNS therapy candidates with ID.

Dietary Treatments

When one or more of the above treatment options (i.e., antiepileptic medications, epilepsy surgery, and VNS) prove to be either ineffective or unsuitable for an individual, many then resort to dietary treatments as a means to manage seizure activity. Physicians and parents of many children also opt for dietary treatments because most antiepileptic medications are not approved by the FDA for young children. The risks involved with surgery or even the simple implantation of the vagus nerve stimulator are heightened in young children as well, making dietary treatments an appealing option.

There is a longstanding history of treating epilepsy with diet regulation. Even Hippocrates wrote of a man becoming seizure free after fasting from all food and drink for a period of time in the fifth century BC (Neal 2012). Today, there are several different dietary approaches that claim to treat epilepsy, including the modified Atkins diet (MAD), the low glycemic index treatment (LGIT), and the ketogenic diet, which is the most commonly used and well-researched option of the dietary treatments.

Ketogenic Diet The ketogenic diet requires individuals to follow a strict regimen of eating foods that are high in fat, moderate in protein, and low in carbohydrates. Usually, the body burns glucose obtained from carbohydrates in order to produce energy. However, when carbohydrates, and thereby glucose, is limited, the body then resorts to burning one's own fat for energy, similar to the body's response during fasting. Once the body's own fat has been depleted, then energy is produced by burning exogenous fats consumed by eating foods that are high in fat content (e.g., butter, oil, cream, and mayonnaise). This process leaves deposits of ketone bodies in the blood which build up over time and results in the body being in a state of *ketosis*. When in a state of ketosis, researchers have shown seizure activity to significantly reduce, and in some cases even stop entirely. However, the precise reason why this diet is effective is still unclear.

In 2013, Li et al. conducted a meta-analysis investigating the success of the ketogenic diet as a means to treat epilepsy. Thirty eight prospective and retrospective studies were included in the meta-analysis. For the purposes of the study, therapeutic success was defined as greater than 50% reduction in seizure frequency. The retrospective studies collectively demonstrated a success rate of 58.4% at 3 months and 30.1% at 12 months. Within the prospective studies, the success rate for patients was 53.9% at 3 months and 55% at 12 months. Diet efficacy decreased as the duration of the diet increased, which may suggest that individuals are less compliant or strict with their dietary regimen over time. There is also a trend of greater success in younger patients simply due to lower storage levels of energy in children (Li et al. 2013).

There has been limited research studying the effects of the ketogenic diet specifically in the ID population. One 2010 study examined the efficacy of the keteogenic diet as a treatment for refractory epilepsy in children with ID (Coppola et al. 2010). Seventy-four percent of the samples also had diagnoses of cerebral palsy. One year following the initiation of the diet, 20 participants of the initial 38 remained on the diet. Eleven of these children (28.9%) had greater than 50% reduction in seizures and the other nine (23.7%) were seizure-free.

There are a number of advantages of choosing the ketogenic diet as a means to control one's epilepsy. First, there are fewer and often times less severe side effects associated with the ketogenic diet compared to antiepileptic medications. Second, some individuals evince seizure freedom within the first few weeks of following the diet, unlike most AEDs, which often only show results after a few months. Third, as previously mentioned, researchers have shown the diet to be somewhat more effective in children, as children can maintain high levels of ketosis for longer periods of time compared to adults (Coppola et al. 2010). Compliance is also less of an obstacle with children, since their diet is usually managed by a parent or caregiver. Fourth, while the ketogenic diet is not intended to improve cognitive functioning, some researchers have shown improvement in intellectual functioning in individuals with frequent myoclonic seizures, which usually cause ongoing cognitive deteriorations (Kossoff et al. 2011). Finally, the ketogenic diet has shown excellent success in persons who receive nutrition via gastrostomy tubes (Coppola et al. 2010). Many individuals with ID present with motor difficulties which impair their ability to eat by mouth; thus, a gastrostomy tube is often inserted to provide nutrition (Kuhn et al. 2007; Trabi et al. 2010). These patients nearly always have guaranteed compliance with the diet. One study investigating the efficacy of the ketogenic diet found that 59 % of the participants with gastrostomy tubes had greater than 90 % reduction in seizure activity within 12 months (Kossoff et al. 2004).

However, this dietary approach is not without some drawbacks that should also be considered. For most, a lack of weight gain is often a problem (Coppola et al. 2010). However, in individuals with ID the opposite can often occur—too much weight gain. Children with ID are commonly less active and as a result burn fewer calories than typically developing children. However, when nutritionists initially calculate each patient's daily caloric intake, they tend to err on the side of overestimation of calories and usually refer to recommended daily allowances of calories based on average children. Since children with ID burn fewer calories, these recommended daily allowances are often too great, requiring these families to later make a cut in their child's daily caloric intake. Kossoff et al. (2011) suggest that nutritionists account for each child's activity level when making these initial dietary calculations, as it is often "psychologically easier for families to add calories or a snack to the diet than to reduce calories" (p. 144).

This diet also requires a great deal of commitment and effort. Some families may opt for medication treatment, simply due to the ease associated with administration and compliance. Usually, the first 3 months of following the ketogenic diet are considered a trial period for the family to discern if this approach will fit within their lifestyle (Kossoff et al. 2011; Li et al. 2013). Individuals on the ketogenic diet must follow a strict meal plan of specific types and quantities of foods. It may also be more difficult for families with specific dietary restrictions due to culture, religion, or allergies to follow the ketogenic diet. Those on the diet should also be careful when using certain beauty/hygiene products (e.g., lipstick, suntan lotion, and soap), as these products often contain ingredients inconsistent with the diet, leading to seizure activity (Kossoff et al. 2011). There are also socialization difficulties to consider (Pfeifer 2012). For example, when in the community with friends or family, individuals on this diet may feel it to be difficult to partake in gatherings that largely revolve around or include food (e.g., lunch in the cafeteria, family picnics, birthday parties, etc.). Other side effects may include: slightly decreased growth, high cholesterol, constipation, gastrointestinal intolerances, gastroesophageal reflux, kidney stones, hypoglycemia, acidosis, and dehydration. Finally, the ketogenic diet has not shown great success in treating those with complex partial seizures (Coppola et al. 2010; Kossoff et al. 2011, 2004).

Modified Atkins Diet The MAD is a diet very similar to the ketogenic diet but recommends fewer fats and more protein and carbohydrates (Magrath et al. 2012). This diet also offers many pre-made, MAD-approved products (e.g., candy bars and shakes). Families also do not typically require the support of a nutritionist, as the diet is much less restrictive compared to the ketogenic diet. Little research has been done to determine the efficacy of MAD in individuals with ID. However, Kossoff et al. (2011) note that this diet may be more amenable for individuals with behavioral problems, since the highly strict-nature of the ketogenic diet may lead to irritability and behavioral issues.

Low Glycemic Index Treatment The LGIT was developed in 2002 after there had been a few reported cases of seizure activity in individuals on the ketogenic diet immediately following the consumption of foods with a high glycemic index value (Kossoff et al. 2011; Pfeifer 2012). Those following this diet are permitted to consume 40–60 g of carbohydrates per day; however, those carbohydrates must have a glycemic index of less than 50. Like the MAD treatment, the LGIT is less restrictive, making it easier for parents to also follow this diet alongside their child. The only reported side effects include: weight loss, acidosis, and constipation (Kossoff et al. 2011). Again, there is a paucity of research regarding this treatment within the ID population. Pfeifer (2012) noted, however, that this treatment has been previously used with success in those with Angelman syndrome and tuberous sclerosis.

Neurobehavioral Approaches

In recent years, there has been a growing interest in the development of educational and neurobehavioral programs for individuals with epilepsy. The literature on neurobehavioral and psychosocial approaches to managing epilepsy and associated problems within the ID population, however, is very limited (Kerr et al. 2009; Martin and Brown 2009). In the general epilepsy population, psychobehavioral therapies have shown to improve psychological well-being, epilepsy knowledge, self-management, self-efficacy, perceived competencies, social skills, contentedness with therapy, medication compliance, and seizure control (Tang et al. 2014). Types of therapies may include: biofeedback, relaxation training, breathing training, reinforcement-based management, exercise programs, cognitive behavioral therapy, mindfulness-based therapy, multimodel educational intervention, and skill-based training (Mostofsky 1993; Tang et al. 2014). There are many similar programs that teach and promote independence, adaptive skills, and methods of coping for children and adults with cognitive impairments with no diagnosis of epilepsy. However, when families search for programs or therapies that individualize this training/therapy specifically for those with epilepsy and ID, the number and availability of programs drop drastically.

Huber and Seidel (2006) developed a psychoeducative program for individuals with epilepsy and mild ID. After 5 years of offering the program, feedback from 165 participants was received and reviewed. Fifty-five percent of the sample reported an improvement in their knowledge of epilepsy, 52 % reported improved coping skills, and 57 % indicated that they had an increased level of independence following the program. Only 3–7 % of responders reported no improvement.

This study is one of the first to indicate that such programs designed for those with comorbid diagnoses of epilepsy and ID can produce promising outcomes. As previously mentioned, those with epilepsy and ID encounter many obstacles cognitively, adaptively, physically, psychologically, socially, and behaviorally. While neurobehavioral, educative, and psychosocial approaches to treatments may not lead to seizure freedom, they can help minimize the deleterious problems associated with these comorbid diagnoses.

Other Alternative Therapies

It is important for both parents and clinicians to know that the four primary treatments for epilepsy include antiepileptic medications, epilepsy surgery, VNS therapy, and the ketogenic diet. All of these methods are supported by empirical research and are the major treatment options suggested by current research and well-informed clinicians. Nevertheless, there are many other alternative therapies available to families. However, the research supporting these therapies remains limited. This is not to say that complementary and alternative medicines (CAMs) will never be supported by research. For example, the ketogenic diet was once considered a CAM; however, with extensive empirical research it is now considered a part of mainstream medicine.

As noted previously, epilepsy is a highly prevalent disorder found in individuals in many different countries. While treatment accessibility is common in the USA, this is not the case in all areas of the world. Unfortunately, many who are diagnosed with the disorder are unable to either afford or access empirically supported treatments (Meinardi et al. 2001). In fact, it has been estimated that 75 % of those with epilepsy live in resource-poor countries with little to no access to medical treatments (Shashi et al. 2014). Some have estimated that 85 % of those diagnosed with epilepsy are either inappropriately treated or not treated at all (Meinardi et al. 2001). When main medical treatments are unavailable, many often then resort to CAMs. Every year, CAMs also become more popular within Western society with the expansion of media outlets (Devinsky et al. 2012).

One example of a CAM for epilepsy includes herbal remedies. Many herbal medicines have shown to affect the central nervous system (CNS) and seizure activity. These may include substances found in plants, foods, vitamins, and animal compounds. Shashi et al. (2014) reviewed several examples of herbal drugs used in the treatment of epilepsy which included: *Nardostachys jatamansi*, *Cotyledon orbiculata*, *Laurus nobilis*, *Bacopa monnieri*, *Rhizoma pinelliae*, *Taxus wallichiana*, *Sutherlandia frutescens*, *Ficus platyphylla*, *Scutellaria baicalensis*, *Harpagophytum procumbens*, *Delphinium denudatum*, *Withania somnifera*, *Leonotis leonurus*, and *Magnolia grandiflora*. When taken appropriately, many of these herbal options are said to have significantly fewer side effects than those associated with antiepileptic medications. Currently, there are no published clinical trials supporting the use of herbal remedies for the treatment of epilepsy (Devinsky et al. 2012).

Osteopathy is another CAM method of treating many disorders by alleviating tension in the skeletal system. Cranial osteopathy is occasionally used as a treatment for epilepsy by relieving tension in the skull and spine through massage to allow the spinal fluid to drain and flow more freely (Baker 2007). There is no evidence, however, that massaging the head or body can improve seizure functioning (Devinsky et al. 2012). Finally, other examples of CAMs for the treatment of epilepsy include, but are not limited to: aromatherapy, vitamins and supplements, craniosacral therapy, chiropractic therapy, transcranial magnetic stimulation, hormonal therapy, and homeopathic medicines (Devinsky et al. 2012).

Psychosocial Impact

Although the comorbidity if ID and epilepsy poses great challenges throughout the assessment and treatment process as described above, these conditions also influence a number of other areas in one's life. The presentation of other comorbid psychiatric conditions is often affected. Other areas of psychosocial impact may include: increased safety concerns, difficulties related to independent living, employment status, and caregiver burden. The ways in which these areas may be adversely influenced by the presence of comorbid diagnoses of epilepsy and ID are discussed below.

Other Comorbid Conditions

While a great deal of research has been conducted regarding psychopathology in individuals with ID and separately in individuals with epilepsy, few studies have specifically investigated psychopathology within the context of co-occurring epilepsy and ID. In one such study, McDermott et al. (2005) found that seizure disorders in individuals with ID is associated with increased psychiatric symptoms and challenging behaviors including mood swings, attention-seeking behaviors, and lack of empathy; these factors likely increase the probability of meeting criteria for a psychiatric disorder. Although symptoms of psychopathology may be expressed differently in individuals with ID compared to those without ID, it is well-established that many types of psychopathology occur at higher rates in the ID population (Matson and Shoemaker 2011). Additionally, challenging behavior (CB; e.g., physical aggression, verbal aggression, property destruction, and other disruptive behavior) is common in individuals with ID (Matson and Neal 2009). CB may or may not be attributable to a psychiatric diagnosis, but nonetheless has a considerable impact on the choice and effectiveness of interventions and overall quality of life. Some disorders which cause both ID and seizures are associated with specific phenotypes that may include an increased probability of particular types of CB or psychopathology. For example, tuberous sclerosis is associated with hyperactivity, challenging behaviors, and stereotypies often seen in individuals with pervasive developmental delay or autism (Curatolo et al. 2004). Rett syndrome is associated with mood and anxiety symptoms (Bebbington et al. 2008), and Lesch–Nyhan syndrome often occurs with repetitive self-injury (Schretlen et al. 2005).

In the general population, research on the relationship between psychopathology and epilepsy is often equivocal. For example, children with epilepsy may not have the same opportunities or obtain the same levels of achievement in education or employment. Some have suggested that medications or seizures cause attention deficits which affect achievement. However, Oostrom et al. (2002) found that school or behavioral difficulties prior to seizure onset as well as maladaptive parent reaction to diagnosis were both related to attention deficits, whereas epilepsy-specific variables were not. Epilepsy is a chronic condition with widely varying severity, etiology, and expression across individuals; the same may also be said of psychopathology in general. However, there are some psychological issues, such as anxiety and depression, which seem to occur at higher rates than others among individuals with epilepsy, and at higher rates than in the general population (Swinkels et al. 2001). In a study of over 200 participants with epilepsy, Piazzini et al. (2001) found significantly higher rates of anxiety and depression as compared to a control group. These same diagnoses are also common in individuals with ID, further highlighting the importance of assessing for possible psychiatric comorbidities in dually diagnosed individuals.

Should psychiatric comorbidities be present, medical professionals may consider the use of psychotropic medications to manage severe symptoms. When prescribing psychotropic medications, careful consideration should be taken to minimize risk by avoiding medications and combinations of drugs most likely to have deleterious side effects within the context of other medical problems or treatments. For a discussion of use of antipsychotic, antidepressant, and other psychotropic drugs in individuals with epilepsy, as well as effects, dosage ranges, and potential interactions, see Alper et al. (2002). Clinicians and caregivers should be aware of the potential side effects of AEDs causing or exacerbating psychiatric symptoms and challenging behavior. For example, tiagabine may have dose-related anxiety effects, lamotrigine may be too stimulating for some individuals with ID and increase challenging behaviors, and vigabatrin has been associated with psychotic symptoms and challenging behaviors (for more detail, see Dolman and Scheepers 2008). In the case of challenging behaviors, greater treatment effects may be seen by use of a carefully designed and implemented behavioral treatment plan, avoiding the need for medication.

However, when medications are used, there are a number of valuable assessment tools available for clinicians, which measure adverse side effects. For example, the *Matson Evaluation of Drug Side-effects* (*MEDS*; Matson 1997) is a useful scale to periodically assess for side effects common to psychotropic medication use in individuals with developmental disabilities. This 93-item scale includes short items (e.g., “excessive hair loss,” “change in appetite,” and “tires easily”) and assesses possible symptoms across nine domains including cardiovascular/hematologic, gastrointestinal, endocrine/genitourinary, eye/ear/noes/throat, skin/allergies/temperature, general CNS, CNS-dystonia, CNS-Parkonsonism/dyskinesia, and CNS-akathasia. The *Scale for the Evaluation and Identification of seizures, Epilepsy, and Anticonvulsant Side effects—B* (*SEIZES-B*; Matson 2000) is a similarly designed caregiver report measure which looks more specifically at side effects of AEDs.

Anxiety and Depression Although historically it was thought that individuals with ID lacked the capacity to develop psychopathology, it is now widely recognized that not only do psychiatric disorders exist among individuals with ID, but they are likely at a greater risk than the general population for developing such disorders (Smith and Matson 2010). Anxiety and mood disorders are especially common (McGillivray and McCabe 2007; Ross and Oliver 2003; Tsiouris 2001). Diagnosis of anxiety and mood disorders in individuals with normal cognitive functioning, including those with epilepsy, typically relies heavily on self-report, standardized self-rating scales, and structured or semi-structured interviews (e.g., Kanner and Palac 2002), but other assessment practices using evidence-based observational or caregiver report measures are often critical in assessing for these disorders in ID (Smith and Matson 2010). Examples of such caregiver report measures include the *Diagnositic Assessment for the Severely Handicapped-II* (*DASH-II*; Matson 1995) for individuals with severe and profound ID, the *Psychopathology Instrument for Mentally Retarded Adults* (*PIMRA*; Matson 1988) for adults with ID, and the *Assessment of Dual Diagnosis* (*ADD*; Matson 1997) to assess for psychopathology in individuals with mild to moderate ID.

Depending on location, seizures affecting the limbic system (e.g., temporal lobe seizures) may give rise to preictal and postictal psychiatric symptoms; most notably, anxiety or fear is the most commonly reported aura in temporal lobe epilepsy. Some researchers have found anxiety disorders including generalized anxiety disorder, panic disorder, phobias, and obsessive-compulsive disorder are especially common in individuals with seizures originating in the temporal lobe, although other studies have yielded conflicting results regarding whether individuals with temporal lobe seizures are more likely to develop interictal mood and anxiety disorders than individuals with extratemporal lobe seizures (Marsh and Rao 2002; Swinkels et al. 2001). Depression occurs at high rates in individuals with epilepsy, with prevalence estimates of approximately 10 % of individuals with controlled seizures but up to 50 % in individuals with recurrent seizures (Barry 2003; Gilliam and Kanner 2002; Kanner 2003). Depression is more common in individuals with chronic disorders generally, but this seems to be over-represented among individuals with neurological disorders including epilepsy (Barry 2003).

It is likely that mood and anxiety disorders in the context of epilepsy are affected by both neurological differences and psychosocial stressors. There may be shared mechanisms involved including a shared genetic predisposition (Kanner and Balabanov 2002; Scheepers and Kerr 2003); additionally, psychosocial factors such as fear of and frequency of seizures, medication side effects, perceived stigma or discrimination, and vocational/social sequelae play a role in the development of psychological disorders, with seizure severity correlated with the severity of self-reported psychosocial problems (de Souza and Salgado 2006; Whitman and Hermann 1986).

Challenging Behaviors Studies of challenging behavior in individuals with and without ID have suggested no significant effect of epilepsy on the likelihood of challenging behaviors, but rather that degree of ID or comorbid psychiatric symptoms may have a greater effect on rates of challenging behavior (Andrews et al. 1999; Espie et al. 2003). Challenging behaviors are common in the ID population, and are a frequent focus of intervention (Matson and Rivet 2008). In a study of over 300 individuals with ID, Matson et al. (1999) found no significant differences in those with and without seizures with regard to CB topography, frequency, or function. Nonetheless, in the context of individuals with epilepsy, challenging behaviors must be carefully assessed to determine whether the challenging behaviors are related to auras, or preictal or postictal phenomena. Treatment planning to address challenging behaviors must take into account the underlying maintaining variables for the behaviors and center around addressing those factors. In a study of children with ID, epilepsy, and challenging behaviors, Lewis et al. (2000) found no significant effect of medication on challenging behavior between children who were and were not taking AEDs; many individuals with ID are unnecessarily given psychotropic medications for behavior management (Matson and Neal 2009). This approach could be particularly problematic for individuals taking AEDs, as some psychotropic medications may lower the seizure threshold. In many cases, challenging behaviors are environmentally maintained and can be treated with the same treatments proven to be effective for individuals with ID and no seizure disorder, such as communication training, social skills training, environmental enrichment, and behavior modification plans (Matson et al. 1999). Useful, brief caregiver report measures for identifying the variables maintaining challenging behaviors include the Questions About Behavior Function (QABF; Matson and Vollmer 1995) and Motivation Assessment Scale (MAS; Durand 1988).

Safety Concerns

Overall, individuals with ID are at a greater risk for injury and accidents than the general population; the same is true for individuals with epilepsy. For individuals with both ID and epilepsy, caregivers should take precautions to avoid unnecessary risk without unduly limiting the individual's freedom and opportunity to participate in normative activities. Special attention should be given to reducing risk for burns, fractures, and drowning.

ID alone does not appear to be a risk factor for burns, perhaps due to a tendency to live and work in more heavily supervised settings (Spitz et al. 1994). Epilepsy does raise the risk for burns in the general population, and individuals with ID are likely at an increased risk for burns in less restrictive settings (e.g., supported independent living). In a study of 134 individuals with epilepsy, Hampton et al. (1988) found 38 % reported having suffered a burn due to a seizure. Common causes of burns include scalding from cooking with hot liquids or oils, or consuming hot beverages; contact with heating appliances or stoves are also common sources of injury (Josty et al. 2000). Simple safety measures such as habitually using the back burners, turning pot handles so they do not hang over the counter edge, and setting water thermostats to a lower temperature to avoid scalding water in the shower can decrease risk of burns either due to seizures or simple accident.

Both ID (Sherrard et al. 2001) and epilepsy (Bell et al. 2008) are associated with an increased risk of drowning, particularly while bathing, although risk is also increased for drowning in pools and open bodies of water. The seizure and cognitive characteristics of an individual as well as his/her bathing routine should be assessed for risk of drowning, perhaps showering instead of bathing to decrease risk. Close supervision by an adult trained to respond appropriately should a seizure occur in the water decreases the risk of drowning to approximately that of the general population (Kemp and Sibert 1993).

Unsurprisingly, individuals with epilepsy are also at greater risk of injury due to falls. Additional factors further impact the likelihood of injury from falls. Some medications, including AEDs and psychotropic medications, can affect bone mineral density and increase risk of osteoporosis. Accordingly, the risk of fractures due to falls can be increased and further impacted by the sedative effects of some medications. Osteopenia is a condition exacerbated by immobility and is common in institutionalized individuals with ID (Jaffe et al. 2005; Ryder et al. 2003). This condition is may be exacerbated by decreased mobility either due to motor problems or daily routines. The bone density of individuals with ID and epilepsy should be regularly monitored. Healthy habits should be instilled including maintaining a nutritionally balanced diet, adequate daily physical activity, and regular exposure to sunlight to promote vitamin D synthesis should be encouraged, particularly for institutionalized individuals. Calcium and vitamin D supplementation may also be considered under guidance from a physician.

Psychosocial Concerns

Over the past 40 years, an increased focus has been placed on providing supports for individuals with ID to live in least-restrictive settings; accordingly, many individuals have moved from residential facilities into group homes and supported independent living arrangements in the community (Braddock et al. 2001). However, individuals with increased needs, especially medical needs, often require additional supports and services that are more readily available in a more restricted setting (Turygin et al. 2014). Even in the general population, an epilepsy diagnosis may limit vocational opportunities. For example, increased severity of seizures is negatively correlated with better employment status, and increased frequency of falls is significantly associated with lower levels of employment (Vickery et al. 2000).

These disadvantages are particularly salient for individuals who dually diagnosed with ID and epilepsy. Placement in more restrictive environments decreases the degree of freedom available to an individual, with limitations on independence subsequently decreasing quality of life (Wehmeyer and Bolding 2001), and further limiting ability to engage in normative activities critical for developing social and adaptive skills. It is, therefore, unsurprising that individuals with ID and seizures tend to have greater deficits in social and adaptive behaviors than individuals with ID but no seizures (Matson et al. 1999). It is critical that clinicians and caregivers periodically assess psychosocial factors for individuals with epilepsy just as they would for individuals with ID, ensuring that individuals are permitted opportunities for self-determination, with efforts to promote community inclusion and participation.

Family Factors

Families with children who have special needs must contend with both the normal challenges of family life and the additional challenges of meeting their child's unique needs. Understandably, receiving a diagnosis of a chronic condition, such as ID or epilepsy, can cause considerable distress to a parent or primary caregiver (Cramm and Nieboer 2011; Rodenburg et al. 2011). Having a child with special needs, whether due to medical needs or developmental disability, often has a significant impact on family functioning, as family routines often must change to accommodate the child's needs (Heiman 2002). Parents may respond to a child's disability with greater levels of anxiety and overprotection, which also impact family relationships (Lardieri et al. 2000), and are more likely to experience greater overall stress, more health problems, increased risk for depression, and encounter greater restrictions on family activities than parents of typically developing children (Heiman 2002). Parents of children with multiple health care needs also often experience frustration with a lack of coordination between different service providers (Freedman and Boyer 2000). These issues are likely compounded when the child has dual disabilities, such as ID and epilepsy, and is likely to be receiving a greater number and variety of services. Siblings are also often affected by worry and concern for a brother or sister who experiences seizures, with many reporting feeling responsible to protect their sibling to the point of altering their own plans and activities (Tsuchie et al. 2006).

Additionally, prolonged or very frequent seizures can incur substantial financial burden, with significant direct costs (e.g., costs incurred with emergency room visits) and indirect costs. For parents and family members, indirect costs may include time away from work or loss of employment (Graves 1998). One consideration with the added clinical benefit of more rapid treatment is to increase availability of at-home emergency medication. Researchers have found that the use of at-home rectal diazepam for emergency treatment of seizures not only reduces seizure severity but also significantly decreases parental stress and financial burden (Kriel et al. 1991;

O'Dell et al. 2005). This treatment option promoted a greater sense of efficacy in managing the disorder, thus allowing for a more normal lifestyle. Parents were more comfortable leaving children with other caregivers, thus adding flexibility to their schedule and enabling some parents cost savings compared to the cost of an emergency room visit, with some researchers estimating a savings of $ 2000 or more per episode (O'Dell et al. 2005).

Some researchers have suggested that the impact of psychosocial factors, including the reactions of caregivers and family members, may actually have a greater impact on quality of life than the clinical aspects of the disorder itself (O'Dell et al. 2007), thus the overall needs of the family should not be overlooked. The *Parenting Stress Index* (*PSI*; Abidin 1990) is a useful self-report scale to measure parent stress. The *Duke Social Support and Stress Scale* (*DUSOCS*; Parkerson 1996) more specifically assesses stressors related to having a family member with a chronic illness or disability. Respite care, consolidated case management, and cognitive behavioral techniques are promising methods for reducing stress in caregivers of individuals with ID (Hastings and Beck 2004); these approaches can also be applied to caregivers of dually diagnosed individuals with ID and epilepsy.

Conclusion

In sum, the comorbidity of ID and epilepsy poses challenges for clinicians, caregivers, and of course the individuals, themselves. Additionally, these comorbid disorders can adversely influence a number of areas, including the assessment process, the treatment of epilepsy, the presence of additional comorbidities, and other psychosocial factors. Given the widespread impact that ID and epilepsy can have, this area continues to deserve further investigation to aid in advancing current clinical practice.

References

Abidin, R. R. (1990). *Parenting stress index (PSI)*. Charlottesville: Pediatric Psychology Press.

Alper, K. R., Barry, J. J., & Balabanov, A. J. (2002). Treatment of psychosis, aggression, and irritability in patients with epilepsy. *Epilepsy & Behavior, 3*(5), 13–18.

Alvarez, N., Besag, F., & Iivanainen, M. (1998). Use of antiepileptic drugs in the treatment of epilepsy with intellectual disability. *Journal of Intellectual Disability Research, 42,* 1–15.

Andrews, T. M., Everitt, A. D., & Sander, J. W. A. S. (1999). A descriptive survey of long-term residents with epilepsy and intellectual disability at the chalfont centre: Is there a relationship between maladaptive behaviour and magnetic resonance imaging findings? *Journal of Intellectual Disability Research, 43*(6), 475–483.

Andriola, M. R., & Vitale, S. A. (2001). Vagus nerve stimulation in the developmentally delayed. *Epilepsy & Behavior, 2,* 129–134.

Arif, H., Buchsbaum, R., Weintraub, D., Pierro, J., & Hirsch, L. J. (2009). Patient-reported cognitive side effects of antiepileptic drugs: Predictors and comparison of all commonly used antiepileptic drugs. *Epilepsy & Behavior, 14*(1), 202–209.

Arshad, S., Winterhalder, R., Underwood, L., Kelesidi, K., Chaplin, E., Kravariti, E., & Tsakanikos, E. (2011). Epilepsy and intellectual disability: Does epilepsy increase the likelihood of co-morbid psychopathology? *Research in Developmental Disabilities, 32,* 353–357.

Arvio, M., & Sillanpaa, M. (2005). Topiramate in long-term treatment of epilepsy in the intellectually disabled. *Journal of Intellectual Disability Research, 49,* 183–189.

Arzimanoglou, A. (1997). The surgical treatment of Sturge–Weber syndrome with respect to its clinical spectrum. *Current Problems IN Epilepsy, 11,* 353–363.

Ashworth, M., Martin, L., & Hirdes, J. P. (2008). Prevalence and correlates of pica among adults with intellectual disability in institutions. *Journal of Mental Health Research in Intellectual Disabilities, 1,* 176–190.

Avbersek, A., & Sisodiya, S. (2010). Does the primary literature provide support for clinical signs used to distinguish psychogenic nonepileptic seizures from epileptic seizures? *Journal of Neurology, Neurosurgery & Psychiatry, 81*(7), 719–725.

Baker, R. (2007). *Meeting special needs: A practical guide to support children with epilepsy.* London: Practical Pre-School Books.

Barry, J. J. (2003). The recognition and management of mood disorders as a comorbidity of epilepsy. *Epilepsia, 44*(s4), 30–40.

Bebbington, A., Anderson, A., Ravine, D., Fyfe, S., Pineda, M., De Klerk, N., & Leonard, H. (2008). Investigating genotype–phenotype relationships in Rett syndrome using an international data set. *Neurology, 70*(11), 868–875.

Bell, G. S., Gaitatzis, A., Bell, C. L., Johnson, A. L., & Sander, J. W. (2008). Drowning in people with epilepsy how great is the risk? *Neurology, 71*(8), 578–582.

Berg, A. T., & Scheffer, I. E. (2011). New concepts in classification of the epilepsies: Entering the 21st century. *Epilepsia, 52,* 1058–1062.

Berg, A. T., Berkovic, S. F., Brodie, M. J., Buchhalter, J., Cross, J. H., Van Emde Boas, W., & Scheffer, I. E. (2010). Revised terminology and concepts for oranization of seizures and epilepsies: Report of the ILAE commission on classification and terminology, 2005–2009. *Epilepsia, 51*(4), 676–685.

Berkovic, S. F. (2000). Paroxysmal movement disorders and epilepsy links across the channel. *Neurology, 55*(2), 169–170.

Bisulli, F., Vignatelli, L., Naldi, I., Licchetta, L., Provini, F., Plazzi, G. & Tinuper, P. (2010). Increased frequency of arousal parasomnias in families with nocturnal frontal lobe epilepsy: A common mechanism? *Epilepsia, 51*(9), 1852–1860.

Bjornaes, H., Stabell, K.E., Hemminghyt, E., Roste, G. K., & Bakke, S. J. (2004). Resective surgery for intractable focal epilepsy in patients with low IQ: Predictors for seizure control and outcome with respect to seizures and neuropsycholgoical and psychosocial functioning. *Epilepsia, 45,* 131–139.

Boon, P., Vonck, K., Vandekerckhove, T., D'have, M., Nieuwenhuis, L., Michielsen, G., & De Reuck, J. (1999). Vagus nerve stimulation for medically refractory epilepsy: Efficacy and cost-benefit analysis. *Acta Neurochirurgica, 141,* 447–452.

Bourgeois, M., Aicardi, J., & Goutières, F. (1993). Alternating hemiplegia of childhood. *The Journal of pediatrics, 122*(5), 673–679.

Bowley, C., & Kerr, M. (2000). Epilepsy and intellectual disability. *Journal of Intellectual Disabilities, 44*(5), 529–543.

Braddock, D., Emerson, E., Felce, D., & Stancliffe, R. J. (2001). Living circumstances of children and adults with mental retardation or developmental disabilities in the United States, Canada, England and Wales, and Australia. *Mental Retardation and Developmental Disabilities Research Reviews, 7*(2), 115–121.

Brodie, M. J., Schachter, S. C., & Kwan, P. (2012). *Fast facts: Epilepsy.* Abingdon: Health Press.

Brylewski, J. E., & Wiggs, L. (1998). A questionnaire survey of sleep and night-time behaviour in a community-based sample of adults with intellectual disability. *Journal of Intellectual Disability Research, 42*(2), 154–162.

Buelow, J. M., & Shore, C. P. (2010). Management challenges in children with both epilepsy and intellectual disability. *Clinical Nurse Specialist, 24,* 313–320.

Carreno, M., Donaire, A., Jiménez, M. P., Agudo, R., Quilez, A., Rumià, J., & Setoain, X. (2005). Complex motor behaviors in temporal lobe epilepsy. *Neurology, 65*(11), 1805–1807.
Castriotta, R. J., Atanasov, S., Wilde, M. C., Masel, B. E., Lai, J. M., & Kuna, S. T. (2009). Treatment of sleep disorders after traumatic brain injury. *Journal of Clinical Sleep Medicine, 5*(2), 137–144.
Charous, S. J., Kempster, G., Manders, E., & Ristanovic, R. K. (2001). The effect of vagal nerve stimulation on voice. *Laryngoscope, 111,* 2028–2031.
Chelune, G., Naugle, R. I., Hermann, B. P., Barr, W. B., Trenerry, M. R., Loring, D. W., & Westerveld, M. (1998). Does presurgical IQ predict seizure outcome after temporal lobectomy? Evidence from the Bozeman epilepsy consortium. *Epilepsia, 39,* 314–318.
Clarke, D. B., Olivier, A., Andermann, F., & Fish, D. (1996). Surgical treatment of epilepsy: The problem of lesion/focus incongruence. *Surgical Neurology, 46*(6), 579–586.
Coppola, G., Verrotti, A., Ammendola, E., Operto, F. F., della Corte, R., Signoriello, G., & Pascotto, A. (2010). Ketogenic diet for the treatment of catastrophic epileptic encephalopathies in childhood. *European Journal of Paediatric Neurology, 14,* 229–234.
Corbett, J. (1993). Epilepsy and mental handicap. In J. Laidlaw, A. Richens, & J. Oxley (Eds.), *A textbook of epilepsy* (3rd ed., pp. 631–636). Edinburgh: Churchill Livingstone.
Cramm, J. M., & Nieboer, A. P. (2011). Psychological well-being of caregivers of children with intellectual disabilities: Using parental stress as a mediating factor. *Journal of Intellectual Disabilities, 15*(2), 101–113.
Crawford, P., Brown, S., & Kerr, M. (2001). A randomized open-label study of gabapentin and lamotrigine in adults with learning disability and resistant epilepsy. *Seizure, 10,* 107–115.
Crompton, D. E., & Berkovic, S. F. (2009). The borderland of epilepsy: Clinical and molecular features of phenomena that mimic epileptic seizures. *The Lancet Neurology, 8*(4), 370–381.
Crow, Y. J., Zuberi, S. M., McWilliam, R., Tolmie, J. L., Hollman, A., Pohl, K., & Stephenson, J. B. (1998). "Cataplexy" and muscle ultrasound abnormalities in Coffin–Lowry syndrome. *Journal of medical genetics, 35*(2), 94–98.
Curatolo, P., Porfirio, M. C., Manzi, B., & Seri, S. (2004). Autism in tuberous sclerosis. *European Journal of Paediatric Neurology, 8*(6), 327–332.
Danielsson, S., Gillberg, I. C., Billstedt, E., Gillberg, C., & Olsson, I. (2005). Epilepsy in young adults with autism: A prospective population-based follow-up study of 120 individuals diagnosed in childhood. *Epilepsia, 46*(6), 918–923.
Davies, R., Baxendale, S., Thompson, P., & Duncan, J. S. (2009). Epilepsy surgery for people with a low IQ. *Seizure, 18,* 150–152.
de Souza, E. A. P., & Salgado, P. C. B. (2006). A psychosocial view of anxiety and depression in epilepsy. *Epilepsy & Behavior, 8*(1), 232–238.
Derry, C. P., Davey, M., Johns, M., Kron, K., Glencross, D., Marini, C., & Berkovic, S. F. (2006). Distinguishing sleep disorders from seizures: Diagnosing bumps in the night. *Archives of neurology, 63*(5), 705–709.
Devinsky, O. (2002). What do you do when they grow up? Approaches to seizures in developmentally delayed adults. *Epilepsia, 43,* 71–79.
Devinsky, O., Schachter, S. C., & Pacia, S. V. (2012). *Alternative therapies for epilepsy.* New York: Demos Medical.
DiMario, F. J. (2001). Prospective study of children with cyanotic and pallid breath-holding spells. *Pediatrics, 107*(2), 265–269.
Dolman, J., & Scheepers, M. (2008). Psychopathology in people with epilepsy and intellectual disabilities. In V. P. Prasher & M. P. Kerr (Eds.), *Epilepsy and intellectual disabilities* (pp. 155–180). London: Springer.
Duchowny, M. S. (1989). Surgery for intractable epilepsy: Issues and outcome. *Pediatrics, 84,* 886–894.
Durand, V. M. (1988). The motivation assessment scale. In M. Hernsen & A. Bellack (Eds.), *Dictionary of behavioral assessment techniques* (pp. 309–310). Tarrytown: Pergamon Press, Inc.
Engel J. Jr. (2006). ILAE classification of epilepsy syndromes. *Epilepsy Research, 70,* 5–10.
Engel, J. (2013). *Seizures and epilepsy.* New York: Oxford University.

Ernst, J. P. (2004). Fever can suppress epilepsy seizures. *Epilepsia, 45,* 199.
Espie, C. A., Watkins, J., Curtice, L., Epsie, A., Duncan, R., Ryan, J. A., & Sterrick, M. (2003). Psychopathology in people with epilepsy and intellectual disability: An investigation of potential explanatory variables. *Journal of Neurology, Neurosurgery, & Psychiatry, 74*(11), 1485–1492.
Fisher, R. S., Boas, W. V. E., Blume, W., Elger, C., Genton, P., Lee, P., & Engel, J. (2005). Epileptic seizures and epilepsy: Definitions proposed by the International League Against Epilepsy (ILAE) and the International Bureau for Epilepsy (IBE). *Epilepsia, 46,* 470–472.
Fitzgerald, B., & Ring, H. (2009). Epilepsy, mental health, adults with learning disability—reviewing the evidence. *Psychiatry, 8,* 422–424.
Forsgren, L., Beghi, E., Oun, A., & Sillanpaa, M. (2005). The epidemiology of epilepsy in Europe—A systematic review. *European Journal of Neurology, 12*(4), 245–253.
Freedman, R. I., & Boyer, N. C. (2000). The power to choose: Supports for families caring for individuals with developmental disabilities. *Health & Social Work, 25*(1), 59–68.
Galván-Manso, M., Campistol, J., Conill, J., & Sanmartí, F. X. (2005). Analysis of the characteristics of epilepsy in 37 patients with the molecular diagnosis of Angelman syndrome. *Epileptic Disorders: International Epilepsy Journal with Videotape, 7*(1), 19–25.
Gastaut, H., Broughton, R., & De Leo, G. (1981). Syncopal attacks compulsively self-induced by the Valsalva manoeuvre in children with mental retardation. *Electroencephalography and Clinical Neurophysiology, 35*(Suppl. 1), S323–S329.
Genton, P., Velizarova, R., & Dravet, C. (2011). Dravet syndrome: The long-term outcome. *Epilepsia, 52*(Suppl. 2), S44–S49.
Gilliam, F., & Kanner, A. M. (2002). Treatment of depressive disorders in epilepsy patients. *Epilepsy & Behavior, 3*(5), 2–9.
Glaxo Smith Kline. (2013). *Lamictal prescribing information.* Research Triangle Park: GlaxoSmithKline.
Glaze, D. G., Schultz, R. J., & Frost, J. D. (1998). Rett syndrome: Characterization of seizures versus non-seizures. *Electroencephalography and Clinical Neurophysiology, 106*(1), 79–83.
Gleissner, U., Clusmann, H., Sassen, R., Elger, C. E., & Helmstaedter, C. (2006). Postsurgical outcome in pediatric patients with epilepsy: A comparison of patients with intellectual disabilities, subaverage intelligence, and average-range intelligence. *Epilepsia, 47,* 406–414.
Goldenberg, M. M. (2010). Overview of drugs used for epilepsy and seizures. *P & T: Journal for Formulary Management, 35*(7), 392–415.
Graves, N. (1998). Pharmacoeconomic considerations in treatment options for acute seizures. *Journal of Child Neurology, 13*(Suppl. 1), S27–S29.
Hampton, K. K., Peatfield, R. C., Pullar, T., Bodansky, H. J., Walton, C., & Feely, M. (1988). Burns because of epilepsy. *British Medical Journal (Clinical Research Edition), 296*(6637), 1659.
Handforth, A., DeGorgio, C. M., Schachter, S. C., Uthman, B. M., Naritoku, D. K., Tecoma, E. S., & Wheless, J. W. (1998). Vagus nerve stimulation therapy for partial onset seizures: A randomized active-control trial. *Neurology, 51,* 48–55.
Hastings, R. P., & Beck, A. (2004). Practitioner review: Stress intervention for parents of children with intellectual disabilities. *Journal of Child Psychology and Psychiatry, 45*(8), 1338–1349.
Heiman, T. (2002). Parents of children with disabilities: Resilience, coping, and future expectations. *Journal of Developmental and Physical Disabilities, 14*(2), 159–171.
Higgins, D., Dix, D., & Gold, M. E. (2010). Vagal nerve stimulation: A case report. *AANA Journal, 78,* 146–150.
Hoefnagels, W. A. J., Padberg, G. W., Overweg, J., Van der Velde, E. A., & Roos, R. A. C. (1991). Transient loss of consciousness: The value of the history for distinguishing seizure from syncope. *Journal of Neurology, 238*(1), 39–43.
Horrocks, I. A., Nechay, A., Stephenson, J. B., & Zuberi, S. M. (2005). Anoxic-epileptic seizures: Observational study of epileptic seizures induced by syncopes. *Archives of Disease in Childhood, 90*(12), 1283–1287.
Huber, B., & Seidel, M. (2006). Psychoeducation in epilepsy with PEPE: Interim results after 5 years. *Z Epileptol, 19,* 251–257.

Huf, R. L., Mamelak, A., & Kneedy-Cayem, K. (2005). Vagus nerve stimulation therapy: 2-year prospective open-label study of 40 subjects with refractory epilepsy and low IQ who are living in long-term care facilities. *Epilepsy & Behavior, 6*, 417–423.

Huttenlocher, P. R., & Hapke, R. J. (1990). A follow-up study of intractable seizures in childhood. *Annals of Neurology, 28*, 699–705.

IASSID Guidelines Group. (2001). Clinical guidelines for the management of epilepsy in adults with an intellectual disability. *Seizure, 10*, 401–409.

Jaffe, J. S., Timell, A. M., Elolia, R., & Thatcher, S. S. (2005). Risk factors for low bone mineral density in individuals residing in a facility for the people with intellectual disability. *Journal of Intellectual Disability Research, 49*(6), 457–462.

Jankovic, J. (1994). Post-traumatic movement disorders: Central and peripheral mechanisms. *Neurology, 44*(11), 2006–2006.

Josty, I. C., Narayanan, V., & Dickson, W. A. (2000). Burns in patients with epilepsy: Changes in epidemiology and implications for burn treatment and prevention. *Epilepsia, 41*(4), 453–456.

Kanemoto, K., Watanabe, Y., Tsuji, T., Fukami, M., & Kawasaki, J. (2001). Rub epilepsy: A somatosensory evoked reflex epilepsy induced by prolonged cutaneous stimulation. *Journal of Neurology, Neurosurgery & Psychiatry, 70*(4), 541–543.

Kanner, A. M. (2003). Depression in epilepsy: Prevalence, clinical semiology, pathogenic mechanisms, and treatment. *Biological Psychiatry, 54*(3), 388–398.

Kanner, A. M., & Balabanov, A. (2002). Depression and epilepsy how closely related are they? *Neurology, 58*(8 suppl. 5), S27–S39.

Kanner, A. M., & Palac, S. (2002). Neuropsychiatric complications of epilepsy. *Current neurology and Neuroscience Reports, 2*(4), 365–372.

Karakis, I., Montouris, G. D., Piperidou, C., Luciano, M. S., Meador, K. J., & Cole, A. J. (2013). The effect of epilepsy surgery on caregiver quality of life. *Epilepsy Research, 107*, 181–189.

Kasteleijn-Nolst Trenité, D. G. (2012). Provoked and reflex seizures: Surprising or common? *Epilepsia, 53*(Suppl. 4), S105–S113.

Kaufmann, W. E., & Moser, H. W. (2000). Dendritic anomalies in disorders associated with mental retardation. *Cerebral Cortex, 10*(10), 981–991.

Kelly, K., Stephen, L. J., Sills, G. J., & Brodie, M. J. (2002). Topiramate in patients with learning disability and refractory epilepsy. *Epilepsia, 43*(4), 399–402.

Kemp, A. M., & Sibert, J. R. (1993). Epilepsy in children and the risk of drowning. *Archives of Disease in Childhood, 68*(5), 684–685.

Kerr, M., Fraser, W., & Felce, D. (1996). Primary health care for people with a learning disability: A keynote review. *British Journal of Learning Disabilities, 24*, 2–8.

Kerr, M. P., Baker, G. A., & Brodie, M. J. (2005). A randomized, double-blind, placebo-controlled trial of topiramate in adults with epilepsy and intellectual disability: Impact on seizures, severity, and quality of life. *Epilepsy & Behavior, 7*, 472–480.

Kerr, M., Turky, A., & Huber, B. (2009). The psychosocial impact of epilepsy in adults with an intellectual disability. *Epilepsy & Behavior, 15*, 26–30.

Kerr, M., Gil-Nagel, A., Glynn, M., Mula, M., Thompson, R., & Zuberi, S. M. (2013). Treatment of behavioral problems in intellectually disabled adult patients with epilepsy. *Epilepsia, 54*, 34–40.

Kersing, W., Dejonckere, P. H., van der Aa, H. E., & Buschman, H. P. J. (2002). Laryngeal and vocal changes during vagus nerve stimulation in epileptic patients. *Journal of Voice, 16*, 251–257.

Khoury, J. S., Winokur, R. S., Tracy, J. I., & Sperling, M. R. (2005). Predicting seizure frequency after epilepsy surgery. *Epilepsy Research, 67*, 89–99.

Koeppen, A. H. (2003). Familial hemiplegic migraine. *Archives of Neurology, 60*(5), 663–664.

Kossoff, E. H., McGrogan, J. R., & Freeman, J. M. (2004). Benefits of an all-liquid ketogenic diet. *Epilepsia, 45*, 1163.

Kossoff, E. H., Freeman, J. M., Turner, Z., & Rubenstein, J. E. (2011). *Ketogenic diets: Treatments for epilepsy and other disorders* (5th ed.). New York: Demos Health.

Krahn, L. E., Lymp, J. F., Moore, W. R., Slocumb, N., & Silber, M. H. (2005). Characterizing the emotions that trigger cataplexy. *Journal of Neuropsychiatry and Clinical Neurosciences, 17*(1), 45–50.

Kriel, R. L., Cloyd, J. C., Hadsall, R. S., Carlson, A. M., Floren, K. L., & Jones-Saete, C. M. (1991). Home use of rectal diazepam for cluster and prolonged seizures: Efficacy, adverse reactions, quality of life, and cost analysis. *Pediatric Neurology, 7*(1), 13–17.

Kuhn, D. E., Girolami, P. A., & Gulotta, C. S. (2007). Feeding disorders. *Internaitonal Review of Research in Mental Retardation, 34,* 387–414.

Kwan, P., & Brodie, M. J. (2000). Early identification of refractory epilepsy. *New England Journal of Medicine, 342,* 314–319.

Lardieri, L. A., Blacher, J., & Swanson, H. L. (2000). Sibling relationships and parent stress in families of children with and without learning disabilities. *Learning Disability Quarterly, 23*(2), 105–116.

Leach, J. P., Stephen, L. J., Salveta, C., & Brodie, M. J. (2006). Which electroencephalography (EEG) for epilepsy? The relative usefulness of different EEG protocols in patients with possible epilepsy. *Journal of Neurology, Neurosurgery & Psychiatry, 77*(9), 1040–1042.

Lempert, T., Bauer, M., & Schmidt, D. (1994). Syncope: A videometric analysis of 56 episodes of transient cerebral hypoxia. *Annals of Neurology, 36*(2), 233–237.

Lennox, N., Taylor, M., Rey-Conde, T., Bain, C., Purdie, D., & Boyle, F. (2005). Beating the barriers: Recruitment of people with intellectual disability to participate in research. *Journal of Intellectual Disability Research, 49,* 296–305.

Leung, H., & Ring, H. (2013). Epilepsy in four genetically determined syndromes of intellectual disability. *Journal of Intellectual Disability Research, 57*(1), 3–20.

Levisohn, P. M. (2000). Epilepsy surgery in children with developmental disabilities. *Seminars in Pediatric Neurology, 7,* 194–203.

Lewis, J. N., Tonge, B. J., Mowat, D. R., Einfeld, S. L., Siddons, H. M., & Rees, V. W. (2000). Epilepsy and associated psychopathology in young people with intellectual disability. *Journal of Paediatrics and Child Health, 36*(2), 172–175.

Li, H., Zou, Y., & Ding, G. (2013). Therapeutic success of the ketogenic diet as a treatment option for epilepsy: A meta-analysis. *Systematic Review, 23,* 613–620.

Lieb, J. P., Rausch, R., Engel, J., & Crandall, P. H. (1980). Complementary prognostic value of EEF and IQ data with respect to surgical outcome in temporal lobe epilepsy. *Soc Neurosci Proc, 6,* 850.

Lieb, J. P., Rausch, R., Engel, J., Brown, W. J., & Crandall, P. H. (1982). Changes in intelligence following temporal lobectomy: Relationship of EEG activity, seizure relief, and pathology. *Epilepsia, 23,* 1–23.

Lowenstein, D. H. (2008). Seizures and epilepsy. In A. S. Fauci, D. L. Kasper, & D. L. Longo (Eds.), *Harrison's principles of internal medicine* (17th ed., pp. 2498–2512). New York: McGraw-Hill.

Magrath, G., Leung, M., & Randall, T. (2012). The modified Atkins diet. In E. Neal (Ed.), *Dietary treatment of epilepsy: Practical implementation of ketogenic therapy.* West Sussex: Wiley.

Malow, B. A. (2004). Sleep deprivation and epilepsy. *Epilepsy Currents, 4*(5), 193–195.

Marsh, L., & Rao, V. (2002). Psychiatric complications in patients with epilepsy: A review. *Epilepsy Research, 49,* 11–33.

Martin, P. (2008). Diagnosis of epilepsy in persons with intellectual disabilities. In V. P. Prasheer & M. P. Kerr (Eds.), *Epilepsy and intellectual disabilities* (pp. 43–60). London: Springer.

Martin, J. P., & Brown, S. W. (2009). Best clinical and research practice in adults with an intellectual disability. *Epilepsy & Behavior, 15,* 64–68.

Martin, P., Schreiner, A., Rettig, K., & Schauble, B. (2009). Topiramate in patients with epilepsy and intellectual disability. *Epilepsy & Behavior, 14,* 496–502.

Mathern, G. W., Giza, C. C., Yudovin, S., Vinters, H. V., Peacock, W. J., Shewmon, D. A., & Shields, W. D. (1999). Postoperative seizure control and antiepileptic drug use in pediatric epilepsy surgery patients: The UCLA experience, 1986–1997. *Epilepsia, 40,* 1740–1749.

Matson J. L. (1988). *Psychopathology instrument for mentally retarded adults* (*PIMRA*). Worthington: International Diagnostic Systems.

Matson, J. L. (1995). *Diagnostic assessment for the severely handicapped revised* (*DASH-II*). Baton Rouge: Disability Consultants, LLC.

Matson, J. L. (1997). *Assessment for dual diagnosis* (*ADD*). Baton Rouge: Disability Consultants, LLC.

Matson, J. L. (1998). *Matson evaluation of drug side-effects* (*MEDS*). Baton Rouge: Disability Consultants, LLC.

Matson, J. L. (2000). *Scale for the evaluation and identification of seizures, epilepsy, and anticonvulsant side effects, B form*. Baton Rouge. Disability Consultants, LLC.

Matson, J. L., & Neal, D. (2009). Psychotropic medication use for challenging behaviors in persons with intellectual disabilities: An overview. *Research in Developmental Disabilities, 30*(3), 572–586.

Matson, J. L., & Rivet, T. T. (2008). Characteristics of challenging behaviours in adults with autistic disorder, PDD-NOS, and intellectual disability. *Journal of Intellectual and Developmental Disability, 33*(4), 323–329.

Matson, J. L., & Shoemaker, M. E. (2011). Psychopathology and intellectual disability. *Current Opinion in Psychiatry, 24*(5), 367–371.

Matson, J. L. & Vollmer, T. (1995). *Questions about behavioral function* (*QABF*). Baton Rouge: Disability Consultants, LLC.

Matson, J. L., Bamburg, J. W., Mayville, E. A., & Khan, I. (1999). Seizure disorders in people with intellectual disability: An analysis of differences in social functioning, adaptive functioning and maladaptive behaviours. *Journal of Intellectual Disability Research, 43*(6), 531–539.

Matson, J. L., Fodstad, J. C., & Dempsey, T. (2009). The relationship of children's feeding problems to core symptoms of autism and PDD-NOS. *Research in Autism Spectrum Disorders, 3,* 759–766.

Matsumoto, A., Kumagai, T., Miura, K., Miyazaki, S., Hayakawa, C., & Yamanaka, T. (1992). Epilepsy in Angelman syndrome associated with chromosome 15q deletion. *Epilepsia, 33*(6), 1083–1090.

McDermott, S., Moran, R., Platt, T., Wood, H., Isaac, T., & Dasari, S. (2005). Prevalence of epilepsy in adults with mental retardation and related disabilities in primary care. *American Journal of Mental Retardation, 110,* 48–56.

McGillivray, J. A., & McCabe, M. P. (2007). Early detection of depression and associated risk factors in adults with mild/moderate intellectual disability. *Research in Developmental Disabilities, 28*(1), 59–70.

McGoldrick, P., & Wolf, S. (2012). Vagus nerve stimulator: Another option for treatment of epilepsy. *Exceptional Parent, 42*(6), 28–31.

McGrother, C., Bhaumik, S., Thorp, C., Hauck, A., Branford, D., & Watson, J. (2006). Epilepsy in adults with intellectual disabilities: Prevalence, associations, and service implications. *Seizure, 15*(6), 376–386.

Meinardi, H., Scott, R. A., Reis, R., & Sander, J. W. A. S. (2001). The treatment gap in epilepsy: The current situation and ways forward. *Epilepsia, 42,* 136–149.

Mendez, O. E., & Brenner, R. P. (2006). Increasing the yield of EEG. *Journal of Clinical Neurophysiology, 23*(4), 282–293.

Mostofsky, D. I. (1993). Behavior modification and therapy in the management of epileptic disorders. In D. I. Mostofsky & Y. Loyning (Eds.), *The neurobehavioral treatment of epilepsy*. Hillsdale: Lawrence Erlbaum Associates.

Musumeci, S. A., Ferri, R., Elia, M., Colognola, R. M., Bergonzi, P., & Tassinari, C. A. (1991). Epilepsy and fragile X syndrome: A follow-up study. *American Journal of Medical Genetics, 38,* 511–513.

Nakken, K. O., Solaas, M. H., Kjeldsen, M. J., Friis, M. L., Pellock, J. M., & Corey, L. A. (2005). Which seizure-precipitating factors do patients with epilepsy most frequently report? *Epilepsy & Behavior, 6*(1), 85–89.

Navarro, V., Adam, C., Petitmengin, C., & Baulac, M. (2006). Toothbrush-thinking seizures. *Epilepsia, 47*(11), 1971–1973.

Neal, E. (2012). Introduction to the ketogenic diet and other dietary treatments. In E. Neal (Ed.), *Dietary treatments of epilepsy: Practical implementation of ketogenic therapy*. West Sussex: Wiley.

Nechay, A., Ross, L. M., Stephenson, J. B. P., & O'Regan, M. (2004). Gratification disorder ("infantile masturbation"): A review. *Archives of Disease in Childhood, 89*(3), 225–226.

Nicolson, A. (2008). Resective surgery for patients with epilepsy and intellectual disabilities. In V. P. Prasher & M. P. Kerr (Eds.), *Epilepsy and intellectual disabilities*. London: Springer.

O'Dell, C., Shinnar, S., Ballaban-Gil, K. R., Hornick, M., Sigalova, M., Kang, H., & Moshé, S. L. (2005). Rectal diazepam gel in the home management of seizures in children. *Pediatric Neurology, 33*(3), 166–172.

O'Dell, C., Wheless, J. W., & Cloyd, J. (2007). The personal and financial impact of repetitive or prolonged seizures on the patient and family. *Journal of Child Neurology, 22*(Suppl. 5), S61–S70.

Oguni, H. (2013). Epilepsy and intellectual and developmental disabilities. *Journal of Policy and Practice of Intellectual Disabilities, 10,* 89–92.

Oostrom, K. J., Schouten, A., Kruitwagen, C. L. J. J., Peters, A. C. B., & Jennekens-Schinkel, A. (2002). Attention deficits are not characteristic of schoolchildren with newly diagnosed idiopathic or cryptogenic epilepsy. *Epilepsia, 43*(3), 301–310.

Parkerson, G. (1996). *Duke social support and stress scale* (*DUSOCS*). Durham: Duke University Medical Center Department of Community and Family Medicine.

Pfeifer, H. H. (2012). The low glycaemic index treatment. In E. Neal (Ed.), *Dietary treatment of epilepsy: Practical implementation of ketogenic therapy*. West Sussex: Wiley.

Piazzini, A., Canevini, M. P., Maggiori, G., & Canger, R. (2001). Depression and anxiety in patients with epilepsy. *Epilepsy & Behavior, 2*(5), 481–489.

Prasher, V. P., & Kerr, M. (2008). *Epilepsy and intellectual disabilities*. London: Springer.

Prasher, V.P., Furlong, E., & Weerasena, L. (2008). Vagus nerve stimulation therapy: An intellectual disabilities perspective. In V. P. Prasher & M. P. Kerr (Eds.), *Epilepsy and intellectual disabilities*. London: Springer.

Rai, D., Kerr, M. P., McManus, S., Jordanova, V., Lewis, G., & Brugha, T. S. (2012). Epilepsy and psychiatric comorbidity: A nationally representative population-based study. *Epilepsia, 53*(6), 1095–1103.

Rausch, R., & Crandall, P. H. (1982). Psychological status related to surgical control of temporal lobe seizures. *Epilepsia, 23,* 191–202.

Reiser, M. F., Hricak, H., & Knauth, M. (2013). *MRI in epilepsy* (H. Urbach Ed.). Berlin: Springer.

Renfroe, J. B., & Wheless, J. W. (2002). Earlier use of adjunctive vagus nerve stimulation therapy for refractory epilepsy. *Neurology, 59,* 26–30.

Robinson, S. J. (2012). Childhood epilepsy and autism spectrum disorders: Psychiatric problems, phenotypic expression, and anticonvulsants. *Neuropsychology Review, 22,* 271–279.

Rodenburg, R., Wagner, J. L., Austin, J. K., Kerr, M., & Dunn, D. W. (2011). Psychosocial issues for children with epilepsy. *Epilepsy & Behavior, 22*(1), 47–54.

Ross, E., & Oliver, C. (2003). The assessment of mood in adults who have severe or profound mental retardation. *Clinical Psychology Review, 23*(2), 225–245.

Ryder, K. M., Williams, J., Womack, C., Nayak, N. G., Nasef, S., Bush, A., & Carbone, L. (2003). Appendicular fractures: A significant problem among institutionalized adults with developmental disabilities. *American Journal of Mental Retardation, 108*(5), 340–346.

Sazgar, M., Carlen, P. L., & Wennberg, R. (2003). Panic attack semiology in right temporal lobe epilepsy. *Epileptic Disorders: International Epilepsy Journal with Videotape, 5*(2), 93–100.

Schaffer, M. J., Szabo, C. A., Jackson, C. E., & Simpson, C. B. (2005). Vagal nerve stimulation: Clinical and electrophysiological effects on vocal fold function. *Annals of Ontology, Rhinology, and Laryngology, 114,* 7–14.

Scheepers, M., & Kerr, M. (2003). Epilepsy and behaviour. *Current Opinion in Neurology, 16*(2), 183–187.

Schretlen, D. J., Ward, J., Meyer, S. M., Yun, J., Puig, J. G., Nyhan, W. L., & Harris, J. C. (2005). Behavioral aspects of Lesch–Nyhan disease and its variants. *Developmental Medicine & Child Neurology, 47*(10), 673–677.

Schulze-Bonhage, A., Kurth, C., Carius, A., Steinhoff, B. J., & Mayer, T. (2006). Seizure anticipation by patients with focal and generalized epilepsy: A multicentre assessment of premonitory symptoms. *Epilepsy Research, 70*(1), 83–88.

Shashi, P., Jangra, M. K., & Yadav, A. K. (2014). Herbal and synthetic approaches for the treatment of epilepsy. *International Journal of Nutrition, 4,* 43–52.

Shaw, G. Y., Sechtem, P., Searl, J., & Dowdy, E. S. (2006). Predictors of laryngeal complications in patients implanted with the cyberonics vagal nerve stimulator. *Annals of Ontology, Rhinology, and Laryngology, 115*(4), 260–267.

Sherrard, J., Tonge, B. J., & Ozanne-Smith, J. (2001). Injury in young people with intellectual disability: Descriptive epidemiology. *Injury Prevention, 7*(1), 56–61.

Shields, W. D. (2004). Management of epilepsy in mentally retarded children using the newer antiepileptic drugs, vagus nerve stimulation, and surgery. *Journal of Child Neurology, 19,* 58–64.

Singh, B. K., & White-Scott, S. (2002). Role of topiramate in adults with intractable epilepsy, mental retardation, and developmental disabilities. *Seizure, 11,* 47–50.

Smith, K. R., & Matson, J. L. (2010). Psychopathology: Differences among adults with intellectually disabled, comorbid autism spectrum disorders and epilepsy. *Research in Developmental Disabilities, 31*(3), 743–749.

Southall, D. P., Johnson, P., Salmons, S., Talbert, D. G., Morley, C. J., Miller, J., & Helms, P. J. (1985). Prolonged expiratory apnoea: A disorder resulting in episodes of severe arterial hypoxaemia in infants and young children. *The Lancet, 326*(8455), 571–577.

Spitz, M. C., Towbin, J. A., Shantz, D., & Adler, L. E. (1994). Risk factors for burns as a consequence of seizures in persons with epilepsy. *Epilepsia, 35*(4), 764–767.

Stafstrom, C. E. (1993). Epilepsy in down syndrome: Clinical aspects and possible mechanisms. *American Journal on Mental Retardation, 98,* 12–26.

Stephenson, J., Breningstall, G., Steer, C., Kirkpatrick, M., Horrocks, I., Nechay, A., & Zuberi, S. (2004). Anoxic-epileptic seizures: Home video recordings of epileptic seizures induced by syncopes. *Epileptic Disorders: International Epilepsy Journal with Videotape, 6*(1), 15–19.

Stephenson, J. B., Hoffman, M. C., Russell, A. J., Falconer, J., Beach, R. C., Tolmie, J. L., & Zuberi, S. M. (2005). The movement disorders of Coffin–Lowry syndrome. *Brain and Development, 27*(2), 108–113.

Sweney, M. T., Silver, K., Gerard-Blanluet, M., Pedespan, J. M., Renault, F., Arzimanoglou, A., & Swoboda, K. J. (2009). Alternating hemiplegia of childhood: Early characteristics and evolution of a neurodevelopmental syndrome. *Pediatrics, 123*(3), e534–e541.

Swinkels, W. A. M., Kuyk, J., De Graaf, E. H., Van Dyck, R., & Spinhoven, P. H. (2001). Prevalence of psychopathology in Dutch epilepsy inpatients: A comparative study. *Epilepsy & Behavior, 2*(5), 441–447.

Swoboda, K. J., Soong, B. W., McKenna, C., Brunt, E. R. P., Litt, M., Bale, J. F., & Ptáček, L. J. (2000). Paroxysmal kinesigenic dyskinesia and infantile convulsions: Clinical and linkage studies. *Neurology, 55*(2), 224–230.

Tang, V., Michaelis, R., & Kwan, P. (2014). Psychobehavioral therapy for epilepsy. *Epilepsy & Behavior, 32,* 147–155.

Tatum, W. O., Johnson, K. D., Goff, S., Ferreira, J. A., & Vale, F. L. (2001). Vagus nerve stimulation and drug reduction. *Neurology, 56,* 561–563.

Trabi, T., Dunitz-Scheer, M., Kratky, E., Beckenbach, H., & Scheer, P. J. (2010). Inpatient tube weaning in children with long-term feeding tube dependency: A retrospective analysis. *Infant Mental Health Journal, 31,* 664–681.

Tsiouris, J. A. (2001). Diagnosis of depression in people with severe/profound intellectual disability. *Journal of Intellectual Disability Research, 45*(2), 115–120.

Tsuchie, S. Y., Guerreiro, M. M., Chuang, E., Baccin, C. E., & Montenegro, M. A. (2006). What about us? Siblings of children with epilepsy. *Seizure, 15*(8), 610–614.

Turygin, N., Matson, J. L., & Adams, H. (2014). Prevalence of co-occurring disorders in a sample of adults with mild and moderate intellectual disabilities who reside in a residential treatment setting. *Research in Developmental Disabilities, 35*(7), 1802–1808.

Vargha-Khadem, F., Isaacs, E., van der Werf, S., Robb, S., & Wilson, J. (1992). Development of intelligence and memory in children with hemiplegic cerebral palsy. The deleterious consequences of early seizures. *Brain: A Journal of Neurology, 115,* 315–329.

Veldhuizen, R., Binnie, C. D., & Beintema, D. J. (1983). The effect of sleep deprivation on the EEG in epilepsy. *Electroencephalography and Clinical Neurophysiology, 55*(5), 505–512.

Vickrey, B. G., Berg, A. T., Sperling, M. R., Shinnar, S., Langfitt, J. T., Bazil, C. W., & Spencer, S. S. (2000). Relationships between seizure severity and health-related quality of life in refractory localization-related epilepsy. *Epilepsia, 41*(6), 760–764.

Wang, D., Pascual, J. M., Yang, H., Engelstad, K., Jhung, S., Sun, R. P., & De Vivo, D. C. (2005). Glut-1 deficiency syndrome: Clinical, genetic, and therapeutic aspects. *Annals of Neurology, 57*(1), 111–118.

Webb, D., Fryer, A., & Osborne, J. (1991). On the incidence of fits and mental retardation in tuberous sclerosis. *Journal of Medical Genetics, 6,* 395–397.

Wehmeyer, M. L., & Bolding, N. (2001). Enhanced self-determination of adults with intellectual disability as an outcome of moving to community-based work or living environments. *Journal of Intellectual Disability Research, 45*(5), 371–383.

Welsh Office. (1995). *Welsh health survey, 1995*. Cardiff: Welsh Office.

Weston, T. M., Baxter, W. H., Felce, D., & Kerr, M. (2008). A general practice-based prevalence study of epilepsy among adults with intellectual disabilities and of its association with psychiatri disorder, behaviour disturbance and carer stress. *Journal of Intellectual Disability Research, 52,* 163–173.

Wethe, J. V., Prigatano, G. P., Gray, J., Chapple, K., Rekate, H. L., & Kerrigan, J. F. (2013). Cognitive functioning before and after surgical resection for hypothalamic hamartoma and epilepsy. *American Academy of Neurology, 81,* 1044–1050.

Whitman, S., & Hermann, B.P. (1986). *Psychopathology in epilepsy: Social dimensions*. New York: Oxford University Press.

Wieling, W., Ganzeboom, K. S., & Saul, J. P. (2004). Reflex syncope in children and adolescents. *Heart, 90*(9), 1094–1100.

Wilcox, J., & Kerr, M. P. (2008). The use of antiepileptic medication in adults with intellectual disabilities. In V. P. Prasher & M. P. Kerr (Eds.), *Epilepsy and intellectual disabilities* (pp. 97–108). London: Springer.

Williams, D., Kirkpatrick-Sanchez, S., Enzinna, C., Dunn, J., & Borden-Karasack, D. (2009). The clinical management and prevention of Pica: A retrospective follow-up of 41 individuals with intellectual disabilities and Pica. *Journal of Applied Research in Intellectual Disabilities, 22,* 210–215.

Yang, M. L., Fullwood, E., Goldstein, J., & Mink, J. W. (2005). Masturbation in infancy and early childhood presenting as a movement disorder: 12 cases and a review of the literature. *Pediatrics, 116*(6), 1427–1432.

Zabara, J. (1985). Peripheral control of hypersynchonous discharge in epilepsy. *Electroencephalography and Clinical Neurophysiology, 61,* 162.

Zalvan, C., Sulica, L., Wolf, S., Cohen, J., Gonzalez-Yanes, O., & Blitzer, A. (2003). Laryngopharyngeal dysfunction from the implant vagal nerve stimulator. *Laryngoscope, 113,* 221–225.

Zuberi, S. M. (2008). Differential diagnosis of epilepsy. In V. P. Prasheer & M. P. Kerr (Eds.), *Epilepsy and intellectual disabilities* (pp. 61–84). London: Springer.

Chapter 8
Dementia

Matthew J. Konst, Lauren W. Rasmussen and Nicole Turygin

Introduction

Dementia in Intellectual Disability

Dementia has been identified as a syndrome that is defined by the presence of deficits in occupational and social performance that result from progressive deficits in cognitive functioning, including memory loss (Cummings 1984; Douglas and Josephson 2014). In addition to the observed decline in memory, dementia is associated with pervasive impairments in intellectual functioning that are acquired rather than congenital and impair multiple capacities (e.g., language, visuospatial skills, cognition, and personality; Cummings 1984; Douglas and Josephson 2014). Dementia expression is associated with multiple neurodegenerative diseases (e.g., Alzheimer's disease [AD] and vascular dementia [VD]). Although AD and dementia with Lewy bodies (DLB) are two of the most prevalent causes of dementia in intellectual disabilities (ID), the onset of dementia may also be associated with the presence of Parkinson's disease, strokes, hypothyroidism, or vitamin (B_{12}) deficiency (Evans 1990). Some conditions leading to dementia are considered reversible. However, Boustani et al. (2003) cautioned that only 1.5 % of mild–moderate cases of dementia are actually reversible. Dementia is most prevalent in elderly populations. Following a systematic review of the literature, Ferri and colleagues (2006) estimated that 23.9 % of the world's population over the age of 60 met the diagnostic cri-

M. J. Konst (✉)
Department of Psychology, Louisiana State University, Baton Rouge, LA 70803, USA
e-mail: mkonst1@tigers.lsu.edu

L. W. Rasmussen
Adjunct Professor of Neuropsychology, Louisiana State University,
Baton Rouge, LA 70803, USA

N. Turygin
Department of Psychiatry, Indiana University School of Medicine, Indianapolis, IW, USA

J. L. Matson, M. L. Matson (eds.), *Comorbid Conditions in Individuals with Intellectual Disabilities,* Autism and Child Psychopathology Series,
DOI 10.1007/978-3-319-15437-4_8

teria for dementia. Based upon the observed prevalence, the authors estimated that there are approximately 4.6 million new cases per year. Schoenburg and colleagues (1987) reported the average annual incidence rate of dementia to be 187.5 new cases/100,000/year; AD being the most common (123.3 new cases/100,000/year).

The presence of neurological deficits, chromosomal abnormalities, and genetic metabolic disorders are considered risk factors for dementia in ID (Durkin et al. 1994). However, to date, age is considered the strongest risk factor for dementia (Boustani et al. 2003). This factor appears to remain consistent regardless of preexisting conditions although the presence of comorbid conditions (i.e., Down syndrome [DS]) may expedite the onset. Researchers have not identified significant differences in the age of onset when comparing those with that of ID (Evenhuis 1997) and the general population (Koopmans et al. 1991). Strydom et al. (2007) reported that although dementia is common in those with ID, prevalence rates are variable and dependent upon the diagnostic criteria employed. Further, the validity of current dementia criteria has not been systematically analyzed in ID populations (Strydom et al. 2007). Aylward et al. (1997) identified the lack of standardized criteria as a significant hurdle impairing the advancement of research and treatment approaches available to those with ID. Given this observation, a diagnosis of dementia in individuals with ID does not currently serve as a prognostic indicator (Aylward et al. 1997).

The heterogeneous presentation observed, in those with dementia in the general population, is exacerbated in populations with impaired cognitive functioning (i.e., ID). Symptoms such as deterioration in self-care skills, daily living skills, and memory are often reported when dementia is present in ID populations. Additional symptoms may include disorganized thinking and periods of confusion (Strydom et al. 2007). Observed deficits for those with dementia are also variable and dependent upon the causal mechanisms associated with dementia onset. Those with VD most often exhibit focal cognitive deficits such as blunted affect, decreased motivation, depressed mood, and motor retardation (Mahler and Cummings 1991; Sultzer et al. 1993) or deficits in executive functioning (e.g., planning, working memory regulation, and response inhibition; Kramer et al. 2002; Román and Royall 1999).

Advancements in the provision of care and services have increased the life expectancy of those with ID (Eyman et al. 1991; Janicki et al. 1985). This makes an increased understanding of dementia in those with ID imperative given the strong association between age and dementia onset. Given the preexisting cognitive impairment associated with ID, a diagnosis of dementia would be indicated by cognitive decline from the individual's baseline of intellectual functioning (Aylward et al. 1997). However, clinicians may be forced to rely on observation and caregiver report for those with significant cognitive deficits which may impede the detection of cognitive decline through standardized testing. Comorbid physical impairments (e.g., mobility and sensory deficits) are a notable factor in ID populations that inhibit social and adaptive functioning and may also hinder the assessment of cognitive decline (Evenhuis 1997).

The presence of ID poses difficulties in diagnosis due to the relatively high floor effects that often fail to distinguish between deficits in dementia and cognitive deficits due to ID. Palmer (2006) used neuropsychological tests in a sample of adults with ID to determine the degree to which a neuropsychological test could distinguish between deficits in ID and dementia. Those with ID and dementia exhibited problems with memory and learning, agnosia, semantic verbal fluency, attention, and executive function relative to those with only ID, but separate cutoffs were needed to distinguish those with dementia, since low scores were observed for all individuals with ID. Deficits in coping mechanisms observed in ID populations suggest that they may be especially vulnerable to dementia when compared to the general population (Evenhuis 1997). This highlights the need for continuous evaluation in ID populations to monitor an individual's functioning. Consideration is also needed relative to the individual's level of functioning (e.g., mild or profound). Given the levels of impairment observed in ID populations, a decline in functioning for someone with profound ID may present differently compared to an individual with mild or moderate ID (Aylward et al. 1997). Further, the decline in cognitive functioning should exceed that typically observed in aging ID populations. However, this area is currently hindered by the dearth of research investigating factors associated with aging in those with ID (Nagdee 2011).

The course of cognitive decline as assessed by tests of cognitive functioning is reported to be approximately 10% each year in the general population with AD or DLB (Ballard et al. 2001; Janicki and Dalton 1999a). Decline in cognitive functioning is not limited to memory and may include abstract reasoning skills (e.g., planning and organizational skills or judgment) and deficits associated with dementia are not limited to cognitive decline. Progressive decline in cognitive functioning and memory may not be readily apparent in those with more severe forms of ID. Apraxia and aphasia may be some of the first cognitive deficits readily observed. For instance, for those with verbal language skills, a decline in the demonstration of verbal skills (aphasia) may be observed (Aylward et al. 1997). On the other hand, those with ID who have developed dementia, commonly exhibit a decline in the ability to carry out self-care and activities of daily functioning (e.g., self-dressing or self-feeding; Strydom et al. 2007) which may be associated with apraxia.

Changes in behavioral presentation other than cognitive decline in ID populations are also common and cause significant distress (Burns et al. 1990; Cooper and Prasher 1998; Ryden 1988). Some variation has been observed in the expression of noncognitive symptoms based upon the underlying etiology of ID manifestation. Those individuals with ID associated with factors other than DS exhibit aggression more frequently than those with ID resulting from DS. However, individuals with ID due to DS exhibit greater rates of sleep disturbance, hyperactivity, and depressed mood than individuals with ID without DS (Cooper and Prasher 1998). Some symptoms are prevalent in ID following onset of dementia regardless of underlying etiology: urinary and fecal incontinence, decreased energy, and difficulty walking (Cooper and Prasher 1998).

Prevalence

When excluding those individuals with comorbid DS, the prevalence of dementia in individuals with ID under age 60 is approximately 13.1% (Strydom et al. 2009). The estimated prevalence rate in the same population over the age of 60 has been reported to range from 6 to 18.3 % (Janicki and Dalton 2000; Strydom et al. 2009). Previous prevalence estimates in similar populations identified similar rates across different age ranges. In an investigation of individuals over the age of 65, Cooper (1997b) reported a prevalence rate of 20.2 %. Patel et al. (1993) examined individuals over the age of 50 and found a prevalence rate of 8.3 %. Some studies have reported that 14 % of individuals with ID over the age of 59 have dementia, this rate increases to 22 % by age 65 (Cooper 1997). To date, no significant differences have been observed for differential prevalence rates based upon the observed level of intellectual functioning (e.g., mild and profound ID; Strydom et al. 2009).

The prevalence of dementia is influenced by those factors associated with its onset. Of the dementia subtypes, AD is the most common in individuals with ID over the age of 60 without comorbid DS (Janicki and Dalton 2000; Strydom et al. 2007). The prevalence of AD in ID populations was observed to be three times higher than that in the general population (Strydom et al. 2007). The estimated prevalence rate of AD in ID populations is 8.6 % (Strydom et al. 2007). Rocca and colleagues (1991) observed a stable prevalence rate of AD in a longitudinal analysis of European populations. When the authors separated the population into age groups, significantly greater prevalence rates were observed as the age increased (Evans 1990; Rocca et al. 1991; Schoenburg et al. 1987). In general, for persons 65 years of age and older, the overall estimated prevalence of AD was 11.3 % (Evans 1990; Pfeffer et al. 1987). Evans (1990) estimated that 4 % of persons between 65 and 74 years of age met the criteria for AD. This rate increased to 16.4 % in individuals aged 75–84, and rose to 47.55 % when individuals were over the age of 85. Researchers caution that prevalence rates are significantly influenced by diagnostic approaches and the criteria used to diagnose AD and dementia in general (Kay et al. 1985; Henderson and Jorm 1987; McKhann et al. 1984).

Neurodegenerative Diseases in ID

For individuals with ID, researchers have previously identified AD as the most commonly occurring subtype of dementia, followed by DLB, frontotemporal dementia, and lastly VD (Strydom et al. 2007). There is currently a dearth of research available that has distinguished between dementia subtypes in ID populations. This may be attributed to differences in presentation due to the presence and variation of cognitive deficits in ID populations, and the influences of comorbid conditions (Strydom et al. 2010). Further impediment may also be associated with variation in the assessments and diagnostic criteria used to diagnose individuals. Given the limited availability of research for ID populations the following is a review of the research available surrounding dementia in ID populations and in the general population regarding each dementia subtype.

Alzheimer's Disorder (AD) The description of AD presented by Alzheimer (1907) was associated with neurological deficits (e.g., neurofibrillary tangles and neuritic plaques), with symptoms of dementia noted to occur most often in middle-aged adults. Neurofibrillary tangles and senile plaques are the structural lesions most often identified in those with AD (Dickson 2002). However, despite increased research efforts surrounding AD, the etiology of the disorder remains unclear (Katzman 1986).

Evans (1990) suggested that AD may be better classified as a heterogeneous category. Some researchers have suggested that the observed heterogeneity in Alzheimer symptom manifestation warrants consideration of AD subtypes. Following a longitudinal analysis, Mayeux et al. (1985) proposed four groups based upon symptom manifestation: typical (slow deterioration of intellectual and functional capabilities); myoclonic (intellectual decline); benign (minimal symptom progression); and extrapyramidal (presence of psychotic symptoms and severe functional and intellectual decline). The heterogeneity of symptoms is likely associated with the observed variance in diagnosis. Researchers have demonstrated that on average the onset of AD symptoms may not lead to clinical diagnosis for 3.5–5.5 years after the initial symptom onset (Heyman et al. 1987; Huff et al. 1987; Knopman et al. 1988).

It has previously been hypothesized that the prevalence of AD is not static and may continue to increase given increases in the average life expectancy (Evans 1990). Aside from age, additional factors are considered to place individuals at risk for AD. Researchers have observed an earlier age of onset for individuals with a family history of AD (Thai et al. 1988). However, this may also be attributed to the increased awareness and willingness to seek services. Further, researchers have demonstrated that having a first-degree relative with AD, or the presence of the apolipoprotein E-ε4 (APOE-ε4) genotype is associated with an increased risk for AD (Blacker and Tanzi 1998; Lautenschlager et al. 1996). Individuals with AD are three times more likely to possess the APOE-ε4 allele than the general population (Boustani et al. 2003). However, the exact role of this genotype is uncertain as Lai and Williams (1989) demonstrated that not all individuals with AD have the allele and persons with the allele do not always develop AD. Gender has also been noted to be a contributing factor, as rates of AD have been observed to be elevated in females (Rocca et al. 1991). Ernst and Hay (1994) reported that women diagnosed with AD tend to live a year longer (4.3 years) on average as compared to men (3.3 years; Barclay et al. 1985; Hier et al. 1989). Researchers have previously suggested that physical activity may serve as a protective factor against AD (Yoshitake et al. 1995).

Multiple researchers have demonstrated moderate reliability for a diagnosis of AD (Blacker et al. 1994; Farrer et al. 1994; Lopez et al. 1999). However, multiple diagnostic criteria have been proposed and analyzed. During a systematic review of proposed criteria for AD, the criteria from the National Institute of Neurologic, Communicative Disorders and Stroke–AD and Related Disorders Association (NINCDS-ADRDA) and the Diagnostic and Statistical Manual of Mental Disorders, 4th Edition (*DSM-IV*) were each observed to demonstrate good sensitivity and moderate specificity (Knopman et al. 2001).

Dementia with Lewy Bodies (DLB) DLB is reported to be the second most common dementia subtype when ID is present (McKeith et al. 2004; Strydom et al. 2007). However, the ascertainment of DLB being more prevalent than VD is dependent upon the population surveyed and the criteria used to identify individuals

(Heidebrink 2002). Within the general population, prevalence estimates are variable and range from 3 to 26.3 % (Chan et al. 2002; Heidebrink 2002; Perry et al. 1990a; Shergill et al. 1994). For ID populations, the prevalence rate of DLB was reported to be similar to that observed in the general population (Strydom et al. 2007).

The presence of Lewy bodies was originally associated with Parkinson's disease and was only later identified as a separate pathology (Kosaka et al. 1980, 1983). Since its initial identification researchers have identified some variation in the manifestation of Lewy bodies. This observation has led to the proposal of three subtypes based upon the location of the Lewy bodies (Kosaka et al. 1980, 1983). The diffuse subtype of DLB impacts multiple areas of the brain (e.g., diencephalic, basal ganglia nuclei, brainstem, and the cortical area). The location of Lewy body manifestation results in differential symptom presentation. For example, the brainstem subtype remains localized and does not transcend to other cerebral areas. The transitional subtype of DLB is associated with a variable and diffuse manifestation of Lewy bodies (e.g., limbic cortices, brainstem, and diencephalic region; Dickson 2002).

The presence of DLB is commonly associated with AD symptomology (Dickson 2002; Hansen et al. 1990). Aside from the expression of Parkinson's disease, those with DLB may also exhibit neuroleptic sensitivity, motor impairment, confusion, and hallucinations (Byrne et al. 1989; McKeith et al. 2004; Perry et al. 1989, 1990). Visual hallucinations are common in individuals with DLB in as many as 46 % of the individuals experiencing them at some point during the course of the disease (McKeith 1998). Although symptoms of hallucinations, delusions, and depression are more prevalent in individuals with DLB, these symptoms are not unique to DLB and are also observed in those with AD (Ballard et al. 1999).

The diagnostic criteria proposed by the Consortium for dementia with Lewy bodies (Consortium for DLB; McKeith et al. 1996) demonstrated high specificity on average, but low sensitivity (Holmes et al. 1999; Litvan et al. 1998; Lopez et al. 1999; Luis et al. 1999; Mega et al. 1996; Verghese et al. 1999). Two central criteria proposed include (a) the presence of recurring detailed visual hallucinations and (b) variations in awareness and attention associated with instability of cognitive abilities (McKeith et al. 1996).

Vascular Dementia (VD) Fratiglioni and colleagues (1999) reported that VD is the second most common form of dementia in the general population. However, in comparison to the general population, there is a decreased prevalence of VD in ID populations. Specifically, FTD and DLB are reportedly more common than VD in those with ID (Strydom et al. 2007). There are three critical components necessary for a diagnosis of VD; the presence of cerebrovascular disease (CVD), dementia, and a clear association or temporal relationship between the two (Chui et al. 1992; Román et al. 1993). Symptom presentation is reportedly variable and dependent upon the location and cause of cerebral damage (Román 2002). Of the two predominate causes, small-vessel disease is often associated with depressed mood, impaired memory, disturbed executive functioning, impaired information processing, parkinsonian features, and urinary disturbances (Kurz 2001; Román and Royall 1999). Small-vessel disease is also associated with diabetes and hypertension and may be evidenced by white matter or basal ganglia lacunae, white matter lesions, or a combination of the two (Erkinjuntti et al. 2004; Román 2002).

The second common cause of cerebral damage, large-vessel disease, is more likely to result in diffuse cortical impairment (Erkinjuntti et al. 2004; Mahler and Cummings 1991; Sultzer et al. 1993). The presence of VD is also associated with transient symptoms, gait disturbances, and incontinence (Thai et al. 1988). Cardiovascular health (e.g., hypertension) and strokes have been identified as risk factors for VD onset (Hofman et al. 1997; Longstreth et al. 1998; Thai et al. 1988). Additional risk factors may include alcohol consumption, age, previous strokes, and elevated blood pressure levels (Yoshitake et al. 1995).

Differing groups have proposed diagnostic criteria specific to VD. They include the California Alzheimer's Disease Diagnostic and Treatment Centers (CAD-DTC; Chui et al. 1992) and the National Institute of Neurological Disorders and Stroke and the Association Internale pour la Recherche et l'Enseignement en Neurosciences (NINDS-AIREN; Román et al. 1993). The criteria proposed by the CAD-DTC are reportedly more sensitive (0.63) but less specific (0.64; Gold et al. 1997) than those proposed by NINDS-AIREN (0.55 and 0.84 sensitivity and specificity, respectively; Gold et al. 2002). In general, a review of the studies investigating each of the diagnostic criteria proposed for VD (i.e., *DSM-IV*, NINDS-AIREN, CAD-DTC, and Hachinski Ischemic Standards) evidence low diagnostic sensitivity, but high specificity (Knopman et al. 2001).

Frontotemporal Dementia (FTD) Frontotemporal dementia (FTD) has previously been separated into three prototypic syndromes; FTD, semantic dementia (SD), and progressive non-fluent aphasia (PA; Mackenzie et al. 2009; Neary et al. 1998). Of the three syndromes, FTD is reportedly the most common (Neary et al. 1998). As implied by its name, FTD is associated with the degeneration of the frontal lobe and is bilateral and symmetric (Englund et al. 1994; Neary et al. 1998). Degeneration in the spinal motor neurons is suggested to be a distinguishing feature of FTD when compared to the other forms of dementia (e.g., AD and VD; Englund et al. 1994). Currently there is limited research investigating the manifestation and prevalence of FTD in ID populations. Strydom and colleagues (2007) observed similar prevalence rates of FTD in individuals with ID when compared to the general population. The average age of onset for FTD in a sample ranging in age from 45 to 64 years was 52.8 years (Ratnavalli et al. 2002). Onset of FTD is associated with a preservation of memory functioning, social disinhibition, significant shifts in personality, stereotyped behavior, and loss of insight (Gustafson 1987; Neary et al. 1998; Snowden et al. 1996). Additional symptoms may include behavioral features (e.g., deficits in personal hygiene, mental rigidity, and disinhibition), physical symptoms (e.g., incontinence and deficits in primitive reflexes), speech disturbances (e.g., stereotypic speech and echolalia), and affective symptoms (e.g., anxiety, depression, and decreased empathy; Gustafson 1987, 1993; Neary et al. 1988; Risberg 1987).

Those with SD may continue to exhibit appropriate speech capabilities while evidencing significant deficits in the comprehension of verbal and nonverbal concepts (Hodges et al. 1992; Neary et al. 1998; Snowden et al. 1989; Snowden et al. 1996). The SD variant is associated with the exhibition of progressive language deficits

(Grossman 2002; Hodges et al. 1992; Snowden et al. 1989). For those with SD neurological insults include bilateral atrophy in the anterior temporal neocortex (Neary et al. 1998). Individuals with PA typically maintain their capability to understand word meanings, but exhibit expressive language deficits to include grammatical and phonological errors, deficits in word retrieval, and effortful speech production (Snowden et al. 1996; Snowden et al. 1992; Weintraub et al. 1990). Neurologic deficits most often include asymmetric atrophy of the left frontotemporal lobes (Neary et al. 1998).

Utilizing autopsy and previous assessments, Varma and colleagues (1999) demonstrated that most patients evidencing neurologic deficits associated with FTD met the diagnostic criteria for AD. Following an autopsy to verify FTD diagnosis and a chart review, Rosen and colleagues (2002) identified five factors that reliably distinguished individuals with FTD from those with AD. Similar to previous research (Miller et al. 1997), features included hyperorality, absence of amnesia, social conduct disorders, and the absence of a perceptual disorder. Researchers have suggested that an interdisciplinary (physiological, behavioral, and neuropsychological) approach was best for distinguishing AD from FTD (Rosen et al. 2002). Advancements in biochemistry, molecular genetics, and neuropathology have further increased the specificity of classification for FTD. Advancements have led to newly proposed criteria that are identified by the proteins associated with neuropathologic diagnosis (see Cairns et al. 2007 and Mackenzie et al. 2009 for a complete review).

Mortality

The factors associated with the onset of dementia have also been associated with an increased risk for mortality. The reported average survival length following onset of dementia is variable and has ranged from 3.3 to 9.3 years (Schoenburg et al. 1987; Wolfson et al. 2001). Researchers have previously reported that individuals with ID live an average of 7.3 years following diagnosis of dementia (Evenhuis 1997). However, Wolfson et al. (2001) cautioned that the estimates of life expectancy following dementia onset may be overestimated. They reported that researchers often fail to consider those with progressive forms of dementia, that may result in death prior to the individual's inclusion in a study. Researchers may also fail to consider the onset of dementia in relation to the participant's inclusion in the study. The onset of dementia is often difficult to pinpoint due to the gradual progression of symptoms and external factors already mentioned (Doraiswamy et al. 1998; Knopman 1998; Ross et al. 1997). These factors along with variations in the criteria and diagnostic approaches across studies likely influence the variability observed. Although dementia is associated with significant decreases in functioning, it is important to note that it is not a significant primary cause of death in ID populations. A longitudinal study identified vascular and respiratory diseases as the two most prevalent causes of mortality for those with ID (Patja et al. 2001). These two diseases accounted for 58 % of the deaths observed.

The presence of comorbid conditions and the causal mechanisms underlying dementia onset are also factors associated with differential mortality outcomes. When dementia was present, Coppus and colleagues (2006) observed a mortality rate of 44.4 % in patients with DS over the age of 60 which was significantly greater than non-demented peers (10.7 %). Individuals with probable AD were noted to be outlived by those with VD and those with a possible AD diagnosis (Wolfson et al. 2001). Onset at a younger age has been associated with increased survival (Diesfeldt et al. 1986; Mölsä et al. 1986). In addition, researchers have also begun examining the contribution of risk- and protective-factors associated with the onset of dementia and mortality. Prognostic factors include comorbid medical or neurological illness, age, severity of pre-morbid intellectual functioning, psychosocial support systems, DS, familial history, and early onset of dementia symptoms (Evenhuis 1997; Harper and Wadsworth 1993; Janicki and Dalton 1999; Janicki and Jacobson 1986; Lin et al. 2014). Presently, controversy remains surrounding the relationship between educational attainment and mortality (Geerlings et al. 1997; Stern et al. 1995; Wolfson et al. 2001).

Comorbid Conditions

Dementia co-occurs at higher rates in individuals with ID (Cooper 1997; Shooshtari et al. 2011; Strydom et al. 2007). Moreover, the neurological deficits inherent in individuals with familial ID may place individuals with ID at increased risk for declines in cognitive function at an earlier age (Zigman et al. 1993). General aging processes have been observed to occur at younger ages in individuals with intellectual and developmental disabilities. The disorder that is most strongly associated with both ID and the increased likelihood of onset of dementia is DS.

Few researchers have examined the degree to which disorders related to ID represent risk factors for dementia. Disorders such as epilepsy, cerebral palsy, autism, DS, and genetic disorders such as Prader–Willi syndrome and Williams syndrome are associated with the presence of ID. The presence of ID has been hypothesized to relate to an increased risk of dementia, as those with ID possess less "reserve capacity" of brain function (Strydom et al. 2013). Thus, the brains of those with ID are likely to be more vulnerable to pathological assault, and are more likely to exhibit earlier symptoms of dementia, relative to those without ID. The presence of comorbid conditions in those with ID has been observed to impact the onset and rates of dementia, especially DS.

Dementia in Down Syndrome

Down syndrome is a disorder that most commonly results from the triplication of the 21st chromosome (HSA21). Approximately 1 in 800 children in the USA is born with the disorder. The vast majority of individuals with DS have an ID. Down syndrome manifests with specific physical features, including epicanthal folds, a flat nasal bridge, protruding tongue, slanted palpebral fissures, heart valve defects, predisposition to leukemia, and cataracts (Visootsak and Sherman 2008). Life expectancy for individuals with DS has dramatically increased over the past century. In 1929 the life expectancy for someone with DS was 9 years, and 12 years in 1949 (Bell et al. 2003). It was estimated that 76 % of individuals with DS survived to age 1 and 65 % survived to age 10 in the 50s and 60s (Bittles and Glasson 2004). In 2002, the life expectancy of individuals with DS has increased to approximately 60 years on average (Glasson et al. 2002).

Cognitive deficits in DS follow general trends. The mean IQ in individuals with DS is 50 and generally ranges from 30 to 70 (Vicari 2004). Vocabulary and adaptive skills generally develop more quickly than memory and executive function, and the overall rate of learning and IQ scores decline with age (Nadel 2003). Remarkably, individuals with DS exhibit more dramatic declines in performance across domains when tasks are very demanding. Deficits are observed in both short-term and long-term memory in individuals with DS. On tasks of implicit memory, children with DS perform at the same level as children without DS. However, they exhibit significant deficits in explicit memory tasks (Contestabile et al. 2010).

Researchers have demonstrated significant differences in the symptom manifestation associated with dementia within ID populations. Specifically, differences in decline are influenced by the presence of DS, and include a gradual decline in long-term memory and verbal language skills (Devenny et al. 1996). Dementia is a very common disorder in individuals with DS. Janicki and Dalton (2000) observed a 3 % prevalence rate in an ID only group over the age of 60. When the authors included individuals with DS and comorbid ID this rate increased to 56 %. In addition to prevalence, the presence of DS in ID populations may also alter the average age of onset. For example, the average age of onset is significantly influenced by the presence or absence of DS. Lai (1992) reported an average age of onset for those with DS between 51 and 54 years of age, whereas individuals with ID without DS are diagnosed after the age of 65 on average (Janicki and Dalton 1993, 2000; Lai and Williams 1989). Behavior change is often observed prior to the observation of cognitive decline (Holland et al. 2000). Adams and colleagues (2008) observed that referral for dementia evaluation for those with DS was triggered by behavioral excess, and the effect of behavioral change on the provision of care (Oliver et al. 2000). Examples of behavioral change include both deficits and excesses (e.g., agitation and restlessness, sleep disturbance, withdrawal; Doody et al. 1995; Petry et al. 1988; Reichman and Negron 2001).

Neuroanatomical studies of individuals with DS have revealed a variety of differences in individuals with the disorder. Although individuals with DS may not exhibit symptoms of dementia (Devenny et al. 1996; Zigman et al. 1996) researchers have suggested that brain lesions typical of AD appear in individuals with DS by 40 years of age (Wisniewski et al. 1985). Post-mortem studies of the brains of individuals with DS have revealed decreased brain volumes which are most apparent in the frontal and temporal areas, and the cerebellum (Bowman et al. 2013). Neuroimaging studies of children with DS have also revealed decreases in hippocampal volume. The ID associated with DS is attributed to these differences in brain volume and architecture. With time, the majority of individuals with DS will develop the beta-amyloid plaques and neurofibrillary tangles characteristic of AD.

Interestingly, there is some belief among researchers that plaques and tangles observed in individuals with DS are distinct from those observed in the brains of individuals with AD and are common among individuals with DS without dementia (Mann 1993; Wisniewski and Rabe 1986). The non-fibrillary nature of these plaques and tangles is believed not to harm the nearby neurons, in contrast to the fibrillary structures observed in AD.

Symptoms of dementia in individuals with DS are numerous. Slowness, apathy, disinterest in activities and social relationships may be noticed and may represent dysfunction of the frontal lobe. It has been reported that adults with DS and a lower mental age often present with clinical depression based on caregiver and self-report measures (Burt et al. 1992). According to Evenhuis (1990), many adults with DS lose the ability to follow complex directions and experience overall slowing. Slowness may manifest through flattening of the voice, hesitation in beginning to speak, and difficulties with comprehension. Affected individuals may nap frequently during the day and sleep less at night, instead wandering or talking to themselves (Evenhuis 1990; Deb and McHugh 2010; Prasher 1995).

Depression

Within the general population, the prevalence of comorbid depression in individuals without ID who are diagnosed with dementia is estimated to range from 24 to 80% (Cummings and Victoroff 1990; Burns et al. 1990; Rubin and Kinscherf 1989). Evenhuis (1997) also noted a high rate of delirium and depressive symptoms in individuals with all levels of ID. Symptoms of depression and dementia have been noted to overlap and impede differential diagnosis given the observed difficultly to distinguish symptom manifestation in aging adults (Strydom et al. 2007). However, some controversy surrounding the expression of affective symptoms is noted in the research. In a study of comorbid neuropsychiatric symptoms, Wetzels et al. (2010) noted that affective symptoms (e.g., anxiety and depression) decreased and that symptoms of apathy tended to increase. The authors reported that irritability, aberrant motor behaviors, and agitation were the most prevalent symptoms (Wetzels et al. 2010). This controversy is likely influenced by the heterogeneity of dementia. Affective symptom expression is reportedly influenced by the diseases associated with the onset of dementia (e.g., VD and AD). Those individuals whose dementia was associated with VD most often exhibited symptoms of depression and aggression (Wetzels et al. 2010). However, symptoms of anxiety and apathy were more prevalent for those with AD when compared to those with VD. Vulnerability to symptoms of delirium in elderly populations has also been attributed to physical illness and some medications and is reportedly exacerbated when dementia is present (Lipowski 1989). It has also been suggested that the presence or absence of DS may alter the presentation of symptoms of dementia in those with ID (Cooper and Prasher 1998). Thorough differential diagnosis is important when depression symptoms are observed.

Identification and Assessment

The diagnosis of dementia is associated with multiple approaches to the development of diagnostic criteria. Most often diagnostic criteria are created relative to the specific disease underlying the onset of dementia (i.e., AD, VD, DLD, and FTD). Given this individualistic approach the research supporting each of the proposed diagnostic criteria is variable. This variability also directly impacts reported prevalence rates. Though this is true in the general population, the observed dearth of diagnostic criteria and research relevant to ID populations is especially salient.

It should be noted that no specific consideration for ID populations was presented in the *DSM-IV-TR* or *ICD-10*. Researchers have advocated for the use of *ICD-10* criteria for the identification of dementia in ID populations (Aylward et al. 1997). The *ICD-10* criteria incorporate functional decline in areas other than cognition and encourage the establishment of a dementia diagnosis before attempting to differentiate its specific form (e.g., AD or VD; Aylward et al. 1997). For individuals with ID, cognitive decline may involve deficits in memory which may include a failure to recognize familiar persons or requiring persistent prompts to carry out tasks they had previously mastered (Aylward et al. 1997). However, universal consensus amongst researchers and clinicians has not been reached and further research is required.

Early Identification

Researchers continue to stress the importance of early identification and diagnosis (Cattel et al. 2000; Moïse et al. 2004) suggesting that early intervention may slow the decline (Bridges-Webb et al. 2003). Early identification and referral may increase treatment efficacy and overall quality of life for individuals and their families.

A significant impairment to early dementia diagnosis remains the dearth of identified symptoms and triggers as early warning signs (Bowers et al. 1990). There remains a significant need for research on individuals with ID surrounding the epidemiology of dementia, including prevention, early indicators, and early intervention. Wilkinson and Janicki (2002) stressed the importance of information dissemination regarding dementia for families and caregivers of individuals with ID. This is especially important given the variety of living situations an individual with ID may be placed in and the increased difficulty of identifying cognitive decline or decreased adaptive functioning in individuals with impaired intellectual functioning. Further, information dissemination is especially important given that symptoms of dementia are most often observed and reported by family members or caregivers (Speechly et al. 2008).

In addition to assessment difficulties researchers have previously identified external factors that further impede a diagnosis of dementia. Primary care physicians are often the frontline for aging individuals (Heagerty and Eskenazi 1994). There is a large variation in the diagnostic practices of medical physicians (Glasser 1993; Rubin et al. 1987; Somerfield et al. 1991). Generally, physicians are more likely to rely on laboratory tests at the exclusion of cognitive and mental status evaluations (Fortinsky et al. 1995). The use of physical examination and review of personal records is not associated with effective identification of dementia. In a systematic review of dementia research, Boustani and colleagues (2003) reported that in a primary care setting 50–60 % of those with dementia are not diagnosed. Researchers have repeatedly demonstrated that more than half of the persons diagnosed with mild to moderate dementia were not identified by a physician (Cooper et al. 1996; Lagaay et al. 1992; O'Connor et al. 1988; Ólafsdóttir et al. 2000).

In a survey of physicians given a diagnostic vignette, Fortinsky and colleagues (1995) observed that 90 % of physicians would provide diagnostic information to a caregiver, as opposed to 50 % reporting that they would also directly tell the patient. The uncertainty of dementia diagnosis is likely a factor impacting such decisions given the heterogeneity of symptom manifestation and prognosis (Moody 1992). The stigma, negative outcomes (deterioration), and prognosis associated with dementia has also been linked to a reluctance to diagnose patients with dementia (Milne et al. 2000; Vernooij-Dassen et al. 2005). Regardless of assets in place for diagnosing dementia, Vernooij-Dassen and colleagues (2005) reported that the negative stigma surrounding dementia is the largest factor impeding early diagnosis. The importance of assessing individuals with ID for dementia should not be tarnished by the bias or stigma associated with prognosis and treatment (Wilkinson and Janicki 2002). It is important to provide services that address the individual's current needs and plan for the future regardless of the individual's level of intellectual functioning (Wilkinson and Janicki 2002). However, a decline in stigma has been associated with increased awareness surrounding dementia and the provision of psychoeducational resources to caretakers, family, general health practitioners, and the general population. Researchers have previously provided a number of suggested targets to decrease the stigma associated with dementia (see Vernooij-Dassen et al. 2005).

Early Indicators

Early indicators for dementia most often include impaired daily living skills, memory, behaviors or personal demeanor, and interpersonal communication (Speechly et al. 2008). For those with ID, symptoms such as irritability, apathy, memory decline, confusion, and emotional lability are frequently reported as early indicators of dementia (Dalton and Crapper-McLachlan 1986; Evenhuis 1990; Lai and Williams 1989; Strydom et al. 2007). De Lepeleire et al. (1998) also suggested that increased need for support, emotional instability, decreased occupational functioning, and daily living skill disturbances may be indicative of dementia onset. Factors such as hospital admission, loss of a caregiver or loved one, and medication changes are factors often highlighting the presence of dementia (De Lepeleire et al. 1998). This was postulated due to the rapid change in the provision of care or level of functioning, which may highlight the accommodations the caregiver or family member had increasingly provided as severity increased.

According to a study conducted by Cooper and Prasher (1998), the earliest signs of dementia among adults with ID include lack of energy, disturbed sleep, difficulty walking, urinary and fecal incontinence, and being uncooperative. Among adults with ID who do not have DS, aggression is among the most common behavioral manifestations of dementia (Cooper and Prasher 1998). Compared to adults with DS and no evidence of progressive dementia, those with suspected dementia perform globally worse on neuropsychological measures of attention, executive functioning, language, and memory (Palmer 2006). Similar findings are cited by Ball et al. 2006, which indicated that adults with DS suspected of having dementia present with early symptoms of decline in executive skills, psychomotor functioning, attention, language, episodic memory, abstract reasoning, visuospatial organization, and reduced empathy and emotional lability.

Gait disturbance is commonly observed in those with dementia (Waite et al. 2000), especially in older individuals (Nutt et al. 1993). Gait disturbance is not noted to be limited to specific dementia subtypes and has been observed in those with VD (Hennerici et al. 1994; Thompson and Marsden 1987) and AD (Ala and Frey 1994; O'Keeffe et al. 1996). However, some researchers have suggested that it may occur later in the course of development of AD (McKhann et al. 1984; Thomas et al. 2002).

Multiple factors have been suggested to impact gait disturbance in demented populations. Thomas and colleagues (2002) observed a reciprocal relationship between cognitive decline and the severity of gait disturbance such that as cognitive decline increased so did gait impairment. The presence of gait disturbance is also associated with the retardation of internal organ system functioning (e.g., respiratory, renal, cardiac; Thomas et al. 2002). In those with ID, gait disturbance may not be readily apparent depending upon premorbid motor functioning.

Assessment

Early identification is currently hampered by the lack of available measures for individuals with ID. At present, the average duration between symptom onset and dementia diagnosis is reported to vary between 12 and 36 months (Cattel et al. 2000; Fiske et al. 2005; Speechly et al. 2008). Whereas some researchers have reported that the average evaluation for dementia is carried out 30 months after symptoms are initially reported (Haley et al. 1992).

Assessment approaches and related criteria for measuring decline in cognitive and adaptive behaviors for ID populations are largely absent (Strydom and

Hassiotis 2003). The utilization of measures such as the *Mini Mental State Examination* that are commonly used to identify dementia in the general population is often inappropriate for individuals with ID (Strydom and Hassiotis 2003; Sturmey et al. 1991). Wilkinson and Janicki (2002) identified the need for the creation of a standardized assessment of dementia in individuals with ID. Assessments should be utilized to create a baseline of functioning that could be used to identify any change in functioning following successive administrations (Burt and Aylward 2000; Wilkinson and Janicki 2002). Aylward and colleagues (1997) advocated for the use of standardized testing procedures after the age of 25 in individuals with ID as a means of establishing a personal baseline of functioning. This approach should be comprehensive and incorporate direct observation and information from persons such as caretakers or family members who have regular interactions with the individual.

Despite the availability of standardized neuropsychological assessments, no criteria surrounding performance decline on such measures has been identified to be indicative of dementia (Aylward et al. 1997). Although researchers advocate for the use of a mental status exam to track cognitive performance, no psychometric properties specific to ID populations are currently available (Aylward et al. 1997). Further, it is necessary to account for the significant variation in intellectual functioning observed within ID populations regarding assessment administration. This is especially true in relation to the assessment of psychological and behavioral functioning. For example, standardized scales are available that are appropriate for individuals with severe and profound ID (*Diagnostic Assessment for the Severely Handicapped II*; Matson 1994) whereas other measures may be more appropriate for mild or moderate ID (Aylward et al. 1997).

Researchers have noted methodological flaws in research that have hindered the development of widely used assessments and criteria (Aylward et al. 1997; Sturmey et al. 1991) including a relative lack of representative longitudinal studies (Evenhuis 1990; Lai and Williams 1989). Strydom and Hassiotis (2003) noted the benefits of longitudinal assessment in ID populations given the acknowledged impairment surrounding the interpretation of singular dementia screenings (McDaniel et al. 1998). A longitudinal approach may be particularly insightful given the relative dearth of information that has been collected surrounding aging in individuals with ID (Nagdee 2011; Silverman et al. 1998).

The direct assessment of dementia symptoms is noted to be especially difficult in ID populations (Strydom and Hassiotis 2003). However, some direct assessment measures have been developed and utilized for individuals with ID. Some researchers have suggested the use of informant-based screeners for those with ID (Deb and Braganza 1999). Screening measures most often focus on one of two domains (i.e., functional assessment and tests of cognition) and may utilize self-report or informant report (Boustani et al. 2003). However, a dual approach (i.e., direct and indirect measures) has proved beneficial in assessing the general population for dementia (Mackinnon and Mulligan 1998). Researchers have suggested that dementia test batteries should also include both direct and indirect measures of dementia for individuals with ID (Burt and Aylward 2000). Further, it is important to note that a single administration of a measure does not satisfy the requirement for documented cognitive decline when diagnosing dementia. As such, longitudinal assessment and monitoring of cognitive and adaptive functioning is necessary. A full review of the available diagnostic measures and screeners for dementia is beyond the scope of the current chapter (for such a review see Zeilinger et al. 2013). Instead, this review will focus largely on those measures that have been evaluated for use in ID populations.

Indirect Assessment

***Dementia Screening Questionnaire for Individuals with Intellectual Disabilities* (*DSQIID*;** Deb et al. 2007). The *DSQIID* is an informant-based rating scale consisting of 53 items which require approximately 15 min to administer. Deb and colleagues (2007) demonstrated excellent test–retest (0.95) and inter-rater reliability (0.9). Furthermore, initial evaluation indicated that the *DSQIID* is both sensitive (0.92) and specific (0.97) for those with ID (Deb et al. 2007). The *DSQIID* is a valid measure of dementia symptomatology regardless of the presence or absence of DS (Deb et al. 2007; Lin et al. 2014).

***Dementia Questionnaire for Mentally Retarded Persons* (*DMR*;** Evenhuis et al. 1990). One instrument with reported psychometric properties specific to ID populations is the *DMR*. This informant-based screening questionnaire contains 50 items and eight subscales (Evenhuis et al. 1990). Researchers have demonstrated its use for individuals with ID with and without DS Evenhuis (1992, 1996). Although Evenhuis (1992, 1996) demonstrated the sensitivity and specificity of the *DMR*, Prasher (1997) reported that it had adequate sensitivity, but poor specificity (47%) and produced a high rate of false-positives (38.5%). The *DMR* is also noted to be biased against dementia subtypes, and may underdiagnose VD. Additionally, the presence of depression, sensory disabilities, or organic illness has been suggested to lead to false positive identification (Evenhuis 1996). However, Prasher (1997) demonstrated that changes to cut-off scores increased the *DMR* specificity and decreased false-positive rates. Therefore, additional analysis may lead to cut-score modification and increase the utility of the *DMR*.

***Short Informant Questionnaire on Cognitive Decline in the Elderly* (*IQCODE*;** Jorm 1994). The utility of the *IQCODE* has also been evaluated for use in ID populations. The *IQCODE* short form is composed of 16 items that were derived from the original 26 item *IQCODE* (Jorm 1994). However, some controversy exists in the literature regarding the scales psychometric properties. Researchers have reported that the *IQCODE* has limited inter-rater reliability and test–retest reliability (Schultz et al. 1998). Jorm (2004) reported that it exhibits high reliability and indicated that it was a valid measure of cognitive decline. The author did note that the *IQCODE* is adversely affected by the informant–subject relationship and the presence of comorbid symptoms (e.g., depression or anxiety). Given the controversy surrounding the reliability of the IQCODE future research is necessary to determine its utility in ID populations.

Early Signs of Dementia Checklist (Visser et al. 1997). The *Early Signs of Dementia Checklist* is another screener for dementia. It contains 37 total items which are used to assess for the early stages of cognitive decline. Researchers have reported that the *Early Signs of Dementia Checklist* has excellent inter-rater reliability and internal consistency (Visser et al. 1997). However, limited additional research on this measure is available at present. Future research in ID populations is necessary to determine the efficacy of this measure as a dementia screener in ID populations.

Down Syndrome Dementia Scale (DSDS; Gedye 1995). The *DSDS* is a 60-item screener developed specifically for individuals with severe or profound ID associated with the presence of DS. It is used to assess decline in cognitive functioning and memory (Aylward et al. 1997). Items measure the manifestation of dementia symptoms and determine whether they are newly developed symptoms or typical of the individual (Deb and Braganza 1999). Items are distributed onto three subscales that aid the clinician in classifying dementia onset into one of four stages (i.e., early, middle, late, and very late) based upon symptom presentation (Nelson et al. 2001). Researchers have demonstrated the utility of the *DSDS* in ID populations when DS is not present (Burt and Aylward 2000) and demonstrated its sensitivity (0.85) and specificity (0.89) in ID populations when DS is present (Deb and Braganza 1999).

Direct Assessment

Test for Severe Impairment (TSI; Albert and Cohen 1992). The *TSI* is a direct measure of cognitive functioning. It contains 24 items which assess three broad areas (memory, knowledge of body parts, and language production) and requires approximately 10 min on average (Albert and Cohen 1992). Cosgrave et al. (2000) demonstrated the validity, test–retest reliability, and inter-rater reliability of the *TSI* in DS populations with comorbid ID. The *TSI* may be especially beneficial for individuals with poor verbal skills as only eight items require verbal responding (Cosgrave et al. 1999).

Severe Impairment Battery (SIB; Saxton et al. 1990). The *SIB* was designed as a direct measure of dementia symptoms (Saxton et al. 2005). Administration of the original *SIB* was noted to take approximately 30 min on average, and prompted researchers to create an abbreviated version. The short form consists of 16 total items and may be administered in half the time of the original *SIB* and has demonstrated validity in populations with severe symptoms of dementia (Saxton et al. 2005). The *SIB* allows for the reliable assessment of change across multiple domains in populations with severe dementia (Schmitt et al. 1997; Wild and Kaye 1998). This is especially useful in research which has previously excluded those with severe dementia due to a decreased ability to monitor change. The *SIB* has also been translated into multiple languages (i.e., Spanish, French, and Italian; Barbarotto et al. 2000; Boller et al. 2002; Panisset et al. 1994; Pippi et al. 1999). Although it is noted to be a reliable assessment of individuals with severe symptoms of dementia, it was originally developed for use in the general population and requires future research demonstrating its validity in populations with ID (Strydom and Hassiotis 2003).

Dual Approach

Researchers have also sought to organize and streamline the assessment approach to dementia by identifying and recommending specific measures for use in ID populations. These batteries reference some of the measures outlined above and some additional measures of domains relevant to dementia. The *Test battery for dementia in ID* is divided into two sections to gain information directly from the individual and from informant report. Informant report is used to assess adaptive skills, problematic behaviors, psychiatric symptoms, and memory and cognitive functioning (Burt and Aylward 2000). Direct assessment is used to measure the individuals cognitive functioning and memory. Although it is not a formalized singular measure, the *Test battery or dementia in ID* outlines multiple measures that have been developed to assess dementia in ID populations. This battery represents an attempt by the American Association on Intellectual and Developmental Disabilities (AAIDD) to help direct and streamline research of dementia in ID populations.

A similar test battery was proposed by Crayton et al. (1998) and is identified as the *Neuropsychological assessment of dementia in adults with ID*. This battery includes measures of adaptive behavior, receptive language, memory, learning, aphasia, agnosia, and apraxia (Oliver et al. 1998). See Crayton and colleagues (1998) and Oliver and colleagues (1998) for a list of the specific measurements included.

interRAI-Intellectual Disability (***interRAI ID***; Martin et al. 2007). The *interRAI ID* is a measure of aggression, depression, cognition, and self-care skills. It consists of 391 items and is reported to demonstrate good internal consistency and reliability (Mor 2004; Morris et al. 2000; Morris et al. 1997). Additional measures are embedded within the *interRAI ID* that assess various areas of functioning (i.e., Cognitive Performance Scale, Activities of Daily Living Hierarchy, Aggressive Behavior Scale, and the Depression Rating Scale; Martin et al. 2007; Morris et al. 2000). Martin and colleagues (2007) demonstrated that the *interRAI ID* is a valid and reliable measure that provides information relative to the quality of life and the provision of services in ID populations. A Chinese version of the *interRai ID* has also been developed (Chan et al. 2013). This measure has also demonstrated high test–retest reliability and internal consistency. Chan and colleagues (2013) also demonstrated the scales concurrent and discriminant validity in ID populations.

Neuroimaging

Historically neuroimaging procedures have been used predominately to identify the etiology and prognosis of those with dementia (Tartaglia et al. 2011). Nagdee (2011) noted that neuroimaging may aid with differential diagnosis but is not always required. Further, despite its utility regarding differential diagnosis, clinical assessment is necessary for a formal diagnosis of dementia (Vitali et al. 2008). However, the revolution in neuroimaging techniques has increased interest in their use as a diagnostic tool (Tartaglia et al. 2011). Researchers have noted that increased knowledge surrounding individual subtypes of dementia (e.g., AD and FTD), and their molecular pathologies may also help to increase the role of neuroimaging (Tartaglia et al. 2011). A decision to use neuroimaging may be related to the observed level of intellectual deficits. In those with severe and profound ID the use of formal diagnostic assessments may be hindered and neuroimaging may be informative (Nagdee 2011). Different neuroimaging processes allow for the analysis of the functional capacity, biochemistry, structure, and metabolic properties (Tartaglia et al. 2011).

Specific modalities include the use of computed tomography (CT) and magnetic resonance imaging (MRI) to inform treatment and aid in differential diagnosis (Knopman et al. 2001). The use of neuroimaging is noted to be particularly advantageous for preliminary assessment and early identification given that the neurological deviations may appear before the onset of overt dementia symptoms (Tartaglia et al. 2011). Wisniewski and colleagues (1985) demonstrated that all individuals with DS begin exhibiting the brain lesions associated with AD around 40 years of age (Janicki and Dalton 1999). However, not all of these individuals immediately display prototypical symptoms of dementia (Devenny et al. 1996; Zigman et al. 1996).

It should be noted that not all types of neuroimaging procedures are advantageous, appropriate, or readily available for ID populations. For instance, the use of electro-encephalographic readings may not be forthcoming as observed abnormalities may be better related to the primary ID diagnosis (Nagdee 2011). Additional considerations include the presence of preexisting medical conditions, behavioral deficits, and physical abnormalities that may also limit the utility of neuroimaging techniques. A full review of the neuroimaging methods utilized to inform dementia diagnosis is beyond the scope of the current chapter. Further, the specific application and utility of neuroimaging for dementia in ID populations has not been extensively evaluated. For a review of neuroimaging procedure please refer to Tartaglia et al. (2011).

Differential Diagnosis

The consideration of multiple factors is paramount when a diagnosis of dementia is suspected, especially in populations with ID. The observation of functional impairment is heterogeneous in those with ID and dependent upon multiple independent factors (e.g., training and education, intellect, and living situation; Aylward et al. 1997). Further, a readily apparent change in memory functioning may only be apparent long after a gradual decline in adaptive behaviors and self-care skills (Nagdee 2011). For those with ID, premorbid deficits in behavior, emotion regulation, and cognition may also mask early indicators of dementia (Deb and Janicki 1995; Janicki and Dalton 1999). Comorbid conditions are known to significantly impact the onset and expression of psychological impairment.

An analysis of secondary factors for individuals with ID should also include consideration of the influences of pharmacotherapy approaches on cognitive decline and routine testing for changes in hearing and vision which may not be self-reported by individuals with ID (Aylward et al. 1997). Knopman and colleagues (2001) insisted that in addition to any screener for dementia, individuals should be assessed for hypothyroidism, B_{12} deficiency, and symptoms of depression. However, a formal assessment for syphilis is not warranted unless neurosyphilis is suspected (Knopman et al. 2001). Given these suggestions, a multidisciplinary approach may be beneficial for the differential diagnosis of dementia.

The observation of mixed dementia forms also impedes differential diagnosis (Román 2002). Kalaria and Ballard (1999) reported that those with VD may exhibit cognitive deficits similar to AD and that vascular lesions have been reported in one-third of those diagnosed with AD. In comparison to "pure" forms of dementia, the presence of AD and vascular lesions is associated with expedited cognitive decline (Pasquier et al. 1998) and increased symptom manifestation (Snowdon et al. 1997).

Treatment and Interventions

With the incidence of dementia increasing among adults with ID, it is imperative that behavioral and pharmacological interventions as well as staff training be investigated and considered in each individual's plan of care. While literature is expanding in this area, most studies are focused on adults with DS who function in the mild or moderate range of ID. Several treatment plans are aimed at early detection and intervention based on annual assessment of mood, adaptive abilities, and neurocognitive functioning. There is some variance in the treatment costs associated with dementia. This is largely dependent upon the type of services sought (e.g., independent living, institutionalization, and assisted living) and the degree of impairment present (Brookmeyer et al. 2007). Researchers have estimated that the average annual cost of care for an individual with AD ranges from $ 12,000 to $ 47,000 (Coughlin and Liu 1989; Ernst and Hay 1994; Hu et al. 1986; Huang et al. 1988; Max et al. 1995; Rice et al. 1993). Based upon previously described deficits, it seems reasonable to develop interventions that target decline in cognition, changes in mood and personality, and decline in functional independence.

Pharmacological Interventions

There has been limited support for the use of pharmacological interventions to slow the progression of dementia in adults with ID. One of the primary issues is difficulty detecting efficacy of the medication based on low premorbid levels of functioning. In a review of the literature conducted by Prasher 2004, donepezil was the only medication found to be consistently efficacious in the treatment of dementia in adults with DS but cautioned that studies were limited to rivastigmine, galantamine, or memantine in this population. A later study examined the use of memantine in a Ts65Dn (TS) mouse experiment (Rueda et al. 2010). The TS mouse is partially trisomic for the region of chromosome 16 and has been shown to exhibit pheonotypic characteristics of people with DS (Rueda et al. 2010). These mice also have biomarkers for AD including amyloid-B protein, impairment in N-methyl-D-aspartate (NMDA) receptors, and vesicular glutamate transporter 1 (VGLUT1) alterations, low levels of which are associated with long-term memory deficits (Rueda et al. 2010). Results of the study suggests that 30 mg/kg/day of memantine treatment for 9 weeks improved water maze performance, grip strength, decreased levels of amyloid-B protein in the hippocampus, and increased VGLUT1 levels in the hippocampus (Rueda et al. 2010). There are several warnings and contraindications for the use of these medications with the ID population, including sick-sinus syndrome, supraventricular conduction abnormalities, peptic ulcers, chronic airway diseases, and hepatic or renal impairment (Prasher 2004). Alternative drug therapies currently under investigation include metal chelators, non-steroidal anti-inflammatories, antioxidants, hormones, herbs, and vitamins (Prasher 2004).

Given the comorbidity of depression and dementia in adults with DS, studies have been aimed at treating the mood component of the presentation and determining the residual cognitive decline to determine presence of dementia versus pseudodementia. In a study conducted by Tsiouris and Patti (1997), adults with DS in the profound, severe, moderate, or mild range of ID were diagnosed with depression as per the *DSM-IV-TR* and were screened for AD. Selective Serotonin Reuptake Inhibitors (SSRIs) were used for treatment and most participants were diagnosed with major depressive disorder (Tsiouris and Patti 1997). Twenty-one of the participants in the study were diagnosed with probable AD. Those treated with SSRIs who had comorbid dementia mostly demonstrated gains in energy level, interest in activities, independence in eating, positive mood and affect, sleep, and a decrease in behavioral outbursts (Tsiouris and Patti 1997). There was also a noted delay in the dementing process reported in four cases when treated for depression, suggesting perhaps that the deflated mood was contributing to observed cognitive and functional decline (Tsiouris and Patti 1997).

Behavioral Interventions

Whereas behavioral interventions are often limited in this population due to their difficulty retaining information and learning new replacement behaviors, there is cited success in a case study using differential reinforcement of other behaviors with an individual dually diagnosed with dementia and DS (Vogl and Rapp 2011). This behavioral technique involves delivery of items known to be reinforcing to the individual contingent on the absence of challenging behaviors (Vogl and Rapp 2011). Results of the study at 2- and 3-month follow-up indicated sustained behavioral change (Vogl and Rapp 2011).

In addition to formal behavior modifications, environmental modifications and recreational enhancements have been attempted with this population. Environmental modifications attempted include separate spaces for occupational and recreational activities, physiotherapeutic bath, and areas for relaxation and other activities (De Vreese et al. 2012). The importance of adequate signage, safety features, welcoming wall colors, floor coverings, air quality, daylight, and soft-indirect lighting are stressed (De Vreese et al. 2012). Use of cameras, calming music, and pet therapies are also recommended (De Vreese et al. 2012). Sustained cognitive and functional abilities, and improvement in mood including reduction of depression and anxiety and improvement in self-esteem and personal control have been measured in adults with mild neurocognitive decline and ID when provided with these environmental modifications compared to those without these interventions (De Vreese et al. 2012). Decline has been noted predominately in individuals with ID and neurocognitive decline, who live in institutionalized rather than personalized settings (De Vreese et al. 2012). The reason given for this differential is the lack of use of a person-centered approach to client management (De Vreese et al. 2012). It is presumed that using a person-centered approach aids in enhancing memory and verbal communication abilities, autonomy, and relational styles (De Vreese et al. 2012). Furthermore, such environmental adaptations provide physical and sensory supports not available in all standard care facilities.

Staff Interventions

Staff training to promote awareness about cognitive decline in the ID population has been an ongoing topic of research. As these individuals experience progressive changes in neurocognitive status and functional independence, they typically also need modifications to their nutritional plans and suffer from comorbid medical illnesses (McCarron et al. 2010). Data obtained from a focus group study, revealed that staff struggled with preparing themselves for end-of-life needs of the individuals, swallowing deficits, and modifying environments to support their needs (McCarron et al. 2010). Other concerns presented from direct care staff include feeling unprepared and unconfident about their ability to work with adults with dementia, burnout, and pain management (Wilkinson et al. 2005). Janicki (2011) highlighted the importance of initial and continued assessment in the areas of staff skill sets, attitudes, and comprehension, need for additional resources provided within the environment, and cognitive assessment of the individuals with ID and dementia for treatment planning. Recommendations for interventions have included modified training programs and shorter shifts given the increasing needs of this population (Wilkinson et al. 2005).

A study conducted by Fahey-McCarthy et al. (2009) sought to assess the need for training of staff supporting adults with ID and dementia, and implementing a training program. A 20-session program was designed that included training on caring for people with ID, caring for people with dementia, culture competency, palliative care, and nutrition, hydration, and pain concerns (Fahey-McCarthy et al. 2009).

The Pearlin Model is a widely utilized framework for understanding and managing caregiver stress when working with adults with AD (McCarron and McCallion 2005). This model proposes four domains for understanding stress of caregivers of individuals with AD including background and contextual factors, primary and secondary strains, mediating factors, and outcomes and manifestations of stress (McCarron and McCallion 2005). McCarron and McCallion (2005) adapted this model for use with adults with ID and dementia. With regard to background and contextual factors, their revised model takes into account not only staff and family caregiver demographics but also duration of caregiving and disease and participation in day services programming. Primary stressors include impact of change in cognition on relationships, behavioral and personality changes, restlessness/wandering, sleep disturbance, incontinence, being uncooperative, and caregiving tasks themselves (McCarron and McCallion 2005). Secondary stressors involve support received from family members regarding their care of the individual supported, limited time for the caregiver to engage in personal recreational activities, not having clear expectations of their job expectancies, staffing ratio issues, and intrapsychic strain (McCarron and McCallion 2005). Mediating factors include coping mechanisms, social support, and training, whereas outcomes involve psychological distress (e.g., depression and anxiety), physical ailments, absenteeism, burnout, and turnover (McCarron and McCallion 2005). The authors proposed that this model will promote a better understanding of stress and coping processes of staff caregivers who work with adults with dementia and ID (McCarron and McCallion 2005).

Given the limited research on interventions for adults with comorbid ID and dementia, future studies are needed in this area. Specific pharmacology trials in this population, extending into the severe and profound classifications of disability, need to be expanded upon and replicated. Staff intervention research is often based around design of programs rather than implementation. While these models offer guidance and structure, there is limited information on their efficacy. Furthermore, behavioral interventions, aside from environmental modifications, are sparse and limited to primarily case studies. Finally, there is little information on promoting maintenance of current abilities and cognitive strategies or reminiscence to enhance orientation and memory retrieval.

Future Directions

Despite the overall prevalence of dementia and the observed increases predicted based upon improved healthcare and longevity, significant deficits surrounding key areas remain. The observed research limitations are exponentially larger in populations with ID. For instance, the prevalence of dementia is variable and largely dependent upon the diagnostic criteria used. Prevalence estimates are also dependent upon the assessments used, the presence of comorbid conditions, and the consideration of mixed forms of dementia. Despite the observation and suggestion of mixed forms of dementia in the general population, this same research is largely nonexistent in ID populations. To date minimal research exists surrounding the prevalence and manifestation of mixed forms of dementia in ID populations.

Despite some preliminary research surrounding the identification of potential prognostic factors associated with dementia, this research remains largely absent with specific regard to ID populations. Researchers have also begun examining the contribution of risk- and protective-factors associated with onset of dementia and mortality. Prognostic factors include comorbid medical or neurological illness, age, severity of premorbid intellectual functioning, psychosocial support systems, DS, familial history, and early onset of dementia symptoms (Evenhuis 1997; Harper and Wadsworth 1993; Janicki and Dalton 1999; Janicki and Jacobson 1986; Lin et al. 2014). Future research is necessary to clarify the relationship between educational attainment and mortality in dementia populations (Geerlings et al. 1997; Stern et al. 1995; Wolfson et al. 2001). Increased efforts are necessary to continue to develop this line of investigation.

The development of measures used to screen and diagnose dementia in ID populations is impaired by the lack of a unified approach to research surrounding the topic. This is influenced ultimately by the heterogeneity of dementia symptoms and its associated neurodegenerative disorders. For general and ID populations this impediment is exasperated by multiple factors to include the use of multiple forms of diagnostic criteria to identify dementia. With regard to ID populations there is a critical need for research surrounding the development and utility of reliable and valid assessment measures. This will require longitudinal research as well as replication of studies. However, these factors alone are not completely responsible for impeding early diagnosis. The observed stigma associated with dementia and a relative lack of early indicators is also responsible for delaying diagnosis and treatment. Increased psychoeducational efforts targeting health practitioners, caretakers, and the general population (e.g., family and friends) may help to increase identification while simultaneously decreasing stigma.

As individuals with ID likely share genetic vulnerabilities towards developing dementia, researchers should consider potential shared biomarkers between the development of dementia and particular genetic disorders. Additional information may help todetermine the prognosis of dementia in different disorders, as well as help to determine the most appropriate treatments and assessments for any declines that may be observed during the course of a disorder. Further, researchers should continue to examine the relationship between the level of ID and the declines that may serve as markers for dementia. This may help to mitigate the current underdiagnosis of dementia in the ID population.

Given the limited research on interventions for adults with comorbid ID and dementia, future studies are needed in this area. Specific pharmacology trials in this population, extending into the severe and profound classifications of disability, need to be expanded upon and replicated. Staff intervention research is often based around the design of programs rather than implementation. While these models offer guidance and structure, there is limited information on their efficacy. Furthermore, behavioral interventions, aside from environmental modifications, are sparse and limited to primarily case studies. Finally, there is little information on promoting maintenance of current abilities and cognitive strategies or reminiscence to enhance orientation and memory retrieval. Music therapy has been tried in adults with dementia in an attempt to promote relaxation, stimulate social and emotional functioning, and reduce anxiety (Vink et al. 2013). Results have been mixed with regard to the effectiveness of this form of treatment but may be of benefit to try in adults with ID. Art therapy has similarly been tried with adults presenting with dementia. In a case study authored by Safar and Press (2011), an individual with previous experience in art showed improvement in sense of self, emotional expression, coping, and feelings of powerlessness. It appears that this form of therapy may be beneficial in an ID population suffering from dementia which otherwise has difficulty with emotional expression and learning, and comprehending coping strategies.

References

Adams, D., Oliver, C., Kalsy, S., Peters, S., Broquard, M., Basra, T., Konstandinidi, E., & McQuillan, S. (2008). Behavioural characteristics associated with dementia assessment referrals in adults with Down syndrome. *Journal of Intellectual Disability Research, 52*(4), 358–368.

Ala, T. A., & Frey, W. H. (1994). Validation of the NINCDS-ADRDA criteria regarding gait in the clinical diagnosis of Alzheimer disease. A clinicopathologic study. *Alzheimer Disease and Associated Disorders, 9*(3), 152–159.

Albert, M., & Cohen, C. (1992). The Test for Severe Impairment: An instrument for the assessment of patients with severe cognitive dysfunction. *Journal of the American Geriatrics Society, 40*(5), 449–453.

Alzheimer, A. (1907). Über eine eigenartige Erkrankung der Hirnrinde. *Allgemeine Z Psychiatrie Psychisch-Gerichtliche Medicine, 64,* 146–148.

Aylward, E. H., Burt, D. B., Thorpe, L. U., Lai, F., & Dalton, A. (1997). Diagnosis of dementia in individuals with intellectual disability*. *Journal of Intellectual Disability Research, 41*(2), 152–164.

Ball, S. L., Holland, A. J., Hon, J., Huppert, F. A., Treppner, P., & Watson, P. C. (2006). Personality and behavior changes mark the early stages of Alzheimer's disease in adults with down's syndrome: Findings from a prospective population-based study. *International Journal of Geriatric Psychiatry, 21,* 661–673.

Ballard, C., Holmes, C., McKeith, I., Neill, D., O'Brien, J., Cairns, N., Lantos, P., Perry, E., Ince, P., & Perry, R. (1999). Psychiatric morbidity in dementia with Lewy bodies: A prospective clinical and neuropathological comparative study with Alzheimer's disease. *American Journal of Psychiatry, 156*(7), 1039–1045.

Ballard, C., O'brien, J., Morris, C. M., Barber, R., Swann, A., Neill, D., & McKeith, I. (2001). The progression of cognitive impairment in dementia with Lewy bodies, vascular dementia and Alzheimer's disease. *International Journal of Geriatric Psychiatry, 16*(5), 499–503.

Barbarotto, R., Cerri, M., Acerbi, C., Molinari, S., & Capitani, E. (2000). Is SIB or BNP better than MMSE in discriminating the cognitive performance of severely impaired elderly patients? *Archives of Clinical Neuropsychology, 15*(1), 21–29.

Barclay, L. L., Zemcov, A., Blass, J. P., & McDowell, F. H. (1985). Factors associated with duration of survival in Alzheimer's disease. *Biological Psychiatry, 20*(1), 86–93.

Bell, R., Rankin, J., & Donaldson, L. J. (2003). Down's syndrome: Occurrence and outcome in the north of England, 1985–1999. *Paediatric Perinatal Epidemiology, 17,* 33–39.

Bittles, A. H., & Glasson, E. J. (2004). Clinical, social, and ethical implications of changing life expectancy in Down syndrome. *Developmental Medicine and Child Neurology, 46,* 282–286.

Blacker, D., & Tanzi, R. E. (1998). The genetics of Alzheimer disease: Current status and future prospects. *Archives of Neurology, 55*(3), 294–296.

Blacker, D., Albert, M. S., Bassett, S. S., Go, R. C., Harrell, L. E., & Folstein, M. F. (1994). Reliability and validity of NINCDS-ADRDA criteria for Alzheimer's disease: The National Institute of Mental Health Genetics Initiative. *Archives of Neurology, 51*(12), 1198.

Boller, F., Verny, M., Hugonot-Diener, L., & Saxton, J. (2002). Clinical features and assessment of severe dementia: A review. *European Journal of Neurology, 9*(2), 125–136.

Boustani, M., Peterson, B., Hanson, L., Harris, R., & Lohr, K. N. (2003). Screening for dementia in primary care: A summary of the evidence for the US Preventive Services Task Force. *Annals of Internal Medicine, 138*(11), 927–937.

Bowers, J., Jorm, A. F., Henderson, S., & Harris, P. (1990). General practitioners' detection of depression and dementia in elderly patients. *The Medical Journal of Australia, 153*(4), 192–196.

Bowman, A. B., Ess, K. C., Kumar, K. K., & Summar, K. L. (2013). Down syndrome. In J. L. R. Rubenstein & P. Rakic (Eds.), *Neural Circuit Development and Function in the Brain* (pp. 547–571). San Diego: Elsevier.

Bridges-Webb, C. W. J., Wolk, J., Pond, D., & Britt, H. (2003). *Care of patients with dementia in general practice Guidelines*. North Sydney: NSW Department of Health.

Brookmeyer, R., Johnson, E., Ziegler-Graham, K., & Arrighi, H. M. (2007). Forecasting the global burden of Alzheimer's disease. *Alzheimer's & Dementia, 3*(3), 186–191.

Burns, A., Jacoby, R., & Levy, R. (1990). Psychiatric phenomena in Alzheimer's disease. IV: Disorders of behaviour. *The British Journal of Psychiatry, 157*(1), 86–94.

Burt, D. B., & Aylward, E. H. (2000). Test battery for the diagnosis of dementia in individuals with intellectual disability. *Journal of Intellectual Disability Research, 44*(2), 175–180.

Burt, D. D., Loveland, K. A., & Lewis, K. R. (1992). Depression and the onset of dementia in adults with mental retardation. *American Journal on Mental Retardation, 96*(5), 502–511.

Byrne, E. J., Lennox, G., Lowe, J., & Godwin-Austen, R. B. (1989). Diffuse Lewy body disease: Clinical features in 15 cases. *Journal of Neurology, Neurosurgery & Psychiatry, 52*(6), 709–717.

Cairns, N. J., Bigio, E. H., Mackenzie, I. R., Neumann, M., Lee, V. M. Y., Hatanpaa, K. J., White, C. L. 3rd, Schneider, J. A., Grinberg, L. T., Halliday, G., Duyckaerts, C., Lowe, J. S., Holm, I. E., Tolnay, M., Okamoto, K., Yokoo, H., Murayama, S., Woulfe, J., Munoz, D. G., Dickson, D. W., Ince, P. G., Trojanowski, J. Q., & Mann, D. M. (2007). Neuropathologic diagnostic and nosologic criteria for frontotemporal lobar degeneration: Consensus of the Consortium for Frontotemporal Lobar Degeneration. *Acta Neuropathologica, 114*(1), 5–22.

Cattel, C., Gambassi, G. A., Zuccala, G., Carbonin, P., & Bernabei, R. (2000). Correlates of delayed referral for the diagnosis of dementia in an outpatient population. *The Journals of Gerontology. Series A, Biological sciences and Medical Sciences, 55*(2), M98–M102.

Chan, S. S., Chiu, H. F., Lam, L. C., & Leung, V. P. (2002). Prevalence of dementia with Lewy bodies in an inpatient psychogeriatric population in Hong Kong Chinese. *International Journal of Geriatric Psychiatry, 17*(9), 847–850.

Chan, C. L., Lai, C., & Chi, I. (2013). A validity and reliability study of a Chinese assessment tool for persons with moderate to severe intellectual disabilities. *Journal of Intellectual Disability-Diagnosis and Treatment, 1*(1), 6–14.

Chui, H. C., Victoroff, J. I., Margolin, D., Jagust, W., Shankle, R., & Katzman, R. (1992). Criteria for the diagnosis of ischemic vascular dementia proposed by the State of California Alzheimer's Disease Diagnostic and Treatment Centers. *Neurology, 42*(3), 473–480.

Contestabile, A., Benfenati, F., & Gasparini, L. (2010). Communication breaks-down: From neurodevelopment defects to cognitive disabilities in Down syndrome. *Progress in Neurobiology, 91,* 1–22.

Cooper, S. A. (1997a). High prevalence of dementia among people with learning disabilities not attributable to Down's syndrome. *Psychological Medicine, 27*(03), 609–616.

Cooper, S. A. (1997b). Psychiatric symptoms of dementia among elderly people with learning disabilities. *International Journal of Geriatric Psychiatry, 12*(6), 662–666.

Cooper, S. A., & Prasher, V. P. (1998). Maladaptive behaviours and symptoms of dementia in adults with Down's syndrome compared with adults with intellectual disability of other aetiologies. *Journal of Intellectual Disability Research, 42*(4), 293–300.

Cooper, B., Bickel, H., & Schaufele, M. (1996). Early development and progression of dementing illness in the elderly: A general-practice based study. *Psychological Medicine, 26*(2), 411–420.

Coppus, A. M., Evenhuis, H., Verberne, G. J., Visser, F., Van Gool, P., Eikelenboom, P., & Van Duijin, C. (2006). Dementia and mortality in persons with Down's syndrome. *Journal of Intellectual Disability Research, 50*(10), 768–777.

Cosgrave, M. P., Tyrrell, J., McCarron, M., Gill, M., & Lawlor, B. A. (1999). Determinants of aggression, and adaptive and maladaptive behaviour in older people with Down's syndrome with and without dementia. *Journal of Intellectual Disability Research, 43*(5), 393–399.

Cosgrave, M. P., Tyrrell, J., McCarron, M., Gill, M., & Lawlor, B. A. (2000). A five year follow-up study of dementia in persons with Down's syndrome: Early symptoms and patterns of deterioration. *Irish Journal of Psychological Medicine, 17*(1), 5–11.

Coughlin, T. A., & Liu, K. (1989). Health care costs of older persons with cognitive impairments. *The Gerontologist, 29*(2), 173–182.

Crayton, L., Oliver, C., Holland, A., Bradbury, J., & Hall, S. (1998). The neuropsychological assessment of age related cognitive deficits in adults with Down's syndrome. *Journal of Applied Research in Intellectual Disabilities, 11*(3), 255–272.

Cummings, J. L. (1984). Dementia: Definition, classification, and differential diagnosis. *Psychiatric Annals, 14*(2), 85–89.

Cummings, J. L., & Victoroff, J. I. (1990). Noncognitive neuropsychiatric syndromes in Alzheimer's disease. *Cognitive and Behavioral Neurology, 3*(2), 140–158.

Dalton, A. J., & Crapper-McLachlan, D. R. (1986). Clinical expression of Alzheimer's disease in Down's syndrome. *The Psychiatric Clinics of North America, 9*(4), 659–670.

De Lepeleire, J., Heyman, J., & Buntinx, F. (1998). The early diagnosis of dementia: Triggers, early signs and luxating events. *Family Practice, 15*(5), 431–436.

De Vreese, L. P., Mantesso, U., De Bastiani, E., Weger, E., Marangoni, A. C., & Gomiero, T. (2012). Impact of dementia-derived nonpharmacological intervention procedures on cognition and behavior in older adults with intellectual disabilities: A 3-year follow-up study. *Journal of Policy and Practice in Intellectual Disabilities, 9*(2), 92–102.

Deb, S., & Braganza, J. (1999). Comparison of rating scales for the diagnosis of dementia in adults with Down's syndrome. *Journal of Intellectual Disability Research, 43*(5), 400–407.

Deb, S., & Janicki, M. P. (1995). Conference report: International colloquium on mental retardation and Alzheimer's disease. *Journal of Intellectual Disability Research, 39,* 149–150.

Deb, S., & McHugh, R. (2010). Dementia among persons with Down syndrome. *International Review of Research in Mental Retardation, 39,* 221–255.

Deb, S., Hare, M., Prior, L., & Bhaumik, S. (2007). Dementia screening questionnaire for individuals with intellectual disabilities. *The British Journal of Psychiatry, 190*(5), 440–444.

Devenny, D. A., Silverman, W. P., Hill, A. L., Jenkins, E., Sersen, E. A., & Wisniewski, K. E. (1996). Normal aging in adults with Down's syndrome: A longitudinal study. *Journal of Intellectual Disability Research, 40,* 208–221.

Dickson, D. W. (2002). Dementia with Lewy bodies: Neuropathology. *Journal of Geriatric Psychiatry and Neurology, 15*(4), 210–216.

Diesfeldt, H. F. A., Houte, L. R., & Moerkens, R. M. (1986). Duration of survival in senile dementia. *Acta Psychiatrica Scandinavica, 73*(4), 366–371.

Doody, R. S., Massman, P., Mahurin, R., & Law, S. (1995). Positive and negative neuropsychiatric features in Alzheimer's disease. *Journal of Neuropsychiatry and Clinical Neurosciences, 7,* 54–60.

Doraiswamy, P. M., Steffens, D. C., Pitchumoni, S., & Tabrizi, S. (1998). Early recognition of Alzheimer's disease: What is consensual? What is controversial? What is practical? *Journal of Clinical Psychiatry, 59*(13), 6–18.

Douglas, V. C., & Josephson, S. A. (2014). Dementia and Systemic Disease. In M. J. Aminoff & S. A. Josephson (Eds.), *Aminoff's Neurology and General Medicine* (5th ed., pp. 1263–1277). London: Elsevier.

Durkin, M. S., Schupf, N., Stein, Z. A., & Susser, M. W. (1994). Epidemiology of mental retardation. In M. Levene & R. Lifford (Eds.), *Fetal and neonatal neurology and neurosurgery* (2nd ed., pp. 689–706). Edinburgh: Churchill Livingston.

Englund, B., Brun, A., Gustafson, L., Passant, U., Mann, D. M. A., Neary, D., & Snowden, J. S. (1994). Clinical and neuropathological criteria for frontotemporal dementia. *Journal of Neurology, Neurosurgery & Psychiatry, 57,* 416–418.

Erkinjuntti, T., Roman, G., Gauthier, S., Feldman, H., & Rockwood, K. (2004). Emerging therapies for vascular dementia and vascular cognitive impairment. *Stroke, 35*(4), 1010–1017.

Ernst, R. L., & Hay, J. W. (1994). The US economic and social costs of Alzheimer's disease revisited. *American Journal of Public Health, 84*(8), 1261–1264.

Evans, D. A. (1990). Estimated prevalence of Alzheimer's disease in the United States. *The Milbank Quarterly, 68*(2), 267–289.

Evenhuis, H. M. (1990). The natural history of dementia in Down's syndrome. *Archives of Neurology, 47,* 369–373.

Evenhuis, H. M. (1992). Evaluation of a screening instrument for dementia in ageing mentally retarded persons. *Journal of Intellectual Disability Research, 36*(4), 337–347.

Evenhuis, H. M. (1996). Further evaluation of the dementia questionnaire for persons with mental retardation (DMR). *Journal of Intellectual Disability Research, 40*(4), 369–373.

Evenhuis, H. M. (1997). The natural history of dementia in ageing people with intellectual disability. *Journal of Intellectual Disability Research, 41*(1), 92–96.

Evenhuis, H. M., Kengen, M. M. F., & Eurlings, H. A. L. (1990). *Dementia questionnaire for mentally retarded persons (DMR): For diagnosis of dementia in mentally retarded people.* Zwammerdam: Hooge Burch.

Eyman, R. K., Call, T. L., & White, J. F. (1991). Life expectancy of persons with Down syndrome. *American Journal on Mental Retardation, 95*(6), 603–612.

Fahey-McCarthy, E., McCarron, M., Connaire, K., & McCallion, P. (2009). Developing an education intervention for staff supporting persons with an intellectual disability and advanced dementia. *Journal of Policy and Practice in Intellectual Disabilities, 6*(4), 267–275.

Farrer, L. A., Cupples, L. A., Blackburn, S., Kiely, D. K., Auerbaeh, S., Growdon, J. H., Connor-Lacke, L., & Kukull, W. A. (1994). Interrater agreement for diagnosis of Alzheimer's disease The MIRAGE study. *Neurology, 44*(4), 652–656.

Ferri, C. P., Prince, M., Brayne, C., Brodaty, H., Fratiglioni, L., Ganguli, M., Hall, K., Hasegawa, K., Hendrie, H., Huang, Y., Jorm, A., Mathers, C., Menezes, P. R., Rimmer, E., & Scazufca, M. (2006). Global prevalence of dementia: A Delphi consensus study. *The Lancet, 366*(9503), 2112–2117.

Fiske, A., Gatz, M., Aadnøy, B., & Pedersen, N. L. (2005). Assessing age of dementia onset: Validity of informant reports. *Alzheimer Disease & Associated Disorders, 19*(3), 128–134.

Fortinsky, R. H., Leighton, A., & Wasson, J. H. (1995). Primary care physicians' diagnostic, management, and referral practices for older persons and families affected by dementia. *Research on Aging, 17*(2), 124–148.

Fratiglioni, L., Launer, L. J., Andersen, K., Breteler, M. M., Copeland, J. R., Dartigues, J. F., Lobo, A., Martinez-Lage, J., Soininen, H., & Hofman, A. (1999). Incidence of dementia and major subtypes in Europe: A collaborative study of population-based cohorts. Neurologic diseases in the elderly research group. *Neurology, 54*(11), 5–10.

Gedye, A. (1995). *Dementia scale for down syndrome.* Manual. Vancouver: Gedye Research and Consulting, Vancouver.

Geerlings, M. I., Deeg, D. J. H., Schmand, B., Lindeboom, J., & Jonker, C. (1997). Increased risk of mortality in Alzheimer's disease patients with higher education? A replication study. *Neurology, 49*(3), 798–802.

Glasser, M. (1993). Alzheimer's disease and dementing disorders: Practices and experiences of rural physicians. *American Journal of Alzheimer's Disease and Other Dementias, 8*(4), 28–35.

Glasson, E. J., Sullivan, S. G., Hussain, R., Petterson, B. A., Montgomery, P. D., & Bittles, A. H. (2002). The changing survival profile of people with Down's syndrome: Implications for genetic counselling. *Clinical Genetics, 62*(5), 390–393.

Gold, G., Giannakopoulos, P., Montes-Paixao, C., Herrman, F. R., Mulligan, R., Michel, J. P., & Bouras, C. (1997). Sensitivity and specificity of newly proposed clinical criteria for possible vascular dementia. *Neurology, 49*(3), 690–694.

Gold, G., Bouras, C., Canuto, A., Bergallo, M. F., Herrmann, F. R., Hof, P. R., Mayor, P. A., Michel, J. P., & Giannakopoulos, P. (2002). Clinicopathological validation study of four sets of clinical criteria for vascular dementia. *American Journal of Psychiatry, 159*(1), 82–87.

Grossman, M. (2002). Frontotemporal dementia: A review. *Journal of the International Neuropsychological Society, 8*(04), 566–583.

Gustafson, L. (1987). Frontal lobe degeneration of non-Alzheimer type. II. Clinical picture and differential diagnosis. *Archives of gerontology and geriatrics, 6*(3), 209–223.

Gustafson, L. (1993). Clinical picture of frontal lobe degeneration of non-Alzheimer type. *Dementia and Geriatric Cognitive Disorders, 4*(3–4), 143–148.

Haley, W. E., Clair, J. M., & Saulsberry, K. (1992). Family caregiver satisfaction with medical care of their demented relatives. *The Gerontologist, 32*(2), 219–226.

Hansen, L., Salmon, D., Galasko, D., Masliah, E., Katzman, R., DeTeresa, R., Thal, L., Pay, M. M., Hofstetter, R., Klauber, M., & Alford, M. (1990). The Lewy body variant of Alzheimer's disease: A clinical and pathologic entity. *Neurology, 40*(1), 1–8.

Harper, D. C., & Wadsworth, J. (1993). A primer on dementia in persons with mental retardation: Conclusions and current findings. In R. J. Fletcher & A. Dosen (Eds.), *Mental health aspects of mental retardation: Progress in assessment and treatment* (pp. 169–198). New York: Lexington.

Heagerty, B., & Eskenazi, L. (1994). A practice and program perspective on family caregiving. *Family Caregiving: Agenda for the Future*, 35–48.

Heidebrink, J. L. (2002). Is dementia with Lewy bodies the second most common cause of dementia?. *Journal of Geriatric Psychiatry and Neurology, 15*(4), 182–187.

Henderson, A. S., & Jorm, A. F. (1987). Is case-ascertainment of Alzheimer's disease in field surveys practicable? *Psychological Medicine, 17*(03), 549–555.

Hennerici, M. G., Oster, M., Cohen, S., Schwartz, A., Motsch, L., & Daffertshofer, M. (1994). Are gait disturbances and white matter degeneration early indicators of vascular dementia? *Dementia and Geriatric Cognitive Disorders, 5*(3–4), 197–202.

Heyman, A., Wilkinson, W. E., Hurwitz, B. J., Helms, M. J., Haynes, C. S., Utley, C. M., & Gwyther, L. P. (1987). Early-onset Alzheimer's disease Clinical predictors of institutionalization and death. *Neurology, 37*(6), 980–984.

Hier, D. B., Warach, J. D., Gorelick, P. B., & Thomas, J. (1989). Predictors of survival in clinically diagnosed Alzheimer's disease and multi-infarct dementia. *Archives of Neurology, 46*(11), 1213–1216.

Hodges, J. R., Patterson, K., Oxbury, S., & Funnell, E. (1992). Semantic dementia progressive fluent aphasia with temporal lobe atrophy. *Brain, 115*(6), 1783–1806.

Hofman, A., Ott, A., Breteler, M., Bots, M. L., Slooter, A. J., van Harskamp, F., van Duijn, C. N., Van Broeckhoven, C., & Grobbee, D. E. (1997). Atherosclerosis, apolipoprotein E, and prevalence of dementia and Alzheimer's disease in the Rotterdam Study. *The Lancet, 349*(9046), 151–154.

Holland, A. J., Hon, J., Huppert, F. A., & Stevens, F. (2000). Incidence and course of dementia in people with Down's syndrome: Findings from a population-based study. *Journal of Intellectual Disability Research, 44*(2), 138–146.

Holmes, C., Cairns, N., Lantos, P., & Mann, A. (1999). Validity of current clinical criteria for Alzheimer's disease, vascular dementia and dementia with Lewy bodies. *The British Journal of Psychiatry, 174*(1), 45–50.

Hu, T. W., Huang, L. F., & Cartwright, W. S. (1986). Evaluation of the costs of caring for the senile demented elderly: A pilot study. *The Gerontologist, 26*(2), 158–163.

Huang, L. F., Cartwright, W. S., & Hu, T. W. (1988). The economic cost of senile dementia in the United States, 1985. *Public Health Reports, 103*(1), 3.

Huff, F. J., Growdon, J. H., Corkin, S., & Rosen, T. J. (1987). Age at onset and rate of progression of Alzheimer's disease. *Journal of the American Geriatrics Society, 35*(1), 27–30.

Janicki, M. P. (2011). Quality outcomes in group home dementia care for adults with intellectual disabilities. *Journal of Intellectual Disability Research, 55*(8), 763–776.

Janicki, M. P., & Dalton, A. J. (1993). Alzheimer disease in a select population of older adults with mental retardation. *The Irish Journal of Psychology, 14*(1), 38–47.

Janicki, M. P., & Dalton, A. J. (1999a). Dementia in intellectual disabilities. In N. Bouras (Ed.), *Psychiatric and behavioural disorders in intellectual disabilities and mental retardation* (pp. 121–153). Cambridge: Cambridge University Press.

Janicki, M. P., & Dalton, A. J. (Eds.). (1999b). *Dementia, aging, and intellectual disabilities: A handbook*. Psychology Press.

Janicki, M. P., & Dalton, A. J. (2000). Prevalence of dementia and impact on intellectual disability services. *Mental Retardation, 38*(3), 276–288.

Janicki, M. P., & Jacobson, J. W. (1986). Generational trends in sensory, physical, and behavioral abilities among older mentally retarded persons. *American Journal of Mental Deficiency, 90*(5), 490–500.

Janicki, M. P., Ackerman, L., & Jacobson, J. W. (1985). State developmental disabilities/aging plans and day-planning for an older developmentally disabled populations. *Mental Retardation, 23,* 297–301.

Jorm, A. F. (1994). A short form of the Informant Questionnaire on Cognitive Decline in the Elderly (IQCODE): Development and cross-evaluation. *Psychological Medicine, 24,* 145–153.

Jorm, A. F. (2004). The Informant Questionnaire on Cognitive Decline in the Elderly (IQCODE): A review. *International Psychogeriatrics, 16*(03), 275–293.

Kalaria, R. N., & Ballard, C. (1999). Overlap between pathology of Alzheimer disease and vascular dementia. *Alzheimer Disease and Associated Disorders, 13,* S115–S123.

Katzman, R. (1986). Alzheimer's disease. *New England Journal of Medicine, 314,* 964–973.

Kay, D. W. K., Henderson, A. S., Scott, R., Wilson, J., Rickwood, D., & Grayson, D. A. (1985). Dementia and depression among the elderly living in the Hobart community: The effect of the diagnostic criteria on the prevalence rates. *Psychological Medicine, 15*(4), 771–788.

Knopman, D. S. (1998). The initial recognition and diagnosis of dementia. *The American Journal of Medicine, 104*(4), 2–12.

Knopman, D. S., Kitto, J., Deinard, S., & Heiring, J. (1988). Longitudinal study of death and institutionalization in patients with primary degenerative dementia. *Journal of the American Geriatrics Society, 36*(2), 108–112.

Knopman, D. S., DeKosky, S. T., Cummings, J. L., Chui, H., Corey–Bloom, J., Relkin, N., Small, G. W., Miller, B., & Stevens, J. C. (2001). Practice parameter: Diagnosis of dementia (an evidence-based review) Report of the Quality Standards Subcommittee of the American Academy of Neurology. *Neurology, 56*(9), 1143–1153.

Koopmans, R. T., Van Hell, M. E., De Jongh, F., Froeling, P. G., van den Hoogen, H. J., & van Weel, C. (1991). The course of Alzheimer's disease in a group of nursing home patients: Epidemiology, (co) morbidity and mortality. *Netherlands Journal of Medicine, 135*(19), 845–850.

Kosaka, K., Matsushita, M., Oyanagi, S., & Mehraein, P. (1980). A cliniconeurophathological study of the "Lewy body disease". *Seishin shinkeigaku zasshi = Psychiatria et neurologia Japonica, 82*(5), 292.

Kosaka, K., Yoshimura, M., Ikeda, K., & Budka, H. (1983). Diffuse type of Lewy body disease: Progressive dementia with abundant cortical Lewy bodies and senile changes of varying degree–a new disease? *Clinical Neuropathology, 3*(5), 185–192.

Kramer, J. H., Reed, B. R., Mungas, D., Weiner, M. W., & Chui, H. C. (2002). Executive dysfunction in subcortical ischemic vascular disease. *Journal of Neurology, Neurosurgery & Psychiatry, 72*(2), 217–220.

Kurz, A. F. (2001). What is vascular dementia? *International Journal of Clinical Practice Supplement, 120,* 5–8.

Lagaay, A. M., Van Der Meij, J. C., & Hijmans, W. (1992). Validation of medical history taking as part of a population based survey in subjects aged 85 and over. *British Medical Journal, 304*(6834), 1091.

Lai, F. (1992). Clinicopathologic features of Alzheimer disease in Down syndrome. *Progress in Clinical and Biological Research, 379,* 15.

Lai, F., & Williams, R. S. (1989). A prospective study of Alzheimer disease in Down syndrome. *Archives of Neurology, 46*(8), 849–853.

Lautenschlager, N. T., Cupples, L. A., Rao, V. S., Auerbach, S. A., Becker, R., Burke, J., Chui, H., Duara, R., Foley, E. J., Glatt, S. L., Green, R. C., Jones, R., Karlinsky, H., Kukull, W. A., Kurz, A., Larson, E. B., Martelli, K., Sadovnick, A. D., Volicer, L., Waring, S. C., Growdon, J. H., & Farrer, L. A. (1996). Risk of dementia among relatives of Alzheimer's disease patients in the MIRAGE study: What is in store for the oldest old? *Neurology, 46*(3), 641–650.

Lin, J. D., Lin, L. P., Hsia, Y. C., Hsu, S. W., Wu, C. L., & Chu, C. M. (2014). A national survey of caregivers' perspective of early symptoms of dementia among adults with an intellectual disability based on the DSQIID scale. *Research in Autism Spectrum Disorders, 8*(3), 275–280.

Lipowski, Z. J. (1989). Current concepts—geriatrics: Delirium in the elderly patient. *The New England journal of medicine, 320,* 578–582.

Litvan, I., MacIntyre, A., Goetz, C. G., Wenning, G. K., Jellinger, K., Verny, M., Bartko, J. J., Jankovic, J., McKee, A., Brandel, J. P., Chaudhuri, K. R., Lai, E. C., D'Olhaberriague, L., Pearce, R. K., & Agid, Y. (1998). Accuracy of the clinical diagnoses of Lewy body disease, Parkinson disease, and dementia with Lewy bodies: A clinicopathologic study. *Archives of Neurology, 55*(7), 969–978.

Longstreth, W. T., Bernick, C., Manolio, T. A., Bryan, N., Jungreis, C. A., & Price, T. R. (1998). Lacunar infarcts defined by magnetic resonance imaging of 3660 elderly people: The Cardiovascular Health Study. *Archives of Neurology, 55*(9), 1217–1225.

Lopez, O. L., Litvan, I., Catt, K. E., Stowe, R., Klunk, W., Kaufer, D. I., Becker, J. T., & DeKosky, S. T. (1999). Accuracy of four clinical diagnostic criteria for the diagnosis of neurodegenerative dementias. *Neurology, 53*(6), 1292–1299.

Luis, C. A., Barker, W. W., Gajaraj, K., Harwood, D., Petersen, R., Kashuba, A., Waters, C., Jimison, P., Pearl, G., Petito, C., Dickson, D., & Duara, R. (1999). Sensitivity and specificity of three clinical criteria for dementia with Lewy bodies in an autopsy-verified sample. *International Journal of Geriatric Psychiatry, 14*(7), 526–533.

Mackenzie, I. R., Neumann, M., Bigio, E. H., Cairns, N. J., Alafuzoff, I., Kril, J., Kovacs, G. G., Ghetti, B., Halliday, G., Holm, I. E., Ince, P. G., Kamphorst, W., Revesz, T., Rozemuller, A. J., Kumar-Singh, S., Akiyama, H., Baborie, A., Spina, S., Dickson, D. W., Trojanowski, J. Q., & Mann, D. M. (2009). Nomenclature for neuropathologic subtypes of frontotemporal lobar degeneration: Consensus recommendations. *Acta neuropathologica, 117*(1), 15–18.

Mackinnon, A., & Mulligan, R. (1998). Combining cognitive testing and informant report to increase accuracy in screening for dementia. *American Journal of Psychiatry, 155*(11), 1529–1535.

Mahler, M. E., & Cummings, J. L. (1991). Behavioral neurology of multi-infarct dementia. *Alzheimer Disease and Associated Disorders, 5*(2), 122–130.

Mann, D. M. (1993). The molecular pathology of dementia. *Current Opinion in Psychiatry, 6,* 549–556.

Martin, L., Hirdes, J. P., Fries, B. E., & Smith, T. F. (2007). Development and psychometric properties of an assessment for persons with intellectual disability—the interRAI ID. *Journal of Policy and Practice in Intellectual Disabilities, 4*(1), 23–29.

Max, W., Webber, P., & Fox, P. (1995). Alzheimer's disease the unpaid burden of caring. *Journal of Aging and Health, 7*(2), 179–199.

Mayeux, R., Stern, Y., & Spanton, S. (1985). Heterogeneity in dementia of the Alzheimer type: Evidence of subgroups. *Neurology, 35*(4), 453–453.

McCarron, M., & McCallion, P. (2005). A revised stress and coping framework for staff carers of persons with intellectual disabilities and dementia. *Journal of Policy and Practice in Intellectual Disabilities, 2*(2), 139–148.

McCarron, M., McCallion, P., Fahey-McCarthy, E., Connaire, K., & Dunn-Lane, J. (2010). Supporting persons with Down syndrome and advanced dementia: Challenges and care concerns. *Dementia, 9*(2), 285–298.

McDaniel, W. F., Foster, R. A., Compton, D. M., & Courtney, A. S. (1998). A strategy for screening memory functions in individuals with mental retardation. *Research in Developmental Disabilities, 19*(4), 317–325.

McKeith, I. G. (1998). Dementia with Lewy bodies: Clinical and pathological diagnosis. *Alzheimers Reports, 1*(2), 83–87.

McKeith, I. G., Galasko, D., Kosaka, K., Perry, E. K., Dickson, D. W., Hansen, L. A., Salmon, D. P., Lowe, J., Mirra, S. S., Byrne, E. J., Lennox, G., Quinn, N. P., Edwardson, J. A., Ince, P. G., Bergeron, C., Burns, A., Miller, B. L., Lovestone, S., Collerton, D., Jansen, E. N., Ballard, C., de Vos, R. A., Wilcock, G. K., Jellinger, K. A., & Perry, R. H. (1996). Consensus guidelines for the clinical and pathologic diagnosis of dementia with Lewy bodies (DLB): Report of the consortium on DLB international workshop. *Neurology, 47*(5), 1113–1124.

McKeith, I., Mintzer, J., Aarsland, D., Burn, D., Chiu, H., Cohen-Mansfield, J., Dickson, D., Dubois, B., Duda, J. E., Feldman, H., Gauthier, S., Halliday, G., Lawlor, B., Lippa, C., Lopez, O. L., Carlos, M. J., O'Brien, J., Reid, W., & Playfer, J. (2004). Dementia with Lewy bodies. *The Lancet Neurology, 3*(1), 19–28.

McKhann, G., Drachman, D., Folstein, M., Katzman, R., Price, D., & Stadlan, E. M. (1984). Clinical diagnosis of Alzheimer's disease Report of the NINCDS-ADRDA Work Group under the auspices of Department of Health and Human Services Task Force on Alzheimer's Disease. *Neurology, 34*(7), 939–944.

Mega, M. S., Masterman, D. L., Benson, D. F., Vinters, H. V., Tomiyasu, U., Craig, A. H., Foti, D. J., Kaufer, D., Scharre, D. W., Fairbanks, L., & Cummings, J. L. (1996). Dementia with Lewy bodies reliability and validity of clinical and pathologic criteria. *Neurology, 47*(6), 1403–1409.

Miller, B. L., Ikonte, C., Ponton, M., Levy, M., Boone, K., Darby, A., Berman, N., Mena, I., & Cummings, J. L. (1997). A study of the Lund-Manchester research criteria for frontotemporal dementia: Clinical and single-photon emission CT correlations. *Neurology, 48*(4), 937–941.

Milne, A. J., Woolford, H. H., Mason, J., & Hatzidimitriadou, E. (2000). Early diagnosis of dementia by GPs: An exploratory study of attitudes. *Aging & Mental Health, 4*(4), 292–300.

Moïse, P., Schwarzinger, M., & Um, M. Y. (2004). *Dementia Care in 9 OECD Countries: A comparative analysis* (No. 13). Paris: OECD Publishing.

Mölsä, P. K., Marttila, R. J., & Rinne, U. K. (1986). Survival and cause of death in Alzheimer's disease and multi-infarct dementia. *Acta Neurologica Scandinavica, 74*(2), 103–107.

Moody, H. R. (1992). A critical view of ethical dilemmas in dementia. In R. H. Binstock (Ed.), *Dementia and aging: Ethics, values, and policy choices* (pp. 86–100). Baltimore: The Johns Hopkins University Press.

Mor, V. (2004). A comprehensive clinical assessment tool to inform policy and practice: Applications of the minimum data set. *Medical Care, 42*(4), 3–50.

Morris, J. N., Fries, B. E., Steel, K., Ikegami, N., Bernabei, R., Carpenter, G. I., Gilgen, R., Hirdes, J. P., & Topinkova, E. (1997). Comprehensive clinical assessment in community setting: Applicability of the MDS-HC. *Journal of the American Geriatrics Society, 45*(8), 1017–1024.

Morris, J. N., Carpenter, I., Berg, K., & Jones, R. N. (2000). Outcome measure for use with home care clients. *Canadian Journal on Aging, 19*, 87–105.

Nadel, L. (2003). Down's syndrome: A genetic disorder in biobehavioral perspective. *Genes, Brains, and Behavior, 2*, 156–166.

Nagdee, M. (2011). Dementia in intellectual disability: A review of diagnostic challenges. *African Journal of Psychiatry, 14*(3), 194–199.

Neary, D., Snowden, J. S., Northen, B., & Goulding, P. (1988). Dementia of frontal lobe type. *Journal of Neurology, Neurosurgery and Psychiatry, 51*(3), 353–361.

Neary, D., Snowden, J. S., Gustafson, L., Passant, U., Stuss, D., Black, S. A., Freedman, M., Kertesz, A., Robert, P. H., Albert, M., Boone, K., Miller, B. L., Cummings, J., & Benson, D. F. (1998). Frontotemporal lobar degeneration: A consensus on clinical diagnostic criteria. *Neurology, 51*(6), 1546–1554.

Nelson, L. D., Orme, D., Osann, K., & Lott, I. T. (2001). Neurological changes and emotional functioning in adults with Down syndrome. *Journal of Intellectual Disability Research, 45*(5), 450–456.

Nutt, J. G., Marsden, C. D., & Thompson, P. D. (1993). Human walking and higher-level gait disorders, particularly in the elderly. *Neurology, 43*(2), 268–279.

O'Connor, D. W., Pollitt, P. A., Hyde, J. B., Brook, C. P., Reiss, B. B., & Roth, M. (1988). Do general practitioners miss dementia in elderly patients? *British Medical Journal, 297*(6656), 1107.

O'Keeffe, S. T., Kazeem, H., Philpott, R. M., Playfer, J. R., Gosney, M., & Lye, M. (1996). Gait disturbance in Alzheimer's disease: A clinical study. *Age and Ageing, 25*(4), 313–316.

Ólafsdóttir, M., Skoog, I., & Marcusson, J. (2000). Detection of dementia in primary care: The Linköping study. *Dementia and Geriatric Cognitive Disorders, 11*(4), 223–229.

Oliver, C., Crayton, L., Holland, A., Hall, S., & Bradbury, J. (1998). A four year prospective study of age-related cognitive change in adults with Down's syndrome. *Psychological Medicine, 28*(6), 1365–1377.

Oliver, C., Crayton, L., Holland, A., & Hall, S. (2000). Cognitive deterioration in adults with Down syndrome: Effects on the individual, caregivers, and service use. *American Journal on Mental Retardation, 105*(6), 455–465.

Paclawskyj, T. R., Matson, J. L., Bamburg, J. W., & Baglio, C. S. (1997). A comparison of the diagnostic assessment for the severely handicapped-II (DASH-II) and the aberrant behavior checklist (ABC). *Research in Developmental Disabilities, 18*(4), 289–298.

Palmer, G. A. (2006). Neuropsychological profiles of persons with mental retardation and dementia. *Research in Developmental Disabilities, 27,* 299–308.

Panisset, M., Roudier, M., Saxton, J., & Boiler, F. (1994). Severe impairment battery: A neuropsychological test for severely demented patients. *Archives of Neurology, 51*(1), 41.

Pasquier, F., Leys, D., & Scheltens, P. (1998). The influence of coincidental vascular pathology on symptomatology and course of Alzheimer's disease. In H.-J. Gertz & Th. Arendt (Eds.), *Alzheimer's disease—From basic research to clinical applications* (pp. 117–127). Vienna: Springer.

Patel, P., Goldberg, D., & Moss, S. (1993). Psychiatric morbidity in older people with moderate and severe learning disability. II: The prevalence study. *The British Journal of Psychiatry, 163*(4), 481–491.

Patja, K., Mölsä, P., & Iivanainen, M. (2001). Cause-specific mortality of people with intellectual disability in a population-based, 35-year follow-up study. *Journal of Intellectual Disability Research, 45*(1), 30–40.

Perry, R. H., Irving, D., Blessed, G., Perry, E. K., & Fairbairn, A. F. (1989). Senile dementia of Lewy body type and spectrum of Lewy body disease. *The Lancet, 333*(8646), 1088.

Perry, R. H., Irving, D., & Tomlinson, B. E. (1990a). Lewy body prevalence in the aging brain: Relationship to neuropsychiatric disorders, Alzheimer-type pathology and catecholaminergic nuclei. *Journal of the Neurological Sciences, 100*(1), 223–233.

Perry, R. H., Irving, D., Blessed, G., Fairbairn, A., & Perry, E. K. (1990b). Senile dementia of Lewy body type: A clinically and neuropathologically distinct form of Lewy body dementia in the elderly. *Journal of the Neurological Sciences, 95*(2), 119–139.

Petry, S., Cummings, J. L., Hill, M. A., & Shapira, J. (1988). Personality alterations in dementia of the Alzheimer type. *Archives of Neurology, 45*(11), 1187.

Pfeffer, R. I., Afifi, A. A., & Chance, J. M. (1987). Prevalence of Alzheimer's disease in a retirement community. *American Journal of Epidemiology, 125*(3), 420–436.

Pippi, M., Mecocci, P., Saxton, J., Bartorelli, L., Pettenati, C., Bonaiuto, S., Cucinotta, D., Masaraki, G., Neri, M., Tammaro, A. E., Vergani, C., Chionne, F., & Senin, U. (1999). Neuropsychological assessment of the severely impaired elderly patient: Validation of the Italian short version of the Severe Impairment Battery (SIB). *Aging Clinical and Experimental Research, 11* (4), 221–226.

Prasher, V. (1995). Age-specific prevalence, thyroid dysfunction, and depressive symptomatology in adults with Down's syndrome and dementia. *International Journal of Geriatric Psychiatry, 10,* 25–31.

Prasher, V. P. (1997). Dementia Questionnaire for Persons with Mental Retardation (DMR): Modified criteria for adults with Down's syndrome. *Journal of Applied Research in Intellectual Disabilities, 10*(1), 54–60.

Prasher, V. P. (2004). Review of donepezil, rivastigmine, galantamine and memantine for the treatment of dementia in Alzheimer's disease in adults with down syndrome: implications for the intellectual disability population. *International journal of geriatric psychiatry, 19*(6), 509–515.

Ratnavalli, E., Brayne, C., Dawson, K., & Hodges, J. R. (2002). The prevalence of frontotemporal dementia. *Neurology, 58*(11), 1615–1621.

Reichman, W. E., & Negron, A. (2001). Negative symptoms in the elderly patient with dementia. *International Journal of Geriatric Psychiatry, 16*(S1), S7–S11.

Rice, D. P., Fox, P. J., Max, W., Webber, P. A., Lindeman, D. A., Hauck, W. W., & Segura, E. (1993). The economic burden of Alzheimer's disease care. *Health Affairs, 12*(2), 164–176.

Risberg, J. (1987). Frontal lobe degeneration of non-Alzheimer type. III. Regional cerebral blood flow. *Archives of Gerontology and Geriatrics, 6*(3), 225–233.

Rocca, W. A., Hofman, A., Brayne, C., Breteler, M., Clarke, M., Copeland, J. R., Dartigues, J. F., Engedal, K., Hagnell, O., Heeren, T. J., & Amaducci, L. (1991). Frequency and distribution of Alzheimer's disease in Europe: A collaborative study of 1980–1990 prevalence findings. *Annals of neurology, 30*(3), 381–390.

Román, G. C. (2002). Defining dementia: Clinical criteria for the diagnosis of vascular dementia. *Acta Neurologica Scandinavica, 106*(s178), 6–9.

Román, G. C., & Royall, D. R. (1999). Executive control function: A rational basis for the diagnosis of vascular dementia. *Alzheimer Disease and Associated Disorders, 13,* S69–S80.

Román, G. C., Tatemichi, T. K., Erkinjuntti, T., Cummings, J. L., Masdeu, J. C., Garcia, J. A., Amaducci, L., Orgogozo, J. M., Brun, A., Hofman, A., & Scheinberg, P. (1993). Vascular dementia diagnostic criteria for research studies: Report of the NINDS-AIREN International Workshop. *Neurology, 43*(2), 250–260.

Rosen, H. J., Hartikainen, K. M., Jagust, W., Kramer, J. H., Reed, B. R., Cummings, J. L., Boone, K., Ellis, W., Miller, C., & Miller, B. L. (2002). Utility of clinical criteria in differentiating frontotemporal lobar degeneration (FTLD) from AD. *Neurology, 58*(11), 1608–1615.

Ross, G. W., Abbott, R. D., Petrovitch, H., Masaki, K. H., Murdaugh, C., Trockman, C., Curb, J. D., & White, L. R. (1997). Frequency and characteristics of silent dementia among elderly Japanese-American men: The Honolulu-Asia aging study. *Journal of the American Medical Association, 277*(10), 800–805.

Rubin, E. H., & Kinscherf, D. A. (1989). Psychopathology of very mild dementia of the Alzheimer type. *The American Journal of Psychiatry, 146*(8), 1017–1021.

Rubin, S. M., Glasser, M. L., & Werckle, M. A. (1987). The examination of physicians' awareness of dementing disorders. *Journal of the American Geriatrics Society, 35*(12), 1051–1058.

Rueda, N., Llorens-Martín, M., Flórez, J., Valdizán, E., Banerjee, P., Trejo, J. L., & Martínez-Cué, C. (2010). Memantine normalizes several phenotypic features in the Ts65Dn mouse model of Down syndrome. *Journal of Alzheimer's Disease, 21*(1), 277–290.

Ryden, M. B. (1988). Aggressive behavior in persons with dementia who live in the community. *Alzheimer Disease & Associated Disorders, 2*(4), 342–355.

Safar, L. T., & Press, D. Z. (2011). Art and the brain: Effects of dementia on art production in art therapy. *Art Therapy, 28*(3), 96–103.

Saxton, J., McGonigle-Gibson, K. L., Swihart, A. A., Miller, V. J., & Boller, F. (1990). Assessment of the severely impaired patient: Description and validation of a new neuropsychological test battery. *Psychological Assessment: A Journal of Consulting and Clinical Psychology, 2*(3), 298.

Saxton, J., Kastango, K. B., Hugonot-Diener, L., Boller, F., Verny, M., Sarles, C. E., Girgis, R. R., Devouche, E., Mecocci, P., Pollock, B. G., & DeKosky, S. T. (2005). Development of a short form of the Severe Impairment Battery. *The American Journal of Geriatric Psychiatry, 13*(11), 999–1005.

Schmitt, F. A., Ashford, W., Ernesto, C., Saxton, J., Schneider, L. S., Clark, C. M., Ferris, S. H., Mackell, J. A., Schafer, K., & Thal, L. J. (1997). The severe impairment battery: Concurrent validity and the assessment of longitudinal change in Alzheimer's disease. *Alzheimer Disease and Associated Disorders, 11,* 51–56.

Schoenburg, B. S., Kokmen, E., & Okazaki, H. (1987). Alzheimer's disease and other dementing illnesses in a defined United States population: Incidence rates and clinical features. *Annals of Neurology, 22*(6), 724–729.

Schultz, J. M., Aman, M. G., & Rojahn, J. (1998). Psychometric evaluation of a measure of cognitive decline in elderly people with mental retardation. *Research in Developmental Disabilities, 19*(1), 63–71.

Shergill, S., Mullan, E., D'ath, P., & Katona, C. (1994). What is the clinical prevalence of Lewy body dementia? *International Journal of Geriatric Psychiatry, 9*(11), 907–912.

Shooshtari, S., Martens, P. J., Burchill, C. A., Dik, N., & Naghipur, S. (2011). Prevalence of depression and dementia among adults with developmental disabilities in Manitoba, Canada. *International Journal of Family Medicine, 2011,* 1–9.

Silverman, W., Zigman, W. B., Kim, H., Krinsky-McHale, S., & Wisniewski, H. M. (1998). Aging and dementia among adults with mental retardation and Down syndrome. *Topics in Geriatric Rehabilitation, 13*(3), 49–64.

Snowden, J. S., Goulding, P. J., & Neary, D. (1989). Semantic dementia: A form of circumscribed cerebral atrophy. *Behavioural Neurology, 2*(3), 167–182.

Snowden, J. S., Neary, D., Mann, D. M. A., Goulding, P. J., & Testa, H. J. (1992). Progressive language disorder due to lobar atrophy. *Annals of Neurology, 31*(2), 174–183.

Snowden, J. S., Neary, D., & Mann, D. M. (1996). *Fronto-temporal lobar degeneration: fronto-temporal dementia, progressive aphasia, semantic dementia.* Edingburgh: Churchill Livingstone.

Snowdon, D. A., Greiner, L. H., Mortimer, J. A., Riley, K. P., Greiner, P. A., & Markesbery, W. R. (1997). Brain infarction and the clinical expression of Alzheimer disease: The Nun Study. *Journal of the American Medical Association, 277*(10), 813–817.

Somerfield, M. R., Weisman, C. S., Ury, W., Chase, G. A., & Folstein, M. F. (1991). Physician practices in the diagnosis of dementing disorders. *Journal of the American Geriatrics Society, 39*(2), 172–175.

Speechly, C. M., Bridges-Webb, C., & Passmore, E. (2008). The pathway to dementia diagnosis. *Medical Journal of Australia, 189*(9), 487–489.

Stern, Y., Tang, M. X., Denaro, J., & Mayeux, R. (1995). Increased risk of mortality in Alzheimer's disease patients with more advanced educational and occupational attainment. *Annals of Neurology, 37*(5), 590–595.

Strydom, A., & Hassiotis, A. (2003). Diagnostic instruments for dementia in older people with intellectual disability in clinical practice. *Aging and Mental Health, 7*(6), 431–437.

Strydom, A., Livingston, G., King, M., & Hassiotis, A. (2007). Prevalence of dementia in intellectual disability using different diagnostic criteria. *The British Journal of Psychiatry, 191*(2), 150–157.

Strydom, A., Hassiotis, A., King, M., & Livingston, G. (2009). The relationship of dementia prevalence in older adults with intellectual disability (ID) to age and severity of ID. *Psychological Medicine, 39*(1), 13.

Strydom, A., Shooshtari, S., Lee, L., Raykar, V., Torr, J., Tsiouris, J., Jokinen, N., Courtenay, K., Bass, N., Sinnema, M., & Maaskant, M. (2010). Dementia in older adults with intellectual disabilities—epidemiology, presentation, and diagnosis. *Journal of Policy and Practice in Intellectual Disabilities, 7*(2), 96–110.

Strydom, A., Chan, T., King, M., Hassiotis, A., & Livingston, G. (2013). Incidence of dementia in older adults with intellectual disabilities. *Research in Developmental Disabilities, 34,* 1881–1885.

Sturmey, P., Reed, J., & Corbett, J. (1991). Psychometric assessment of psychiatric disorders in people with learning difficulties (mental handicap): A review of measures. *Psychological Medicine, 21*(1), 143–155.

Sultzer, D. L., Levin, H. S., Mahler, M. E., High, W. M., & Cummings, J. L. (1993). A comparison of psychiatric symptoms in vascular dementia and Alzheimer's disease. *American Journal of Psychiatry, 150,* 1806–1812.

Tartaglia, M. C., Rosen, H. J., & Miller, B. L. (2011). Neuroimaging in dementia. *Neurotherapeutics, 8*(1), 82–92.

Thai, L. J., Grundman, M., & Klauber, M. R. (1988). Dementia Characteristics of a referral population and factors associated with progression. *Neurology, 38*(7), 1083–1090.

Thomas, V. S., Vandenberg, E. V., & Potter, J. F. (2002). Non-neurological factors are implicated in impairments in gait and mobility among patients in a clinical dementia referral population. *International Journal of Geriatric Psychiatry, 17*(2), 128–133.

Thompson, P. D., & Marsden, C. D. (1987). Gait disorder of subcortical arteriosclerotic encephalopathy: Binswanger's disease. *Movement Disorders, 2*(1), 1–8.

Tsiouris, J. A., & Patti, P. J. (1997). Drug treatment of depression associated with dementia or presented as 'pseudodementia' in older adults with Down syndrome. *Journal of Applied Research in Intellectual Disabilities, 10*(4), 312–322.

Varma, A. R., Snowden, J. S., Lloyd, J. J., Talbot, P. R., Mann, D. M. A., & Neary, D. (1999). Evaluation of the NINCDS-ADRDA criteria in the differentiation of Alzheimer's disease and frontotemporal dementia. *Journal of Neurology, Neurosurgery and Psychiatry, 66*(2), 184–188.

Verghese, J., Crystal, H. A., Dickson, D. W., & Lipton, R. B. (1999). Validity of clinical criteria for the diagnosis of dementia with Lewy bodies. *Neurology, 53*(9), 1974–1982.

Vernooij-Dassen, M. J., Moniz-Cook, E. D., Woods, R. T., Lepeleire, J. D., Leuschner, A., Zanetti, O., de Rotrou, J., Kenny, G., Franco, M., Peters, V., & Iliffe, S. (2005). Factors affecting timely recognition and diagnosis of dementia across Europe: From awareness to stigma. *International Journal of Geriatric Psychiatry, 20*(4), 377–386.

Vicari, S. (2004). Memory development and intellectual disabilities. *Acta Pediatrica Supplement, 93,* 60–63.

Vink, A. C., Zuidersma, M., Boersma, F., Jonge, P., Zuidema, S. U., & Slaets, J. P. J. (2013). The effect of music therapy compared with general recreational activities in reducing agitation in people with dementia: A randomised controlled trial. *International Journal of Geriatric Psychiatry, 28*(10), 1031–1038.

Visootsak, J., & Sherman, S. L. (2008). Trisomy 21: Causes and consequences. *International Review of Research in Mental Retardation, 36,* 61–90.

Visser, F. E., Aldenkamp, A. P., Van Huffelen, A. C., & Kuilman, M. (1997). Prospective study of the prevalence of Alzheimer-type dementia in institutionalized individuals with Down syndrome. *American Journal on Mental Retardation, 101*(4), 400–412.

Vitali, P., Migliaccio, R., Agosta, F., Rosen, H. J., & Geschwind, M. D. (2008). Neuroimaging in dementia. *Seminars in Neurology, 28*(4) 467–483.

Vogl, M., & Rapp, J. T. (2011). Differential reinforcement of other behavior and extinction to reduce loitering and stealing for an adult with an intellectual disability and dementia. *Clinical Case Studies, 10*(3), 229–235.

Waite, L. M., Broe, G. A., Grayson, D. A., & Creasey, H. (2000). Motor function and disability in the dementias. *International Journal of Geriatric Psychiatry, 15*(10), 897–903.

Weintraub, S., Rubin, N. P., & Mesulam, M. (1990). Primary progressive aphasia: Longitudinal course, neuropsychological profile, and language features. *Archives of Neurology, 47*(12), 1329.

Wetzels, R. B., Zuidema, S. U., de Jonghe, J. F., Verhey, F. R., & Koopmans, R. T. (2010). Course of neuropsychiatric symptoms in residents with dementia in nursing homes over 2-year period. *The American Journal of Geriatric Psychiatry, 18*(12), 1054–1065.

Wild, K. V., & Kaye, J. A. (1998). The rate of progression of Alzheimer's disease in the later stages: Evidence from the Severe Impairment Battery. *Journal of the International Neuropsychological Society, 4*(05), 512–516.

Wilkinson, H., & Janicki, M. P. (2002). The Edinburgh Principles with accompanying guidelines and recommendations. *Journal of Intellectual Disability Research, 46*(3), 279–284.

Wilkinson, H., Kerr, D., & Cunningham, C. (2005). Equipping staff to support people with an intellectual disability and dementia in care home settings. *Dementia, 4*(3), 387–400.

Wisniewski, H. M., & Rabe, A. (1986). Discrepancy between Alzheimer-Type Neuropathology and Dementia in Persons with Down's Syndrome. *Annals of the New York Academy of Sciences, 477*(1), 247–260.

Wisniewski, K. E., Wisniewski, H. M., & Wen, G. Y. (1985). Occurrence of neuropathological changes and dementia of Alzheimer's disease in Down's syndrome. *Annals of neurology, 17*(3), 278–282.

Wolfson, C., Wolfson, D. B., Asgharian, M., M'Lan, C. E., Østbye, T., Rockwood, K., & Hogan, D. B. (2001). A reevaluation of the duration of survival after the onset of dementia. *New England Journal of Medicine, 344*(15), 1111–1116.

Yoshitake, T., Kiyohara, Y., Kato, I., Ohmura, T., Iwamoto, H., Nakayama, K., Ohmori, S., Nomiyama, K., Kawano, H., Ueda, K., & Fujishima, M. (1995). Incidence and risk factors of vascular dementia and Alzheimer's disease in a defined elderly Japanese population: The Hisayama Study. *Neurology, 45*(6), 1161–1168.

Zeilinger, E. L., Stiehl, K. A., & Weber, G. (2013). A systematic review on assessment instruments for dementia in persons with intellectual disabilities. *Research in Developmental Disabilities, 34*(11), 3962–3977.

Zigman, W. B., Schupf, N., Zigman, A., & Silverman, W. (1993). Aging and Alzheimer Disease in people with mental retardation. *International Review of Research in Mental Retardation, 19,* 41–70.

Zigman, W. B., Schupf, N., Sersen, E., & Silverman, W. (1996). Prevalence of dementia in adults with and without Down syndrome. *American Journal on Mental Retardation, 100*(4), 403–412.

Chapter 9
Obesity

Amanda Faith Casey and Roy Rasmussen

Introduction

One of the main goals of Healthy People (2010) was to eradicate health disparities associated with various populations in the USA (United States Department of Health and Human Services 2000). However, figures suggest that the obesity 'epidemic' continues to rise and pose a serious threat to public health on an individual and societal level regardless of race, class, gender or, as we will discuss, presence of disability (Flegal et al. 2002; Haslam and James 2005; Haslam et al. 2005; Ogden et al. 2012; Popkin et al. 2012). Research underlines that body mass index (BMI) across the general population increased in men and women by 0.4 kg/m^2 and 0.5 kg/m^2, respectively, between 1980 and 2008 (Finucane et al. 2011). This trend is particularly troubling as obesity contributes to a variety of serious medical conditions, including hypertension, diabetes, heart disease, arthritis, stroke, stress and respiratory diseases (Daniels 2006; Daniels et al. 2005; Eckel 1997). Moreover, research connects total and regional body fat with conditions such as insulin resistance, glucose metabolism, serum lipid concentrations, and abnormal blood pressure (Williams et al. 1992).

Prevalence of Obesity Amongst Individuals with Intellectual Disability (ID)

A growing number of studies indicate that incidences of obesity (BMI $\geq$30 kg/m^2) and extreme obesity (BMI $\geq$40 kg/m^2) remain consistently high for youth and adults with various types of intellectual disability (ID), including individuals with

A. F. Casey (✉) · R. Rasmussen
Department of Human Kinetics, St. Francis Xavier University, Antigonish, NS B2G 2W5, Canada
e-mail: acasey@stfx.ca

J. L. Matson, M. L. Matson (eds.), *Comorbid Conditions in Individuals with Intellectual Disabilities*, Autism and Child Psychopathology Series,
DOI 10.1007/978-3-319-15437-4_9

no clearly diagnosed syndrome, Down syndrome, Duane syndrome, Prader–Willi syndrome and even developmental disabilities such as autism spectrum disorder (Emerson 2005; Rimmer and Yamaki 2006; Rubin et al. 1998; Stewart et al. 2009). It is extremely difficult to generalize findings within such a heterogeneous population; however, there is now a strong enough evidence base to suggest that obesity is as great, if not greater, a concern for individuals with ID than it is for individuals without ID (Melville et al. 2005; Yamaki 2005). This is particularly prescient for individuals belonging to certain subcategories of ID who remain at increased risk for becoming obese. Age (Moran et al. 2005; Stancliffe et al. 2011), gender (Lloyd, Temple and Foley 2012), race/nationality (Lloyd et al. 2012), poverty (Yamaki and Fujiura 2002), living arrangements (Rimmer et al. 1993) level of functioning (Robertson et al. 2000) and genetic cause of ID (Dudley et al. 2008; Melville et al. 2005; Rimmer and Wang 2005; Rubin et al. 1998) are all probable determinants for obesity in individuals with ID.

Age Until recently, most studies exploring rates of obesity had centered on adult rather than pediatric populations with ID (Foley et al. 2014; Lloyd et al. 2012; Maiano 2011). Little evidence existed to document the prevalence of obesity and related concerns in youth with ID on an international level (Allerton et al. 2011; Emerson and Robertson 2010; Harris et al. 2003; Takeuchi 1994). More studies now seem to demonstrate, however, that BMI status acts as a significant indicator of adiposity-based health risk. Maiano's review (2011) found that obesity ranges varied from 7–36 % in children and adolescents with ID. This compared unfavorably to work carried out by Janssen et al. (2005) which showed obesity to be present in only 0.4–7.9 % of the general pediatric population. Recent work by Lloyd et al. (2012–2014), focusing on BMI-based data in Special Olympics athletes, also offered greater insight into the dangers of obesity for youth with ID across the world, finding approximately 30 % of the international sample with ID to be obese despite previous participation in Special Olympics competitions.

This literature also supports previous studies that suggest that an individual with ID may be increasingly likely to become overweight or obese with age (Emerson 2005; Lloyd et al. 2012; Maiano 2011; Temple et al. 2014). This remains an important area of study as individuals with ID are living longer than ever before and therefore experiencing increased health complications to go with it (Draheim 2006). Although pediatric obesity amongst children aged 8–12 years with ID may be at similar levels to those of children without ID (Foley et al. 2014; Janssen 2005), rates are far higher in adolescents with ID (45 %) in comparison to adolescents without ID (Ogden et al. 2010, 2012; Telama et al. 2005).

Substantial levels of obesity have also been reported in adult populations (Sohler et al. 2009; Stedman and Leland 2010; Temple, et al. 2014). Numerous findings illustrate that the prevalence of obesity in adults with ID is equal to or above that of adults without ID (Emerson 2005; Frey and Rimmer 1995), with high incidences documented during midlife (Yamaki 2005) and for the aging population with ID (De Winter et al. 2012). Yamaki (2005) examined annual survey data from 1985 to 2000 and showed that rates of obesity amongst 3499 adults with ID remained significantly above that of adults without ID at each of the 4-year evaluation periods.

In support, Rimmer and Wang (2005) found that, in their US sample, rates of obesity were double (60 vs. 30 %) that of adults without ID while extreme obesity was two and a half times as high (12.1 vs. 4.7 %).

Gender The majority of studies have found clear discrepancies in obesity rates based on gender as well (Bhaumik et al. 2008; Melville et al. 2005; Sohler et al. 2009). With a few exceptions (Dudley et al. 2008; Foley et al. 2014), most population-level data have shown that girls (Lloyd et al. 2012) and women (Emerson 2005; Stancliffe et al. 2011) may be more overweight/obese than boys and men who have ID. An early study by Rimmer et al. (1993) explored prevalence amongst adults with ID in institutions as well as in family and community-based facilities, revealing obesity to be much more common in women (58.8 %) than men (27.5 %). Melville and his fellow collaborators' (2005) case-control study also found women with Down syndrome to be more likely to be obese than matched pairs (odds ratio = 2.17). Finally, Lloyd et al. (2012) demonstrated that girls (54 %) were more at risk for obesity than boys (47 %).

Race/Nationality Overall, North America possesses the highest rates of obesity according to large studies sampling both youth and adults who displayed various impairments in intellectual functioning (Foley et al. 2013; Temple et al. 2014). Harris et al. (2003) reported that US Special Olympians (65 %) remained significantly more overweight and obese than non-US Special Olympians. Within North America itself, black people experience higher rates of obesity and extreme obesity than white people (Jones and Sinclair 2008; Rimmer et al. 2010c). For adults, Temple et al. (2014) emphasized that rates of overweight/obesity remained high for adult males and females from North America but lower for men from Africa, North Africa as well as the Middle East and Latin America. In support, Lloyd et al.'s (2012) data on children showed obesity to be lower in East Asia, Asia Pacific and Latin America even though the prevalence of obesity still remained above that recorded for children without ID in those regions.

Poverty As with the general population (Ezzati et al. 2002), research suggests that obesity may be associated with lower income levels based on the large number of people with ID who originate from poorer backgrounds (Fujiura and Yamaki 1997; Yamaki and Fukiura 2002). Lloyd et al. (2012) reported obesity levels to be high (27.9–34.3 %) amongst youth with ID in Africa, North Africa and the Middle East and these findings concur with recently documented obesity epidemics in the developing world (Popkin et al. 2012).

Living Arrangements The majority of adults with ID now live in the community (Prouty and Lakin 2006) and are finding themselves more likely to be overweight and/or obese than adults who live in more restrictive, institutional based settings (Bryan et al. 2000; Frey and Rimmer 1995). Research documenting the movement of individuals from institutions to supported community arrangements has noted significant weight changes and increased weight-related incapacities (Bryan et al. 2000; Gabre et al. 2002; Seekins et al. 2005; Temple and Walkley, 2003). Studies carried out by Rimmer et al. (1993) and Lewis et al. (2002), for example, both showed that individuals with ID who were in a less restrictive, family-based environment, reported the highest rates of obesity, ahead of peers living in community-based residential facilities and far ahead of individuals from institutional settings.

Level of Disability Individuals diagnosed with mild or moderate ID, or those who are considered 'more able', experience more incidences of being overweight and obesity than do adults with profound ID (Molteno et al. 2000; Robertson et al. 2000). Similarly, adults with ID, who have relatively higher IQs and score higher on nutrition knowledge tests, are shown to experience higher rates of obesity (Golden and Hatcher 1997).

Genetic Disposition Individuals with certain genetic causes of ID may also be more likely to be obese (Dudley et al. 2008; Melville et al. 2005). Disabilities associated with Down syndrome and Prader–Willi syndrome are recognized to have high levels of obesity unless there are large levels of support in place to manage energy intake and output. Rimmer and Wang (2005) found obesity to be 10 % higher amongst adults with Down syndrome (70.7 %) compared to adults with ID who did not have Down syndrome. The same study showed that 19 % of adults with Down syndrome were extremely obese. Similarly, Rubin et al. (1998) reported that 45 % of men and 56 % of women with Down syndrome were overweight. Using a criterion measurement, air displacement plethysmography (ADP), Usera and colleagues (2005) measured percentage body fat to be 43 % across a sample of participants with Down syndrome against 20.5 % in participants without Down syndrome. In Prader–Willi syndrome, Dudley et al. (2008) found that adult participants with ID had significantly high rates of obesity across the world, especially in France.

Measuring Obesity

There remains the worrying possibility that these high levels of obesity are over or underestimated (Casey 2013; Humphries et al. 2009b; Rimmer and Yamaki 2006). Individuals with ID may have been excluded from samples because they live in group homes, or simply because various populations with ID are frequently omitted from health surveillance initiatives (Center for Disease Control 2008). It is also possible that individuals with ID may have made errors when documenting their own weight using self-report (Rimmer et al. 2010c), as inaccurate estimates of obesity are often the result of people overestimating height and underestimating weight (Ogden et al. 2010). For example, Rimmer and Wang (2005) used actual BMI measurements and documented much higher levels of obesity among individuals with disabilities than had been noted in two previously published reports which relied upon self-report data. Many other studies may also have been unrepresentative of populations with ID. Bryan et al. (2000) explained that 15 % of their own participants did not have their weight assessed because of a lack of suitable, accessible scales in community settings. Additionally, some of the largest available samples featured only Special Olympics athletes who may or may not have been more

Consequences of Obesity

It is absolutely essential to uncover reliable ways to measure adiposity amongst individuals with ID because, as with the general population, obesity remains an important indicator of health in this population (van Schrojenstein Lantman-de Valk et al. 2007). Indeed, due to a reduced health threshold, ever-growing research suggests that obesity may contribute towards a greater number of obesity-related conditions among individuals with ID compared to peers without ID (Havecamp et al. 2003; Turk 2006). Health concerns include cardiovascular disease (Draheim 2006), reduced social and physical functioning (Seekins et al. 2005), decreased quality of life (Hughes et al. 2007), challenges in forming peer relationships (Koplan et al. 2005) as well as larger propensity for depression, stigma (Daniels, 2006) and reduced opportunities for community integration (Rimmer et al. 1993). More specifically, individuals with ID who possess abdominal obesity are also approximately ten times as likely to have elevated biological risk factors including hypertension, hypertriglyceridemia, hyperinsulinemia, and low high-density lipoprotein (good) cholesterol levels when compared to people who are not abdominally obese (Draheim et al. 2002).

Young people with ID who are obese remain at increased risk of exhibiting obesity-related physical, psychological, social and/or emotional conditions (e.g., conditions not linked to the primary disability) in comparison to individuals with ID who are not obese (Rimmer et al. 2011). Such conditions may have a negative impact on an individual's health and functional ability. Rimmer et al. (2010) followed 14 health conditions associated with individuals with ID, and revealed that youth who were overweight or obese had significantly higher rates in 11 of these conditions whereas individuals with ID who were of healthy weight had higher incidences in only 3 out of 14 conditions. Overall, individuals with ID who were overweight or obese were far more likely to experience asthma, high blood pressure, high blood cholesterol, type II diabetes mellitus, depression, fatigue as well as preoccupation with weight and pressure sores. For individuals with Down syndrome, research suggests that their unique body fat distribution may increase the potential for insulin resistance (Fonseca et al. 2005) and type II diabetes mellitus (Magge et al. 2008). All of these obesity-related conditions may interrupt and/or reduce work and social activities (Pain and Wiles 2006) in this population as well as add to the strain placed on various health care systems across the world, exemplified by one qualitative study which suggests that people with disabilities who are obese require more care and pay more for assistive devices in comparison to people without disabilities (Pain and Wiles 2006).

Causes of Obesity: Genetics versus Environmental Factors

Genetics For individuals with ID, researchers used ordinarily to connect secondary health concerns such as obesity and related conditions to the primary disability itself (Marge, 1988; Rimmer, 1999). Indeed, certain researchers argue that genetics plays a more important role than environmental factors in the presence of obesity. Genetic factors are well documented to impact how much weight is gained in people with and without disabilities (Haslam and James 2005). One study by Traci et al. (2001) demonstrated that adults with ID with a known family history of weight and obesity-related concerns possessed substantially higher BMIs than individuals without a documented history of difficulties. For certain sub-categories of ID, the genetic argument has scientific support related to physiological and/or metabolic differences. Biological reasons are attributed to why women may be more obese than men in people with and without disabilities (James et al. 2004). Moreover, unusual body composition which features disproportionately high fat and irregular fat distribution may be common in both Prader–Willi and Down syndrome (Brambilla et al. 1997; Gonzalez-Aguero et al. 2011). Indeed, for individuals with Down syndrome, Guijjaro et al. (2007) found body fat to be more truncal, indicating elevated levels of abdominal and visceral fat stores.

However, genetics alone cannot explain the global obesity epidemic experienced by people with and without ID (Haslam and Janes 2005). An increasing number of researchers in the field of ID instead relate high rates of obesity to personal and environmental factors (Rimmer et al. 2011) citing regular medication (Merriman et al. 2005) as well as poor eating habits and an overwhelmingly sedentary lifestyle (Binkley et al. 2000; Swinburn and Egger 2002; Bowman and Vinyard 2004). As Temple et al. (2014) explain, in countries with middle to low income, researchers have characterized this development as a 'nutrition transition' (Popkin 2002; Prentice 2006; Finucane et al. 2011) marked by an uptake in the consumption of energy-dense diets, sweetened foods, edible oils and animal source foods as well as diminished participation in work and leisure-related physical activity (Prentice 2006; Popkin et al. 2012).

Medication Research highlights that an increasing number of drugs may lead to weight gain and obesity in people with and without ID (Haslam 2005). Intake of psychotropic drugs may produce increased weight gain (Hellings et al. 2001) and/or higher BMI amongst people with ID in comparison to people with ID who are not taking such drugs (Merriman et al. 2005). A recent study by De Winter et al. (2012) also documented higher rates of obesity amongst individuals taking antipsychotic drugs. The reasons behind these developments are not fully documented by the research community (Blackburn 2000), and current interventions such as calorie restriction do not appear to control weight gain effectively (Cohen et al. 2001).

Physical Inactivity Strong evidence suggests that individuals with ID do not partake in enough physical activity to garner certain health benefits including decreased obesity (Fernhall and Pitetti 2001; Frey et al. 2005; 2008; Graham and Reid 2000; Van de Vliet et al. 2006). The American College of Sports Medicine (2009) guidelines recommend that individuals with ID undertake at least 30 mins of moderate intensity exercise on most, if not all, days of the week. However, Draheim et al. (2002) found that no adults with ID over thirty participated in any vigorous activity while Stanish et al. (2006) revealed that less than one-third of individuals with ID stay physically active for 30 mins on most or all days of the week. This trend has been echoed in studies focusing on youth and adults with Down syndrome who are shown to engage in less vigorous physical activity than their peers without Down syndrome (Balic et al. 2000; Shields et al. 2009; Whitt-Glover et al. 2006).

Researchers have underlined that physical inactivity may be linked to a variety of barriers associated with the natural and built environment, transportation, physical health (e.g., reduced physical fitness), cost, mental health (e.g., emotional/psychological issues), discriminatory attitudes, policies as well as a lack of trained professionals, adapted equipment and information (Rimmer and Marques 2012; Rimmer et al. 2004). Furthermore, parents have reported that many programs that do exist are not meeting either the cognitive or physical needs of their children, or are too short in duration for their children to become successful (Menear 2007). In short, it appears that individuals with ID must overcome considerable barriers in order to reverse this pattern of physical inactivity and avoid the substantial health consequences associated with a sedentary lifestyle including obesity-related concerns (Rimmer et al. 2011; Rimmer et al. 2012).

Nutrition Research suggests that nutrition and food habits may be at least partially responsible for high levels of obesity found in populations with ID (Braunschweig et al. 2004; Bryan et al. 2000; Draheim et al. 2002a; Humphries et al. 2009b; Rubin et al. 1998). Satisfactory nutrition is essential in regulating obesity and preventing further health conditions amongst people of all ages with ID (Humphries et al. 2009; Draheim et al. 2007). Yet, research underlines that individuals with ID are a nutritionally vulnerable population and it remains a challenge to monitor dietary intake due to difficulties arising from memory, comprehension, dexterity, literacy and communication, which make recalling, recording and quantifying food consumption complicated (Draheim et al. 2002; Humohries et al. 2008 2009). These same concerns mean that individuals with ID may not always be able to foresee health complications arising from obesity in the future (Rimmer and Yamaki 2006; Spitalnik and White-Scott 2001). As such, individuals with ID are likely to have eating dysfunctions (Hove 2004) and make unhealthy eating choices when unsupervised, including consuming insufficient micronutrients (Adolfsson et al. 2008) and eating excessively throughout the day (Bertoli et al. 2006; Starr and Mardsen 2008). Indeed, foods with higher energy density including many rich in fats, extracted sugars and refined starches are being eaten in large quantities on a reoccurring basis with such items often being used as a reward for good behavior (Casey et al. 2012). The daily diet of individuals with ID who live in group home settings has also been shown to include nutrient-poor foods and dietary fats while staff supporting individuals with ID may not have the requisite knowledge or training with regards to food and nutrition (Humphries et al. 2004). With approximately two-thirds of the population in the United States now living in community-based group homes as opposed to larger institutions, this remains an area of great concern (Prouty and Lakin 2006).

Research emphasizes that certain individuals with Prader–Willi syndrome may eat in an inappropriate manner, including practices such as overeating, stealing and hoarding grocery items (Holland et al. 1995), pica (Dykens 2000) and digesting contaminated foods (Dykens 2000). All of these choices may compound the genetic risk for obesity in this sub-population (Dudley et al., 2008).

Reduction Measures

Given the outlandishly high rates of obesity identified, it is necessary for researchers to explore measures to prevent and manage these concerns in populations with ID through diverse means as underlined by numerous reviews (Biswas et al. 2010; Casey and Rasmussen 2013; Hamilton et al. 2007; Heller et al. 2011; Maı¨ano et al. 2014; Spanos et al. 2013). Reviewers underline that interventions have focused overwhelmingly on nonsurgical measures including behavior, exercise (e.g., energy expenditure), diet (energy intake) and various combinations of the three. Options such as bariatric (weight loss) surgery have remained largely unexplored with the exception of one recent case study (Heinberg and Schauer 2014). This is possibly due to ethical concerns associated with working with people who have disabilities (Spanos et al. 2013), as well as participants displaying certain contraindications for weight loss surgery including eating disorders (Dykens 2000), depression and schizophrenia (Rimmer et al. 2010a).

Behavioral Interventions Spanos et al. (2013) explain in their review that certain behavior change interventions introduced for adults with ID have largely centered on the comprehensive behavioral self-control approach advocated by Rotari and Fox (1981). Behaviorists have attempted to change eating and physical activity patterns in adults with ID through various teaching strategies related to increasing self-awareness and controlling overeating, snacking and physical activity participation through self-monitoring and reinforcement (Fox et al. 1985; McCarron and Andrasik 1990). The aforementioned studies have also incorporated a weight loss maintenance intervention, although just one study produced a statistically significant weight loss (McCarron and Andrasik 1990) with certain participants gaining weight at long-term follow-up (Fox et al. 1985).

Exercise Interventions Increasing physical activity may represent a more viable alternative to behavioral interventions alone, while offering a consistent routine to improve the health of individuals with ID. Regular exercise has been documented to manage levels of body fat in individuals without ID (Gutin 2011; Gutin et al. 2005; Ross and Janssen 2001) with research suggesting that young people who carry out more vigorous physical activity than their peers become leaner over a longer period of time (Moore et al. 2003; Stevens et al. 2007). Certain behavioral interventionists have therefore seen it as advantageous to include an aerobic exercise component in order to successfully induce a weight loss in their participants (Fox et al. 1984; Fisher 1986; Heller et al. 2004).

Interventions focusing solely on exercise training have incorporated many different modes of activity including walking, aquatics, rowing, jogging, dancing as well as circuit and treadmill exercises (Casey and Rasmussen 2013; Maı¨ano et al. 2014; Melville et al. 2005; Spanos et al. 2013). Some of these activities have produced weight loss in various samples with ID including amongst adults (Wu et al. 2010), children (Singh et al. 2008) as well as individuals with Down syndrome (Rimmer et al. 2004a). Certain changes were statistically significant (Elmahgoub et al. 2009; Elmahgoub et al. 2011; Ordonez et al. 2006) while others were maintained at 6-month follow-up (Wu et al. 2010). Researchers have documented positive change in waist circumference (Elmahgoub et al. 2009, 2011) and also BMI (Moss 2009) including amongst individuals with Down syndrome (Rimmer et al. 2004a). Secondary health benefits have also been noted, including improved walking performance, cardio-respiratory fitness, muscle strength, mental health and increased levels of physical activity across various samples (Elmahgoub et al. 2009, 2011; Mendonca and Pereira 2009; Mendonca et al. 2011; Moss 2009; Rimmer et al. 2004a).

It is important to note, however, that significant changes in weight and BMI have not been reported universally across studies adopting an energy expenditure approach (Casey et al. 2010; González-Aguero et al. 2011; Mendonca et al. 2011). In addition, no studies focusing on adults produced a clinical weight loss of greater than 5 % when 10–15 % has been recommended (Spanos et al. 2013). Results with regards to changes in body fat percentage following periods of exercise training also remain far from definitive. A minority of studies have produced statistically significant positive changes in body fat (Ordonez et al. 2006; Wu 2010) and lean mass (Elmahgoub et al. 2009; 2011), but the majority of studies have resulted in no change in samples featuring children, adults as well as individuals with Down syndrome (Casey et al. 2010; Ozmen et al. 2007; Pitetti and Tan 1991; González-Aguero et al. 2011). It is possible that in these studies caloric expenditure did not exceed caloric intake, suggesting that exercisers with ID were unable to strike a successful balance between calories burnt and consumed throughout the different intervention studies.

Nutrition Interventions Individuals with ID may well benefit from more sustained dietary monitoring (Humphries et al. 2009a). However, limited nutrition specific interventions have been conducted in this area (Spanos et al. 2013) and there still remains little evidence of success in pediatric populations with ID. Past interventions have mostly targeted the type and amount of food and drink adults consumed in order to achieve and maintain a hypocaloric energy intake. An early example by Antal et al. (1988) introduced a reduced calorie diet (1000–1100 kcal) to adults with ID who were obese through the use of a 30 day rotating menu in an institutional setting. This resulted in significant weight loss at 9 months in both women and men. Bertoli et al. (2006) offered nutritional counseling and assessments to a small community sample through a medical practitioner and dietician in order to facilitate healthier living. Despite a 65 % dropout rate, this study also led to a significant decrease in weight and BMI in six participants after 1 year. Humphries et al.'s (2009) study sought to change food systems in group homes through the implementation of MENU-AIDDs (Materials Supporting Education and Nutrition for Adults with Intellectual or Developmental Disabilities). Greater menu planning and dietary adequacy was achieved but changes in direct outcomes were not forthcoming.

Multicomponent Interventions Overall, multicomponent interventions that have featured a combination of exercise, diet and/or behavioral elements (Bergstrom et al. 2013; Bradley 2005; Chapman et al. 2005; Chapman, Craven and Chadwick, 2008; Croce, 1990; Hinckson et al. 2013; Melville et al. 2011; Messersmith et al. 2008; Singh et al. 2008) have been somewhat more consistent at achieving primary reduction outcomes than single component interventions (Casey and Rasmussen 2013; Maı"ano et al. 2014; Spanos et al. 2013).

Several studies have adopted healthy lifestyle components for adults and children with ID, that seek to promote health education through various educational techniques and different methods of physical activity (Bergstrom et al. 2013; Bradley 2005; Casey et al. 2012; Chapman et al. 2005; Croce 1990). For example, Hinckson et al. (2013) combined physical activity sessions with health promotion class sessions centered on teaching children with ID about healthy eating in a motivational climate. Similarly, Singh et al. (2008) combined walking with the promotion of food and self-awareness.

Additional studies have included energy deficit diets in their intervention regimen. An early study by Croce (1990) introduced a caloric restriction diet (along with behavioral techniques) to three participants who were obese, requiring 3500 kcal weekly reduction below what is required to maintain body weight in tandem with an exercise program three times per week. Messersmith et al.'s (2008) case study added a low calorie diet (600–800 calories per day) to regular aerobic activities and behavioral reinforcement strategies to an adolescent with Prader–Willi syndrome. Also working with Prader–Willi syndrome, Descheemaeker et al. (1994) adopted a personalized low calorie diet in an intervention also aimed at the development of motor skills and beneficial food intake behavior across different generations. Melville et al.'s (2011) individualized diet plan aimed to facilitate an energy deficit of 600 Kcal (2510 kJ) each day for a targeted weight loss of 0.5 kg–1 kg/week. Similarly, Saunders et al. (2011) introduced a low-calorie diet (1200–1300 kcal per day) that supported the consumption of high volume foods in order to give off the feeling of fullness. The latter two studies both promoted the importance of participation in regular physical activity through educational means.

Findings suggest that multiple component interventions may lead to weight loss (Bradley 2005; Croce 1990; Descheemaeker et al. 1994; Singh et al. 2008) which may be both statistically significant (Chapman 2005, 2008; Melville et al. 2011; Saunders et al. 2011) and retained at long-term follow-up (Chapman 2005, 2008; Singh et al. 2008). According to Spanos et al. (2013), energy deficit interventions that offer opportunities for increased energy expenditure seemingly produce the most weight loss (Melville et al. 2011; Saunders et al. 2011). BMI and, to a lesser degree, body fat (Croce 1990) have also been documented to change following multicomponent interventions (Ewing et al. 2004; Messersmith et al. 2008; Singh et al. 2008; Melville et al. 2011; Saunders et al. 2011).

In terms of secondary outcomes, multicomponent interventions have contributed to increased physical activity (Bergstrom et al. 2013), and cardiovascular fitness (Croce 1990; Messersmith et al. 2008) as well as a reduction in sedentary behavior (Melville et al. 2011), hospital visits and the consumption of unhealthy foods (Hinckson et al. 2013). However, it is evident that not all multicomponent studies have provided a significant decrease in BMI, waist circumference or body fat (Bergstrom et al. 2013; Casey et al. 2012; Ewing et al. 2004; Hinckson et al. 2013). Certain interventions have also increased obsessive compulsive behavior (Descheemaeker et al. 1994) and failed to reduce anxiety amongst youth with Prader–Willi syndrome (Messersmith et al. 2008).

Limitations of Findings

Researchers continue to explore the reasons behind these somewhat inconsistent findings across all intervention studies (Casey and Rasmussen 2013; Maiano et al. 2014; Spanos et al. 2013). Some have emphasized a lack of stringent study design and follow-up (Wu 2010), small heterogeneous sample sizes (Bertoli et al. 2006; Casey et al. 2010, 2012; Messersmith et al. 2008) as well as inconsistent methods of measurement (Ozmen et al. 2008). Spanos et al. (2013) suggest that clinical guidelines recommending exercise training interventions include 225–300 mins of moderate activity per week in order to treat obesity have seldom been met (National Institute for Health and Clinical Excellence 2006). It is also evident that few studies have featured a control group (Bergstrom et al. 2013; Elmahgoub et al. 2009; Mendonca et al. 2011; Rimmer et al. 2004a). Moreover, designs have rarely been replicated, possibly because certain activities, whether related to behavioral techniques, physical activity or exercise, have not been adequately described or have merely provided advice (rather than direct intervention), all of which make replication in the clinical setting extremely challenging (Bradley 2005; Chapman 2005, 2008; Melville et al. 2011) and reduces their potential effectiveness in community settings (Rimmer et al. 2010b).

Recommendations for Clinical Practice

This chapter has reviewed the prevalence, determinants, causes and reduction measures implemented on individuals who have ID in order to promote more effective and sustainable methods to combat the elevated levels of obesity identified in this population. Our review of the literature on obesity and individuals with ID reveals that the following should be taken into consideration when working to try and prevent or manage obesity in individuals with ID:

1. Ensure individuals with ID are included in local, national and international population surveillance data so that practitioners have a more accurate indication of the magnitude of the effects of the obesity epidemic on this population.
2. Adults and pediatric populations across the globe, including many who are experiencing the 'nutrition transition' in developing and low-income countries, are in need of priority (early) intervention. Interventions should target at least a 5–10 % clinically significant weight loss in individuals with ID who are either overweight or obese.
3. Increased efforts required to reduce the high rates of obesity in certain subcategories of ID including women, group home residents and people who have Prader–Willi syndrome or Down syndrome. Each syndrome should be treated as its own disability for the purposes of identification, measurement and management.
4. Practitioners should seek to understand the effects of obesity on related secondary health conditions in populations with ID (e.g., asthma, high blood pressure, high blood cholesterol, type II diabetes mellitus, depression, fatigue, etc.).

5. Careful consideration should be given to the choice of measurement tools used to assess adiposity-based health risk in individuals with ID. In particular, caution should be used when determining whether BMI rather than body composition remains the most reliable gauge of obesity across heterogeneous populations with ID.
6. Alternative field measures such as BIA, skinfold thickness and waist circumference should also be considered on a case-by-case basis especially as skinfold thickness, in particular, has met with a fair degree of noncompliance in past studies.
7. Population specific regression equations are important when using certain anthropometric methods. Until this is achieved, more complex measurement equipment such as DXA and ADP should be prioritized for individuals with ID in order to gain a better understanding as to the effectiveness of reduction measures and the prevalence of obesity.
8. Increasing physical activity levels in populations with ID remains an essential priority as many participate in far less activity than peers without ID. Individuals with ID have demonstrated good trainability in structured interventions across a variety of different activities (e.g., Walking, swimming, treadmill, gym, etc.). Clinical guidelines recommend at least 225–300 min of moderate to vigorous physical activity per week. Blood pressure, heart rate (e.g., Down syndrome) and other potential contraindications to exercise should be monitored especially in instances where individuals are already overweight or obese.
9. Assistance may be required so that individuals with ID may overcome a wide range of personal and environmental barriers for physical activity related to physical health, transportation, resource availability, adapted equipment as well as social and psychological concerns.
10. Practitioners need to take into account the nutritional behavior and/or diet of individuals with ID who have been shown to make poor food choices when unmonitored. Consideration should be given to the fact that there remain few valid and reliable methods to assess dietary intake in this population.
11. Dietary recommendations include the incorporation of a diet with 600–1000 kcal per day deficit or low energy content by reducing fat intake. Educational support and counseling to people with ID as well as family/workers in group settings may be necessary in order to promote a healthier lifestyle especially as individuals with ID are living longer and continue to move away from larger, more restrictive, institutional settings.
12. Overall, a greater emphasis should be placed upon multicomponent interventions. A strong evidence base exists to show that combined behavioral strategies, physical activity and diet may act as a catalyst for decreased obesity (weight, BMI and body composition) in individuals with ID. Energy deficit interventions in tandem with regular physical activity have produced the most weight loss.
13. A single case study shows that bariatric surgery may represent a potential option in critical situations for certain individuals with ID who are extremely obese, especially when other intervention strategies have not worked (e.g.,

noncompliance). However, careful attention should be paid to the presence of contraindications for weight loss surgery including eating disorders and certain forms of mental illness.

14. Further attention should be paid to the effects of reduction measures on obesity-related secondary conditions (e.g., physical, psychological, social and emotional) as well.
15. Interventions should consist of larger and more homogeneous samples or, in special circumstances, should be in the form of a rigorous single-subject design with adequate follow-up based on the heterogeneity that presents itself within the population.

Conclusion

This chapter has emphasized that the obesity epidemic remains an even greater concern for individuals with ID than it does for the general population. This is especially true for adults, women, North Americans, group home and low income residents as well as individuals with ID caused by Down syndrome and Prader–Willi syndrome. Research suggests the health related concerns caused by obesity and extreme obesity are only increasing in populations with ID who are living longer than ever. Most worryingly, rates of physical activity and healthy eating are particularly low which may greatly exacerbate the problem moving forward. Furthermore, the omission of individuals with ID from population survey data and inconsistent methods of measuring adiposity may mean we do not know the true scale of obesity and related health risk in this population especially within the developing world.

Greater efforts are required to prevent and manage high levels of obesity. Reduction measures should center on changes in body composition as well as weight and BMI. It is apparent that methods to date have produced largely inconsistent results, and this limits their potential use in clinical and community settings. Multicomponent interventions show the most promise in terms of decreasing obesity, yet further collaborative interventions are recommended in order to have a better understanding of the roles, behavior, physical activity and diet play in reducing obesity and related secondary health conditions in populations with ID across the world.

References

Adolfsson, P., Sydner, Y. M., Fjellstrom, C., Lewin, B., & Andersson, A. (2008). Observed dietary intake in adults with intellectual disability living in the community. *Journal of Food and Nutrition Research, 52,* 10.

Allerton, L. A., Welch, V., & Emerson, E (2011). Health inequalities experienced by children and young people with intellectual disabilities: A review of literature from the United Kingdom. *Journal of Intellectual Disabilities, 15,* 269–278.

Antal, M., Zajkas, G., Rajhathy, B., Nagy, K., Szanto, E., Thur, M., Dworschák, E., Gergely, A., Bedő, M., & Bíró, G. (1988). Longitudinal examinations in the course of dietotherapy of mentally retarded obese in-patients. Z Ernahrungswiss, *27,* 101–108.

Balic, M. G., Mateos, E. C., Blasco, C. G., & Fernhall, B. (2000). Physical fitness levels of physically active and sedentary adults with Down syndrome. *Adapted Physical Activity Quarterly, 17*(3), 310–321.

Bergström, H., Hagströmer, M., Hagberg, J., & Elinder, L. S. (2013). A multi-component universal intervention to improve diet and physical activity among adults with intellectual disabilities in community residences: A cluster randomised controlled trial. *Research in Developmental Disabilities, 34*(11), 3847–3857.

Bertoli, S., Battezzat, A., Merati, G., Margonato, V., Maggioni, M., Testolin, G., et al. (2006) Nutritional status and dietary patterns in disabled people. *Nutrition Metabolism and Cardiovascular Disease, 16,* 100–112.

Bhaumik, S., Watson, J. M., Thorp, C. F., Tyrer, F., & McGrother, C. W. (2008). Body mass index in adults with intellectual disability: Distribution, associations and service implications: A population-based prevalence study. *Journal of Intellectual Disability Research, 52,* 287–298.

Binkley, J., K., Eales, J., & Jekanowski, M. (2000). The relation between dietary change and rising US obesity. *International Journal of Obesity Related Metabolism Disorders, 24,* 1032–1039.

Biswas, A., B., Vahabzadeh, A., Hobbs, T., & Healy, J. M. (2010). Obesity in people with learning disabilities: Possible causes and reduction interventions. *Nursing Times, 106,* 16–18.

Blackburn, G. L. (2000). Weight gain and antipsychotic medication. *Journal of Clinical Psychiatry,* 61(Suppl.), 36–41.

Bowman, S. A., & Vinyard, B. T. (2004). Fast food consumption of U.S. adults: Impact on energy and nutrient intakes and overweight status. *Journal of American College of Nutrition, 23,* 163–168.

Bradley, S. (2005). Tackling obesity in people with learning disability. *Learning Disability Practice, 7,* 10–14.

Rambillo, P. Bosio, L., Monzoni, P., Pietrobelli A., Beccaria L., & Chiomello L. (1997). Peculiar body composition in patients with Prader-Labhart-Willi syndrome. American Jounral of Clinical Nutrition, 65, 1369–1374.

Braunschweig, C., Gomez, S., Sheean, P., Tomey, K., Rimmer, J., & Heller, T. (2004). Nutritional status and risk factors for chronic disease in urban-dwelling adults with Down syndrome. *American Journal of Mental Retardation, 109,* 186–193.

Bryan, F., Allan, T., & Russell, L. (2000). The move from a long-stay learning disabilities hospital to community homes: A comparison of clients' nutritional status. *Journal of Human Nutrition and Dietetics, 13,* 265–270.

Casey, A. F. (2013). Measuring body composition in individuals with intellectual disability: A scoping review. *Journal of Obesity.* doi:10.1155/2013/628428.

Casey, A. F., & Rasmussen, R. (2013). Reduction measures and percent body fat in individuals with intellectual disabilities: A scoping review. *Disability and Health Journal, 6*(1), 2–7.

Casey, A. F., Rasmussen, R., MacKenzie, S., & Glenn, J. (2010). Dual-energy X-ray absorptiometry to measure the influence of a sixteen-week community-based swim training program on body fat in children and adolescents with intellectual disabilities. *Archives of Physical Medicine and Rehab, 91*(7), 1064–1069.

Casey, A. F., Boyd, J., Mackenzie, S., & Rasmussen, R. (2012). Dual-energy X-ray absorptiometry to measure the effects of a 13-week aquatic exercise and diet intervention on body fat in adults with intellectual disability from group home settings. *Journal of Human Kinetics, 32,* 221–229.

Centers for Disease Control and Prevention. (2008). *Youth risk behavior surveillance—United States, 2007. Morbidity and mortality weekly report 57* (S. 4). Atlanta: Centers for Disease Control and Prevention.

Chapman, M. J., Craven, M. J., & Chadwick, D. D. (2005). Fighting fit? An evaluation of health practitioner input to improve healthy living and reduce obesity for adults with learning disabilities. *Journal of Intellectual Disabilities, 9,* 131–144.

Chapman, M. J., Craven, M. J., & Chadwick, D. D. (2008). Following up fighting fit: The long term impact of health practitioner input on obesity and BMI amongst adults with intellectual disabilities. *Journal of Intellectual Disabilities, 12,* 309–323.

Cohen, S., Glazewski, R., Khan, S., & Khan, A. (2001). Weight gain with resperidone among patients with mental retardation: Effects of calorie restriction. *Journal of Clinical Psychiatry, 62,* 114–116.

Croce, R. V. (1990). Effects of exercise and diet on body composition and cardiovascular fitness in adults with severe mental retardation. *Education and Training in Mental Retardation, 25,* 176–187.

Daniels, S. R. (2006). The consequences of childhood overweight and obesity. *The Future of Children, 16,* 47–67.

Daniels, S. R., Arnett, D., Eckel, R. H., Gidding, S. S., Hayman, L. L., Kumanyika, S., et al. (2005). Overweight in children and adolescents. Pathophysiology, consequences, prevention, and treatment. *Circulation, 111,* 1999–2012.

De Winter, C. F., Bastiaanse, L. P., Hilgenkamp, T. I. M., Evenhuis, H. M., & Echteld, M. A. (2012). Overweight and obesity in older people with intellectual disability. *Research in Developmental Disabilities, 33,* 398–405.

Descheemaeker, M. J., Swillen, A., Plissart, L., Borghgraef, M., Rasenberg, S., Curfs, L. M. G., & Fryns, J. P. (1994). The Prader-Willi syndrome: A self supporting program for children, youngsters and adults. *Genetic Counseling, 5,* 199–205.

Deurenberg, P. (1995). Limitations of the bioelectrical impedance method for the assessment of body fat in severe obesity. *American Journal of Clinical Nutrition, 64*(3), 449–452.

Draheim, C. C. (2006). Cardiovascular disease prevalence and risk factors of persons with mental retardation. *Mental Retardation and Developmental Disabilities Research Reviews, 12,* 3–12.

Draheim, C. C., McCubbin, J. A., & Williams, D. P. (2002). Differences in cardiovascular disease risk between nondiabetic adults with mental retardation with and without Down syndrome. *American Journal of Mental Retardation, 107,* 201–211.

Draheim, C. C., Williams, D. P., & McCubbin, J. A. (2002a). Prevalence of physical inactivity and recommended physical activity in community-based adults with mental retardation. *Mental Retardation, 40,* 436–444.

Draheim, C. C., Williams, D. P., & McCubbin, J. A. (2003). Cardiovascular disease risk factor differences between special Olympians and non-special Olympians. *Adapted Physical Activity Quarterly, 20,* 118–133.

Draheim, C. C., Stanish, H. I., Williams, D. P., & McCubbin, J. A. (2007). Dietary intake of adults with mental retardation who reside in community settings. *American Journal of Mental Retardation, 112,* 392–400.

Dudley, O., McManus, B., Vogels, A., Whittington, J., & Muscatelli, F. (2008). Cross-cultural comparisons of obesity and growth in Prader-Willi syndrome. *Journal of Intellectual Disability Research, 52,* 426–436.

Dykens, E. M. (2000). Contaminated and unusual food combinations: What do people with Prader-Willi syndrome choose? *Mental Retardation, 38,* 163–171.

Eckel, R. H. (1997). Obesity and heart disease: A statement for healthcare professionals from the Nutrition Committee, American Health Association. *Circulation, 96,* 3248–3250.

Eisenkolbl, J., Kartasurya, M., & Widhalm, K. (2001). Under-estimation of percentage fat mass measured by bioelectrical impedance analysis compared to the dual-energy X-ray absorpiometry in obese children. *European Journal of Clinical Nutrition, 55,* 423–429.

Elmahgoub, S. M., Lambers, S., Stegen, S., Van Laethem, C., Cambier, D., Calders, P. (2009). The influence of combined exercise training on indices of obesity, physical fitness and lipid profile in overweight and obese adolescents with mental retardation. *European Journal of Pediatrics, 168*(11), 1327–1333.

Elmahgoub, S., Calders, P., Lambers, S., Stegen, S. M., Van Laethem, C., Cambier, D.C. (2011). The effect of combined exercise training in adolescents who are overweight or obese with intellectual disability: the role of training frequency. *Journal of Strength Conditioning Research, 25*(8), 2274–2282.

Emerson, E. (2005). Underweight, obesity and exercise among adults with intellectual disabilities in supported accommodation in Northern England. *Journal of Intellectual Disability Research, 49,* 134–143.

Emerson, E., & Robertson, J. (2010). Obesity in young children with intellectual disabilities or borderline intellectual functioning. *International Journal of Pediatric Obesity, 5,* 320–326.

Ewing, G., McDermott, S., Thomas-Koger, m., Whitney, W., & Pierce, K. (2004). Evaluation of a cardiovascular health program for participants with mental retardation. Health Education and Behaviour, 31, 77–87.

Ezzati, M., Lopez, A. D., Rodgers, A., Vander Hoorn, S., & Murray, C. J. (2002). Selected major risk factors and global and regional burden of disease. *Lancet, 360,* 1347–1360.

Fegan, P. (2009). Intellectual disabilities. In J. L. Durstine, G. E. Moore, P. L. Painter, & S. O. Roberts (Eds.), *American college of sports medicine exercise management for persons with chronic diseases and disabilities* (2nd ed., pp. 359–367). Champaign: Human Kinetics.

Fernhall, B., & Pitetti, K. (2001). Limitations to physical work capacity in individuals with mental retardation. *Clinical Exercise Physiology, 3,* 176–185.

Finucane, M. M., Stevens, G. A., Cowan, M. J., Danaei, G., Lin, J. K., & Paciorek, C. J., et al. (2011). National, regional, and global trends in body-mass index since 1980: Systematic analysis of health examination surveys and epidemiological studies with 960 country-years and 9.1 million participants. *Lancet, 377,* 557–567.

Fisher, E. (1986). Behavioral weight reduction program for mentally retarded adult females. *Perceptual Motor Skills, 62,* 359–362.

Flegal, K. M., Carroll, M. D., & Ogden, C. L., et al. (2002). Prevalence and trends in obesity among US adults 1999–2000. *Journal of American Medical Association, 288,* 1723–1727.

Foley, J. T., Lloyd, M., & Temple, V. A. (2013). Body mass index trends among adult U.S. Special Olympians, 2005–2010. *Adapted Physical Activity Quarterly, 30,* 373–386.

Foley, J. T., Lloyd, M., Vogel, D., & Temple, V. A. (2014). Obesity trends of 8–18 year old Special Olympians: 2005–2010. *Research in Developmental Disabilities, 35,* 705–710.

Fonseca, C. T., Amaral, D. M., Ribeiro, M. G., Beserra, I. C. R., & Guimaraes, M. G. (2005). Insulin resistance in adolescents with Down syndrome: A cross-sectional study. *BMC Endochrin Disorders, 5*(6), 1–6.

Fox, R. A., Haniotes, H., & Rotatori, A. (1984). A streamlined weight loss program for moderately retarded adults in a sheltered workshop setting. *Applied Research in Mental Retardation, 5,* 69–79.

Fox, R. A., Rosenberg, R., & Rotatori, A. F. (1985). Parent involvement in a treatment program for obese retarded adults. *Journal of Behavioural Therapy and Experimental Psychiatry, 16,* 45–48.

Frey, B., & Rimmer, J. H. (1995). Comparison of body composition between German and American adults with mental retardation. *Medicine and Science in Sports and Exercise, 27,* 1439–1443.

Frey, G. C., Buchanan, A. M., & Rosser Sandt, D. D. (2005). I'd rather watch TV: An examination of physical activity in adults with mental retardation. *Mental Retardation, 43,* 241–254.

Frey, G. C., Stanish, H. I., & Temple, V. A. (2008). Physical activity of youth with intellectual disability: Review and research agenda. *Adapted Physical Activity Quarterly, 25*(2), 95–117.

Fujiura, G. T., & Yamaki, K. (1997). Analysis of ethnic variations in developmental disability prevalence and household economic status. *Mental Retardation, 35,* 286–294.

Gabre, P., Martinsson, T., & Gahnberg, L. (2002). Move of adults with intellectual disability from institutions to community-based living: Changes of food arrangements and oral health. *Swedish Dental Journal, 26,* 81–88.

Golden, E., & Hatcher, J. (1997). Nutrition knowledge and obesity of adults in community residences. *Mental Retardation, 35,* 177–184.

Gonzalez-Aguero, A.G., Vicente-Rodriguez, I., Ara, L.A., Moreno, J.A., & Casajus, JA. (2011). Accuracy of prediction equations to assess percentage of body fat in children and adolescents with Down syndrome compared to air displacement plethysmography. *Research in Developmental Disabilities, 32,* 1764–1769.

Graham, A., & Reid, G. (2000). Physical fitness of adults with an intellectual disability: A 13-year follow-up study. *Research Quarterly for Exercise and Sport, 71*(2), 152–161.

Guijarro, M., Valero, C., Paule, B., Gonzalez-Macias, J., & Riancho, J. A. (2007). Bone mass in young adults with Down syndrome. *Journal of Intellectual Disability Research, 52*(3), 182–189.

Gutin, B. (2011). Diet vs exercise for the prevention of pediatric obesity: The role of exercise. *International Journal of Obesity, 35,* 29–32.

Gutin, B., Yin, Z., Humphries, M. C., & Barbeau, P. (2005). Relations of moderate and vigorous physical activity to fitness and fatness in adolescents. *American Journal of Clinical Nutrition, 81*(4), 746–750.

Hames, K. C., Anthony, S. J., Thornton, J. C., Gallagher, D., & Goodpaster, B. H. (2014). Body composition analysis by air displacement plethysmography in normal weight to extremely obese adults. *Obesity, 22,* 1078–1084. doi:10.1002/oby.20655.

Hamilton, S., Hankey, C. A., Miller, S., Boyle, S., & Melville, C. A. (2007). A review of weight loss interventions for adults with intellectual disabilities. *Obesity Review, 8,* 339–345.

Harris, N., Rosenberg, A., Jangda, S., O'Brien, K., & Gallagher, M. L. (2003). Prevalence of obesity in International Special Olympic athletes as determined by body mass index. *Journal of the American Dietetic Association, 103,* 235–237.

Haslam, D. W., & James, W. P. (2005). Obesity. *Lancet, 366,* 1197–1209.

Haslam, D., Sattar, N., & Lean, M. (2005). ABC of obesity. Obesity-time to wake up. *British Medical Journal, 33,* 640–642.

Havecamp, S., Scandlin, D., & Roth, M. (2003). Health disparities among adults with developmental disabilities, adults with other disabilities, and adults not reporting disability in North Carolina. *Public Health Reports, 119,* 418–426.

Heinberg, L. J., & Schauer, P. R. (2014). Intellectual disability and bariatric surgery: A case study on optimization and outcome. Surgery for Obesity and Related Diseases . Official Journal of the American Society for Bariatric Surgery, 1–4. doi:10.1016/j.soard.2014.01.014

Heller, T., Hsieh, K., & Rimmer, J. H. (2004). Attitudinal and psychosocial outcomes of a fitness and health education programme on adults with Down syndrome. *American Journal of Mental Retardation, 109,* 175–185.

Heller, T., McCubbin, J. A., Drum, C., & Peterson, J. (2011). Physical activity and nutrition health promotion interventions: what is working for people with intellectual disabilities? *Intellectual and Developmental Disabilities, 49,* 26–36.

Hellings, J. A., Zarcone, J. R., Crandall, K., Wallace, D., & Schroeder, S. R. (2001). Weight gain in a controlled study of resperidone in children, adolescents, and adults with mental retardation and autism. *Journal of Child and Adolescent Psychopharmacology, 11,* 229–238.

Heymsfield, S. B., Lohman, T. G., Wang, Z., & Going, S. B. (2005). *Human body composition.* Champaign: Human Kinetics Ltd.

Heyward, V. H., & Stolarczyk, L. M. (1996). *Applied body composition assessment.* Champaign: Human Kinetics.

Hinckson, E. A., Dickinson, A., Water, T., Sands, M., & Penman, L. (2013). Physical activity, dietary habits and overall health in overweight and obese children and youth with intellectual disability or autism. *Research in Developmental Disabilities, 34,* 1170–1178.

Holland, A. J., Treasure, J., Coskeran, P., & Dallow, J. (1995). Characteristics of the eating disorder in Prader-Willi syndrome: Implications for treatment. *Journal of Intellectual Disability Research, 39,* 373–381.

Hove, O. (2004). Prevalence of eating disorders in adults with mental retardation living in the community. *American Journal on Mental Retardation, 109,* 501–506.

Hughes, A. R., Farewell, K., Harrid, D., & Reilly, J. J. (2007). Quality of life in a clinical sample of obese children. International Journal of Obesity, 31, 39–44.

Humphries, K., Traci, M. A., & Seekins, T. (2004). A preliminary assessment of the nutrition food-system environment of adults with intellectual disabilities living in supported arrangements in the community. *Ecology of Food and Nutrition, 43,* 517–532.

Humphries, K., Traci, M., & Seekins, T. (2008). Food on film: Pilot test of an innovative method for recording food intake of adults with intellectual disabilities living in the community. *Journal of Applied Research in Intellectual Disabilities, 21,* 168–173.

Humphries, K., Pepper, A., Traci, M., Olson, J., & Seekins, T. (2009a). Nutrition intervention improves menu adequacy in group homes for adults with intellectual or developmental dis abilities developmental disabilities residing in group homes: MENU-AIDDs. *Disability and Health Journal, 2*(3), 136–144.

Humphries, K., Traci, M. A., & Seekins, T. (2009b). Nutrition and adults with intellectual or developmental disabilities: Systematic literature review results. *Intellectual and Developmental Disabilities, 47*(3), 163–185.

James, W. P. T., Rigby, N., & Leach, R. (2004). The obesity epidemic, metabolic syndrome and future prevention strategies. *European Journal of Cardiovascular Prevention and Rehabilitation, 11,* 3–8.

Janssen, I., Katzmarzyk, P. T., Boyce, W. F., Vereecken, C., Mulvihill, C., Roberts, C., et al. (2005). Comparison of overweight and obesity prevalence in school-aged youth from 34 countries and their relationships with physical activity and dietary patterns. *Obesity Reviews, 6,* 123–132.

Jones, G., & Sinclair, L. B. (2008). Multiple health disparities among minority adults with mobility limitations: An application of the ICF framework and codes. *Disability and Rehabilitation, 30,* 901–915.

Kelly, L. E., & Rimmer, J. H. (1987). A practical method for estimating percent body fat of adult mentally retarded males. *Adapted Physical Activity Quarterly, 4,* 117–125.

Koplan, J. P., Liverman, C. T., & Kraak, V. I. (2005). Preventing childhood obesity: Health in the balance: Executive summary. *Journal of the American Dietetic Association, 105,* 131–138.

Lazzer, S., Bedogni, G., Agosti, F., De Col, A., Mornati, D., & Sartorio, A. (2008). Comparison of dual-energy x-ray absorpiometry, air displacement plethysmography and bioelectrical impedance analysis for the assessment of body composition in severely obese Caucasian children and adolescents. *British Journal of Nutrition, 100,* 918–924.

Lewis, M. A., Lewis, C. E., & Leake, B., et al. (2002). The quality of health care for adults with developmental disabilities. *Public Health Reports, 117,* 174–184.

Liusuwan, A., Widman, L., Abresch, R. T., & McDonald, C. M. (2004). Altering body composition affects resting energy expenditure and interpretation of body mass index in children with spinal cord injury. *Journal of Spinal Cord Medicine, 27,* 24–28.

Lloyd, M., Temple, V. A., & Foley, J. T. (2012). International BMI comparison of children and youth with intellectual disabilities participating in Special Olympics. *Research in Developmental Disabilities, 33*(6), 1708–1714.

Lopes, T. de S., Ferreira, D. M., Pereira, R. A., Veiga, G.V. da., & Marins, V. M. R. de. (2008). Assessment of anthropometric indexes of children and adolescents with Down syndrome. *Jornal de Pediatria, 84*(4), 350–356. Accessed 28 April 2014. http://www.scielo.br/scielo.php?script=sci_arttext&pid=S002175572008000400011&lng=en&tlng=en.

Magge, S. N., O'Neill, K. L., Shults, J., Stallings, V. A., & Stettler, N. S. (2008). Leptin levels among prepubertal children with Down syndrome compared to their siblings. *Journal of Pediatrics, 152*(3), 321–326.

Maı"ano, C. (2011). Prevalence and risk factors of overweight and obesity among children and adolescents with intellectual disabilities. *Obesity Reviews, 12*(3), 189–197.

Mai ano, C., Normand, C. L., Aime, A., & Begarie, J. (2014). Lifestyle interventions targeting changes in body weight and composition among youth with an intellectual disability: A systematic review. Research in Developmental Disabilities, 35, 1914–1926.

Marge, M. (1988). Health promotion for persons with disabilities: Moving beyond rehabilitation. *American Journal of Health Promotion, 2,* 29–44.

McCarran, M. S., & Andrasik, F. (1990). Behavioral weight-loss for multiply handicapped adults: Assessing caretaker involvement and measures of behavior change. *Addictive Behaviour, 15,* 13–20.

Melville, C. A., Cooper, S. A., McGrother, C. W., Thorp, C. F., & Collacott, R. (2005). Obesity in adults with Down syndrome: A case control study. *Journal of Intellectual Disability Research, 49,* 125–133.

Melville, C. A., Boyle, S., Miller, S., Macmillan, S., Penpraze, V., Pert, C., Spanos, D., Mathews, L., Robinson, N., Murray, H., & Hankey, C. R. (2011). An open study of the effectiveness of a multi-component weight-loss intervention for adults with intellectual disabilities and obesity. *British Journal of Nutrition, 105,* 1553–1562.

Mendonca, G. V., & Pereira, F. D. (2009). Influence of long-term exercise training on submaximal and peak aerobic capacity and locomotor economy in adult males with Down's syndrome. *Medicine and Science Monitor, 15*(2), CR33–CR39.

Mendonca, G. V., Pereira, F. D., & Fernhall, B. (2011). Effects of combined aerobic and resistance exercise training in adults with and without Down syndrome. *Archives of Physical Medicine and Rehabilitation, 92,* 37–45.

Menear, K. S. (2007). Parents perceptions of health and physical activity needs of children with Down syndrome. *Down syndrome Research and Practice, 12*(1), 60–68.

Merriman, S., Haw, C., Kirk, J., & Stubbs, J. (2005). Risk factors for coronary heart disease among inpatients who have mild intellectual disability and mental illness. *Journal of Intellectual Disability Research, 49,* 309–316.

Messersmith, N. V., Slifer, K. J., Gómez-Cabello, A., Pulbrook-Vetter, V., & Bellipanni, K. (2008). Interdisciplinary behavioral intervention for life-threatening obesity in an adolescent with Prader-Willi syndrome—A case report. *Journal of Developmental & Behavioral Pediatrics, 29,* 129–134.

Molteno, C., Smit, I., Mills, J., & Huskisson, J. (2000). Nutritional status of patients in a long-stay hospital for people with mental handicap. *South African Journal of Clinical Nutrition, 13,* 145–149.

Moore, L., DiGao, A., Bradlee, M., Cupples, L., Sundarajan-Ramamurti, A., & Proctor, M., et al. (2003). Does early physical activity predict body fat change throughout childhood? *Preventive Medicine, 37,* 10–17.

Moran, R., Drane, W., McDermott, S., Dasari, S., Scurry, J. B., & Platt, T. (2005). Obesity among people with and without mental retardation across adulthood. *Obesity Research, 13,* 342–349.

Moss, S. J. (2009). Changes in coronary heart disease risk profile of adults with intellectual disabilities following a physical activity intervention. *Journal of Intellectual Disability Research, 53,* 735–744.

National Institute for Health and Clinical Excellence. (2006). *Obesity: The prevention, identification, assessment and management of overweight and obesity in adults and children.* London: NICE.

Ogden, C. L., Carroll, M. D., Curtin, L. R., Lamb, M. M., & Flegal, K. M. (2010). Prevalence of high body mass index in US children and adolescents, 2007–2008. *Journal of the American Medical Association, 303*(3), 242–249.

Ogden, C. L., Carroll, M. D., Kit, B. K., & Flegal, K. M. (2012). Prevalence of obesity and trends in body mass index among US children and adolescents, 1999–2010. *Journal of the American Medical Association, 307*(5), 483–490.

Ordoñez, R. J., Rosety, M., & Rosety-Rodriquez, M. (2006). Influence of 12-week exercise training on fat mass percentage in adolescents with Down syndrome. *Medicine and Science Monitor, 12*(10), 416–419.

Ozmen, T., Yildirim, N. U., Yuktasir, B., & Beets, M. W. (2007). Effects of school-based cardiovascular-fitness training in children with mental retardation. *Pediatric Exercise Science, 19,* 171–178.

Pain, H., & Wiles, R. (2006). The experience of being disabled and obese. *Disability and Rehabilitation, 28*(19), 1211–1220.

Pitetti, K. H., & Tan, D. M. (1991). Effects of a minimally supervised exercise program for mentally retarded adults. *Medicine and Science in Sports and Exercise, 23*(5), 594–601.

Popkin, B. M. (2002). Part II. What is unique about the experience in lower-and middle-income less industrialised countries compared with the very-high income industrialised countries? *Public Health Nutrition, 5,* 205–214.

Popkin, B. M., Adair, L. S., & Ng, S. W. (2012). Global nutrition transition and the pandemic of obesity in developing countries. *Nutrition Reviews, 70,* 3–21.

Prentice, A. M. (2006). The emerging epidemic of obesity in developing countries. *International Journal of Epidemiology, 35,* 93–99.

Prior, B. M., Cureton, K. J., Modlesky, C. M., Evans, E. M., Sloniger, M. A., & Saunders, M., et al. (1997). In vivo validation of whole body composition estimates from dual-energy X-ray absorptiometry. *Journal of Applied Physiology, 83*(2), 623–630.

Prouty, R. W., & Lakin, K. C. (2006). *Residential services for persons with developmental disabilities: Status and trends through 2005.* Minneapolis: University of Minnesota Research and Training Center on Community Living.

Rieken, R., Goudoever, J. V. B., Schierbeek, H., Willemsen, W. P., Calis, W. C. A., Tibboel, D., Evenhuis, H. M., & Penning, C. (2011). Measuring body composition and energy expenditure in children with severe neurologic impairment and intellectual disability. *American Journal of Clinical Nutrition, 94,* 759–766.

Rimmer, J. H. (1999). Health promotion for people with disabilities: The emerging paradigm shift from disability prevention to prevention of secondary conditions. *Physical Therapy, 79,* 495–502.

Rimmer, J. H. (2005). The conspicuous absence of people with disabilities in public fitness and recreation facilities: Lack of interest or lack of access? *American Journal of Health Promotion, 19,* 327–329.

Rimmer, J. H., & Marques, A. C. (2012). Physical activity for people with disabilities. *Lancet, 380,* 193–195.

Rimmer, J. H., & Wang, E. (2005). Obesity prevalence among a group of Chicago residents with disabilities. *Archives of Physical Medicine and Rehabilitation, 86,* 1461–1464.

Rimmer, J. H., & Yamaki, K. (2006). Obesity and intellectual disability. *Mental Retardation and Developmental Disabilities Research Reviews, 12*(1), 22–27.

Rimmer, J. H., Kelly, L. E., & Rosentswieg, J. (1987). Accuracy of anthropometric equations for estimating body composition of mentally retarded adults. *American Journal of Mental Deficiencies, 91,* 626–632.

Rimmer, J. H., Braddock, D., & Fujiura, G. (1993). Prevalence of obesity in adults with mental retardation: Implications for health promotions and disease prevention. *Mental Retard, 31,* 105–110.

Rimmer, J. H., Heller, T., Wang, E., & Valerio, I. (2004a). Improvements in physical fitness in adults with Down syndrome. *American Journal of Mental Retardation, 109*(2), 165–174.

Rimmer, J. H., Riley, B., Wang, E., Rauworth, A., & Jurkowski, J. (2004b). Physical activity participation among persons with disabilities: Barriers and facilitators. *American Journal of Preventive Medicine, 26,* 419–425.

Rimmer, J., Yamaki, K., Davis, B., Lowry, B. M., Wang, E., & Vogel, L. C. (2010a). Obesity and obesity-related secondary conditions in adolescents with intellectual/developmental disabilities. *Journal of Intellectual Disability Research, 45,* 787–794.

Rimmer, J. H., Chen, M. D., McCubbin, J. A., Drum, C., & Peterson, J. (2010b). Exercise intervention research on persons with disabilities: What we know and where we need to go. *American Journal of Physical Medicine and Rehabilitation, 89,* 249–263.

Rimmer, J. H., Wang, E., Yamaki, K., & Davis, B. (2010c). *Documenting disparities in obesity and disability. FOCUS Technical Brief.* Austin: SEDL.

Rimmer, J. H., De-Chen, M., & Hsieh, K. (2011). A conceptual model for identifying, preventing and managing secondary conditions in people with disabilities. *Physical Therapy Journal, 91,* 1728–1739.

Rimmer, J., Schiller, W., & Chen, M.-D. (2012). Effects of disability-associated low energy expenditure deconditioning syndrome. *Exercise and Sport Scientific Review, 40,* 22–29.

Robertson, J., Emerson, E., Gregary, N., Hatton, C., Rutner, S., Kessissoglou, S., & Hallam, A. (2000). Lifestyle related risk factors for poor health in residential settings for people with intellectual disabilities. *Research in Developmental Disabilities, 21,* 469–486.

Ross, R., & Janssen, I. (2001). Physical activity, total and regional obesity: Dose-response considerations. *Medicine and Science in Sports and Exercise, 33*(6), 521–527.

Rotatori, A. F., & Fox, R. (1981). *Behavioral weight reduction program for mentally handicapped persons: A self-control approach.* Baltimore: University Park Press.

Rubin, S., Rimmer, J., Chicoine, B., Braddock, D., & McGuire, D. (1998). Overweight prevalence in persons with Down syndrome. *Mental Retardation, 36,* 175–181.

Saunders, R. R., Saunders, M. D., Donnelly, J. E., Smith, B. K., Sullivan, D. K., Guilford, B., & Rondon, M. F. (2011). Evaluation of an approach to weight loss in adults with intellectual or developmental disabilities. *Intellectual and Developmental Disabilities, 49,* 103–112.

Schutz, Y., Kyle, U. U., & Pichard, C. (2006). Fat-free mass index and fat mass index percentiles in Caucasians aged 18-98 years. *International Journal of Obesity Related Metabolism Disorders, 26,* 953–960.

Seekins, T., Traci, M., Bainbridge, D., & Humphries, K. (2005). Secondary conditions risk appraisal for adults. In W. Nehring (Ed.), *Health promotion for persons with intellectual and developmental disabilities: The state of scientific evidence* (pp. 325–342). Washington, DC: American Association on Mental Retardation.

Shields, N., Dodd, K. J., & Ablitt, C. (2009). Do children with Down syndrome perform sufficient physical activity to maintain good health? A pilot study. *Adapted Physical Activity Quarterly, 26,* 307–320. http://journals.humankinetics.com/apaq.

Singh, N. N., Lancioni, G. E., Singh, A. N., Winton, A. S. W., Singh, J., McAleavey, K. M., & Adkins, A. D. (2008). A mindfulness-based health wellness program for an adolescent with Prader-Willi syndrome. *Behavior Modification, 32,* 167–181.

Slaughter, M. H., Lohman, T. G., & Boileau, R. A., et al. (1988). Skinfold equations for estimations of body fatness in children and youth. *Human Biology, 60*(5), 709–723.

Sohler, N., Lubetkin, E., Levy, J., Soghomonian, C., & Rimmerman, A. (2009). Factors associated with obesity and coronary heart disease in people with intellectual disabilities. *Social Work in Health Care, 48*(1), 76–89.

Spanos, D., Melville, C. A., & Hankey, C. R. (2013). Weight management interventions in adults with intellectual disabilities and obesity: A systematic review of the evidence. *Nutrition Journal, 12,* 132.

Spitalnik, D. M., & White-Scott, S. (2001). Access to health services: Improving the availability and quality of health services for people with mild cognitive limitations. In A.J. Tymchuk, K.C. Lakin, & R. Luckasson (Eds.), The forgotten generation: The status and challenges of adults with mild cognitive limitations. Baltimore: Brookes.

Stancliffe, R. J., Lakin, K. C., Larson, S., Engler, J., Bershadsky, J., & Taub, S., et al. (2011). Overweight and obesity among adults with intellectual disabilities who use intellectual disability/developmental disability services in 20 U.S. States. *American Journal on Intellectual and Developmental Disabilities, 116,* 401–418.

Stanish, H., Temple, V., & Frey, G. (2006). Health-promoting physical activity of adults with mental retardation. *Mental Retardation and Developmental Disabilities Research Review, 12,* 13–21.

Starr, J. M., & Mardsen, L. (2008). Characterisation of user-defined health status in older adults with intellectual disabilities. *Journal of Intellectual Disability Research, 52*(6), 483–489.

Stedman, K. V., & Leland, L. S. (2010). Obesity and intellectual disability in New Zealand. *Journal of Intellectual and Developmental Disability, 35*(2), 112–115.

Stevens, S., Murray, D., Baggett, C., Murray, D., Baggett, C., Elder, J., et al. (2007). Objectively assessed associations between physical activity and body composition in middle-school girls. The trial of activity for adolescent girls. *American Journal of Epidemiology, 166,* 1298–1305.

Stewart, L., Van de Ven, L., Katsarou, V., Rentziou, E., Doran, M., & Jackson, P., et al. (2009). High prevalence of obesity in ambulatory children and adolescents with intellectual disability. *Journal of Intellectual Disability Research, 53*(10), 882–886.

Sung, R. Y. T., Sung, Lau, P., Lam, P. K. W., & Nelson, E. A. S. (2001). Measurement of body fat using leg to leg impedance. *Archives of Disease in Childhood, 85,* 263–267.

Swinburn, B., & Egger, G. (2002). Preventive strategies against weight gain and obesity. *Obesity Reviews, 3,* 289–301.

Takeuchi, E. (1994). Incidence of obesity among school children with mental retardation in Japan. *American Journal of Mental Retardation, 99*(3), 283–288.

Telama, R., Yang, X., Viikari, J., Valimaki, I., Wanne, O., & Raitakari, O. (2005). Physical activity from childhood to adulthood: A 21-year tracking study. *American Journal of Preventive Medicine, 28,* 267–273.

Temple, V. A., & Walkley, J. (2003). Living arrangements and training influences on participation in physical activity among intellectually disabled adults. *Medicine and Science in Sports and Exercise, 35,* 66.

Temple, V. A., Walkley, J. W., & Greenway, K. (2010). Body mass index as an indicator of adiposity among adults with intellectual disability. *Journal of Intellectual & Developmental Disability, 35,* 116–120.

Temple, V. A., Foley, J. T., & Lloyd, M. (2014). Body mass index of adults with intellectual disability participating in Special Olympics by world region. *Journal of Intellectual Disability Research, 57,* 277–284.

Traci, M., Geurts, S., Seekins, T., Burke, R., Humphries, K., & Brennan, L. (2001). *Health status of adult Montanans in supported and semi-independent living arrangements: Overall summary of the secondary conditions surveillance report.* Missoula: University of Montana Rural Institute.

Turk, M. (2006). Secondary conditions and disability. In M. J. Field, A. M. Jette, & L. Martin (Eds.), *Based on a workshop of the committee on disability in America: A new look* (pp. 185–193). Washington, DC: The National Academies Press.

United States Department of Health and Human Services. (2000). *Healthy people 2010.* Washington, DC: U.S. Government Printing Office.

Usera, P. C., Foley, J. T., & Yun, J. (2005). Cross-validation of field based assessments of body composition for individuals with Down syndrome. *Adapted Physical Activity Quarterly, 22*(2), 198.

Van de Vliet, P., Rintala, P., Frojd, K., Verellen, J., Van Houtte, S., Daly, D. J., & Vanlandewijck, Y. C. (2006). Physical fitness profile of elite athletes with intellectual disability. *Scandinavian Journal of Medicine and Science in Sports, 16,* 417–425.

van Schrojenstein Lantman-de Valk, H., Linehan, C., Kerr, M., & Noonan-Walsh, P. (2007). Developing health indicators for people with intellectual disabilities. The method of the Pomona project. *Journal of Intellectual Disability Research, 51*(6), 427–434.

Verstraelen, C. J. F., Maaskant, M. A., Van Kniijff- Raeven, A. G. M., Curfs, L. M. G., Van Schrojenstein Lantman-de Valk, H. M. J (2009). Weighting the weights: Agreement among Anthropometric indicators identifying the weight status of people with intellectual disabilities. *Journal of Applied Research in Intellectual Disability, 22,* 307–313.

Waninge, A., van der Weide, W, Evenhuis, I. J., van Wijck, R., & van der Schans, C. P. (2009). Feasibility and reliability of body composition measurements in adults with severe intellectual and sensory disabilities. *Journal of Intellectual Disability Research, 53,* 377–388.

Warner, J. T., Cowan, F. J., Dunstan, F. D. J., & Gregory, J. D. (1997). The validity of body mass index for the assessment of adiposity in children with disease states. *Annals of Human Biology, 24*(3), 209–215.

Whitt-Glover, M. C., O'Neill, K. L., & Stettler, N. (2006). Physical activity patterns in children with and without Down syndrome. *Pediatric Rehabilitation, 9*(2), 158–164.

Williams, D. P., Going, S. B., & Lohman, T. G., et al. (1992). Body fatness and risk for elevated blood pressure, total cholesterol, and serum lipoprotein ratios in children and adolescents. *American Journal of Public Health, 82,* 358–363.

World Health Organization (1995). The use and interpretation of anthropomtry. WHO, Geneva.

Wu, C. L., Lin, J. D., Hu, J., Yen, C. F., Yen, C. T., Chou, Y. L., & Wu, P. H. (2010). The effectiveness of healthy physical fitness programs on people with intellectual disabilities living in a disability institution: Six-month short-term effect. *Research in Developmental Disabilities, 31,* 713–717.

Yamaki, K. (2005). Body weight status among adults with intellectual disability in the community. *Mental Retardation, 43,* 1–10.

Yamaki, K., & Fujiura, G. T. (2002). Employment and income status of adults with developmental disability disabilities living in the community. *Mental Retardation, 40,* 132–141.

Chapter 10
Pain

Meir Lotan and Joav Merrick

Introduction

Pain

Pain is defined by the International Association for the Study of Pain (IASP) as "an unpleasant sensory or emotional experience associated with actual or potential tissue damage or described in terms of such damage" (Latham and Davis 1994). Pain can have a negative effect on the individual's functional ability, mobility, emotional status, ability to work, interpersonal relationships, and social activities, leading to increased use of health care services and an accompanying increase in health care costs (Merskey and Bogduk 1992). Unequal access to pain relief and failure to treat pain is viewed as poor medicine, unethical practice, and an abrogationof fundamental human rights (Brennan et al. 2007). Yet in some populations, such as children with intellectual and developmental disabilities (IDD), evaluation and management of pain presents a real challenge for the clinician, since those children suffering from pain, cannot voice or present their discomfort in normative manners.

M. Lotan (✉)
Faculty of Health Sciences, Department of Physical Therapy, Ariel University Center of Samana, Ariel, Israel
e-mail: ml_pt_rs@netvision.net.il

J. Merrick
Division of Pediatrics, Hadassah Hebrew University Medical Center, Jerusalem, Israel

J. Merrick
Kentucky Children's Hospital, University of Kentucky, Lexington, USA

J. Merrick
Center for Healthy Development, School of Public Health, Georgia State University, Atlanta, GA, USA

J. L. Matson, M. L. Matson (eds.), *Comorbid Conditions in Individuals with Intellectual Disabilities,* Autism and Child Psychopathology Series,
DOI 10.1007/978-3-319-15437-4_10

Health Status of Children with IDD

Children with IDD often have multiple and sometimes complicated medical problems (Prater and Zylstra 2006). The medical problems diagnosed in this population are diverse, ranging from limb contractures and scoliosis (Berven and Bradford 2002; Thacker et al. 2002) to spasticity (Pfister et al. 2003) and osteoporosis, particularly among non-weight-bearing and immobile patients (Henderson et al. 2002; Tyler et al. 2000). Such findings highlight the need for intense and specifically tailored medical coverage for individuals with IDD. However, as a minority group largely lacking empowerment and advocacy, they are constantly challenged by unmet health care needs. Several investigations (Beange et al. 1995; Fisher 2004; Kerr et al. 1996; Whitfield et al. 1996) have suggested that the health mismanagement of this population has a severe impact on mortality (Bittles et al. 2002; Durvasula and Beange 2001; Hollins et al. 1998); morbidity (Beange et al. 1995; Janicki et al. 1999); and quality of life (Hensel et al. 2002). Many of these medical conditions may cause the child with IDD pain, yet due to their inability to convey their pain and to present their suffering, they are doomed to experience delayed diagnosis and management of painful medical conditions, causing setbacks in hospitalization and even death (Carter and Jancar 1984; Mata 1960; Roy and Simon 1987).

Pain in Children with IDD

The prevalence of pain in the IDD population is unclear; mainly due to communication challenges that make the recognition of pain difficult (Reid et al. 2003). Children with IDD are vulnerable to the same range of pain-inflicting procedures as the non-IDD population, but, in addition, they are also vulnerable to experiencing pain from falls, leg braces, and ill-fitting wheelchairs (Regnard et al. 2003). A study investigating the frequency, duration, intensity, and location of pain, as well as the interference of pain with activities, in adults with cerebral palsy (CP) and IDD, found that pain was a significant problem for the majority of participants (Schwartz et al. 1999). Of the 93 participants (with an average age of 38), the majority had quadriplegia (84 %)[1] and were nonambulatory (94 %). One or more areas of chronic pain (minimum of 3 months' duration) was reported by 67 % of the participants, and 53 % experienced moderate to severe pain on an almost daily basis. Lower extremity pain (66 %) and back pain (63 %) were the most common complaints. The duration of pain ranged from a mean of 7.5 years for upper extremity pain to a mean of 20 years for hip or buttock pain. Likewise, McGrath et al. (2000) investigated the pain experience of 64 children with IDD and found that they suffered pain on a regular basis, with 83 % suffering constant pain at a level higher than 3 on a 10-point scale.

Thus, the accumulating evidence suggests that children with IDD suffer from more pain incidents than the general population and can be considered as a population at risk in regards to pain. Most researchers recommend that additional

[1] CP which affects all four limbs

research is needed to carefully examine how pain can be better managed in children with IDD and multiple disabilities (Schwartz et al. 1999). However, it is clear that better pain management should start with proper pain evaluation and that it is essential for the clinician to use reliable evaluation tools to initiate the pain assessment and intervention processes.

Types of Pain Assessment in IDD

Pain is a subjective and multidimensional phenomenon (Abu-Saad 2000). It can be assessed using a variety of modalities, including self-report, behavioral observation, or physiological measures, depending on the individual client and his or her communication capabilities. The adequacy of pain assessment through different modalities will be presented and discussed within the context of the children with IDD.

Self-Report

Given that pain is a subjective experience, "self-report" is usually considered to be the criterion standard or the "gold standard" in pain assessment (McCaffery and Beebe 1989). There are many psychometric instruments available that translate the subjective experiences of patients into meaningful data which can be used to assist health care providers with pain diagnosis and treatment. Simple pain assessment tools, such as the visual analogue scale (VAS), the numeric rating scale (NRS), and the verbal descriptor scale (VDS), are unidimensional and refer only to intensity of pain. There are also multidimensional tools, such as the McGill Pain Questionnaire (MPQ; Melzack 1975) and the Multidimensional Pain Inventory (MPI; Kerns et al. 1985).

Yet, self-report scales can only be used in individuals old enough or cognitively competent to provide valid information regarding location, quality, intensity, and tolerability of the painful experience (American Academy of Pediatrics and American Pain Society 2001; Johnston 1998). Even children with mild or moderate levels of IDD were found unable to submit reliable self-reports regarding their pain experience (Abu-Saad 2000; Devies and Evans 2001; Fanurik et al. 1998). Therefore, such instruments may be inadequate and ineffective for individuals who use nonconventional forms of communication or who lack the cognitive sophistication to convert their internal experiences into a conventional, standardized expressed language.

Physiological Pain Assessment

There are a number of physiological measures of pain in use, including vagal tone (Gunnar et al. 1995), heart rate (Cohen et al. 1999), blood pressure (Marchette et al. 1991), salivary amylase activity (Yamaguchi et al. 2006), and intracranial pressure

(Stevens and Johnson 1994). Although physiological measures may be viewed as free of response bias and therefore more conducive to objectivity, no single physiological index has been shown to be ideal and specific enough for measuring pain. Moreover, many physiological measures vary not only in accordance with the level of pain (but also in accordance with emotional states, temperature of the environment, body movement, and other extraneous factors). Many are invasive and can be impractical in terms of the time and costs associated with their use. In light of these limitations, physiological measures cannot be considered as suitable for detection of pain in children with IDD.

Behavioral Pain Assessment

Individuals with cognitive and verbal deficits may be unable to describe their feelings of pain or physical discomfort in a conventional manner (Abu-Saad 2000), thus rendering valid self-report as infeasible. In such cases, observation of behavior can be used as an acceptable alternative (McGrath 1998; McGrath et al. 1985; Stevens 1998). Behavioral indicators, such as facial expressions, crying, and body movements, are used to estimate the presence and intensity of pain in nonverbal or preverbal children (Lawrence et al. 1993; Hunt et al. 2004). Behavioral pain measures have been successfully used in the past to assess individuals with IDD (Hadjistavropoulos et al. 2001) and therefore should be the preferred method of pain assessment for children with IDD.

The Importance of Pain Assessment for Children with IDD

Assessing pain in children with IDD is a challenging task and can become extremely difficult at the levels of severe and profound IDD, where the ability to verbally communicate pain experience being severely compromised (Lachapelle et al. 1999). Without objective assessment, pain can be misinterpreted or underestimated, which might lead to inadequate management and undermine quality of life (Malviya et al. 2001).

Available findings suggest that pain in children with severe intellectual disability is common, yet rarely actively treated (Stallard et al. 2001). Children with severe or profound levels of IDD are more likely to have additional disabling conditions or multiple complex medical problems coupled with communication difficulties. Such medical problems, whether directly or indirectly linked to the disability, often necessitate painful procedures, including physical therapy treatments and various medical interventions. Recent data reveal that "sick days" in this population were associated with higher levels of pain and discomfort than "well days" (Carr et al. 2007) and that children with severe cognitive impairments and low communication abilities are likely to experience the most pain over time (Breau et al. 2003). The current situation puts children with IDD at a constant impediment to their quality of life, and therefore there is an urgent need to develop proper pain measures for this population. Yet, there are some objective difficulties in assessing pain in this population.

The Complexity of Assessing Pain in Children with IDD

Given the constant hindrance of pain to quality of life among children with IDD, there is an urgent need to develop a proper pain assessment tool for this population. However, the scientific world has lagged behind when it comes to pain assessment in children with IDD, and there are several reasons for this situation. First, many children with IDD have neurological problems that may affect their ability to comprehend and effectively communicate pain, thus complicating evaluation of the qualitative and quantitative aspects of their pain experience (Oberlander et al. 1999). Typical cognitive difficulties among this population involve reduced level of abstract thinking and spatial orientation. Therefore, children with IDD may be unable to give valid reports of the features of their pain sensation, such as location, intensity, or quality of their pain. They may not be able to respond to questions about their pain or they may respond in a way that is not meaningful to caregivers (Breau et al. 2004). These circumstances make pain measurement in these patients highly difficult or in some cases impossible (Mafrica et al. 2006). Thus, due to this reduced ability to verbally communicate pain, the gold standard of pain assessment, namely self-report, cannot be used with this population.

Second, individuals with IDD often have multiple handicaps and form an extremely heterogeneous group in terms of functional and behavioral repertoires. Functional limitations, such as paralysis and inability to move, may also mask expressions of pain (McGrath et al. 1998). To further complicate the issue of unclear communicative signals, challenging behaviors such as aggression, self-abuse, and tantrums can be observed in this population (Carr et al. 2007). Such behaviors have been connected with painful medical problems (De Lissovoy 1962; Hart et al. 1984), but can also mask pain in children with IDD (Clements 1992). This makes it difficult to ascertain whether the behavior is attributable to pain or another source of distress or whether it is simply part of the individual's regular aberrant behavior.

Third, behavioral indicators of pain in the general population, such as facial grimaces, groaning, or altered sleep patterns (Bodfish et al. 2001), may well appear in children with IDD at times when they are not in pain (McGrath et al. 1998). It is, therefore, not surprising that such behaviors are attributed to the intellectual level of the individual rather than to his pain (Mason and Scior 2004), probably resulting in under-diagnosing of pain in this population.

Finally, assessing and managing pain in children with IDD can be complicated by the effects of medication (Turk and Melzack 2001), as well as the lack of appropriate pain assessment tools. Despite the increased research attention focused on expressive behavior related to pain in children with IDD (Carter et al. 2002; Donovan 2002; Fanurik et al. 1999; Oberlander and O'Donnell 2001; Stallard et al. 2001; Stallard et al. 2002a), research on this topic is still scarce and there are, but few pain assessment scales available for use in this specific population.

Existing Pain Scales

Several scales for pain assessment in children with IDD have been developed, the majority over recent years. The following scales are listed chronologically.

1. *The Evaluation Scale for Pain in Cerebral Palsy* (*ESPCP*; Giusiano et al. 1995)

The ESPCP consists of 22 items of pain behaviors derived from physicians' reports of cues considered to be indicative of pain during medical examination. The items included various facial expressions: crying, movements, and posture (increase in muscular tone and/or involuntary movements, analgesic postures); protective reactions (movement toward painful areas), and social behaviors (e.g., reduced interest in surroundings). Although there appears to be a common set of pain behaviors in children with cerebral palsy and severe intellectual disabilities, the importance of the different items in determining pain is dependent on the individual's level of development.

Using the ESPCP, Collignon et al. (1997) developed a ten-item observational scale to evaluate pain and facilitate therapeutic decision making in children with severe handicaps and adults with CP. Collignon and Giusiano (2001) then further developed the tool to better fit an adolescent population with IDD. These researchers investigated pain behaviors in 100 individuals, ranging in age from 2 to 33 years (mean 16 years), with multiple physical disabilities and profound IDD and without speech or any means of communication ability through symbols. Pain could only be detected by observing global behavioral changes, rather than by the presence of a single sign. In addition, each combination of disabilities appeared to evoke a specific set of behaviors. For instance, behaviors associated with the voluntary protection of painful areas were more likely to occur in individuals with a lesser degree of motor impairment. This tool was not investigated further for psychometric properties.

2. *The Noncommunicating Children's Pain Checklist* (*NCCPC*; Breau et al. 2000)

The collection of pain items for this scale was initiated by McGrath and associates (McGrath et al. 1998). This group of researchers interviewed 20 parents or caregivers of cognitively impaired children, ranging in age from 6 to 29 years, regarding cues they considered to be indicative of pain in their children. The interviews included instances of short, sharp pain, such as needle pain, as well as long-lasting pain, such as headache or injury. A list of 31 cues was elicited. While specific behaviors often differed from one child to another, classes of behaviors (vocal, eating/sleeping, social/personality, facial expressions, body and limbs activity, and physiological reactions) were common to almost all children.

The NCCPC was developed from this initial study (Breau et al. 2000). It was comprised of 30 items and was to be tested in a home setting. Parents and caregivers assessed whether the pain cues were "present" or "absent" in four situations: acute pain, long-term pain, a nonpainful but distressing situation, and a nonpainful, calm situation. On the average, more than four times as many pain cues were present in painful situations than in calm (no-pain) situations. The total number of present cues did not differ between painful and distressed states, but scores for the "eating/sleeping" and "body/limb" subscales were higher during acute pain than during distress.

A second version of the NCCPC checklist, the NCCPC-PV (PV = Postoperative Version), was evaluated in a postoperative setting (Breau et al. 2002a). In this study, items related to eating and sleeping were omitted and each of the remaining items was scored on a four-point ordinal scale according to frequency of occurrence. Twenty-four children, ranging in age from 3 to 19 years, were each observed by one of their caregivers and one of the researchers for 10 min both before and after surgery. When available, nurses also provided their assessments. Each observer completed the NCCPC-PV independently in addition to giving a global rating of the intensity of the child's pain using a VAS. The NCCPC-PV was found to show very high internal consistency (Cronbach's alpha = 0.91) and good inter-rater reliability (ICC 0.78–0.82). A moderate correlation (from 0.39 to 0.53) was observed preoperatively between scores on the NCCPC-PV and global assessments of the child's pain through the VAS. A score of 11 on the NCCPC-PV provided 0.88 % sensitivity and 0.81 % specificity for classifying children who were rated at a moderate-severe level of pain on a verbal rating scale (VRS).

A third revised version of this scale, the NCCPC-R (R = revised), used ordinal ratings according to frequency of occurrence as above, but this time included the items related to eating and sleeping. This version was evaluated in home settings (Breau et al. 2002b). Using the NCCPC-R, 55 caregivers of 71 children with severe cognitive impairments, ranging in age from 3 to 18 years, conducted observations of their children during a time of pain and a time without pain. The NCCPC-R was found to have high internal consistency (Cronbach's alpha = 0.93), as well as a moderate correlation with the pain intensity ratings provided by caregivers (Pearson's r = 0.46). Sensitivity (0.84) and specificity (0.77) for pain were optimized at a cut-off point of 7 out of a possible total score of 90.

3. *The Pain Indicator for Communicatively Impaired Children* (*PICIC*; Stallard et al. 2002b)

The PICIC uses six core items to assess the expression of chronic pain in noncommunicative children with significant IDD. A significant relationship was demonstrated between five of the six core items and the presence and severity of pain (Stallard et al. 2002b). However, further research is needed before the PICIC can be established as a tool holding proper psychometric values.

4. *The Pediatric Pain Profile* (*PPP*; Hunt et al. 2004)

The PPP is a 20-item behavior rating scale designed to assess pain in children with severe neurological and cognitive disability. The validity and reliability of the scale was assessed in 140 children, ranging in age from 1 to 18 years, who were unable to communicate through speech or augmentative communication. Parents used the PPP to retrospectively rate their child's behavior when "at their best" and when in pain. Children were found to display significantly higher scores when in pain than in a nonpain situation, and their scores increased in line with global evaluations of pain.

In order to assess inter-rater reliability, two raters concurrently observed and individually rated each child's behavior. Inter-rater reliability by ICC values was found to range between 0.74 and 0.89. In order to assess the construct validity and responsiveness of the scale, the behavior of 41 children was rated before and 4 h after the administration of an analgesic. The PPP scores were found to be significantly higher before than after analgesic administration ($p < 0.001$). As part of this process, the behavior of 30 children was rated before and 5 days after surgery. Internal consistency ranged from 0.75 to 0.89 (Cronbach's alpha), and sensitivity (1.00) and specificity (0.91) were optimized at a cut-off point of 14 on a 60-point scale. Although there was no significant difference between the mean preoperative and postoperative scores, the highest PPP score occurred in the first 24 h after surgery in 14 (47%) children. Yet, the authors claim that the PPP should be considered as reliable and valid and suggest that it has potential for both clinical and research purposes.

Despite such claims, it seems that more rigorous psychometric properties need to be established for the PPP and that further research is required in order to evaluate the acceptability, feasibility, and usefulness of the PPP as a tool in clinical settings for children with severe to profound neurological and cognitive disabilities. Further validation as an evaluative tool is also required. Finally, it has yet to be determined whether the PPP is also useful for pain assessment in adults with similar degrees of disability (Hunt et al. 2004).

5. *The Body Posture Pain Scale*

A new scale recently developed (Zabalia et al. 2014) which looks at body postures of children aged 6–16. Despite the fact that this scale was specifically developed for children with sickle cell disease (SCD), this self-report pain scale needs further development but might be found useful in achieving valid pain reports from children with chronic diseases.

The Use of Proxy Observer

Although self-report of pain and symptoms is always preferable, that option is not available for many children with IDD. While it is possible for some children with neurological and cognitive impairment to use certain forms of self-report (Fanurik et al. 1998; Ferrell et al. 1995; Parmelee 1996), those unable to report their pain must remain dependent on their caregivers' observational skills. Due to the cognitive and communication difficulties presented by children with IDD, a designated external evaluator is usually assigned to perform the assessment. This person should have close knowledge of the observed child and is termed a proxy observer. When communication is difficult, assumptions by health care professionals about the meaning of any individual's painful experience should be made with caution. Since expression of pain reflects a complex mixture of physical and emotional states, coping style, and family and cultural expectations, it can be misinterpreted by health care professionals (American Academy of Pediatrics and American Pain Society 2001).

Past reports on the use of proxy observers in regards to abstract concepts, such as quality of life, have been contradictory. Some studies found that relatives and clinicians have a tendency to underestimate the well-being of the child with IDD (Britto et al. 2004; Ennett et al. 1991), while others showed that caregiver ratings were significantly higher than the ratings of the child with IDD (Schwartz and Rabinovitz 2003). Still others found substantial positive correlations between the two ratings and no significant difference between self-reports of children with IDD and caregiver reports (Stancliffe 1999). When pain reports are in question, recent studies have shown that caregivers' reports provided the best alternative for self-reports in research aimed at understanding and alleviating pain of children with IDD (Breau et al. 2004). When a group of children with IDD with good communication abilities was investigated the use of caregivers as proxy observers of pain experience has been found to correspond with the reports made by the children experiencing pain themselves, both in regards to acute pain (Schneider and LoBiondo Wood 1992) and long-lasting pain (Miller 1996). Therefore, most of the existing evidence suggests that the translation of health-related nonverbal communication by proxy observers familiar with the patient does accurately reflect and facilitate the monitoring of health problems and pain in this population.

Management of Pain in Children with IDD

The lack of proper management of pain in children with IDD can be explained by several factors. This uncertainty is partly due to the scarcity of pharmacological studies, which limits understanding of the pharmacodynamics of analgesic medication in this group of clients. The optimal treatment in these patients is mostly experienced-based. The clinician taking care of the child with IDD must make decisions on type and dosage of analgesia without clear knowledge of the impact of those drugs on their patients, as well as the mutual effects several drugs taken together might achieve. This lack of knowledge extends among the range of health professionals who work with people with dementia, including nurses and pharmacists. It is likely that this results in both undertreatment and overtreatment. Efficacy studies of analgesics in children with IDD are challenging but feasible and there is an urgent need for more research in this area. The low dosage of pain medication seems to occur consistently in residential, nursing home, and hospital care (Closs et al. 2004).

Point to Consider When Managing Pain in Children with IDD

Assessment

- Use a standardized tool to assess pain intensity (the list of existing scales is reported in the previous part of this chapter).
- In some cases, a very simple communication board can be used as a way to understand the child's pain experience.
- Ask family or usual caregivers as to whether the child's current behavior (e.g., crying out, restlessness, agitation or withdrawal) is different from their

customary behavior—this change in behavior may signal pain, and most caregivers can decipher these signs and are able to know when the child is in pain.
- Integrating a multiprofessional team experienced in pain management and children with IDD could help in managing a holistic view of the child's condition and therapeutic needs, and applying the best suited pain management.

Applying Medication

- Changes to rule out other causes. Coexisting medical conditions must be considered—verify that none of the existing medical conditions and the medication taken by the child do not collide.
- Other comorbidities such as constipation, lack of appetite, insomnia, and depression must be considered before administering the child's pain management.
- Medications should be individually tailored and dosage should be carefully considered—administer low-level painkillers in low dosage and gradually increase. If not effective, change the medication you are using, to slightly more potent ones.
- If pain is suspected, consider a time-limited trial of an appropriate type and dose of an analgesic agent. Thoroughly investigate behavioral changes and change medication appropriately.

Suggesting Alternative Intervention

- Different, nonpharmaceutical interventions can be applied if medication is not advised. Such interventions can include physical intervention such as:

  - isotonic strengthening exercises, aerobic exercise and other exercise according to the child's cognitive, communicative and physical abilities
  - Transcutaneous electrical nerve stimulation (TENS) should be considered for the effective management of persistent pain.
  - Cold or hot packs can be tried as local pain relief techniques.
  - Massage therapy might be found effective in reducing muscle tone, thereby effecting high muscle tone, when it is the cause for pain experienced by the child.
  - Snoezelen (a multisensory environment) intervention has been found effective in individuals with chronic pain (Schofield et al. 1998; Schofield 1996)
  - In other populations, chiropractic care was found effective in reducing musculoskeletal (Kopansky-Giles et al. 2014).
  - Music was found as a destructor which relaxes the listener, reduces anxiety as well as his subjective perception of pain. Music which the child is familiar with might reduce the child suffering while experiencing pain (Guéguen and Jacob 2014).
  - Some evidence exist to the efficiency of Shiatsu and Acupressure as beneficial for alleviating pain in different populations (Robinson et al. 2011).

Follow Up

- If possible use self-report and observational pain measures to evaluate the pain before and after administering the analgesic.
- The constant collection of accurate and valid clinical data (appropriate to the child's condition and abilities) and the collaboration between caregivers and medical team will provide a good basis for continuous quality management.
- Ensure family/caregivers/health care providers are informed before initiating change in medication and make sure to get proper reports from staff members involved in caring for the child regarding any changes in behavior.

Conclusions

For many years, clinicians did not fully grasp the phenomenon of pain behavior assessment and management in children with IDD. Without a substantial knowledge base, practitioners were left to rely on their own subjective judgments. These were fraught with inconsistencies and personal biases, which typically led to under treatment of pain. Now that the old "myths" have been refuted by solid research data (Schechter 1989; Schechter et al. 1993), it becomes obvious that practitioners should provide care that reflects current advancement of knowledge in the field. Poor assessment and management of pain in children with IDD could be overcome through better education on specific aspects of pain management and through more effective facilitation of pain assessment. It has long been established that inaccurate beliefs and poor knowledge and training of staff and management in long-term care are important barriers to high-quality care. Guidelines for the assessment and treatment of pain are being published to educate and direct the health care professionals (Agency for Health Care Policy and Research 1992; American Pain Society 1992; Berde et al. 1990; Zeltzer et al. 1990), and these must be implemented in everyday practice.

It is, therefore, imperative that each individual caregiver feel the personal responsibility to attend to and alleviate symptoms of pain and distress. This would include the careful assessment of pain and ongoing management to assure that discomfort is minimal. With new scientific data available, including the body of knowledge gathered and developed within the current investigation, both scientific and ethical standards demand that the under treatment of pain be rejected as substandard practice for children with IDD at all ages and at all levels of IDD.

Perspective Toward Future Research

In past years, the clinical and academic milieus have progressed beyond the traditional understanding that the absence of verbalized complaints of pain do not equate to the absence of pain. The health care professional now recognizes the strong influence that physical limitations, life experiences, level of education and cognitive status has on patients' ability to clearly report and accurately describe their pain experiences.

Education of health personnel in regards to IDD, pain in children with IDD with emphasis on improved competency in distinguishing pain behaviors from other behavioral symptoms are crucial at this point (Tousignant-Laflamme et al. 2012).

Further research is warranted in order to identify more characteristics of pain behavior in this population, which in turn could be used in diagnostic profiles or clinical diagnosis of pain in children with IDD. This could be especially relevant in children with profound and severe levels of IDD, where common ways of communication are almost completely absent. This group of clients also presents multiple medical conditions and possible sources of pain, which can result in delays in identifying the current cause of pain, causing untreated illness and suffering for the child with IDD. Despite progress in the last years in the assessment of pain for children with IDD, many with IDD are receiving a multitude of drugs, and therefore clinicians are still afraid to overdose the child with IDD, suspected of pain, thereby preventing proper care adapted to his suffering. Further work is needed to construct appropriate guidelines for the assessment and management of pain in children with IDD, with the aim of reducing their pain and improving their quality of life.

References

Abu-Saad, H. H. (2000). Challenge of pain in the cognitively impaired. *Lancet, 356,* 1867–8.

Agency for Health Care Policy and Research (1992). Acute pain management: Operative or medical procedures and trauma. Rockville, MD

American Academy of Pediatrics Committee on Psychosocial Aspects of Child and Family Health & American Pain Society. Task Force on Pain in Infants, Children and Adolescents (2001). The assessment and management of acute pain in infants, children, and adolescents. *Pediatrics, 108*(3), 793–797.

American Pain Society (1992). *Principles of analgesic use in the treatment of acute pain and cancer pain* (3rd ed.). Skokie: American Pain Society.

Beange, H., McElduff, A., & Baker, W. (1995). Medical disorders of adults with mental retardation: A population study. *American Journal of Mental Retardation, 99,* 595–604.

Berde, C., Ablin, A., Glazer, J., Miser, A., Shapiro, B., Weisman, S., & Zeltzer, P. (1990). Report of the Subcommittee on disease-related pain in childhood cancer. *Pediatrics, 86,* 818–825.

Berven, S., & Bradford, D. S. (2002). Neuromuscular scoliosis: Causes of deformity and principles for evaluation and management. *Seminars in Neurology, 22,* 167–178.

Bittles, A. H., Petterson, B. A., Sullivan, S. G., Hussain, R., Glasson, E. J., & Montgomery, P. D. (2002). The influence of intellectual disability on life expectancy. *The Journals of Gerontology. Series A, Biological Sciences and Medical Sciences, 57,* M470–M472.

Bodfish, J. W., Harper, V. N., Deacon, J. R., & Symons, F. J. (2001). Identifying and measuring pain in persons with developmental disabilities: A manual for the Pain and Discomfort Scale (PADS). Western Carolina Center Research Reports.

Breau, L. M., McGrath, P. J., Camfield, C., Rosmus, C., & Finley, G. A. (2000). Preliminary validation of an observational pain checklist for persons with cognitive impairments and inability to communicate verbally. *Developmental Medicine and Child Neurology, 42,* 609–616.

Breau, L. M., Finley, G. A., McGrath, P. J., & Camfield, C. S. (2002a). Validation of the non-communicating children's pain checklist-postoperative version. *Anesthesiology, 96,* 528–535.

Breau, L. M., McGrath, P. J., Camfield, C. S., & Finley, G. A. (2002b). Psychometric properties of the non-communicating children's pain checklist-revised. *Pain, 99,* 349–357.

Breau, L. M., Camfield, C. S., McGrath, P. J., & Finley, A. (2003). The incidence of pain in children with severe cognitive impairments. *Archives of Pediatrics and Adolescent Medicine, 157,* 1219–1226.

Breau, L. M., Camfield, C. S., McGrath, P. J., & Finley, G. A. (2004). Risk factors for pain in children with severe cognitive impairments. *Developmental Medicine and Child Neurology, 46,* 364–371.

Brennan, F., Carr, D. B., & Cousins, M. (2007). Pain management: A fundamental human right. *Anesthesia and Analgesia, 105,* 205–221.

Britto, M. T., Kotagal, U. R., Chenier, T., Tsevat, J., Atherton, H. D., & Wilmott, R. W. (2004). Differences between adolescents' and parents' reports of health-related quality of life in cystic fibrosis. *Pediatric Pulmonology, 37,* 165–171.

Carr, E. G., Jamie, Æ, & Owen-DeSchryver, S. (2007). Physical illness, pain, and problem behavior in minimally verbal people with developmental disabilities. *Journal of Autism and Developmental Disorders, 37,* 413–424.

Carter, G., & Jancar, J. (1984). Sudden death in the mentally handicapped. *Psychological Medicine, 14,* 691–695.

Carter, B., McArthur, E., & Cunliffe, M. (2002). Dealing with uncertainty: Parental assessment of pain in their children with profound special needs. *Journal of Advanced Nursing, 38,* 449–457.

Clements, J. (1992). I can't explain… "Challenging behaviour": Towards a shared conceptual framework. *Clinical Psychology Forum, 39,* 29–37.

Closs, S. J., Barr, B., & Briggs, M. (2004). Cognitive status and analgesic provision in nursing home residents. *The British Journal of General Practice: The Journal of the Royal College of General Practitioners, 54*(509), 919–921.

Cohen, L. L., Blount, R. L., Cohen, R. J., Schaen, E. R., & Zaff, J. (1999). Comparative study of distraction versus topical anesthesia for pediatric pain management during immunizations. *Health Psychology: Official Journal of the Division of Health Psychology, American Psychological Association, 18,* 591–598.

Collignon, P., & Giusiano, B. (2001). Validation of a pain evaluation scale for patients with severe cerebral palsy. *European Journal of Pain (London, England), 5,* 433–442.

Collignon, P., Giusiano, B., Boutin, A. M., & Combes, J. C. (1997). Utilisation d'une échelle d'hétéroévaluation de la doleur chez le sujet sévérement polyhandicapé. *Douleur et Analgesie, 1,* 27–32.

De Lissovoy, V. (1962). Head banging in early childhood. *Child Development, 33,* 43–56.

Devies, D., & Evans, L. (2001). Assessing pain in people with learning disabilities. *British Journal of Nursing* (Mark Allen Publishing), *10*(8), 513–516.

Donovan, J. D. (2002). Learning disability nurses' experiences of being with clients who may be in pain. *Journal of Advanced Nursing, 38,* 458–466.

Durvasula, S., Beange, H. (2001). Health inequalities in people with intellectual disability: Strategies for improvement. *Health Promotion Journal of Australia, 11,* 27–31.

Ennett, S. T., DeVellis, B. M., Earp, J. A., Kredich, D., Warren, R. W., & Wilhelm, C. L. (1991). Disease experience and psychosocial adjustment in children with juvenile rheumatoid arthritis: Children's versus mothers' reports. *Journal of Pediatric Psychology, 16,* 557–568.

Fanurik, D., Koh, J. L., Harrison, R. D., Conrad, T. M., & Tomerlin, C. (1998). Pain assessment in children with cognitive impairment. An exploration of self-report skills. *Clinical Nursing Research, 7,* 103–124.

Fanurik, D., Koh, J. L., Schmitz, M. L., Harrison, D., Roberson, P. K., & Killebrew, P. (1999). Pain assessment and treatment in children with cognitive impairment: A survey of nurses' and physicians beliefs. *The Clinical Journal of Pain, 15,* 304–312.

Ferrell, B. A., Ferrell, B. R., & Rivera, L. (1995). Pain in cognitively impaired nursing home patients. *Journal of Pain and Symptom Management, 10,* 591–598.

Fisher, K. (2004). Health disparities and mental retardation. *Journal of Nursing Scholarship: An Official Publication of Sigma Theta Tau International Honor Society of Nursing/Sigma Theta Tau, 36,* 48–53.

Giusiano, B., Jimeno, M. T., Collignon, P., & Chau, Y. (1995). Utilization of neural network in the elaboration of an evaluation scale for pain in cerebral palsy. *Methods of Information in Medicine, 34,* 498–502.

Guéguen, N., & Jacob, C. (2014). The influence of music on temporal perception and pain in a dental clinic. In J. Merrick, P. Schilfiled, & M. Murad (Eds.), *Pain: International research in pain management* (pp. 297–300). New York: Nova.

Gunnar, M. R., Porter, F. L., Wolf, C. N., Rigaruso, J., & Larson, M. C. (1995). Neonatal stress reactivity: Prediction to later emotional temperament. *Child Development, 66,* 1–13.

Hadjistavropoulos, T., Von Baeyer C., Craig, K. D. (2001). Pain assessment in persons with limited ability to communicate. In DC Turk & R Melzack (Eds.), *Hand book of pain assessment* (2nd ed., pp. 134–52). New York: The Gilford press.

Hart, H., Bax, M., & Jenkins, S. (1984). Health and behavior in preschool children. *Child: Care, Health and Development, 10,* 1–16.

Henderson, R. C., Lark, R. K., Gurka, M. J., Worley, G., Fung, E. B., Conaway, M., Stallings, V. A., & Stevenson, R. D. (2002). Bone density and metabolism in children and adolescents with moderate to severe cerebral palsy. *Pediatrics, 110(1 pt 1)*, e5.

Hensel, E., Rose, J., Kroese, B. S., & Banks-Smith, J. (2002). Subjective judgments of quality of life: A comparison study between people with an intellectual disability and those without a disability. *Journal of Intellectual Disability Research, 46,* 95–107.

Hollins, S., Attard, M. T., von Fraunhofer N., McGuigan, S., & Sedgwick, P. (1998). Mortality in people with learning disability: Risks, causes, and death certification findings in London. *Developmental Medicine and Child Neurology, 40,* 50–56.

Hunt, A., Goldman, A., Seers, K., Crichton, N., Mastroyannopoulou, K., Moffat, V., Oulton, K., & Brady, M. (2004). Clinical validation of the paediatric pain profile. *Developmental Medicine and Child Neuorology, 46*(1), 9–18.

Janicki, M. P., Dalton, A. J., Henderson, C. M., & Davidson, P. W. (1999). Mortality and morbidity among older adults with intellectual disability: Health services considerations. *Disability and Rehabilitation, 21,* 284–294.

Johnston, C. C. (1998). Psychometric issues in the measurement of pain. In G. A. Finley & J. McGrath (Eds.), *Measurement of pain in infants and children* (pp. 5–20), (Progress in pain research and management, Vol. 10). Seattle: IASP Press.

Kerns, R. D., Turk, D. C., & Rudy, T. E. (1985). The West Haven-Yale Multidimensional Pain Inventory (WHYMPI). *Pain, 23*(4), 345–356.

Kerr, M., Fraser, W., & Felce, D. (1996). Primary health care for people with a learning disability: A keynote review. *British Journal of Learning Disabilities, 24,* 2–8.

Kopansky-Giles, D., Vernon, H., Boon, H., Steiman, I., Kelly, M., & Kachan, N. (2014). Management of musculoskeletal pain in an integrative, inner city, hospital-based primary care setting: Inclusion of chiropractic care. In J. Merrick, P. Schilfiled, & M. Murad (Eds.), *Pain: International research in pain management* (pp. 279–296). New York: Nova.

Lachapelle, D. L., Hadijistavropoulos, R., & Craig, K. D. (1999). Pain measurement in persons with intellectual disability. *The Clinical Journal of Pain, 15,* 13–23.

Latham, J., & Davis, B. D. (1994). The socio-economic impact of chronic pain. *Disability and Rehabilitation, 16*(1), 39–44.

Lawrence, J., Alcock, D., McGrath, P., Kay, J., MacMurray, S. B., & Dulberg, C. (1993). The development of a tool to assess neonatal pain. *Neonatal Network, 12,* 59–66.

Mafrica, F., Schifilliti, D., & Fodale, V. (2006). Pain in Down's syndrome. *TheScientificWorld Journal, 6,* 140–147.

Malviya, S., Voepel-Lewis, T., Trait, A. R., Merkel, S., Lauer, A., Munro, H., & Farley, F. (2001). Pain management in children with and without cognitive impairment following spine fusion surgery. *Pediatric Anesthesia, 11,* 453–458.

Marchette, L., Main, R., Redick, E., Baggs, A., & Leatherland, J. (1991). Pain reduction interventions during neonatal circumcisions. *Nursing Research, 40,* 241–244.

Mason, J., & Scior, K. (2004). Diagnostic overshadowing amongst clinicians working with people with intellectual disabilities in the UK. *Journal of Applied Research in Intellectual Disabilities, 17,* 85–90.

Mata, A. C. (1960). Management of acute abdomen it the mentally retarded. *Virginia Medical Monthly, 96,* 732–733.

McCaffery, M., & Beebe, A. (1989). *Pain clinical manual for nursing practice*. St. Louis: Mosby.

McGrath, P. J. (1998). Behavioral measures of pain. In G. A. Finley & P. J. McGrath (Eds.), Measurement of pain in infants and children (pp. 83–102). (Progress in pain research and management, Vol. 10). Seattle, IASP Press.

McGrath, P. J., Johnson, G., Goodman, J. T., Schillinger, J., Dunn, J., & Chapman, J. (1985) CHEOPS: A behavioral scale for rating postoperative pain in children. In HL Fields, R Dubner, & F. Cervero (Eds.), Advances in pain research and therapy (Vol. 9, pp. 395–402). New York, Raven Press.

McGrath, P. J., Rosmus, C., Canfield, C., Campbell, M. A., & Hennigar, A. (1998). Behaviours caregivers use to determine pain in nonverbal, cognitively impaired individuals. *Developmental Medicine and Child Neuorology, 40,* 340–343.

McGrath, P. J., Breau, L. M., Camfield, C., & Finley, G. A. (2000). Caregivers management of pain in cognitively impaired children with severe speech impairments. Poster presented at the 5th international symposium on pediatric pain. London, England. June 18–21, 2000.

Melzack, R. (1975). The McGill pain questionnaire: Major properties and scoring methods. *Pain, 1,* 119–133.

Merskey, H., Bogduk, N. (1992). *Taxonomy of chronic pain.* Seattle: IASP Press.

Miller, D. (1996). Comparisons of pain ratings from postoperative children, their mothers, and their nurses. *Pediatric Nursing, 22,* 145–149.

Oberlander, T. F., O'Donnell, M. E., & Montgomery, C. J. (1999). Pain in children with significant neurological impairment. *Journal of Developmental and Behavioral Pediatrics, 20,* 235–243.

Oberlander, T. F., & O'Donnell, M. E. (2001). Beliefs about pain among professionals working with children with significant neurological impairment. *Developmental Medicine and Child Neurology, 43,* 136–140.

Parmelee, P. A. (1996). Pain in cognitively impaired older persons. *Clinics in Geriatric Medicine, 12,* 473–487.

Pfister, A. A., Roberts, A. G., Taylor, H. M., Noel-Spaudling, S., Damian, M. M., & Charles, P. D. (2003). Spasticity in adults living in a developmental center. *Archives of Physical Medicine and Rehabilitation, 84,* 1808–1812.

Prater, C. D., & Zylstra, R. G. (2006). Medical care of adults with mental retardation. *American Family Physician, 73*(12), 2175–83.

Regnard, C., Mathews, D., Gibson, L., & Clarke, C. (2003). Difficulties in identifying distress and its causes in people with severe communication problems. *International Journal of Palliative Nursing, 9,* 173–176.

Reid, B. C., Chenette, R., & Macek, M. D. (2003). Prevalence and predictors of untreated caries and oral pain among special olympic athletes. *Special Care in Dentistry: Official Publication of the American Association of Hospital Dentists, the Academy of Dentistry for the Handicapped, and The American Society for Geriatric Dentistry, 23,* 139–142.

Robinson, N., Lorenc, A., & Liao, X. (2011). The evidence for Shiatsu: A systematic review of Shiatsu and acupressure. *BMC Complementary and Alternative Medicine, 11,* 88.

Roy, A., & Simon, G. B. (1987). Intestinal obstruction as a cause of death in the mentally handicapped. *Journal of Mental Deficiency Research, 31,* 193–197.

Schechter, N. L. (1989). The under treatment of pain in children: An overview. *Pediatric Clinics of North America, 36,* 781–794.

Schechter, N. L., Berde, C. B., & Yaster, M. (1993). Pain in infants, children, and adolescents: An overview. In N. L. Schechter, C. B. Berde, & M. Yaster (Eds.), *Pain in infants, children, and adolescents* (pp. 3–9). Baltimore: Williams & Wilkins.

Schneider, E. M., & LoBiondo Wood, G. (1992). Perceptions of procedural pain: Parents, nurses, and children. Special issue: Measurement issues with child-subjects. *Children's Health Care, 21,* 157–162.

Schofield, P. (1996). Snoezelen: Its potential for people with chronic pain. *Complement Therapies in Nursing and Midwifery, 2*(1), 9–12.

Schofield, P., Davies, B., Hutchinson, R. (1998). Evaluating the use of Snoezelen and chronic pain: the findings of an investigation into its use (Part II). *Complement Therapies in Nursing and Midwifery, 4*(5), 137–43.

Schwartz, C., & Rabinovitz, S. (2003). Life satisfaction of people with intellectual disability living in community residences: Perceptions of the residents, their parents and staff members. *Journal of Intellectual Disability Research, 47,* 75–84.

Schwartz, L., Engel, J. M., & Jensen, M. P. (1999). Pain in persons with cerebral palsy. *Archives of Physical Medicine and Rehabilitation, 80,* 1243–1246.

Stallard, P., Williams, L., Lenton, S., & Velleman, R. (2001). Pain in cognitively impaired, non-communicating children. *Archives of Disease in Childhood, 85,* 460–462.

Stallard, P., Williams, L., Velleman, R., Lenton, S., & McGrath, P. J. (2002a). Brief report: Behaviors identified by caregivers to detect pain in noncommunicating children. *Journal of Pediatric Psychology, 27,* 209–214.

Stallard, P., Williams, L., Velleman, R., Lenton, S., McGrath, P. J., & Taylor, G. (2002b). The development and evaluation of the pain indicator for communicatively impaired children (PICIC). *Pain, 98,* 145–149.

Stancliffe, R. J. (1999). Proxy respondents and the reliability of the quality of life questionnaire empowerment factor. *Journal of Intellectual Disability Research, 43,* 185–193.

Stevens, B. (1998). Composite measures of pain. In GA Finley & PJ McGrath (Eds), *Measurement of pain in infants and children* (pp. 161–178). (Progress in pain research and management, Vol. 10). Seattle: IASP Press.

Stevens, B. J., & Johnson, C. (1994). Physiological responses of premature infants to a painful stimulus. *Nursing Research, 43,* 226–231.

Thacker, M., Hui, J. H., Wong, H. K., Chatterjee, A., & Lee, E. H. (2002). Spinal fusion and instrumentation for paediatric neuromuscular scoliosis: Retrospective review. *Journal of Orthopaedic Surgery (Hong Kong), 10,* 144–151.

Tousignant-Laflamme, Y., Tousignant, M., Lussier, D., et al. (2012). Educational needs of health care providers working in long-term care facilities with regard to pain management. *Pain Research & Management, 17*(5), 341–346.

Turk, D. C., & Melzack, R. (Eds.). (2001). Handbook of pain assessment, (2nd ed.). New York: Guildford Press.

Tyler, C. V. Jr., Snyder, C. W., & Zyzanski, S. (2000). Screening for osteoporosis in community-dwelling adults with mental retardation. *Mental Retardation, 38,* 316–321.

Whitfield, M., Langan, J., & Russell, O. (1996). Assessing general practitioners' care of adult patients with learning disability: Case-control study. *Qual Health Care, 5,* 31–35.

Yamaguchi, M., Takeda, K., Onishi, M., Deguchi, M., & Higashi, T. (2006 Jan-Feb). Non-verbal communication method based on a biochemical marker for people with severe motor and intellectual disabilities. *The Journal of International Medical Research, 34*(1), 30–41.

Zabalia, M., Braeu, L., & Marie-Moustapha, C. (2014). The body posture pain scale. In J. Merrick, P. Schilfiled, & M. Murad (Eds.), *Pain: International research in pain management* (pp. 75–82). New York: Nova.

Zeltzer, L. K., Altman, A., Cohen, D., & LeBaron, S. (1990). Report of the subcommittee on the management of pain associated with procedures in children with cancer. *Pediatrics, 86*(5), 826–831.

Part IV
Motor Movement Problems

Chapter 11
Gait and Balance

Dimitrios Patikas

Introduction

Intellectual disability (ID) is defined as any significant limitation in mental-intellectual function and impairments in adaptive behavior (skills of daily living) established before the age of 18 years. According to Sparrow and Cicchetti (1985), in order to have a global view of the disease, intellectual functioning should be evaluated in the fields of communication, daily living, social and motor skills.

Despite the fact that people with ID have rather heterogeneous motor behavior (Cleaver et al. 2009), it would be quite safe to state that they are in general slower and more "clumsy," and they tend to require more time during motor learning processes compared to their nondisabled counterparts (Davis and Van Emmerik 1995). Studies indicated that children with ID are retarded by 2–4 years in most motor tasks (Rarick et al. 1970). This could be attributed to environmental, maturational, and learning factors. Furthermore, the intelligence level or mental age is related to the motor proficiency of people with ID, probably due to the cognitive demands or complexity of the task (Groden 1969; Kioumourtzoglou et al. 1994). Hence, fine and gross motor problems are endemic among persons with ID and are related to their behavior.

Gait and balance represent two of the most important human motor capacities required for mobility. Any impairment on the development of these motor skills reduces the level of independence and increases the need for permanent support to perform daily activities. Proficiency on these tasks drastically determines the quality of life of an individual, as they are necessary in numerous household and everyday tasks. Therefore, the documentation of such deficits along with their possible causes is very important.

D. Patikas (✉)
Department of Physical Education and Sport Science at Serres, Aristotle University, Thessaloniki, Greece
e-mail: dpatikas@auth.gr

J. L. Matson, M. L. Matson (eds.), *Comorbid Conditions in Individuals with Intellectual Disabilities,* Autism and Child Psychopathology Series,
DOI 10.1007/978-3-319-15437-4_11

Both gait and balance require efficiency, endurance and spatiotemporal accuracy. They belong to the basic gross motor skills that every person should attain during the first years of development. This might be hindered by the presence of ID, regardless whether there is a direct motor debility or not. In many occasions, physical activity is not reduced by the intellectual disorder per se, but due to environmental reasons and the attitude of the individual.

Besides, the maintenance of balance and normal gait is not only mediated by complex neural pathways but might also be affected by multiple skeletomuscular, behavioral, or metabolic causes. Physiological deviation in any of these factors results in a disadvantage for performance, reduced independence, tendency to immobility, and contributes to the final clinical picture (Janicki and Jacobson 1986; Kapell et al. 1998). For this reason limitations in mobility, reflected in gait and balance deficits, may be common in people with ID, ranging from 3 to 63 % depending on the sample characteristics (prevalence of other disabilities, age, gender, level of ID, etc.) and the definition of mobility vs. impaired mobility (Cleaver et al. 2009).

This chapter focuses on the basic motor skills of gait and balance and covers definitions, important issues, prevalence, causes, and interventions related to impaired motor function.

Physical Fitness and Motor Deficits Related to Gait and Balance

Muscle coordination, strength and power, as well as physical fitness in general are some important factors that affect gait and balance. There is a significant body of literature related to these issues regarding persons with ID, which is presented below.

Physical Fitness

Physical fitness is important to promote health and well-being of persons with ID (Fernhall et al. 1988). There are numerous studies showing that people with ID demonstrate physical fitness deficit compared nonsymptomatic peers. In a 13-year follow-up study, it was shown that physical fitness comprised of cardiovascular endurance, muscular strength, muscular endurance, flexibility, and body composition measurements, was lower in adults with ID compared to people without disability, and the rate of the decline in fitness through the ageing process was greater in people with ID (Graham and Reid 2000). Even elite athletes with ID may perform worse than age-matched university students in terms of balance, strength, speed, and aerobic fitness (Van De Vliet et al. 2006). Regarding aerobic fitness, people with ID also show limited capacity (Fernhall 1993; Fernhall et al. 1996a; Fernhall et al. 1998; Pitetti and Fernhall 1997; Pitetti et al. 2001; Yanardag et al. 2013).

Reduced physical fitness has been shown in children with ID as well. In younger ages, children (8–10 years old), early adolescents (11–14 years old), and late adolescents (15–18 years old) with ID demonstrate lower aerobic capacity than age-matched counterparts without ID and this difference increased gradually with age (Pitetti et al. 2001). Young women with ID (mean age: 22.2 years old), compared to age-matched peers without ID (mean age: 23.2 years old), had significantly lower fitness level in terms of balance, cardiovascular and muscular endurance (Yanardag et al. 2013).

Coordination

In general, people with ID demonstrate deficits in motor performance compared to the age-matched counterparts. These deficits are linked to coordination and muscle activation patterns during movement which are different in persons with ID (Cuesta-Vargas and González-Sánchez 2013; Lotan et al. 2009; Van De Vliet et al. 2006; Zafeiridis et al. 2010). The extent of deficits in motor performance depends on the severity of the disease (Vuijk et al. 2010).

It has been previously shown that the presence of even mild ID results in fine and gross motor control deficits (Carmeli et al. 2008), "clumsiness," reduced coordination on the upper extremities (Arnold et al. 2005; Latash et al. 2002) and poor hand-eye coordination (Carmeli et al. 2008). There are also indications which suggest that with increasing severity of ID, these deficits would only be exacerbated (Carmeli et al. 2008).

Compared to persons without ID, they have longer decision and movement times (Baumeister and Kellas 1968; Wade et al. 1978). Several studies have shown that people with ID require longer periods to process and respond to a sensory input (Brewer and Smith 1990; Carmeli et al. 2008; Inui et al. 1995; LeClair et al. 1993).

Another typical characteristic of persons with ID is the increased intraindividual variability (Bruininks 1974; Dobbins and Rarick 1977; Inui et al. 1995; Parker and Bronks 1980; Rarick 1973) and the in accuracy in precision (Brewer and Smith 1990; Carmeli et al. 2008; Shinkfield et al. 1997; Sparrow and Day 2002) when reproducing a movement. These issues are related to inadequate coordination, which is linked to difficulties in manual dexterity (Vuijk et al. 2010) and poor skill performance in general (Horvat et al. 2012; Skowronski et al. 2009). The increased variability is reflected in neuromuscular activation as well, as revealed from electromyographic recordings that appear more variable in persons with ID (Davis et al. 1991).

Muscle Strength and Power

Low physical activity may lead to sarcopenia, decrease in muscle strength and increased risk for falling (Carmeli et al. 2012b). In older people, sarcopenia is a good predictor for risk of falls, hospitalizations, decreased quality of life and mortality (Fielding et al. 2011). In general, muscle strength is assumed to be an important factor that may contribute to balance (Wolfson et al. 1995). This is supported by findings showing that muscle weakness correlates with impaired balance control and greater risk of falls in elderly people (Bhatt et al. 2011). Furthermore, rapid leg movements, which require adequate amounts of power (strength and speed), are crucial in prohibiting falls, when an external perturbation occurs. Thus, strength and power are two components crucial for balance maintenance.

According to the literature, muscle strength and power are reduced in people with ID when compared with nondisabled peers (Angelopoulou et al. 1999; Carmeli et al. 2002a; Carmeli et al. 2013; Pitetti et al. 1992). Moreover, muscle strength does not improve significantly between the ages of 10 and 17 in the presence of ID, and this could be a limiting factor for the endurance, as measured by maximum oxygen uptake in people with ID (Fernhall and Pitetti 2000; Pitetti and Fernhall 1997).

Carmeli et al. (2002a) and Angelopoulou et al. (1999) state that intellectually disabled adults with Down syndrome present inferior performance in knee isokinetic force compared to nondisabled age-matched adults. Besides, the presence of ID within the group of people with Down syndrome revealed resulted in further deterioration in torque output (Angelopoulou et al. 1999), indicating the strong effect the ID may have on force production. For the same muscle group, Pitetti et al. (1992) have shown that adults with Down syndrome and without ID achieve higher forces than adult with Down syndrome and ID, which reinforces the relationship between the presence of ID and strength. Similar strength deficits in people with ID, when compared to nonsymptomatic age-matched peers, have been also indicated in hand grip isometric force (Carmeli et al. 2013), and elbow flexors (Pitetti et al. 1992). This deficit in muscle force is probably due to a low level of physical activity (Carmeli et al. 2012c).

Along similar lines, muscle power, as tested with the Wingate test, in people with ID is reduced (Croce et al. 1996; Horvat et al. 1999; Horvat et al. 1997). Furthermore, jumping ability, which is directly related to power output, is also reduced in people with ID. More particularly, standing long-jump distance (Guidetti et al. 2010; Skowronski et al. 2009), squat jump height (Hassani et al. 2013), and countermovement jump height (Hassani et al. 2014) are reduced in individuals with ID. This deficit in power output could be attributed to lack of stiffness regulation and to deficits in strength, and to impaired learning, coordination, and neuromuscular activation (Hassani et al. 2013; Hassani et al. 2014; Skowronski et al. 2009).

In elderly people, reduced strength of the upper limbs could be related to the presence of adverse health outcomes, and to reduced participation in activities of daily living (Sayer et al. 2006). Previous studies in older adults have shown that decreased lower or upper limb muscle strength is associated with balance control (Lin and Woollacott 2005; Wennie Huang et al. 2010). Therefore, there are extrinsic (environmental) and intrinsic (balance control) factors related to falls due to muscle weakness (Jerome et al. 2000). More specifically, when controlling for age, strength is the best predictor for static balance (Lin and Woollacott 2005). Additionally, tests regarding physical performance can at best predict the onset of attenuation in activities of daily living, including gait and balance control (Wennie Huang et al. 2010).

However, little is known about the relationship between strength and balance in individuals with ID (Carmeli et al. 2003; Carmeli et al. 2002b; Fernhall 1993). In a recent study, a similar relationship, as with nondisabled adults, has been observed for the upper limb muscles in patients with ID (Carmeli et al. 2013). More particularly, performance in hand-grip strength test was correlated with body sway rate (Carmeli et al. 2013). This also indicates that strength decline is not limited to the lower limb muscles that contribute to balance maintenance, but instead a universal decline in strength might have occurred (Stenholm et al. 2012).

On the other hand, and as suggested by Carmeli et al. (2013), the cause and effect could be reversed, i.e., balance decrease might have result in reduced functional ability, social isolation, physical inactivity and deterioration in force output. However, strength deficits, which start approximately during the fifth decade of life, precede the decline in balance, which occurs later in life, when the sensory input (vision, proprioception, and vestibular system) is more profoundly affected.

Gait

Although walking is an apparently simple and natural task, it requires unique and complex motor behavior to propel the body forward, maintaining balance, and adapting constantly to the environment (i.e., obstacle avoidance, perturbations, and ground surface irregularities). It also includes maneuvers that are required to avoid an obstacle, to climb stairs, to walk uphill or downhill, to change directions, etc. This is achieved by an advanced level of cooperation between the sensory (vision, proprioception and vestibular input) and motor systems, under the supervision and influence of numerous supraspinal and spinal centers.

Walking in particular, is one of the most common activities performed among people with ID (Draheim et al. 2002b) and represents their primary mode of transportation (Draheim 2006). It also represents one of the most frequently used motor skills in endurance training interventions for physically active individuals with ID (Stanish and Draheim 2005; Temple and Walkley 2003). Furthermore, many employment tasks performed by people with ID are often physical in nature, and part of them involve elevated levels of walking during the workday (Draheim 2006).

As mentioned above, people with ID have decreased performance in movement accuracy, reaction time, and speed of movement. Under these constraints they produce gait patterns that may differ from the ones of people without ID or any other neuromuscular or musculoskeletal disorder. On the other hand, deviations from typical gait patters in people with ID may be attributed to symptoms that coexist with the disease, such as hypotonia (Croce et al. 1996; Horvat et al. 2003), muscle strength deficits (Pitetti et al. 1992), impairments in the function of the cerebellum (Pinter et al. 2001), joint laxity (Livingstone and Hirst 1986), and reduced plantar flexion moments (Cioni et al. 2001; Cipriani et al. 2012; Ulrich et al. 2004).

As far as it concerns the walking ability of persons with ID, the vast majority of the body of research investigated children with Down syndrome. The only study that compared people with ID and controls is the one from Sparrow et al. (1998), which showed that adults (24–48 years old) with ID demonstrated increased cadence compared to adults without ID, and furthermore, the females in the ID group had shorter stride length when compared to the females of the control group (Sparrow et al. 1998).

Similar findings have been observed in studies that involved people with Down syndrome. It has been shown that they walk slower, with higher cadence, shorter step length, wider base of stance width and longer double support phase (Cioni et al. 2001; Galli et al. 2008a; Kubo and Ulrich 2006a; Kubo and Ulrich 2006b; Parker and Bronks 1980; Parker et al. 1986; Smith et al. 2007; Smith and Ulrich 2008; Ulrich et al. 2004; Virji-Babul and Brown 2004). The reduced walking speed is also reflected in the decreased ground reaction forces during the push off phase (Cioni et al. 2001; Galli et al. 2008a; Kubo and Ulrich 2006a; Smith et al. 2007; Smith and Ulrich 2008). Furthermore, persons with Down syndrome show increased head movement and increased variability in step length, base of stance width and kinematic patterns (Parker and Bronks 1980).

In addition, children and adults with Down syndrome demonstrate a general picture of walking characterized by reduced stability, as reflected by displacements of their center of mass (Agiovlasitis et al. 2009a; Black et al. 2007; Buzzi and Ulrich 2004; Kubo and Ulrich 2006a; Kubo and Ulrich 2006b; Parker and Bronks 1980; Smith and Ulrich 2008). More specifically, the reduced stability shown in adults with Down syndrome is documented by the increased variability in the base of stance width and step length (Agiovlasitis et al. 2009a; Smith and Ulrich 2008), by the increased mediolateral variability of the center of mass, and by the higher mediolateral range of motion of the center of mass (Agiovlasitis et al. 2009a; Buzzi et al. 2002; Kubo and Ulrich 2006a; Kubo and Ulrich 2006b), especially at higher walking speeds (Agiovlasitis et al. 2009a). Similar findings and conclusions have also been shown in studies investigating children with ID during walking (Buzzi and Ulrich 2004; Kubo and Ulrich 2006a; Kubo and Ulrich 2006b).

When increasing walking speed, step length increases and step time decreases in people with (Agiovlasitis et al. 2009a) and without ID (Õunpuu 1994). However, the significantly higher increase in mediolateral variability of the center of mass as a function of walking speed that is observed in individuals with ID compared to asymptomatic peers, is not always compensated by an increase in base of stance width (Smith and Ulrich 2008). Especially in younger people, an increase in walking speed is accompanied by a reduction in step duration as well (Agiovlasitis et al. 2009a).

Interestingly, at higher speeds the vertical displacement of the center of mass stops increasing with speed in people with Down syndrome after a certain threshold, in contrast with people without Down syndrome, who show further increase at similar walking speeds (Agiovlasitis et al. 2009a). This indicates that movement is reorganized for persons with ID at a lower speed threshold, probably to anticipate for the transition from walking to running (Farley and Ferris 1998), which is affected in people with ID (Agiovlasitis et al. 2008).

The investigation of perturbed gait, during obstacle crossing or stair climbing is important to understand the mechanisms of increased falling rates in people with

ID. It seems that persons with ID use different anticipation adjustments and strategies to step over an obstacle. More particularly, the selected strategy to cross the obstacle varies from trial to trial (Virji-Babul and Brown 2004) and there is often hesitation prior to obstacle crossing. Furthermore, they need more time to anticipate the obstacle (Smith and Ulrich 2008; Sparrow et al. 1998; Wu et al. 2008) and therefore, as early as three steps before the obstacle, they may increase the base of stance width and reduce walking speed, cadence, and step length (Wu et al. 2008). Regarding the distance of the foot from the obstacle Smith and Ulrich (2008) reported a decrease in people with Down syndrome which makes obstacle crossing more dangerous for tripping. In contrast, Sparrow et al. (1998) revealed an increase in the distance of the foot from the obstacle which provides a larger safety margin.

Energy Cost

In the general population, there are several gait patterns which could result in increased energy cost. For instance, fluctuations in braking and propulsion forces, as captured by the anterior–posterior velocity of the center of mass during walking, reflect an increased energy cost (Farley and Ferris 1998). Other indications for an increased metabolic cost are increased mediolateral displacement of the center of mass (Donelan et al. 2001; Donelan et al. 2004; Kuo 2007), greater variability in base of stance width, higher step frequency, and shorter step duration (Dean et al. 2007; Doke et al. 2005; Donelan et al. 2001; Donelan et al. 2002a; Donelan et al. 2002b; Donelan et al. 2004; Kuo 2007).

With the exception of the anterior–posterior velocity of the center of mass (Agiovlasitis et al. 2009a), all of the above parameters are affected in people with ID (Agiovlasitis et al. 2009a; Kubo and Ulrich 2006a; Parker and Bronks 1980; Smith and Ulrich 2008; Ulrich et al. 2004). Therefore, such changes in the gait pattern do not only have the potential to reduce stability, but also increase energy cost (Agiovlasitis et al. 2009a; Agiovlasitis et al. 2009b; Buzzi and Ulrich 2004; Kubo and Ulrich 2006a; Ohwada et al. 2005; Ulrich et al. 2004).

As suggested and speculated on in previous studies (Cioni et al. 2001; Parker and Bronks 1980; Ulrich et al. 2004), it has been shown that people with ID consumed 15–38% more oxygen than adults without ID for a certain walking speed on a treadmill (Agiovlasitis et al. 2009b). Similar findings were obtained in over-ground walking (Agiovlasitis et al. 2011) and when accounting for step frequency instead of gait speed (i.e., for a given step frequency, persons with ID showed higher energy expenditure than those without ID) (Agiovlasitis et al. 2012). These findings have important implications in the selection of the intensity of exercise, and suggests that it should be adapted to the requirements of the disability (Agiovlasitis et al. 2012; Agiovlasitis et al. 2009b).

A possible mechanism that could contribute to the increased energy cost during gait is the increased level of antagonist co-contraction (Hassani et al. 2013; Hassani et al. 2014; Latash 2000; Ulrich et al. 2004). A recent study has shown that the level of co-contraction of the leg muscle, especially during the swing phase, is increased during gait in people with Down syndrome (Gontijo et al. 2008). As a result, they adopt a stiffer gait pattern, with reduced range of motion and the hip and knee joints are more flexed through the gait cycle (Galli et al. 2008a; Parker and Bronks 1980; Parker et al. 1986; Ulrich et al. 2004). A further mechanism that contributes to increased energy cost is increased activation of the upper body muscles (McArdle et al. 2007; Winter 2005) and movement of the head (Parker and Bronks 1980) which reflect a compensatory response to imbalance.

All the above suggest that the energy cost increases due to adaptations of the neuromuscular system to compensate for instability. High energy cost in turn, might have adverse effects in mobility, since better endurance is required to achieve the same task within the same timeframe. Thus, another reason for the higher energy cost might be the lower aerobic fitness of people with ID (Fernhall et al. 1996b). On the other hand, high energy cost and the need for energy conservation, might be the cause for the lower walking speed observed in people with ID (Smith and Ulrich 2008). Hence, the issues of energy cost with the level of fitness and the ability to walk are interconnected.

Balance

Balance is an essential motor skill which requires body awareness, fine motor control, bilateral coordination, and motor planning (Kurtz 2008). Performance in balance is determined by two basic components: static and dynamic. Static balance refers to the ability of a person to maintain the vertical projection of the center of gravity within the base of support, while the body position remains stationary. On the other hand, dynamic balance is the ability to maintain body equilibrium during movement, while the base of support changes. This definition closely associates dynamic balance with gait. Impaired stepping ability destabilizes the body's center of mass and reduces the ability to respond to external postural perturbations during walking and therefore increases the risk of falling (Fasano and Bloem 2013). This issue, due to its importance, is covered in the next section.

In ID, balance deficits are related to age, which is influenced by the development of the motor reflex pathways regulating muscle tone and posture (Kokubun and Koike 1995). Earlier studies have shown that children with mild ID are markedly inferior compared to nonhandicapped children when performing one foot static balance test (Howe 1959). As analyzed below, more recent studies verify that individuals with ID have a significantly deteriorated balance capacity and reduced ability to respond to external balance perturbations (Carvalho and Almeida 2009; Dellavia et al. 2009; Enkelaar et al. 2012; Galli et al. 2011; Gomes and Barela 2007; Hale et al. 2007; Hale et al. 2009; Ko et al. 1992; Kokubun et al. 1997; Lahtinen et al. 2007; Okuzumi et al. 1997; Rigoldi et al. 2011; Smith and Ulrich 2008; Suomi and Koceja 1994; Van De Vliet et al. 2006; Van Emmerik et al. 1993; Vuijk et al. 2010; Webber et al. 2004; Yanardag et al. 2013).

According to Lahtinen et al. (2007) adolescents and adults with ID showed impaired static balance as measured by the stork stance balance test. Carvalho and Almeida (2009), measuring the time on seesaw of persons with Down syndrome 21 years younger than control counterparts (i.e., 28 vs. 49 years old, respectively), found no difference between the groups. Similarly, people with ID (Okuzumi et al. 1997) and Down syndrome (Galli et al. 2008b) showed decreased performance in the single leg stance test. Furthermore, people with ID (Hale et al. 2007) or Down syndrome (Smith and Ulrich 2008) scored better in Berg Balance Scale compared to nonsymptomatic peers.

Posturography measurements have shown that persons with ID (Dellavia et al. 2009; Ko et al. 1992; Kokubun et al. 1997; Suomi and Koceja 1994; Van Emmerik et al. 1993) or Down syndrome (Dellavia et al. 2009; Galli et al. 2008b; Gomes and Barela 2007; Kokubun et al. 1997; Webber et al. 2004) have increased sway amplitude and variability when compared to controls, and their strategy to balance was based on shifting the body weight mediolateraly (Galli et al. 2008b; Suomi and Koceja 1994; Van Emmerik et al. 1993).

Comparing people with ID, Down syndrome and controls, the group with ID had significantly more body sway than the Down syndrome and control group, and the Down syndrome group differed significantly with the control group (Dellavia et al. 2009). Furthermore, a significant correlation of the increased sway with the severity of the disease was observed (Suomi and Koceja 1994). In contrast with this finding, a more recent study has shown that the severity of the disease has a negative effect on static and dynamic balance in children with ID (Vuijk et al. 2010). Therefore, this issue remains controversial.

Rigoldi et al. (2011) tested balance ability by means of posturography in three different age groups with and without Down syndrome. They showed that depending on the age group, different strategies were used. More specifically, children with Down syndrome (9–11 years old) increased the range of motion of the center of pressure (COP) on the anterior–posterior and mediolateral axes and increased the trajectory length of the COP. Teenagers with Down syndrome (12–19 years old) revealed increased frequency in the anterior–posterior and mediolateral deviation of the COP and increased range of motion of the COP on the anterior–posterior axis. Finally, adults with Down syndrome (22–46 years old) demonstrated increased range of motion of the COP on the anterior–posterior and mediolateral axes and increased frequency in the deviation of the COP on the anterior–posterior axis (Rigoldi et al. 2011).

Regarding the importance of visual cues on balance, as revealed by the amount of deterioration in balance when eyes are closed (Butterworth and Cicchetti 1978), there is controversy in the literature. Suomi and Koceja (1994) and Webber et al. (2004) showed that people with ID (Suomi and Koceja 1994) or Down syndrome (Virji-Babul and Brown 2004) demonstrate larger increase in body sway when eyes were closed compared to controls. In contrast, this was not supported by Dellavia et al. (2009) and Gomes and Barela (2007).

Another issue that could influence balance is the increased variability in movement mentioned above. More specifically, increased variability in movement patterns could reflect greater responsiveness of the neural postural control system to produce larger and faster corrections, especially in situations of instability (England and Granata 2007). This adaptive process has been observed in several pathologies that affect movement control, with ID being one of them (Agiovlasitis et al. 2009a; Parker and Bronks 1980). This could be reflected by increased body sway velocity during posture observed in persons with Down syndrome (Galli et al. 2008b; Kokubun et al. 1997; Webber et al. 2004) or variations in muscle activation. In line with the latter hypothesis, a recent study has shown that ID has a significant effect on the muscle activation patterns during the sit-to-stand task (Cuesta-Vargas and González-Sánchez 2013).

Regarding dynamic balance, backward and forward translations of the support surface while standing on both feet, showed that persons with ID had delayed reactive response (Hale et al. 2007; Hale et al. 2009). This increased latency in reflex or premotor response may have implications in fall prevention. The delayed response could be attributed to reduced physical activity (Jaffe et al. 2005), that is related to the inability to respond skillfully to balance perturbations. This fact in turn, could induce anxiety, and increased demands on cognitive attention. Another compensatory mechanism that could cope the instability and improve safety is the increased co-contraction observed in people with ID under different circumstances when balance is challenged (Carvalho and Almeida 2009; Hassani et al. 2013; Hassani et al. 2014; Latash 2000; Ulrich et al. 2004).

Risk of Falling

Falling is by definition connected to the ability to perform gait and balance tasks adequately, with minimal physical or cognitive effort, and resisting the adverse effects of fatigue. Therefore, gait and balance problems are among the well-established risk factors for falling (Tinetti et al. 1988). It is indicative that the most common causes for falls in elderly with dementia are the "inadequate (use of) materials, stumbling, or slipping" and "gait and equilibrium disturbances" (van Dijk et al. 1993).

The risk of falling may be exacerbated in the presence of ID, especially in elderly people (Carmeli et al. 2002c; Hsieh et al. 2001). Adults with ID experience significantly more falls compared to their age-matched nondisabled counterparts, and the increasing frequency of falling incidents appears at earlier age of life (Cox et al. 2010; Finlayson et al. 2010; Haynes and Lockhart 2012). Furthermore, this high rate in falling is often accompanied with increased risk of fall-related injuries (Cox et al. 2010; Hale et al. 2007; Hsieh et al. 2001; Sherrard et al. 2001).

It has been reported that 25% (n = 952) to 34% (n = 114) of people with ID older than 18 years old (18–83 and 18–65 years of age, respectively), fell at least once over a period of 12 months (Cox et al. 2010; Hsieh et al. 2012). This value may rise to 57% (n = 338) if the incidence of falling is measured over a period of 33 months (Wagemans and Cluitmans 2006) and to 70% (n = 114) over a period of 5 years (Grant et al. 2001). In a larger scale study (n = 1370), 10% of the adults with ID (40 to 79 years old) were injured due to a fall in the past 12 months

(Janicki et al. 2002). Other studies have shown that 20 % of the falls may require medical assistance and 30–58 % of the fallers are actually recurrent fallers (Hsieh et al. 2001; Wagemans and Cluitmans 2006). Along similar lines, a survey that included 700 people with ID, showed that 31 % of the external injuries were associated with falling, and 45 % of the severe injuries were due to falling (Bray et al. 2002). Other studies have shown that more than 50 % of the injuries that occurred in people with developmental disabilities were due to falls (Hsieh et al. 2001). It is also important to underline that the increased risk of falling is not restricted to elderly people exclusively, but has been shown in younger (5–29 years of age) persons with ID as well (Sherrard et al. 2001).

The risk of falling and the falling rate are important issues for the quality of life of a person. Injuries induced by falling may have various consequences, ranging from slight contusion to fractures or even death (Speechley and Tinetti 1991). Fractures are 1.7–3.3 times more often in individuals with ID than age-matched nonsymptomatic individuals (Lohiya et al. 1999; Tannenbaum et al. 1989). These findings are supported by studies that showed low bone mineral density in people with ID (Center et al. 1998; Jaffe et al. 2005; Janicki et al. 1999; Srikanth et al. 2011).

Although aging plays an important role in the rate of falls there are many other factors that may influence this phenomenon. Regarding the fallers with ID multiple factors have been identified (Chiba et al. 2009; Cox et al. 2010; Grant et al. 2001; Hale et al. 2007; Hsieh et al. 2001; Hsieh et al. 2012; Wagemans and Cluitmans 2006; Willgoss et al. 2010). Such factors, apart from age, include the presence of seizures, epilepsy, arthritis and paretic conditions (Chiba et al. 2009; Cox et al. 2010; Hsieh et al. 2001; Hsieh et al. 2012; Willgoss et al. 2010), the intake of anxiolytics, antipsychotics, anticonvulsants, more than four medicaments and medication in general (Chiba et al. 2009; Cox et al. 2010; Hale et al. 2007; Hsieh et al. 2001; Hsieh et al. 2012; Wagemans and Cluitmans 2006), the existence of past fractures (Cox et al. 2010), the level of disability and mobility (Grant et al. 2001; Hale et al. 2007; Hsieh et al. 2012; Wagemans and Cluitmans 2006; Willgoss et al. 2010), the existence of behavioral problems (Hale et al. 2007; Hsieh et al. 2001; Willgoss et al. 2010), the sex (Grant et al. 2001; Hsieh et al. 2012), the place of residence (home or institution) (Grant et al. 2001), the context and environment of falling (Hale et al. 2007), and the physical condition (Hale et al. 2007; Hsieh et al. 2012). Furthermore, fallers with ID have prominent characteristics during gait such as greater base of stance width, shorter step length, and lower walking speed compared to non-fallers with ID (Chiba et al. 2009).

The incidence of falling might be influenced by intrinsic factors, such as seizures, poor balance, inadequate function of optokinetic nystagmus and vestibulo-ocular reflexes (Costa 2011), inappropriate balance strategy (Hale et al. 2007), and extrinsic factors, such as slippery surfaces and use of walking aids (Hsieh et al. 2012).

The increased incidence of falling in people with ID may also be linked to significant functional deficits that are related to the disorder (Enkelaar et al. 2012). Hale et al. (2007) attempted to identify possible reasons for the increased risk of falling in people with ID, but were inconclusive. The only commonality between patients that tend to fall was the abnormal gait pattern (Hale et al. 2007).

The development of dementia may play a role in the risk of falling. Dementia appears in elderly people and in the presence of ID the prevalence is increased (12–20 %) compared to the prevalence observed in the general population (5 %) (Lin et al. 2014). Studies have shown that when ageing is accompanied by cognitive impairment and dementia, the risk of falls leading to injury doubles (Jensen et al. 2003; Tinetti et al. 1988) and increases with the severity of dementia (van Dijk et al. 1993). Furthermore, 37 % of people with ID and dementia walk unsteadily and lose balance, 11 % walk with aid, and 53 % walk slowly (Lin et al. 2014).

Finally, the consumption of some drugs may increase the risk of falling. Earlier studies have showed that the tendency for falling and injury risk are related to destructive behavior and the use of antipsychotic drugs and a history of seizures (Hsieh et al. 2001). Moreover, antiepileptic drugs, such as phenytoin, are also implicated in adverse effects on balance (Iivanainen 1998).

Causes for Gait and Balance Deficits

Although ID is mainly a cognitive disease, it has multiple effects on motor function. Low performance in several motor skills, including gait and balance is well documented and has multiple intrinsic and extrinsic causes. For instance, causes for impaired balance could be a potential deficit in muscle strength (Pitetti et al. 1992), hypotonia (Croce et al. 1996; Horvat et al. 2003), and joint laxity (Livingstone and Hirst 1986). Beyond motor diseases that are often coherent to ID, inadequate development of the central nervous system, the level of physical activity, and premature aging are some of causes which are analyzed below.

Central Nervous System Dysfunctions

People with ID need more time and effort to learn and improve a task compared to age-matched peers due not only to cognitive constraints, but also to possible impairments in the function of cerebellum (Pinter et al. 2001), which is involved in the process of learning, (Davis and Van Emmerik 1995; Newell 1997). Another possible mechanism leading to such motor deficits could damage in the integrity of the corticospinal tract and changes in morphometry of the frontal and paretial cortex that have been detected in people with ID (Haier et al. 2004; Yu et al. 2008).

Regarding the balance deficits observed in individuals with ID a possible mechanism that may contribute to this could be suboptimal function of the vestibulocerebellum (Pritchard and Alloway 2007). In support to this hypothesis, cerebellum dysfunctions have been detected in patients with Down syndrome (Pinter et al. 2001).

Abnormal function of the central nervous system, related to the motor output, has been shown examining issues of laterality. More specifically, unilateral limb dominance is a typical indication of the specialization of brain hemispheres to perform certain tasks (Nebes 1990; Sperry 1990). People with ID have difficulties discriminating between left and right sides and do not show a preference for one side (Arnold et al. 2005; Carmeli et al. 2008). Hence, there are indications that no interhemispheric specialization has taken place yet, reflecting a motor development setback (Carmeli et al. 2008). These observations document how closely cognitive and motor responses are linked and reveals that there might be an interaction between them.

Low Level of Physical Activity

There is evidence that balance ability may deteriorate due to inactivity. More specifically, a comparison between physically active and inactive adults with ID, showed superior balance skills in the active group (Guidetti et al. 2010). Therefore, the lower performance in movement skills in general could be, at least partially, attributed to a less physically active life-style (Horvat and Franklin 2001). It has been reported that of 17.5–33 % of persons with ID participate in physical activities five or more times a week and although these are apparently high percentages, they are probably overestimates (Stanish et al. 2006). On the other hand, there are several reports that indicate a high prevalence of low level of physical activity for adults with ID residing in community settings (Draheim et al. 2002b; Hall and Thomas 2008; Stanish and Draheim 2005), and on some occasions this prevalence is higher than the general population (Temple and Walkley 2003). In general, findings on this issue are mixed, with studies indicating that persons with ID have either lower, similar, or higher physical activity levels than peers without disabilities (Frey et al. 2008).

The reasons for reduced physical activity could be related to fewer opportunities to practice motor skills or even to the over-protectiveness of parents, friends, relatives, and the surrounding environment in general. All these environmental factors should be considered for people with ID as well. Other possible drawbacks to participation in regular physical activity are the sedentary lifestyle, low motivation, and other psychological and physiological factors (Lotan et al. 2009), as well as the limited opportunities to participate in physical activities that are available to their peers without ID (Horvat and Franklin 2001).

Particularly for elderly people with ID, low level of physical fitness results in premature loss of functioning and health problems (Hilgenkamp et al. 2012). Due to the low physical fitness, there is evidence of enhanced predisposition to development of psychiatric problems (Day and Jancar 1994; Nottestad and Linaker 1999), osteoporosis (Center et al. 1998; Jaffe et al. 2005; Janicki et al. 1999; Srikanth et al. 2011), thyroid disorders, cardiovascular diseases (Draheim 2006), various forms of sensory impairment (Kapell et al. 1998), and early onset of dementia (Janicki and Dalton 2000). In addition, there are several common age-related chronic diseases, such as obesity, hypertension, osteoporosis, diabetes, arthritis, and constipation that also contribute to social isolation.

Considering the above it is not hard to understand that elderly individuals (with or without ID) have difficulties getting involved in some physical activities. This limitation in engagement in exercise- and health-related behaviors, may lead to further deconditioning, functional decline and morbidity (Ashman and Suttie 1996).

On the other hand, a low level of physical activity has numerous consequences for health. Several symptoms have been identified in people with ID, as also found in the general population, such as hyperlipidaemia (Draheim et al. 2002a; Draheim et al. 2002b; Draheim et al. 2003; Rimmer et al. 1994; Yanardag et al. 2013), hypertension (Draheim et al. 2002a; Draheim et al. 2002b, 2003; Rimmer et al. 1994), overweight and obesity (Draheim et al. 2002a; Draheim et al. 2002b, 2003; Horvat and Franklin 2001; Pitetti et al. 2001; Rimmer and Yamaki 2006; Stanish and Draheim 2006; Yanardag et al. 2013). The symptoms that occur more frequently in people with ID could be related to the level of physical activity and could explain why they have higher prevalence in cardiovascular diseases (Draheim 2006).

The former hypothesis is supported by findings showing that physically active athletes that participated in Special Olympics have lower systolic and diastolic blood pressure, triglycerides, and fasting insulin than others who were not physically active (Draheim et al. 2003). On the other hand, there are studies which show no significant differences between people with ID that walk less than 5000 steps per day and more than 10,000 steps per day, in terms of blood pressure, body composition, body mass, and abdominal fat (Stanish and Draheim 2006).

It has to be underlined though that the findings of the above studies are based on cross-sectional studies. This means that in the study of Draheim et al. (2003), the Special Olympic athletes with ID could have been predisposed to be healthier and in the study of Stanish and Draheim (2006), the group that walked more steps per day could have been overweight or obese people with ID that were involved in endurance training for weight loss. Therefore, more longitudinal studies are required to conclude on this issue.

In general, a low level of physical activity and its impact in health could have negative consequence in functional tasks, such as gait and balance. This could be one of the reasons why persons with ID demonstrate advanced and premature aging (Ashman and Suttie 1996; Carmeli et al. 2012a; Schonknecht et al. 2005; Temple and Walkley 2007), which is characterized by health problems, and by deficits in balance due to decline in muscle strength, and deficits in sensory (visual, proprioceptive, vestibular) input. This is especially important if we consider the increased life expectancy observed during the last decades in people with ID (Janicki et al. 1991; Janicki et al. 1999), and the increased number and frequency of age-related diseases, such as cardiovascular diseases (Draheim 2006).

Gait and Balance Assessment

The assessment of gait and balance in patients with ID is very important. Apart from the fact that assessment is a unique tool in research, it may help in diagnosis by detecting impairments and by quantifying the contribution of specific skills to the disability. Furthermore, it can evaluate interventions and document their benefits or drawbacks. This evaluation will have a positive impact on both the establishment and development of current and future interventions. Finally, using specific assessment methods provides the means to identify individuals with potential danger to fall.

Tests are often developed for a specific study, for a singular purpose, or as part of a test battery. There are multiple assessments used for the general populations (Creel et al. 2001; Tang et al. 1998). However, common gait and balance field tests, such as Berg balance scale (Berg et al. 1989) and timed up-and-go, have limited applicability in patients with ID (Bruckner and Herge 2003; Carmeli et al. 2003; Hale et al. 2007; Sackley et al. 2005). This is a result not only of the difficulty of the requested task, but also due to the patient's inherent inability to comprehend and follow the instructions. Other tests that have been used in people with ID are the functional reach test (Carmeli et al. 2005; Hale et al. 2007), the single leg stance test (Hale et al. 2007; Kokubun et al. 1997; Lahtinen et al. 2007), the tree-minute walk test (Carmeli et al. 2004), and the beam-walking test (Boswell 1991; DePaepe and Ciccaglione 1993; Hale et al. 2007; Smith et al. 2007; Wang and Ju 2002). Some tests, such as dynamic gait index (Shumway-Cook and Woollacott 2001), the four-step balance scale (Guralnik et al. 1994), the tandem stance test (Frzovic et al. 1994), or the balance subsection of the Bruininks–Oseretsky Test of Motor Proficiency (Bruininks, 1978) are not applicable in individuals with ID at all (Hale et al. 2007). Therefore, measuring balance performance in people with ID is challenging and needs to be adapted to the patients' requirements. Despite the difficulties in assessing some of these tests, the persons with ID who managed to get a score have on average lower performance than peers without ID (Bruckner and Herge 2003; Carmeli et al. 2004; Carmeli et al. 2005; Chiba et al. 2009; Duncan et al. 1990; Hale et al. 2007; Isles et al. 2004; Smith et al. 2007; Smith and Ulrich 2008; Steffen et al. 2002; Tinetti 1986; Tinetti et al. 1986; Vereeck et al. 2008; Verghese et al. 2009).

Carmeli et al. (2003) underlined the necessity of evaluating balance with more than one test to reduce possible discrepancies between the patient's performance and the assessor's interpretation. Thus, they examined individuals with ID and compared the following five balance tests which determine different properties of static and dynamic balance: one-legged standing (for the assessment of stability with reduced support area), timed up-and-go test (TUG; for the assessment of anticipation and preparation during dual tasks) (Podsiadlo and Richardson 1991), sit-to-stand (or Czuka test, for the assessment of the lower limb muscle strength), forward reach (for the assessment of the postural sway), and full turn (for the assessment of the lower limb coordination during postural adjustments). Significant high correlations were detected between the TUG and full turn tests and between forward reach and one-legged standing and therefore, the authors suggested to use one test of each pair to avoid redundancy. On the other hand, the reliability of the TUG test assessed in people with ID has been shown to be poor (Bruckner and Herge 2003).

Hale et al. (2007) applied a battery of ten balance tests to people with ID, including instrumented posturography. Data could be captured in six tests only. Out of 20 participants with ID, nine completed the computerized posturography (EquiTest®), eight the TUG test (Podsiadlo and Richardson 1991), seven the Berg Balance Scale

(Berg et al. 1989), six the functional reach test (Duncan et al. 1990), three the Clinical Test for Sensory Interaction in Balance (Shumway-Cook and Horak 1986), and three the single leg stance test (Frzovic et al. 1994). Hale et al. (2007) suggest to evaluate gait and balance capacity using observational tools, such as the activities-specific balance confidence scale (Powell and Myers 1995), which is a questionnaire that quantifies the confidence to balance during daily tasks and the gait abnormality rating Scale (Wolfson et al. 1990), which quantifies walking quality. More particularly regarding the former scale, the evaluator watches a videotape of the patient walking, and rates his/her ability according to a modified Gait Abnormality Rating Scale (Hale et al. 2010).

Furthermore, video recording when performing common tasks (stair climbing, obstacle avoidance, etc.) can be useful for documentation and can be watched, replayed in slow-motion and scored later (Hale et al. 2007). Recently, the same research group presented the balance scale for persons with intellectual disabilities (BSID), which is a video-based evaluation tool (Hale and Donovan 2014). BSID includes seven common and already familiar motor tasks, related to daily activities that challenge balance. The person performs the task just once, while being videotaped for later evaluation by the assessor. Each task is graded according to detailed guidelines given to the assessor, and the sum of each score gives a composite BSID score (Hale and Donovan 2014). The test has excellent reliability and is correlates well with the Tinetti score (Tinetti et al. 1986) and the gait abnormality rating scale (Wolfson et al. 1990).

BSID was a product of observations and discussions with persons with ID and their caregivers. The tasks chosen to be tested were (1) sit-to-stand-to-sit, (2) walking on a flat surface, (3) walking over an unstable surface, (4) picking up an object off the floor and reaching to place it on a table, (5) turning 180 degrees, (6) being distracted while walking, and (7) stair climbing (Hale and Donovan 2014). This collection of seven tasks fulfilled certain criteria: (1) they were similar to daily activities, (2) challenged balance capabilities at different levels, (3) required minimal explanation and (4) required minimal equipment (Hale and Donovan 2014). Similar evaluation tools for people with ID could be created in the future using such criteria.

According to Chiba et al. (2009), the Tinetti score could discriminate fallers with ID from non-fallers with ID. The Tinetti Test, or Performance Oriented Mobility Assessment (POMA) consists of two parts that evaluate components of static and dynamic balance, respectively (Tinetti et al. 1986). An evaluator scores nine static and eight dynamic tasks performed by the patient. The sum of scores classifies the patient as low-, moderate- or high-risk for falls person. A score of 25 or lower could identify a faller from a non-faller with 88.9 % sensitivity and 91.9 % specificity (Chiba et al. 2009). Contrary to the Tinetti Test, the TUG test was not sensitive enough to distinguish between fallers and non-fallers (Bruckner and Herge 2003).

Static posturography is commonly used for the assessment of static balance. It measures and quantifies objectively the position of the COP, as measured by force platforms and evaluates the movement of the human body (body sway) during quiet upright standing (Webber et al. 2004). This method has been used successfully in populations with ID (Dellavia et al. 2009; Gomes and Barela 2007; Ko et al. 1992; Suomi and Koceja 1994; Van Emmerik et al. 1993).

Concerning dynamic conditions, balance tests captured with computerized posturography involve unexpected brief forward–backward translations and record the motor anticipatory responses (Hale et al. 2009). Although this test gives insights into the reflexive and premotor responses which tend to be highly repeatable in people with impaired motor functions (Diever et al. 1988), some patients with ID do not cope with it (Hale et al. 2007).

Importance of Physical Activity Interventions

Although individuals with ID have a shorter life expectancy, which is related to the severity of the disease (Bittles et al. 2002), there is a trend for increasing life span, and there are increasingly many peers with ID who live as long as the typical population (Bittles et al. 2002; Janicki et al. 1991; Janicki et al. 1999). This indicates that extrinsic factors may determine not only the quality of life but also longevity. More explicitly, overall improved health status (adequate medical care, health facilities, nutrition, and exercise), and access to new interventions contribute to this change.

Prevention of the functional decline is very important. The increased life expectancy in people with ID (Janicki et al. 1991; Janicki et al. 1999), and the increased number and prevalence of age-related diseases (Draheim 2006) implies that physical activity in combination with a balanced diet—low in cholesterol, saturated fats, trans-fats, and sodium and high in vegetables, fruit, whole grains, and legumes—could be beneficial for prevention of these diseases (Draheim 2006).

Beyond general preventive approaches, such as medical screening for diabetes, hypertension, and hyperlipidaemia, there are several treatment interventions suggested to prevent and overcome motor deficits which occur in people with ID. Physical and occupational therapists are responsible for determining and evaluating motor deficits and treating them accordingly (Turner and Moss 1996). Such interventions are strengthening, stretching, gait education, and adoption of strategies to prevent falls and facilitate balance (Hocking et al. 2014). The promotion of physical activity as an intervention is of particular importance, because people with ID have similar adaptation responses after training programs as their counterparts without ID (Carmeli et al. 2005; Hemayattalab and Movahedi 2010).

Currently, it is accepted that physical fitness can be improved with regular exercise in people with ID (Guidetti et al. 2010). Regular training has positive and significant effects on their muscular endurance, cardiovascular endurance and strength (Chanias et al. 1998). Furthermore, Hinckson et al. (2013) have shown that children involved in training programs were able to manage their weight.

Young individuals with ID demonstrate significant gains in strength and endurance after a 3-week supervised resistance training program (Stopka et al. 1998). Gains in strength accompanied by improvement in balance have been observed after a 12-week (Tsimaras and Fotiadou 2004) or a 6-month (Carmeli et al. 2005) training program in people with ID. During a 9-month period, basketball athletes with ID showed significant gains in muscle strength and endurance, balance and TUG test, whereas inactive individuals with ID showed decrease in TUG test

(Guidetti et al. 2010). Furthermore, it has been suggested that gains in strength might be beneficial for endurance in people with ID (Fernhall and Pitetti 2000). However, people with ID have increased rates of sensory impairment (Janicki et al. 2002), and therefore exercise should be adapted to each patient's requirements.

Walking is one of the most common modes of exercise aimed to improve physical fitness. Persons with ID participate mostly in walking and other low-intensity activities, rather than in more vigorous activities (Stanish and Draheim 2005; Temple and Walkley 2003). Adults with ID may find less intense activities more enjoyable compared to activities that require a high level of physical stamina (Stanish and Draheim 2005). Hence, in this population low-to-moderate intensity activities are often reported (Draheim et al. 2003; Stanish and Draheim 2005) and rates of optional participation in low-to-moderate physical activity programs are high (Stanish et al. 2001). In any case, exercises implemented should be enjoyable and should include motivational strategies to ensure long-term participation. However, more information is required to design and apply effective training programs that include the appropriate exercises, which should be adapted to each individual's requirements.

Balance Improvement

The deficits in balance registered in people with ID imply that balance exercises should be a part of their training programs. There is convincing evidence that physical training programs in the general population not only improve balance but also reduce the risk of falling (Gillespie et al. 2009). Despite the relatively large body of literature, such clear evidence does not exist for people with ID, mostly due to the lack of well-designed randomized clinical trials (Enkelaar et al. 2012). This implies the necessity of further research in this field.

The available randomized clinical trials include people with Down syndrome, treated to improve gait and balance with treadmill training protocols (Angulo-Barroso et al. 2008; Carmeli et al. 2002c; Ulrich et al. 2001; Wu et al. 2007; Wu et al. 2008). Carmeli et al. (2002c) have shown that TUG test performance, as well as knee flexion and extension strength, improved significantly for the experimental group of adults (57–65 years old) with ID after 6 months of training.

Other randomized clinical trials have been applied in infants with Down syndrome and revealed an earlier onset of independent sitting (Ulrich et al. 2001) and walking (Ulrich et al. 2001; Wu et al. 2007; Wu et al. 2008), and longer stride length (Wu et al. 2007). Furthermore, infants with ID responded better to a high compared to a low-intensity treadmill program, by increasing walking speed, cadence, by decreasing double support duration (Angulo-Barroso et al. 2008) and by being able to walk over an obstacle at higher rates within a 6-month training period (Wu et al. 2008).

It has been suggested that gait and balance training could improve standing and postural sway (Gustafson et al. 2000). Therefore, treadmill walking and dynamic ball activities have been used in the past to improve balance and functional independence (Carmeli et al. 2003). After 6 months intervention only minor improvements were detected in two out of five balance tests. This unexpected finding could be attributed to the low number of participants ($n = 15$). Further, it cannot be excluded that the sensitivity of the tests was not high enough to detect any improvement, because of cognitive difficulties of the subjects to acquire the task of the tests (Etnier and Landers 1998). Despite these findings, it is common practice for clinicians to train their patients with treadmill walking and dynamic ball activities. This is because there is a close relationship between balance, muscle strength, well-being and physical training, which underlines the importance of physical training to the improvement of locomotion and perception of well-being among people with ID (Carmeli et al. 2005).

In addition to the above, there are several nonrandomized studies that have shown positive effects on balance after interventions involving physical exercise (Boswell 1991, 1993; Carmeli et al. 2005; Tsimaras and Fotiadou 2004; Wang and Ju 2002). Among the interventions that had positive effects on balance, are exercise programs including 3- (Tsimaras and Fotiadou 2004) or 6-month (Carmeli et al. 2005) strength training, 8-week creative dance training (Boswell 1991, 1993), or 6-week jump training (Wang and Ju 2002).

A cross-sectional study has also shown that involvement in sports may have a positive effect in the reaction time (Un and Erbahceci 2001). Moreover, in a longitudinal study design, a 6-month specific balance and strength training induces improvement in locomotor performance, but this positive effect is not known if they are retained after the end of the intervention (Carmeli et al. 2005).

Fall Prevention

Although fall prevention programs have been proven to be effective in elderly people, this result cannot be generalized for elderly with cognitive impairments or dementia or even for younger individuals with ID (van Dijk et al. 1993; Shaw et al. 2003).

In order to improve gait and balance and keep fall-related injuries to a minimum, it has been suggested that environmental safety, careful medical management and exercise interventions may play an important role (Willgoss et al. 2010). Moreover, adoption of a multimodal approach to fall prevention has been suggested, including supervised exercise, home hazard modification and appropriate medical, ophthalmic, and pharmacological interventions (Hale et al. 2007). Hence, apart from interventions for balance improvement, children with ID and their parents require adoption of injury prevention programs, aiming to learn and implement home and everyday safety strategies that will be useful for their future life (Sherrard et al. 2001). Additionally, it has been suggested that the delayed motor responses to balance perturbations shown in adults with ID and a history of falling, should be treated with physiotherapy interventions aiming to improve balance properties and preventing falls (Hale et al. 2009).

Mental Well-Being

It is important to underline that, apart from benefits in gait and balance control, exercise might have a positive influence on mental health and psychological well-being (mood, confidence, self-esteem, and life satisfaction). This issue is well documented not only in healthy adults (Atlantis et al. 2004; Boutcher 2000; Callaghan 2004) but also in children (Dykens et al. 1998; Maiano et al. 2001; Ninot et al. 2000) and adults (Carmeli et al. 2005; Gabler-Halle et al. 1993; McAuley et al. 2000) with ID. This observation is especially important if we consider that ID induces psychological and behavioral changes (Deci et al. 1999; Matson et al. 2003; Urv et al. 2003) which may lead to anxiety, depression, and lack of motivation (Dagnan and Sandhu 1999).

Exercise and success in motor functions by setting goals may also help to improve some intellectual functions (Carmeli et al. 2008). Further psychosocial benefits are reported as well, including self-efficacy, more positive expected outcomes, fewer cognitive–emotional barriers, improved life satisfaction, and marginally lower depression (Heller et al. 2004).

It is essential to note that any functional debility or psychological stress leads to a vicious cycle of sedentary life style, lack of confidence, requirement of external support, fear, and further functional decline. Besides, prophylactic health practices could delay the onset or minimize the occurrence of life threatening diseases. Therefore, management of the disease and adoption of prevention strategies that attain functional performance, and prohibit the development of additional diseases and disabilities are very important for the quality of the patient's life. Such strategies have significantly improved the health status of people with ID over the past few years (Janicki et al. 2002).

Closing Remarks

People with ID tend to lose independence more often and eventually become institutionalized and fully dependent. In their lifespan, they might be able to function in daily activities with external support ranging from none to extensive. This implies the necessity of developing and implementing effective intervention strategies and training programs. For children with ID, such programs should be instilled into the educational system throughout the school years. For adults with ID, an increase in the level of activity could help delaying the aging process. With intervention approaches it is likely to significantly improve the overall health and quality of life of most persons with ID. In order to achieve this goal a detailed description of the motor deficits and their underlying mechanisms is required. Hence, further studies in these areas are necessary in the future.

It must be remembered that any limitation in movement might coexist with exceptional attributes that can be exploited. For instance, a person with internal motivation has more chances to improve motor abilities and therefore improve function, provided the existence of support from family and health professionals.

Thus, motivational strategies and strategies that encourage lifelong participation should be included in the programs. However, motivational and adherence strategies for physical activity programs are understudied areas for persons with ID and should be a focus of future research.

Screening tests for gait and balance may help to identify patients with ID that have a higher risk of falling (Hale et al. 2007). Thus, early detection of potential functional impairments may improve the prognosis of the disease. Furthermore, since the negative consequences of inactivity on the quality of life of people with ID are well documented (Carmeli et al. 2012b), it is important to evaluate and objectively quantify the performance of muscle function and to use this assessment as a diagnostic tool.

Finally, the education and training of staff that supports people with ID (Wark et al. 2014) is crucial, especially when patients reach an advanced age, as comorbid diseases may appear and it is more probable that their parents have died. A series of training priorities for staff assisting the elderly with an ID has been suggested (Wark et al. 2014). This will help to modify existing and create generic interventions that are economical and efficient.

Summary

According to the current literature balance and gait capacities are affected in people with ID. The decline in motor performance appears in early age and leads to a premature aging process. Compared to their nondisabled counterparts, children and adults with ID demonstrate greater static and dynamic instability, greater energy cost and higher risk of falling. These motor deficits can be attributed not only to the pathophysiology of the disease but also to the level of physical activity. There are several studies suggesting that systematic exercise in individuals with ID may reverse the adverse effects of the disease in terms of efficiency in gait and balance and fall prevention. However, more well-designed randomized clinical trials, case-control and cohort studies are required to understand the mechanisms of the motor deficits that occur with ID, and the effects of training protocols aimed at improving the motor performance of persons with ID.

References

Agiovlasitis, S., Yun, J., Pavol, M. J., & McCubbin, J. A. (2008). Gait transitions of persons with and without intellectual disability. *Research Quarterly for Exercise and Sport, 79*(4), 487–494.

Agiovlasitis, S., McCubbin, J. A., Yun, J., Mpitsos, G., & Pavol, M. J. (2009a). Effects of Down syndrome on three-dimensional motion during walking at different speeds. *Gait & Posture, 30,* 345–350.

Agiovlasitis, S., McCubbin, J. A., Yun, J., Pavol, M. J., & Widrick, J. (2009b). Economy and preferred speed of walking in adults with and without Down syndrome. *Adapted Physical Activity Quarterly, 26,* 118–130.

Agiovlasitis, S., Motl, R. W., Ranadive, S. M., Fahs, C. A., Yan, H., Echols, G. H., Rossow, L., & Fernhall, B. (2011). Energetic optimization during over-ground walking in people with and without Down syndrome. *Gait & Posture, 33*(4), 630–634.

Agiovlasitis, S., Beets, M. W., Motl, R. W., & Fernhall, B. (2012). Step-rate thresholds for moderate and vigorous-intensity activity in persons with Down syndrome. *Journal of Science and Medicine in Sport, 15,* 425–430.

Angelopoulou, N., Tsimaras, V., Christoulas, K., Kokaridas, D., & Mandroukas, K. (1999). Isokinetic knee muscle strength of individuals with mental retardation, a comparative study. *Perceptual and Motor Skills, 88,* 849–855.

Angulo-Barroso, R. M., Wu, J., & Ulrich, D. A. (2008). Long-term effect of different treadmill interventions on gait development in new walkers with Down syndrome. *Gait & Posture, 27,* 231–238.

Arnold, G., Boone, K. B., Lu, P., Dean, A., Wen, J., Nitch, S., & McPherson, S. (2005). Sensitivity and specificity of finger tapping test scores for the detection of suspect effort. *Clinical Neurophysiology, 19*(1), 105–120.

Ashman, A. F., & Suttie, J. N. (1996). The medical health status of older people with mental retardation in Australia. *Journal of Applied Gerontology, 15,* 57–73.

Atlantis, E., Chow, C. M., Kirby, A., & Singh, M. F. (2004). An effective exercise-based intervention for improving mental health and quality of life measures: A randomized controlled trial. *Preventive Medicine, 39,* 424–434.

Baumeister, A. A., & Kellas, G. (1968). Reaction time and mental retardation. *International review of research in mental retardation* (Vol. 2, pp. 163–192). New York: Academic Press.

Berg, K., Wood-Dauphine, S., Williams, J. I., & Gayton, D. (1989). Measuring balance in the elderly: Preliminary development of an instrument. *Physiotherapy Canada, 41,* 304–311.

Bhatt, T., Espy, D., Yang, F., & Pai, Y. C. (2011). Dynamic gait stability, clinical correlates, and prognosis of falls among community-dwelling older adults. *Archives of Physical Medicine and Rehabilitation, 92,* 799–805.

Bittles, A. H., Petterson, B. A., Sullivan, S. G., Hussain, R., Glasson, E. J., & Montgomery, P. D. (2002). The influence of intellectual disability on life expectancy. *Journal of Gerontology, 57A*(7), M470–M472.

Black, D. P., Smith, B. A., Wu, J., & Ulrich, B. D. (2007). Uncontrolled manifold analysis of segmental angle variability during walking: Preadolescents with and without Down syndrome. *Experimental Brain Research, 183,* 511–521.

Boswell, B. (1991). Comparison of two methods of improving dynamic balance of mentally retarded children. *Perceptual and Motor Skills, 73,* 759–764.

Boswell, B. (1993). Effects of movement sequences and creative dance on balance of children with mental retardation. *Perceptual and Motor Skills, 77,* 1290.

Boutcher, S. H. (2000). Cognitive performance fitness and ageing. In S. J. H. Biddle, K. R. Fox & S. H. Boutcher (Eds.), *Physical activity and psychological well-being* (pp. 118–129). London: Routledge.

Bray, A., Gates, S., Vautier, S., Simpson, J., Firth, H., Narbey, C., & Forsyth, H. (2002). *Safe lives for people with intellectual disabilities: a community injury prevention project. Final report to ACC.* Dunedin N.Z.: Donald Beasley Institute.

Brewer, N., & Smith, G. A. (1990). Processing speed and mental retardation: Deadline procedures indicate fixed and adjustable limitations. *Memory & Cognition, 18,* 443–450.

Bruckner, J., & Herge, E. A. (2003). Assessing the risk of falls in elders with mental retardation and developmental disabilities. *Topics in Geriatric Rehabilitation, 19,* 206–211.

Bruininks, R. H. (1974). Physical and motor development of retarted persons. In N. R. Ellis (Ed.), International review of research in mental retardation (Vol. 7, pp. 209–261). New York: Academic Press.

Bruininks, R. H. (1978). *Bruininks-Oseretsky test of motor proficiency: Examiner's manual.* Circle Pines: American Guideance Service.

Butterworth, G., & Cicchetti, D. (1978). Visual calibration of posture in normal and motor retarded Down's syndrome infants. *Perception, 7,* 513–525.

Buzzi, U. H., & Ulrich, B. D. (2004). Dynamic stability of gait cycles as a function of speed and system constraints. *Motor Control, 8,* 241–254.

Buzzi, U. H., Stergiou, N., Kurz, M. J., Hageman, P. A., & Heidel, J. (2002). Nonlinear dynamics indicate aging affects variability during gait. *Clinical Biomechanics, 18*(5), 435–443.

Callaghan, P. (2004). Exercise: A neglected intervention in mental health care? *Journal of Psychiatric and Mental Health Nursing, 11,* 476–483.

Carmeli, E., Barchad, S., Lenger, R., & Coleman, R. (2002a). Muscle power, locomotor performance and flexibility in aging mentally-retarded adults with and without Down's syndrome. *Journal of Musculoskeletal and Neuronal Interactions, 2*(5), 457–462.

Carmeli, E., Barchad, S., Lenger, R., & Coleman, R. (2002b). Muscle strength, locomotor performance and flexibility in aging mentally-retarded adults with and without Down's syndrome. *Journal of Musculoskeletal and Neuronal Interactions, 2,* 457–462.

Carmeli, E., Kessel, S., Coleman, R., & Ayalon, M. (2002c). Effects of a treadmill walking program on muscle strength and balance in elderly people with Down syndrome. *Journals of Gerontology Series A Biological Sciences and Medical Sciences, 57A,* M106–M110.

Carmeli, E., Bar-Chad, S., Lotan, M., Merrick, J. & Coleman, R. (2003). Five clinical tests top assess balance following ball exercises and treadmill training in adult persons with intellectual disability. *Journal of Gerontology, 58A,* 767–772.

Carmeli, E., Kessel, S., Bar-Chad, S., & Merrick, J. (2004). A comparison between older persons with Down syndrome and a control group: Clinical characteristics, functional status and sensorimotor function. *Down's Syndrome, Research and Practice, 9,* 17–24.

Carmeli, E., Zinger-Vaknin, T., Morad, M., & Merrick, J. (2005). Can physical training have an effect on well-being in adults with mild intellectual disability? *Mechanisms of Ageing and Development, 126,* 299–304.

Carmeli, E., Bar-Yossef, T., Ariav, C., Levy, R., & Lieberman, D. G. (2008). Perceptual motor coordination in persons with mild intellectual disability. *Disability and Rehabilitation, 30*(5), 323–329.

Carmeli, E., Imam, B., Bachar, A., & Merrick, J. (2012a). Inflammation and oxidative stress as biomarkers of premature aging in persons with intellectual disability. *Research in Developmental Disabilities, 33,* 369–375.

Carmeli, E., Imam, B., & Merrick, J. (2012b). The relationship of presarcopenia (low muscle mass) and sarcopenia (loss of muscle strength) with functional decline in individuals with intellectual disability (ID). *Archives of Gerontoloy and Geriatrics, 55,* 181–185.

Carmeli, E., Merrick, J., & Imam, B., Levy, R. (2012c). Exercises and sports participation in health older adults with intellectual disability? A pilot study. *Health, 4,* 769–774.

Carmeli, E., Imam, B., Levi, R., & Merrick, J. (2013). Hand grip strength is associated with body sway rate among older adults with intellectual disability. *Journal of Policy and Practice in Intellectual Disabilities, 10*(4), 321–325.

Carvalho, R. L., & Almeida, G. L. (2009). Assessment of postural adjustments in persons with intellectual disability during balance on the seesaw. *Journal of Intellectual Disability Research, 53,* 389–395.

Center, J., Beange, H., & McElduff, A. (1998). People with mental retardation have an increased prevalence of osteoporosis: A population study. *American Journal of Mental Retardation, 103,* 19–28.

Chanias, A. K., Reid, G., & Hoover, M. L. (1998). Exercise effects on health-related physical fitness of individuals with an intellectual disability: A metaanalysis. *Adapted Physical Activity Quarterly, 15,* 119–140.

Chiba, Y., Shimada, A., Yoshida, F., Keino, H., Hasegawa, M., Ikari, H., Miyake, S., & Hosokawa, M. (2009). Risk of fall for individuals with intellectual disability. *American Journal on Intellectual and Developmental Disabilities, 114*(4), 225–236.

Cioni, M., Cocilovo, A., Rossi, F., Paci, D., & Valle, M. S. (2001). Analysis of ankle kinetics during walking in individuals with Down syndrome. *American Journal of Mental Retardation, 106,* 470–478.

Cipriani, D. J., Terry, M. E., Haines, M. A., Tabibnia, A. P., & Lyssanova, O. (2012). Effect of strength frequency and sex on the rate of gain and rate of loss in muscle flexibility during a hamstring-stretching program: A randomized single-blind longitudinal study. *Journal of Strength and Conditioning Research, 26*(8), 2119–2129.

Cleaver, S., Hunter, D., & Ouellette-Kuntz, H. (2009). Physical mobility limitations in adults with intellectual disabilities: A systematic review. *Journal of Intellectual Disability Research, 53,* 93–105.

Costa, A. C. (2011). An assessment of the vestibulo-ocular reflex (VOR) in persons with Down syndrome. *Experimental Brain Research, 214,* 199–213.

Cox, C. R., Clemson, L., Stancliffe, R. J., Durvasula, S., & Sherrington, C. (2010). Incidence of and risk factors for falls among adults with an intellectual disability. *Journal of Intellectual Disability Research, 54,* 1045–1057.

Creel, G. L., Light, K. E., & Thigpen, M. T. (2001). Concurrent and construct validity of scores on the timed movement battery. *Physical Therapy, 81,* 789–798.

Croce, R. V., Pitetti, K. H., Horvat, M., & Miller, J. (1996). Peak torque, average power, and hamstrings/quadriceps ratios in nondisabled adults and adults with mental retardation. *Archives of Physical Medicine and Rehabilitation, 77*(4), 369–372.

Cuesta-Vargas, A. I., & González-Sánchez, M. (2013). Differences in muscle activation patterns during sit to stand task among subjects with and without intellectual disability. *BioMed Research International, 2013,* 173148. doi:10.1155/2013/173148.

Dagnan, D., & Sandhu, S. (1999). Social comparison, self-esteem and depression in people with intellectual disability. *Journal of Intellectual Disability Research, 43,* 372–379.

Davis, W. E., & Van Emmerik, R. E. A. (1995). An ecological task analysis approach for understanding motor development in mental retardation: Philosophical and theoretical underpinnings. In M. Hebbelinck, R. J. Shephard, A. Vermeer & W. E. Davis (Eds.), Physical and motor development in mental retardation (Vol. 40, pp. 1–32). Basel: Karger.

Davis, W. E., Sparrow, W. A., & Ward, T. (1991). Fractionated reaction times and movement times of Down syndrome and other adults with mental retardation. *Adapted Physical Activity Quarterly, 8,* 221–233.

Day, K., & Jancar, J. (1994). Mental and physical health and ageing in mental handicap: A review. *Journal of Intellectual Disability Research, 38,* 241–256.

Dean, J. C., Alexander, N. B., & Kuo, A. D. (2007). The effect of lateral stabilization on walking in young and old adults. *IEEE Transactions on Biomedical Engineering, 54,* 1919–1926.

Deci, E. L., Koestner, R., & Ryan, R. M. (1999). A meta-analytic review of experiments examining the effects of extrinsic rewards on intrinsic motivation. *Psychological Bulletin, 125,* 627–668.

Dellavia, C., Pallavera, A., Orlando, F., & Sforza, C. (2009). Postural stability of athletes in Special Olympics. *Perceptual and Motor Skills, 108,* 608–622.

DePaepe, J. L., & Ciccaglione, S. (1993). A dynamic balance measure for persons with severe and profound mental retardation. *Perceptual and Motor Skills, 76,* 619–627.

Diever, H. C., Horak, F. B., & Nasher, L. M. (1988). Influence of stimulus parameters on human postural responses. *Journal of Neurophysiology, 59,* 1888–1895.

Dobbins, A. D., & Rarick, L. G. (1977). The performance of intellectually normal and educable mentally retarded boys on tests of throwing accuracy. *Journal of Motor Behavior, 9,* 23–28.

Doke, J., Donelan, J. M., & Kuo, A. D. (2005). Mechanics and energetics of swinging the human leg. *The Journal of Experimental Biology, 208,* 439–445.

Donelan, J. M., Kram, R., & Kuo, A. D. (2001). Mechanical and metabolic determinants of the preferred step width in human walking. *Proceedings. Biological sciences/ The Royal Society, 168,* 1985–1992.

Donelan, J. M., Kram, R., & Kuo, A. D. (2002a). Mechanical work for step-to-step transitions is a major determinant of the metabolic cost of human walking. *The Journal of Experimental Biology, 205,* 3717–3727.

Donelan, J. M., Kram, R., & Kuo, A. D. (2002b). Simultaneous positive and negative external mechanical work in human walking. *Journal of Biomechanics, 35,* 117–124.

Donelan, J. M., Shipman, D. W., Kram, R., & Kuo, A. D. (2004). Mechanical and metabolic requirements for active lateral stabilization in human walking. *Journal of Biomechanics, 37,* 827–835.

Draheim, C. C. (2006). Cardiovascular disease prevalence and risk factors of persons with mental retardation. *Mental Retardation and Developmental Disabilities Research Reviews, 12*(1), 3–12.

Draheim, C. C., Williams, D. P., & McCubbin, J. A. (2002a). Physical activity, dietary intake, and the insulin resistance syndrome in non-diabetic adults with mental retardation. *American Journal of Mental Retardation, 107,* 361–375.

Draheim, C. C., Williams, D. P., & McCubbin, J. A. (2002b). Prevalence of physical inactivity and recommended physical activity in community-based adults with mental retardation. *Mental Retardation, 40*(6), 436–444.

Draheim, C. C., Williams, D. P., & McCubbin, J. A. (2003). Cardiovascular disease risk factor differences between Special Olympians and Non-Special Olympians. *Adapted Physical Activity Quarterly, 20,* 118–134.

Duncan, P., Weiner, D. K., Chandler, J., & Studenski, S. (1990). Functional reach: A new clinical measure of balance. *Journal of Gerontology, 45,* M192–M197.

Dykens, E. M., Rosner, B. A., & Butterbaugh, G. (1998). Exercise and sports in children and adolescents with developmental disabilities: Positive physical and psychosocial effects. *Child and Adolescent Psychiatric Clinics of North America, 7,* 757–771.

England, S. A., & Granata, K. P. (2007). The influence of gait speed on local dynamic stability of walking. *Gait & Posture, 25,* 172–178.

Enkelaar, L., Smulders, E., van Schrojenstein Lantman-de Valk, H., Geurts, A. C., & Weerdesteyn, V. (2012). A review of balance and gait capacities in relation to falls in persons with intellectual disability. *Research in Developmental Disabilities, 33,* 291–306.

Etnier, J. L., & Landers, D. M. (1998). Motor performance and motor learning as a function of age and fitness. *Research Quarterly for Exercise and Sport, 69,* 136–146.

Farley, C. T., & Ferris, D. P. (1998). Biomechanics of walking and running: Center of mass movements to muscle action. *Exercise and Sport Sciences Reviews, 26,* 253–285.

Fasano, A., & Bloem, B. R. (2013). Gait disorders. *Continuum, 19*(5), 1344–1382.

Fernhall, B. (1993). Physical fitness and exercise training of individuals with mental retardation. *Medicine and Science in Sports and Exercise, 25,* 442–450.

Fernhall, B., & Pitetti, K. H. (2000). Leg strength related to endurance run performance in children and adolescents with mental retardation. *Pediatric Exercise Science, 12,* 324–333.

Fernhall, B., Tymeson, G. T., & Webster, G. E. (1988). Cardiovascular fitness of mentally retarded individuals. *Adapted Physical Activity Quarterly, 5*(1), 12–28.

Fernhall, B., Pitetti, K., Stubbs, N. B., Stadler, L., & Stadler, L. J. (1996a). Validity and reliability of the 1/2 mile run-walk as an indicator of aerobic fitness in children with mental retardation. *Pediatric Exercise Science, 8,* 130–142.

Fernhall, B., Pitetti, K. H., Rimmer, J. H., McCubbin, J. A., Rintala, P., Millar, A. L., Kittredge, J., & Burkett, L. N. (1996b). Cardiorespiratory capacity of individuals with mental retardation including Down syndrome. *Medicine and Science in Sports and Exercise, 28,* 366–371.

Fernhall, B., Pitetti, K. H., Vukovich, M. D., Stubbs, N., Hensen, T., Winnick, J. P., & Short, F. X. (1998). Validation of cardiovascular fitness field tests in children with mental retardation. *American Journal of Mental Retardation, 102*(6), 602–012.

Fielding, R. A., Rejeski, W. J., Blair, S., Church, T., Espeland, M. A., Gill, T. M., Guralnik, J. M., Hsu, F. C., Katula, J., King, A. C., Kritchevsky, S. B., McDermott, M. M., Miller, M. E., Nayfield, S., Newman, A. B., Williamson, J. D., Bonds, D., Romashkan, S., Hadley, E., Pahor, M., & LIFE Research Group. (2011). The lifestyle interventions and independence for elders study: Design and methods. *Journals of Gerontology Series A Biological Sciences and Medical Sciences, 66*(11), 1226–1237.

Finlayson, J., Morrison, J., Jackson, A., Mantry, D., & Cooper, S.-A. (2010). Injuries, falls and accidents among adults with intellectual disabilities: Prospective cohort study. *Journal of Intellectual Disability Research, 54,* 966–980.

Frey, G. C., Stanish, H. I., & Temple, V. A. (2008). Physical activity of youth with intellectual disability: Review and research agenda. *Adapted Physical Activity Quarterly, 25*(2), 95–117.
Frzovic, D., Morris, M. E., & Vowels, L. (1994). Clinical tests of standing balance: Performance of persons with multiple sclerosis. *Archives of Physical Medicine and Rehabilitation, 49,* M85–M94.
Gabler-Halle, D., Halle, J. W., & Chung, Y. B. (1993). The effects of aerobic exercise on psychological and behavioral variables of individuals with developmental disabilities: A critical review. *Research in Developmental Disabilities, 14,* 359–386.
Galli, M., Rigoldi, C., Brunner, R., Virji-Babul, N., & Giorgio, A. (2008a). Joint stiffness and gait pattern evaluation in children with Down syndrome. *Gait & Posture, 28,* 502–506.
Galli, M., Rigoldi, C., Mainardi, L., Tenore, N., Onorati, P., & Albertini, G. (2008b). Postural control in patients with Down syndrome. *Disability and Rehabilitation, 30*(17), 1274–1748.
Galli, M., Cimolin, V., Vismara, L., Grugni, G., Camerota, F., Celletti, C., Albertini, G., Rigoldi, C., & Capodaglio, P. (2011). The effects of muscle hypotonia and weakness on balance: A study on Prader-Willi and Ehlers-Danlos syndrome patients. *Research in Developmental Disabilities, 32,* 1117–1121.
Gillespie, L. D., Robertson, M. C., Gillespie, W. J., Lamb, S. E., Gates, S., Cumming, R. G., & Rowe, B. H. (2009). Interventions for preventing falls in older people living in the community. *Cochrane Database System Review, 15*(2), CD007146. doi: 10.1002/14651858.CD007146.pub2.
Gomes, M. M., & Barela, J. A. (2007). Postural control in Down syndrome: The use of somatosensory and visual information to attenuate body sway. *Motor control, 11,* 224–234.
Gontijo, A. P., Mancini, M. C., Silva, P. L., Chagas, P. S., Sampaio, R. F., Luz, R. E., & Fonseca, S. T. (2008). Changes in lower limb co-contraction and stiffness by toddlers with Down syndrome and toddlers with typical development during the acquisition of independent gait. *Human Movement Science, 27,* 610–621.
Graham, A., & Reid, G. (2000). Physical fitness of adults with an intellectual disability: A 13-year follow-up study. *Research Quarterly for Exercise and Sport, 71*(2), 152–161.
Grant, H. J., Pickett, W., Lam, M., O'Connor, M., & Ouellette-Kuntz, H. (2001). Falls among persons who have developmental disabilities in institutional and group home settings. *Journal on Developmental Disabilities, 8*(1), 57–73.
Groden, G. (1969). Relationships between intelligence, simple and complex motor proficiency. *American Journal of Mental Deficiency, 74,* 373–375.
Guidetti, L., Franciosi, E., Gallotta, M. C., Emerenziani, G. P., & Baldari, C. (2010). Could sport specialization influence fitness and health of adults with mental retardation? *Research in Developmental Disabilities, 31,* 1070–1075.
Guralnik, J. M., Simonsick, E. M., Ferrucci, L., Glynn, R. J., Berkman, L. F., Blazer, D. G., Scherr, P. A., Wallace, R. B. (1994). A short physical performance battery assessing lower extremity function: association with self-reported disability and prediction of mortality and nursing home admission. *Journal of Gerontology, 49,* M85–M94.
Gustafson, A. S., Noaksson, L., Kronhed, A. C., Moller, M., & Moller, C. (2000). Changes in balance performance in physically active elderly people aged 73-80. *Scandinavian Journal of Rehabilitation and Medicine, 32,* 168–172.
Haier, R. J., Jung, R. E., Yeo, R. A., Head, K., & Alkire, M. T. (2004). Structural brain variation and general intelligence. *NeuroImage, 23*(1), 425–433.
Hale, L., & Donovan, K. (2014). A video-based balance measure for people with intellectual disability. *Journal of Intellectual and Developmental Disability.* doi:10.3109/13668250.2014.898743.
Hale, L., Bray, A., & Littmann, A. (2007). Assessing the balance capabilities of people with profound intellectual disabilities who have experienced a fall. *Journal of Intellectual Disability Research, 51*(4), 260–268.
Hale, L., Miller, R., Barach, A., Skinner, M., & Gray, A. (2009). Motor control test responses to balance perturbations in adults with an intellectual disability. *Journal of Intellectual and Developmental Disability, 34*(1), 81–86.

Hale, L., McIlraith, L., Miller, C., Stanley-Clarke, T., & George, R. (2010). The interrater reliability of the modified gait abnormality rating scale for use with people with intellectual disability. *Journal of Intellectual Disability Research, 35*(2), 77–81.

Hall, J. M., & Thomas, M. J. (2008). Promoting physical activity and exercise in older adults with developmental disabilities. *Topics in Geriatric Rehabilitation, 24,* 64–73.

Hassani, A., Kotzamanidou, M. C., Fotiadou, E., Patikas, D., Evagelinou, C., & Sakadami, N. (2013). Neuromuscular differences between pubescent boys with and without mental retardation during squat jump. *Research in Developmental Disabilities, 34,* 2856–2863. doi:10.1016/j.ridd.2013.05.046.

Hassani, A., Kotzamanidou, M. C., Tsimaras, V., Lazaridis, S., Kotzamanidis, C., & Patikas, D. (2014). Differences in counter-movement jump between boys with and without intellectual disability. *Research in Developmental Disabilities, 35*(7), 1433–1438. doi:10.1016/j.ridd.2014.03.034.

Haynes, C. A., & Lockhart, T. E. (2012). Evaluation of gait and slip parameters for adults with intellectual disability. *Journal of Biomechanics, 45,* 2337–2341.

Heller, T., Hsieh, K., & Rimmer, J. H. (2004). Attitudinal and psychological outcomes of a fitness and health education program on adults with Down syndrome. *American Journal of Mental Retardation, 109,* 175–185.

Hemayattalab, R., & Movahedi, A. (2010). Effects of different variations of mental and physical practice on sport skill learning in adolescents with mental retardation. *Research in Developmental Disabilities, 31,* 81–86.

Hilgenkamp, T. I., van Wijck, R., & Evenhuis, H. M. (2012). Low physical fitness levels in older adults with ID: Results of the HA-ID study. *Research in Developmental Disabilities, 33,* 1148–1158.

Hinckson, E. A., Dickinson, A., Water, T., & Sands, M., Penman, L. (2013). Physical activity, dietary habits and overall health in overweight and obese children and youth with intellectual disability or autism. *Research in Developmental Disabilities, 34*(4), 1170–1178.

Hocking, J., Pearson, A., & McNeil, J. (2014). Physiotherapy to improve gross motor skills in people with intellectual disability: A systematic review protocol. *JBI Database of Systematic Reviews and Implementation Reports, 11*(12), 94–108. doi:10.11124/jbisrir-2013-1180.

Horvat, M., & Franklin, C. (2001). The effects of the environment on physical activity patterns of children with mental retardation. *Research Quarterly for Exercise and Sport, 72*(2), 189–195.

Horvat, M., Pitetti, K. H., & Croce, R. J. (1997). Isokinetic torque, average power, and flexion/extension ratios in nondisabled adults and adults with mental retardation. *Journal of Orthopaedic and Sports Physical Therapy, 25,* 395–399.

Horvat, M., Croce, R., Pitetti, K. H., & Fernhall, B. (1999). Comparison of isokinetic peak force and work parameters in youth with and without mental retardation. *Medicine and Science in Sports and Exercise, 31,* 1190–1195.

Horvat, M., Ramsey, V., Amestoy, R., & Croce, R. (2003). Muscle activation and movement responses in youth with and without mental retardation. *Research Quarterly for Exercise and Sport, 74,* 319–323.

Horvat, M., Croce, R., Zagrodnik, J., Brooks, B., & Carter, K. (2012). Spatial and temporal variability of movement parameters in individuals with Down syndrome. *Perceptual and Motor Skills, 114*(3), 774–782.

Howe, C. E. (1959). A cmoparison of motor skills of mentally retarded and normal children. *Council for Exceptional Children, 25,* 352–354.

Hsieh, K., Heller, T., & Miller, A. B. (2001). Risk factors for injuries and falls among adults with developmental disabilities. *Journal of Intellectual Disability Research, 45*(1), 76–82.

Hsieh, K., Rimmer, J., & Heller, T. (2012). Prevalence of falls and risk factors in adults with intellectual disability. *American Journal on Intellectual and Developmental Disabilities, 117*(6), 442–454.

Iivanainen, M. (1998). Phenytoin: Effective but insidious therapy for epilepsy in people with intellectual disability. *Journal of Intellectual Disability Research, 42*(suppl. 1), 24–31.

Inui, N., Yamanishi, M., & Tada, S. (1995). Simple reaction times and timing of serial reactions of adolescents with mental retardation, autism, and Down syndrome. *Perceptual and Motor Skills, 81,* 739–745.

Isles, R. C., Choy, N. L., Steer, M., & Nitz, J. C. (2004). Normal values of balance tests in women aged 20-80. *Journal of the American Geriatrics Society, 52,* 1367–1372.

Jaffe, J. S., Timell, A. M., Elolia, R., & Thatcher, S. S. (2005). Risk factors for low bone mineral density in individuals residing in a facility for the people with intellectual disability. *Journal of Intellectual Disability Research, 49*(Part 6), 457–462.

Janicki, M. P., & Dalton, A. J. (2000). Prevalence of dementia and impact on intellectual disability services. *Mental Retardation, 38,* 276–288.

Janicki, M. P., & Jacobson, J. W. (1986). Generational trends in sensory, physical and behavioral abilities among older mentally retarded persons. *American Journal of Mental Deficiency, 90*(5), 490–500.

Janicki, M. P., Dalton, A. J., Henderson, C. M., & Davidson, P. W. (1991). Mortality and morbidity among older adults with intellectual disability: Health services considerations. *Disability and Rehabilitation, 21*(5–6), 284–294.

Janicki, M. P., Dalton, A. J., Henderson, C. M., & Davidson, P. W. (1999). Mortality and morbidity among older adults with intellectual disability: Health service considerations. *Disability and Rehabilitation, 21,* 284–294.

Janicki, M. P., Davidson, P. W., Henderson, C. M., McCallion, P., Taets, J. D., Force, L. T., Sulkes, S. B., Frangenberg, E., & Ladrigan, P. M. (2002). Health characteristics and health services utilization in older adults with intellectual disability living in community residences. *Journal of Intellectual Disability Research, 46*(4), 287–298.

Jensen, J., Nyberg, L., Gustafson, Y., & Lundin-Olsson, L. (2003). Fall and injury prevention in residential care—effects in residents with higher and lower levels of cognition. *Journal of the American Geriatrics Society, 51,* 627–635.

Jerome, L. B., Boyette, L. W., Gaasch, D. A., & Lloyd, A. (2000). Effects of lower extremity strength training on functional mobility in older adults. *Journal of Aging and Physical Activity, 8*(3), 214–227.

Kapell, D., Nightingale, B., Rodriguez, A., Lee, J. H., Zigman, W. B., & Schupf, N. (1998). Prevalence of chronic medical conditions in adults with mental retardation: Comparison with the general population. *Mental Retardation, 36,* 269–279.

Kioumourtzoglou, E., Batsiou, S., Theodorakis, Y., & Mauromatis, G. (1994). Selected motor skills of mentally retarded and nonretarded individuals. *Perceptual and Motor Skills, 78,* 1011–1015.

Ko, Y. G., Van Emmerik, R. E., Sprague, R. L., & Newell, K. M. (1992). Postural stability, tardive dyskinesia and developmental disability. *Journal of Intellectual Disability Research, 36*(4), 309–323.

Kokubun, M., & Koike, T. (1995). Problems in balance performance in mental retardation. In A. Vermeer & W. E. Davis (Eds.), Physical and motor development in mental retardation (Vol. 40, pp. 191–197). Basel: Karger.

Kokubun, M., Shinmyo, T., Ogita, M., Morita, K., Furuta, M., Haishi, K., Okuzumi, H., & Koike, T. (1997). Comparison of postural control of children with Down syndrome and those with other forms of mental retardation. *Perceptual and Motor Skills, 84*(2), 499–504.

Kubo, M., & Ulrich, B. (2006a). Coordination of pelvis-HAT (head, arms and trunk) in anterior-posterior and medio-lateral directions during treadmill gait in preadolescents with/without Down syndrome. *Gait & Posture, 23,* 512–518.

Kubo, M., & Ulrich, B. D. (2006b). Early stage of walking: Development of control in mediolateral and anteroposterior directions. *Journal of Motor Behavior, 38*(3), 229–237.

Kuo, A. D. (2007). The six determinants of gait and the inverted pendulum analogy: A dynamic walking perspective. *Human Movement Science, 26,* 617–656.

Kurtz, L. A. (2008). *Understanding motor skills in children with dyspraxia, ADHD, autism, and other learning disabilities*. London: Jessica Kingsley Publishers.

Lahtinen, U., Rintala, P., & Malin, A. (2007). Physical performance of individuals with intellectual disability: A 30-year follow up. *Adapted Physical Activity Quarterly, 24,* 125–143.

Latash, M. L. (2000). Motor coordination in Down syndrome: The role of adaptive changes. In D. J. Weeks, R. Chua, & D. Elliott (Eds.), *Perceptual-motor behavior in Down syndrome* (pp. 199–223). Champaign: Human Kinetics.

Latash, M. L., Kang, N., & Patterson, D. (2002). Finger coordination in persons with Down syndrome: Atypical patterns of coordination and the effects of practice. *Experimental Brain Research, 146,* 345–355.

LeClair, D. A., Pollock, B. J., & Elliott, D. (1993). Movement preparation in adults with and without Down syndrome. *American Journal of Mental Retardation, 97,* 628–633.

Lin, S. I., & Woollacott, M. (2005). Association between sensorimotor function and functional and reactive balance control in the elderly. *Age and Ageing, 34,* 558–563.

Lin, J.-D., Lin, L.-P., Hsia, Y.-C., Hsu, S.-W., Wu, C.-L., & Chu, C. M. (2014). A national survey of caregivers' perspective of early symptoms of dementia among adults with an intellectual disability based on the DSQIID scale. *Research in Autism Spectrum Disorders, 8,* 275–280.

Livingstone, B., & Hirst, P. (1986). Orthopedic disorders in school children with Down's syndrome with special reference to the incidence of joint laxity. *Clinical Orthopaedics and Related Research, 207,* 74–78.

Lohiya, G. S., Crinella, F. M., Tan-Figueroa, L., Caires, S., & Lohiya, S. (1999). Fracture epidemiology and control in a developmental center. *The Western Journal of Medicine, 170,* 203–209.

Lotan, M., Yalon-Chamovitz, S., & Weiss, P. L. (2009). Improving physical fitness of individuals with intellectual and developmental disability through a virtual reality intervention program. *Research in Developmental Disabilities, 30,* 229–239.

Maiano, C., Ninot, G., & Errais, B. (2001). Effects of alternate sport competition in perceived competence for adolescent males with mild to moderate mental retardation. *International Journal of Rehabilitation Research, 24,* 51–58.

Matson, J. L., Mayville, S. B., & Laud, R. B. (2003). A system of assessment for adaptive behavior, social skills, behavioral function, medication sideeffects, and psychiatric disorders. *Research in Developmental Disabilities, 24,* 75–81.

McArdle, W. D., Katch, F. I., & Katch, V. L. (2007). *Exercise physiology: Energy, nutrition, and human performance*. Baltimore: Lippincott Williams & Wilkins.

McAuley, E., Blissmer, B., Katula, J., Duncan, T. E., & Mihalko, S. L. (2000). Physical activity, self-esteem, and self-efficacy relationships in adults: A randomized controlled trial. *Annals of Behavioral Medicine, 22*(2), 131–139.

Nebes, R. D. (1990). Hemispheric specialization in the aged brain. In C. Threvarthen (Ed.), *Brain circuits and functions of the mind. Essays in honor of Roger W. Sperry*. New York: Cambridge University Press.

Newell, K. M. (1997). Motor skills and mental retardation. In W. E. MacLean, Jr. (Ed.), *Ellis'handbook of mental deficiency: Psychological theory and research* (pp. 275–308). Mahwah: Erlbaum.

Ninot, G., Bilard, J., & Sokolowski, M. (2000). Athletic competition: A mean of improving the self-image of mentally retarded adolescent? *International Journal of Rehabilitation Research, 23,* 111–117.

Nottestad, J. A., & Linaker, O. M. (1999). Psychiatric health needs and services before and after complete deinstitutionalization of people with intellectual disability. *Journal of Intellectual Disability Research, 43,* 523–530.

Ohwada, H., Nakayama, T., Suzuki, Y., Yokoyama, T., & Ishimaru, M. (2005). Energy expenditure in males with mental retardation. *Journal of Nutritional Science and Vitaminology, 51,* 68–74.

Okuzumi, H., Tanaka, A., & Haishi, K. (1997). Relationship between age and head movement during stepping in place by nonhandicapped children and persons with mental retardation. *Perceptual and Motor Skills, 85,* 375–381.

Õunpuu, S. (1994). The biomechanics of walking and running. *Clinics in Sports Medicine, 13*(4), 843–863.

Parker, A. W., & Bronks, R. (1980). Gait of children with Down syndrome. *Archives of Physical Medicine and Rehabilitation, 61,* 345–351.

Parker, A. W., Bronks, R., & Snyder, C. W., Jr (1986). Walking patterns in Down's syndrome. *Journal of Mental Deficiency Research, 30*(4), 317–330.
Pinter, J. D., Eliez, S., Schmitt, J. E., Capone, G. T., & Reiss, A. L. (2001). Neuroanatomy of Down's syndrome: A high-resolution MRI study. *American Journal of Psychiatry, 158,* 1659–1665.
Pitetti, K., & Fernhall, B. (1997). Aerobic capacity as related to leg strength in youths with mental retardation. *Pediatric Exercise Science, 9,* 223–236.
Pitetti, K. H., Climstein, M., Mays, M. J., & Barrett, P. J. (1992). Isokinetic arm and leg strength of adults with Down syndrome: A comparative study. *Archives of Physical Medicine and Rehabilitation, 73,* 847–850.
Pitetti, K. H., Yarmer, D. A., & Fernhall, B. (2001). Cardiovascular fitness and body composition of youth with and without mental retardation. *Adapted Physical Activity Quarterly, 18,* 127–141.
Podsiadlo, D., & Richardson, S. (1991). The 'Timed up and Go': A test of basic functional mobility for frail elderly persons. *Journal of the American Geriatrics Society, 39,* 142–148.
Powell, L. E., & Myers, A. M. (1995). The Activities-specific Balance Confidence (ABC) scale. *Journal of Gerontology, 50A,* M28–M34.
Pritchard, T. C., & Alloway, K. D. (2007). *Medical neuroscience* (2nd ed.). Raleigh: Hayes Barton Press.
Rarick, G. L. (1973). Motor perfomance of mentally retarded children. In G. L. Rarick (Ed.), *Physical activity: Human growth and development* (pp. 225–256). New York: Academic Press.
Rarick, G. L., Widdop, J. H., & Broadhead, G. (1970). The physical fitness and motor performance of educable mentally retarded children. *Council for Exceptional Children, 36*(7), 509–519.
Rigoldi, C., Galli, M., Mainardi, L., Crivellini, M., & Albertini, G. (2011). Postural control in children, teenagers and adults with Down syndrome. *Research in Developmental Disabilities, 32,* 170–175.
Rimmer, J. H., & Yamaki, K. (2006). Obesity and intellectual disability. *Mental Retardation and Developmental Disabilities Research Reviews, 12,* 22–27.
Rimmer, J. H., Braddock, D., & Fujiura, G. (1994). Cardiovascular disease risk factors in adults with mental retardation. *American Journal of Mental Retardation, 98,* 510–518.
Sackley, C., Richardson, P., McDonnell, K., Ratib, S., & Dewey, M. (2005). The reliability of balance, mobility and self-care measures in a population of adults with a learning disability known to a physiotherapy service. *Clinical Rehabilitation, 19,* 216–223.
Sayer, A. A., Syddall, H. E., Martin, H. J., Dennison, E. M., Roberts, H. C., & Cooper, C. (2006). Is grip strength associated with healthrelated quality of life? Findings from the Hertfordshire Cohort Study. *Age and Ageing, 35,* 409–415.
Schonknecht, P., Pantel, J., Kruse, A., & Schroder, J. (2005). Prevalence and natural course of aging-associated cognitive decline in a population-based sample of young-old subjects. *American Journal of Psychiatry, 162,* 2071–2077.
Shaw, F. E., Bond, J., Richardson, D. A., Dawson, P., Steen, I. N., McKeith, I. G., & Kenny, R. A. (2003). Multifactorial intervention after a fall in older people with cognitive impairment and dementia presenting to the accident and emergency department: Randomised controlled trial. *British Medical Journal, 326,* 73–79.
Sherrard, J., Tonge, B. J., & Ozanne-Smith, J. (2001). Injury in young people with intellectual disability: Descriptive epidemiology. *Injury Prevention: Journal of the International Society for Child and Adolescent Injury Prevention, 7*(1), 56–61.
Shinkfield, A. J., Sparrow, W. A., & Day, R. H. (1997). Visual discrimination and motor reproduction of movement by individuals with mental retardation. *American Journal of Mental Retardation, 102,* 172–181.
Shumway-Cook, A., & Horak, F. (1986). Assessing the influence of sensory interaction on balance. *Physical Therapy, 66,* 1545–1550.
Shumway-Cook, A., & Woollacott, M. (2001). *Motor Control: Theory and Practical Applications* (2nd ed.). Baltimore: Lippincott Co.

Skowronski, W., Horvat, M., Nocera, J., Roswal, G., & Croce, R. (2009). Eurofit Special: European fitness battery score variation among individuals with intellectual disabilities. *Adapted Physical Activity Quarterly, 26,* 54–67.

Smith, B. A., & Ulrich, B. D. (2008). Early onset of stabilizing strategies for gait and obstacles: Older adults with Down syndrome. *Gait & Posture, 28,* 448–455.

Smith, B. A., Kubo, M., Black, D. P., Holt, K. G., & Ulrich, B. D. (2007). Effect of practice on a novel task-walking on a treadmill: Preadolescents with and without Down syndrome. *Physical Therapy, 87,* 766–777.

Sparrow, S. S., & Cicchetti, D. V. (1985). Diagnostic use of the Vineland Adaptive Behavior Scales. *Journal of Pediatric Psychology, 10,* 215–225.

Sparrow, W. A., & Day, R. H. (2002). Perception and action in mental retardation. In L. M. Glidden (Ed.), *International review of research in mental retardation* (Vols. 241–278). San Diego: Academic Press.

Sparrow, W. A., Shinkfield, A. J., & Summers, J. J. (1998). Gait characteristics in individuals with mental retardation: Unobstructed level-walking, negotiating obstacles, and stair climbing. *Human Movement Science, 17,* 167–187.

Speechley, M., & Tinetti, M. (1991). Falls and injuries in frail and vigorous community elderly persons. *Journal of the American Geriatrics Society, 39,* 46–52.

Sperry, R. W. (1990). Forebrain commissurotomy and conscious awareness. In C. Threvarthen (Ed.), *Brain circuits and functions of the mind. Essays in honor of Roger W. Sperry.* New York: Cambridge University Press.

Srikanth, R., Cassidy, G., Joiner, C., & Teeluckdharry, S. (2011). Osteoporosis in people with intellectual disabilities: A review and a brief study of risk factors for osteoporosis in a community sample of people with intellectual disabilities. *Journal of Intellectual Disability Research, 55,* 53–62.

Stanish, H. I., & Draheim, C. C. (2005). Physical activity assessment using pedometer and questionnaire in adults with mental retardation. *Adapted Physical Activity Quarterly, 22,* 136–145.

Stanish, H. I., & Draheim, C. C. (2006). Walking activity, body composition and blood pressure in adults with intellectual disabilities. *Journal of Applied Research in Intellectual Disabilities, 20*(3), 183–190.

Stanish, H. I., McCubbin, J. A., Draheim, C. C., & van der Mars, H. (2001). Participation of adults with mental retardation in a video- and leader-directed aerobic dance program. *Adapted Physical Activity Quarterly, 18,* 142–155.

Stanish, H. I., Temple, V. A., & Frey, G. C. (2006). Health-promoting physical activity of adults with mental retardation. *Mental Retardation and Developmental Disabilities Research Reviews, 12,* 13–21.

Steffen, T. M., Hacker, T. A., & Mollinger, L. (2002). Age- and gender-related test performance in community-dwelling elderly people: Six-minute walk test, Berg Balance Scale, timed up & go test, and gait speeds. *Physical Therapy, 82,* 128–137.

Stenholm, S., Tiainen, K., Rantanen, T., Sainio, P., Heliövaara, M., Impivaara, O., & Koskinen, S. (2012). Long-term determinants of muscle strength decline: Prospective evidence from the 22-year mini-Finland follow-up survey. *Journal of the American Geriatrics Society, 60*(1), 77–85.

Stopka, C. B., Zambito, K. L., Suro, D. G., Pearson, K. S., Siders, R. A., & Goff, B. H. (1998). Muscular endurance and physical capacity to perform work of adolescents with mental retardation. *Journal of Sport Rehabilitation, 7,* 197–205.

Suomi, R., & Koceja, D. M. (1994). Postural sway patterns of normal men and women and men with mental retardation during a two-legged stance test. *Archives of Physical Medicine and Rehabilitation, 75,* 205–209.

Tang, P. F., Moore, S., & Woollacott, M. H. (1998). Correlation between two clinical balance measures in older adults: Functional mobility and sensory organization test. *Journals of Gerontology Series A Biological Sciences and Medical Sciences, 53,* M140–M146.

Tannenbaum, T. N., Lipworth, L., & Baker, S. (1989). Risk of fractures in an intermediate care facility for persons with mental retardation. *American Journal of Mental Retardation, 93,* 444–451.

Temple, V., & Walkley, J. (2003). Physical activity of adults with intellectual disability. *Journal of Intellectual Disability Research, 28,* 342–352.
Temple, V. A., & Walkley, J. W. (2007). Perspectives of constraining and enabling factors for health promoting physical activity by adults with intellectual disability. *Journal of Intellectual and Developmental Disability, 32*(1), 28–38.
Tinetti, M. E. (1986). Performance-oriented assessment of mobility problems in elderly patients. *Journal of the American Geriatrics Society, 34,* 119–126.
Tinetti, M. E., Williams, T. F., & Mayewski, R. (1986). Fall risk index for elderly patients based on number of chronic disabilities. *American Journal of Medicine, 80*(3), 429–434.
Tinetti, M. E., Speechley, M., & Ginter, S. F. (1988). Risk factors for falls among elderly persons living in the community. *The New England Journal of Medicine, 319,* 1701–1707.
Tsimaras, V. K., & Fotiadou, E. G. (2004). Effect of training on the muscle strength and dynamic balance ability of adults with Down syndrome. *Journal of Strength and Conditioning Research, 18,* 343–347.
Turner, S., & Moss, S. (1996). The health needs of adults with learning disabilities and the health of the nation strategy. *Journal of Intellectual Disability Research, 40,* 438–450.
Ulrich, D. A., Ulrich, B. D., Angulo-Kinzler, R. M., & Yun, J. (2001). Treadmill training of infants with Down syndrome: Evidence-based developmental outcomes. *Pediatrics, 108,* E84.
Ulrich, B. D., Haehl, V., Buzzi, U. H., Kubo, M., & Holt, K. G. (2004). Modeling dynamic resource untilization in populations with unique constraints: Preadolescents with and without Down syndrome. *Human Movement Science, 23,* 133–156.
Un, N., & Erbahceci, F. (2001). The evaluation of reaction time on mentally retarded children. *Pediatric Rehabilitation, 4,* 17–20.
Urv, T. K., Zigman, W. B., & Silverman, W. (2003). Maladaptive behaviors related to adaptive decline in aging adults with mental retardation. *American Journal of Mental Retardation, 108,* 327–339.
Van De Vliet, P., Rintala, P., Fröjd, K., Verellen, J., van Houtte, S., Daly, D. J., & Vanlandewijck, Y. C. (2006). Physical fitness profile of elite athletes with intellectual disability. *Scandinavian Journal of Medicine and Science in Sports, 16*(6), 417–425.
van Dijk, P. T., Meulenberg, O. G., van de Sande, H. J., & Habbema, J. D. (1993). Falls in dementia patients. *The Gerontologist, 33*(2), 200–204.
Van Emmerik, R. E., Sprague, R. L., & Newell, K. M. (1993). Quantification of postural sway patterns in tardive dyskinesia. *Movement disorders: Official Journal of the Movement Disorder Society, 8,* 305–314.
Vereeck, L., Wuyts, F., Truijen, S., & Van de Heyning, P. (2008). Clinical assessment of balance: Normative data, and gender and age effects. *International Journal of Audiology, 47,* 67–75.
Verghese, J., Holtzer, R., Lipton, R. B., & Wang, C. (2009). Quantitative gait markers and incident fall risk in older adults. *Journals of Gerontology Series A Biological Sciences and Medical Sciences, 64,* 896–901.
Virji-Babul, N., & Brown, M. (2004). Stepping over obstacles: Anticipatory modifications in children with and without Down syndrome. *Experimental Brain Research, 159,* 487–490.
Vuijk, P. J., Hartman, E., Scherder, E., & Visscher, C. (2010). Motor performance of children with mild intellectual disability and borderline intellectual functioning. *Journal of Intellectual Disability Research, 54*(11), 955–965.
Wade, M. G., Newell, K. M., & Wallace, S. A. (1978). Decision time and movement time as a function of response complexity in retarded persons. *American Journal of Mental Deficiency, 83,* 135–144.
Wagemans, A., & Cluitmans, J. (2006). Falls and fractures: A major health risk for adults with intellectual disabilities in residential settings. *Journal of Policy and Practice in Intellectual Disabilities, 3,* 136–138.
Wang, W. Y., & Ju, Y. H. (2002). Promoting balance and jumping skills in children with Down syndrome. *Perceptual and Motor Skills, 94,* 443–448.
Wark, S., Hussain, R., & Edwards, H. (2014). The training needs of staff supporting individuals ageing with intellectual disability. *Journal of Applied Research in Intellectual Disabilities, 27*(3), 273–288.

Webber, A., Virji-Babul, N., Edwards, R., & Lesperance, M. (2004). Stiffness and postural stability in adults with Down syndrome. *Experimental Brain Research, 155,* 450–458.

Wennie Huang, W. N., Perera, S., VanSwearingen, J., & Studenski, S. (2010). Performance measures predict onset of activity of daily living difficulty in community-dwelling older adults. *Journal of the American Geriatrics Society, 58*(5), 844–852.

Willgoss, T. G., Yohannes, A. M., & Mitchell, D. (2010). Review of risk factors and preventative strategies for fall-related injuries in people with intellectual disabilities. *Journal of Clinical Nursing, 19,* 2100–2109.

Winter, D. A. (2005). *Biomechanics and motor control of human movement.* Hoboken: Wiley.

Wolfson, L. M., Whipple, R., Amerman, P., & Tobin, J. N. (1990). Gait assessment in the elderly: A gait abnormality rating scale and its relation to falls. *Journal of Gerontology, 45,* M12–M19.

Wolfson, L., Judge, J., Whipple, R., & King, M. (1995). Strength is a major factor in balance, gait, and the occurrence of falls. *Journals of Gerontology Series A Biological Sciences and Medical Sciences, 50,* 64–67.

Wu, J., Looper, J., Ulrich, B. D., Ulrich, D. A., & Angulo-Barroso, R. M. (2007). Exploring effects of different treadmill interventions on Walking onset and gait patterns in infants with Down syndrome. *Developmental Medicine and Child Neurology, 49,* 839–845.

Wu, J., Ulrich, D. A., Looper, J., Tiernan, C. W., & Angulo-Barroso, R. M. (2008). Strategy adoption and locomotor adjustment in obstacle clearance of newly walking toddlers with Down syndrome after different treadmill interventions. *Experimental Brain Research, 186,* 261–272.

Yanardag, M., Arikan, H., Yilmaz, I., & Konukman, F. (2013). Physical fitness levels of young adults with and without intellectual disability. *Kinesiology: International Journal of Fundamental and Applied Kinesiology, 45*(2), 233–240.

Yu, C., Li, J., Liu, Y., Qin, W., Li, Y., Shu, N., & … Li, K. (2008). White matter tract integrity and intelligence in patients with mental retardation and healthy adults. *NeuroImage, 40,* 1533–1541.

Zafeiridis, A., Giagazoglou, P., Dipla, K., Salonikidis, K., Karra, C., & Kellis, E. (2010). Muscle fatigue during intermittent exercise in individuals with mental retardation. *Research in Developmental Disabilities, 31,* 388–396.

Chapter 12
An Overview of Cerebral Palsy

Matthew J. Konst and Johnny L. Matson

Cerebral Palsy (CP)

A universal definition for CP has not yet been agreed upon (Morris 2007). The description proposed by Bax (1964) remains one of the most prevalently cited in the literature and identifies CP as "a disorder of posture and movement due to a defect or lesion in the immature brain." It is important to note that in its simplicity Bax's definition also excludes disorders of posture and movement that are due exclusively to mental deficiency, a progressive disease, or were exhibited for a short period of time. However, researchers criticize this definition because it underemphasizes the consequences of brain damage acquired after birth and neglects other impairments that are observed in individuals with defect or lesion induced movement and posture disorders (i.e., sensory, behavioral, and cognitive impairments; Rosenbaum et al. 2007).

More recently, researchers have suggested that CP be conceptualized as an umbrella term that encompasses multiple components: (a) permanent but not static deficits; (b) impaired movement, posture, and motor functioning; and (c) that is the result of a nonprogressive abnormality, interference, or lesion in the developing brain (Mutch et al. 1992; Surveillance of Cerebral Palsy in Europe 2000). Himmelmann et al. (2006) observed that half of those with CP mainly evince impaired motor functioning, while the remaining half have additional major impairments (e.g., cognitive and/or sensory deficits) adding to the disability and negatively impacting activity level and participation (Rosenbaum et al. 2007; World Health Organization 2001). Although the debate surrounding the definition of CP continues, it does not create controversy surrounding current prevalence rate estimates.

M. J. Konst (✉)
Clinical Psychology, Department of Psychology, Louisiana State University, Baton Rouge, LA, USA
e-mail: mkonst1@lsu.edu

J. L. Matson
Department of Psychology, Louisiana State University, Baton Rouge, LA, USA

J. L. Matson, M. L. Matson (eds.), *Comorbid Conditions in Individuals with Intellectual Disabilities,* Autism and Child Psychopathology Series,
DOI 10.1007/978-3-319-15437-4_12

Prevalence

Despite disagreement surrounding a universally accepted definition of CP, researchers consistently report that CP affects 2–3 per 1000 live births and that it is one of the most common causes of severe physical disability in children (Himmelmann et al. 2005; Surveillance of Cerebral Palsy in Europe 2000). Eight European countries orchestrated the construction of the Surveillance of Cerebral Palsy in Europe (SCPE). This created a network of countries that identified diagnostic criteria for CP in order to estimate the prevalence of CP among their respective areas. These rates (2–3 per 1000) are similar to those observed in other parts of the world such as Australia (2.0–2.5 per 1000; Reddihough and Collins 2003), China (1.6 per 1000; Liu et al. 1999), and the USA (2.12 per 1000; Haerer et al. 1984).

Persons with intellectual disability (ID) are known to be at an increased risk for exhibiting health problems (Schrojenstein Lantman-de Valk et al. 1997). Further, within ID populations, those with severe and profound levels of ID are suggested to be at elevated risk for developing health problems in comparison to higher functioning individuals with ID (Moss et al. 1993). In a review of research investigating premature and low birth weight infants, ID was the most common disability (14%) while CP was the second most frequent (8–12%; Lorenz et al. 1998). Coinciding with the increased prevalence of ID in comparison to CP, researchers have demonstrated their common co-occurrence. An epidemiological study of CP in England and Scotland observed prevalence rates similar to those already presented. Further, of the 1649 infants identified as having CP, nearly one quarter ($n=381$) were identified as having an IQ less than 50 (Pharoah et al. 1998). In a longitudinal study of 909 individuals with CP, 44% had an IQ less than 70, and 26% had an IQ less than 50 (Dolk et al. 2006). The results of an international study of CP reported that 23–44% of the CP population studied had an IQ less than 70 (Cans, 2000). Currently, the estimated prevalence of ID in CP populations ranges from 50 to 70% (Boyle and Lary 1996; Fennel and Dikel 2001; Green and Hurvitz 2007; Hodapp 1998; Liptak and Accardo 2004; Nordmark et al. 2001). Conversely, the estimated prevalence rate of CP in ID populations ranges from 8.4 to17% (Boyle and Lary 1996; Christianson et al. 2002).

Contributing Factors

To date, no individual cause of CP has been identified. It is generally agreed that it may result from a variety of prenatal, perinatal, and postnatal causes (e.g., periventricular and intraventricular hemorrhagic lesions, cerebrovascular malformations, intrauterine infections, hypoxia-ischemia lesions, defects early in fetal development, and CNS infections; Lou, 1998). Researchers suggest that approximately half of all CP cases identified may be accounted for by congenital factors and that another 10–14% may be due to asphyxiation at birth (Tomlin 1995; Torfs et al. 1990).

Increase in the prevalence of CP have been attributed to increased survival rates of low birth weight infants following improvements in neonatal care (Beckung et al. 2007; Hagberg et al. 1989). Specifically, the likelihood of CP has been demonstrated to increase as birth weight decreases. In comparison to the rates of CP overall (2–3 per 1000; Himmelmann et al. 2005; SCPE 2000), Dolk et al. (2006) observed a prevalence rate of 44.5 per 1000 live births when infants weighed less than 1500 g. Some researchers have also identified socioeconomic status (SES) as a significant factor in CP prevalence (Brooks-Gunn et al. 1996; Yeargin-Allsopp et al. 1995). A study in the United Kingdom identified significantly lower rates of CP (2.08 per 1000) in high SES families when compared to low SES families (3.33 per 1000; Dolk et al. 2001; Dowding and Barry 1990). Ethnicity has also been identified as a risk-factor and is associated with the presence of both ID and CP. Although this disparity may be related to differences in SES, researchers have also observed higher rates of CP and ID in African American children (Boyle and Lary 1996; Haerer et al. 1984; Murphy et al. 1995; Torfs et al. 1990). Torrey et al. (2000) have additionally suggested a correlation between birth season and the prevalence of CP. The authors proposed that rates of CP were higher among those born in the summer given the negative effect of maternal infection occurring during the winter and spring seasons.

The genetic factors surrounding the development and exhibition of CP remain controversial and unclear. For instance, in a pilot study of very preterm infants, Nelson et al. (2005) identified several single nucleotide polymorphisms (SNPs) that may be linked with CP development. However, they noted that these associations were variable and largely dependent upon multiple factors to include ethnicity. Further, although the rates of familial inheritance among siblings is low (Bundey and Brett 1985), it is noted to be significantly greater than that observed in the general population (Petterson et al. 1990). Further, the concordance rate of CP is reportedly significantly greater in monozygotic twins when compared to dizygotic twins (Petterson et al. 1990). This observation suggests that there may be an underlying genetic vulnerability. However, researchers continue to recognize that multiple contributing factors are present (Nelson et al. 2005; Petterson et al. 1990). Despite the observed increase in prevalence of CP in monozygotic twins and increased risk among families, little research surrounding genetic contributions has been carried out (Nelson et al. 2005).

Mortality

The negative relationship between impaired mobility and life expectancy is well documented (Eyman et al. 1990; Eyman et al. 1987; Roboz 1972). Profound motor impairments are a significant predictor of early mortality. In a large population-based study of persons with CP in Western Australia, Blair et al. (2001) noted a mortality rate of 1 % per year for the first 5 years of life. A slight decrease in the observed mortality rate was reported up until approximately 15 years of age where it is suggested to remain steady at approximately 0.35 %.

While analyzing mortality rates in CP populations, Blair et al. (2001) reported that the presence of ID was the single strongest predictor of mortality. Additional research has demonstrated that specific factors significantly increase mortality rates in populations with both ID and CP. The most prevalent predictors of mortality are deficits in mobility, severity level of ID, and self-care skills (e.g., toileting and feeding; Eyman et al. 1987; Eyman et al. 1988; Eyman et al. 1989; Miller and Eyman 1978). Tarjan et al. (1968) observed a positive correlation between the severity of ID and physical handicaps and death by respiratory infections. Mortality rates were significantly related to the observed level of ID such that only 50 % of children with IQ/DQ scores less than 20 survived to adulthood. Survival rates increased to 76 % when IQ/DQ scores ranged from 20–34 and 92 % for those with higher scores. Researchers continue to identify respiratory problems as a common cause of death in CP populations. For example, an analysis of individuals in Western Australia with CP across 36 years (1958–1994) suggested that 59 % of deaths were related to respiratory problems (Liptak and Accardo 2004).

Classification

There are multiple classification schemas used for diagnosis, treatment, and research purposes surrounding CP. The selection of various criteria is often influenced by the researcher or clinician's background and/or purpose (e.g., neurosurgeons, pediatricians, and orthopedic surgeons). Regardless of the approach selected, the classification of CP should generally include a description and consideration of four broad areas: motor abilities, neuro-imaging and anatomical observations, comorbid impairments, and consideration of causation and timing (Rosenbaum et al. 2007). Classification of the impairments associated with CP is often based upon factors such as motor functioning, topographical distribution of the deficits observed, and severity level. Similar to the four-part classification system for ID, the classification of the severity of CP utilizes three descriptors: mild, moderate, and severe. These descriptors are used to communicate the impairments observed and those supports necessary for an individual to carry out daily activities. For example, mild CP is used when the individual's participation in daily activities is not impaired by their movement capabilities. Individuals requiring medications, adaptive technology, and braces to carry out daily activities are classified as moderately impaired. The severe level indicates that the individual experiences significant deficits in completing daily activities and requires assistive devices (e.g., wheelchair) to move about.

A topographical classification of CP is used to communicate the location and type of motor impairments present. The term *plegia* identifies the presence of muscular paralysis, while *paresis* is used to indicate muscular weakness. These terms are used in conjunction with prefixes to identify the locus of impairment. The prefix *hemi* (hemiplegia) indicates that one arm and one leg along the same side of the body are affected. In a similar manner, *diplegia* is used to communicate that impairment is present in both legs. The terms *quadriplegia/quadriparesis* are utilized to communicate that all four limbs are affected.

To increase the accuracy and communication of their research, researchers commonly incorporate both topographical and motor functioning classification systems. This two-part classification communicates where and how the impairments affect the individual. Three common classifications of CP include spastic cerebral palsies, extrapyramidal cerebral palsies, and hypotonic cerebral palsies (Fennel and Dikel 2001).

Spastic Cerebral Palsy

The presence of spasticity is linked with upper motor neuron paralysis, which includes the exhibition of inappropriate and excessive involuntary motor movements (McLellan 1991). Spasticity is generally associated with deficits in neurophysiological and musculoskeletal functioning (Flett 2003). From a musculoskeletal standpoint it is associated with irregular muscle and bone growth and alterations of the accompanying connective tissue (Flett 2003). Neurophysiological deficits include hyperreflexia, persistence of primitive reflexes, and increased muscle tone (Flett 2003; Tomlin 1995). The presence of muscular spasticity is also associated with the presence of pain, abnormal movement, and deformity (Voerman et al. 2005). Abnormal neurological functioning is also frequently observed. Abnormal brain CT findings are observed in approximately 70 % of individuals with spastic CP (Odding et al. 2006).

Based upon survey response, Menkes and Sarnat (2000) identified spastic CP as one of the most prevalent forms of CP affecting approximately 66–82 % of CP cases. Similar to classification of CP in general, spastic CP is further separated into three subgroups based upon the location of the physical impairments observed. Researchers have recently questioned the utility of these classification distinctions due to low reliability across studies (Colver and Sethumadhavan 2003; Rosenbaum et al. 2007; Yeargin-Allsopp et al. 2008). However, given their prevalence in research, a brief description will be provided.

Spastic Diplegia Spastic diplegia is associated with bilateral spasticity, with spasticity being less prevalent in the upper torso of the individual than the lower torso. This is the most prevalent form of spasticity and accounts for nearly 70 % of spastic CP cases (Yeargin-Allsopp et al. 2008). The presence of spastic diplegia is linked to specific gait and postural patterns and presentations (Rodda and Graham 2001). These deficits are often the target of intervention. Most often, classification systems utilized by researchers are based upon the observed pattern of knee involvement (Sutherland and Davids 1993). Those gait patterns commonly observed include true equinus, apparent equinus, crouch gait, and jump knee (Rodda and Graham 2001). Equinus is noted to be one of the most prevalent deformities occurring in CP populations (Goldstein and Harper 2001). This deformity is noted to impact an individual's gait and/or standing pattern. Equinus is associated with a disparity in muscle and tendon length relative to skeletal growth which negatively effects dorsiflexion during the gait cycle (Craig and Van Vuren 1976). See Rodda and Graham (2001) for an in-depth review and depiction of common gait patterns.

Cohen and Duffner (1981) reported that one-quarter of those with spastic diplegia experience seizures. Although neurological impairment is common, specific deficits may vary dependent upon multiple factors. Results of magnetic resonance imaging (MRI) investigations often indicate periventricular leukomalacia (PVL) with infarction in the vascular border zone of the thalamus and internal capsule in preterm infants with spastic diplegia (Lou 1998). PVL is most common in preterm and low birth-weight infants and is associated with impaired blood flow causing white matter damage. However, infants with spastic diplegia that are carried to term also commonly evidence PVL, micropolygyria (i.e., impaired neuronal migration), and porencephaly lesions (Menkes and Sarnat 2000). Porencephaly lesions are the result of a congenital disorder which negatively impacts CNS functioning and development (Douzenis et al. 2010).

Spastic Hemiplegia Symptoms associated with spastic hemiplegia are characterized by unilateral spasticity of the leg and arm contralateral to the brain lesion observed. Spastic hemiplegia is the second most common form of spasticity and may account for 26–34 % of spastic CP cases (Yeargin-Allsop et al. 2008). Gait disruption is also commonly observed when spastic hemiplegia is present. A common classification system utilized to describe gait impairment is that suggested by Winters et al. (1987). The authors present a comprehensive review of four commonly observed gait presentations and the underlying musculoskeletal abnormalities observed. The heterogeneity of impairment and musculoskeletal systems impacted by spastic hemiplegia requires a variety of considerations for treatment approaches (Rodda and Graham 2001).

Regarding etiology for spastic hemiplegia, Lou (1998) reported that common perinatal factors associated with spastic hemiplegia include anomalous fetal circulation, maternal infection, placental emboli, and maternal hemodynamic disturbances. Postnatal etiologic factors include vascular accidents, bacterial meningitis, and viral meningoencephalitis (Lou 1998; Menkes and Sarnat 2000).

Spastic Quadraplegia Due to the involvement of both lower and upper extremities, spastic quadriplegia is suggested to be the most impairing form of bilateral CP. In addition to the observed increases in motor functioning impairment, those with spastic quadriplegia evince significantly greater rates of ID and seizure disorders (Fennell and Dikel 2001). Etiologic factors for spastic quadriplegia are variable and dependent upon pregnancy. For example, preterm infants most often exhibit PVL (Fennell and Dikel 2001). However, Lou (1998) reported that cortical lesions disrupting the proliferation of cerebral vessels are commonly observed in those infants carried to term. Finally, polymicrogyria and cystic lesions are most commonly observed in those infants with spastic quadriplegia that were carried to full-term (Fennell and Dikel 2001).

Extrapyramidal Cerebral Palsy

Extrapyramidal CP is also commonly identified as non-spastic CP. It is associated with fluctuating or decreased muscle tone and often involves involuntary motor movements. The involuntary movements accompanying extrapyramidal CP are variable, but are often repetitive and/or rhythmic. Observed deficits commonly include impairments in muscle tone and coordinated movement regulation (Menkes and Sarnat 2000). Estimates of extrapyramidal CP prevalence rates are variable and suggest that it accounts for 5–22% of CP cases. Fennel and Dikel (2001) indicated that investigations utilizing MRIs in individuals with extrapyramidal CP reveal hypoxic-ischemic or kernicterus damage causing lesions in the basal ganglia. Dyskinetic CP is the most prevalent form of extrapyramidal CP and is separated into two groups (athetoid and dystonic) based upon the impairment observed. Athetoid CP is identified when the impairments are present in the limbs and include involuntary motor movements. Dystonic CP is used to describe individuals whose motor impairments primarily involve core or trunk muscle groups resulting in abnormal postures.

Hypotonic Cerebral Palsy

In general, this classification is used to describe the individual's muscle tone and the extent to which separate muscle groups' work in conjunction with each other. The prefix *hypo* indicates decreased muscle tone and the presence of flimsy limbs or poor motor control. Hypotonic CP is characterized by diffuse decreases in muscle tone, which are not directly attributable to a muscle or peripheral nerve disease (Fennel and Dikel 2001). The prevalence of hypotonic CP is reportedly low, accounting for 2.6% of CP cases in a recent study (Yeargin-Alssops et al. 2008). Ataxia is also associated with hypotonic CP and affects coordinated movements such as balance, posture, and fine motor skills. Symptoms include gait disturbances, impaired behavioral deployment, and coordination deficits. Etiological factors associated with hypotonic CP are unclear, but may include abnormalities such as enlarged ventricles, gyral atrophy, or delayed development of the cerebellum (Menkes and Sarnat 2000).

Comorbid Symptoms and Disorders

The manifestation of CP symptoms does not always occur in isolation and may include multiple comorbid conditions. For example, researchers have previously reported a fivefold increase in the exhibition of challenging behaviors when CP is present (Odding et al. 2006). Comorbid sensory impairment, ID, epilepsy, and visuoperceptual impairments are also commonly observed in CP populations (Beckung et al. 2007). Further, the presence of these conditions may exacerbate symptom manifestation. For those with CP, the presence of ID, visual impairment, infantile hydrocephalus, and epilepsy are associated with increased restrictions on mobility and adversely affect an individual's quality of life (Beckung and Hagberg 2002). SCPE (2000) estimated that 31% of children with CP have severe ID, 21% have epilepsy, and 11% have visual disabilities. Additional researchers have demonstrated similar rates of visual impairment (17%) and hearing impairment (4%) in populations with CP (Boyle and Lary 1996).

Intellectual Disability

Despite their common co-occurrence, relatively little is known about the manifestation of ID in CP populations. To date, researchers have been unable to identify a relationship between the location of brain damage and IQ and memory functioning (Vargha-Khadem et al. 1992). Schrojenstein Lantman-de Valk et al. (1997) reported that individuals with severe or profound ID were significantly more likely to have CP than persons with mild ID. Additional factors have been identified that may serve as protective factors as the authors noted that individuals with comorbid ID and Downs syndrome (DS) were significantly less likely to have CP. Regardless of level of ID the presence of comorbid CP in ID populations is associated with an increased risk for additional impairments external to either condition.

With regard to specific forms of CP, researchers suggest that high rates of cognitive impairment occur in those with spastic tetraplegia (Pruitt and Tsai 2009). However, Pruitt and Tsai (2009) suggested that it is difficult to identify the relationship between cognitive functioning and CP due to the heterogeneity of impairments observed in CP populations. Further, the use of intelligence tests are impeded by those impairments commonly observed in CP populations (i.e., auditory, speech, and motor) and may underestimate intellectual capacity (Fennell and Dikel 2001).

Pain

Increased levels of pain are a prevalent and persistent factor observed in CP populations (Engel et al. 2000; Schwartz et al. 1999). Over one-quarter of adults with CP report experiencing chronic pain, with back pain being the most prevalent form (Jahnsen et al. 2004). Survey responses have previously demonstrated that just over half (53 %) of adults reported experiencing moderate to severe levels of pain (Schwartz et al. 1999). The frequency and severity of pain reported has previously been demonstrated to be variable and related to the location and severity of the observed motor impairment (Houlihan et al. 2004). Chronic pain is associated with multiple negative factors (e.g., poor physical role functioning, deterioration of functional skills, and low quality of life; Jahnsen et al. 2004). Further, elevated pain experiences have been shown to negatively impact participation in preferred activities and are positively associated with the presence of depressive symptoms in populations with CP (Engel et al. 2000). Although the presence of pain may be linked to core symptoms of CP, the presence of elevated levels of pain may also occur due to secondary variables such as the presence of a gastrotomy tube (Houlihan et al. 2004). Despite the observed prevalence of pain symptoms, Oberlander (2001) reported that little research has investigated the negative impact these factors have on the individuals and their families.

A general factor impeding further research may be the subjective nature of pain, making the assessment of pain a difficult practice to standardize and measure reliably (Franck et al. 2000; Houlihan et al. 2004; St-Laurent-Gagnon et al. 1999). The assessment of pain in ID populations with CP is exponentially more difficult given the observed deficits in verbal and nonverbal communication. Measures previously developed to assess pain intensity in cognitively impaired populations include the *Children's Hospital of Eastern Ontario Pain Scale* (Harbeck and Peterson 1992) and the *Visual Analogue Scale* (Franck et al. 2000). However, researchers have questioned the validity and reliability of the use of self-report and direct observation measures to monitor pain in ID populations (Chambers et al. 1998; Fanurik et al. 1999).

Speech and Sensory Impairment

Verbal language deficits commonly co-occur with CP and ID (Arvio and Sillanpää 2003). Odding et al. (2006) suggested that as much as 80% of individuals with CP evince some form of speech impairment. The severity of impairment associated with CP and ID may influence the rate and severity of the observed verbal communication deficit. For example, researchers reported that 62% of individuals with severe and profound ID exhibit deficits in verbal communication (Arvio and Sillanpää 2003). Flett and Saunders (1993) also identified a strong correlation between speech deficits and the exhibition of specific motor impairments. Specifically, they observed that those with diplegic forms of CP exhibited the least amount of speech impairments and those with a dyskinetic form of CP exhibited the most. Although the occurrence of aphasia has been documented, dysarthria is the most common speech impairment observed in CP populations (Flett and Saunders 1993). Dysarthria is an umbrella term utilized when speech deficits (e.g., variable speech rate, imprecise consonants, reduced stress, and variation in pitch and loudness) are present and are the result of speech-organ motor control impairment (Darley et al. 1969; Pinto et al. 2004).

Given the importance of language development (Bilenker et al. 1983; Molnar 1985) it is important that audiological examinations and an evaluation of language skills be conducted. The provision of medical evaluations (e.g., hearing and vision) is a necessary area that is often overlooked in ID and CP populations (Kerr et al. 2003). Kerr et al. (2003) noted the difficulty associated with routine hearing and vision assessments in ID populations. However, their analysis revealed a gross disagreement between hypothesized level of functioning and the results of formal assessment. For 506 individuals with ID who had reportedly adequate vision, 47% were noted to have reduced vision following formal assessment (Kerr et al. 2003). Further assessment revealed that only 11% of individuals had adequate hearing, with 61% having mild hearing loss. Speech therapy should be introduced immediately after the identification of any deficits (Bilenker et al. 1983). Interventions may also incorporate nonverbal communication techniques (e.g., picture exchange) when language deficits are present to facilitate communication and decrease challenging behaviors (Bilenker et al. 1983; Redford 1986).

In addition to communication deficits, sensory impairments are also commonly observed in CP populations. Sixty percent of children with CP exhibit some degree of ophthalmic impairment (Edebol-Tysk et al. 1989; Henderson 1961; Weir et al. 1992) with 70% of children exhibiting low visual acuity. Schenk-Rootlieb et al. (1992) suggested the possibility of a cerebral visual disturbance given the inability of ophthalmological examinations to identify causal factors associated with the observed rates of low visual acuity. Visual impairments have been suggested to negatively affect the acquisition of motor skills (Molnar 1991). Researchers have demonstrated that sensory deficits are variable and are often dependent upon the type of CP present. For example, researchers have noted that severe visual impairments are observed in half of those with ID and tetraplegic CP (Edebol-Tysk 1989). Aside from visual impairments, other forms of sensory deficits have been noted. Yekutiel and Jariwala (1994) reported that deficits in stereognosis and in two-point discrimination are commonly observed in half of those with CP. Researchers have suggested that the manifestation of sensory deficits may vary dependent upon the motor impairments observed. For example, 90% of children with hemiplegic CP exhibit bilateral sensory deficits (Cooper et al. 1995).

Seizure Activity

The prevalence of seizures in individuals with CP is variable and dependent upon the type of CP and the manifestation of comorbid disorders (i.e., ID; Pruitt and Tsai 2009). Current estimates of the universal prevalence rate of any seizure disorder in individuals with CP range from 15 to 55% (Odding et al. 2006; Singhi et al. 2003; Wallace 2001). Researchers investigating the prevalence of epilepsy in CP populations have reported that 35–40% of those with CP have been diagnosed with epilepsy (Beckung and Hapberg 2002; Turk et al. 2001). Factors such as co-occurring ID may elevate the prevalence of seizure activity. Hadjipanayis et al. (1997) suggested that the prevalence of seizure activity may be as high as 71% when CP and ID co-occur. However, research reporting the prevalence of seizure disorders in those with ID and comorbid CP has been scant. Future research surrounding this population is important given that the presence of a seizure disorders are also a risk factor for decreased cognitive functioning (Vargha-Khadem et al 1992; Zafeiriou et al. 1999).

Specific risk factors associated with seizure disorders include family history and the presence of neonatal seizures (Kwong et al. 1998; Verrotti et al. 2006). Some researchers have reported that nearly three quarters of those later diagnosed with epilepsy had a seizure within the first year of life (Verrotti et al. 2006; Zafeiriou et al. 1999). Although improved neonatal care has reduced mortality rates surrounding neonatal seizures, it has not reduced the negative neurologic implications associated with their occurrence (Ronen et al. 2007; Tekgul et al. 2006). The presence of neonatal seizures is associated with an increased risk for the development of CP, epilepsy, and global developmental delay (Garfinkle and Shevell 2011). Specific indicators associated with the development of CP include 5-min Apgar scores, the type and onset of the seizure observed, and the findings observed during electroencephalographic investigations (Garfinkle and Shevell 2011).

With regard to specific forms of epilepsy occurring in CP populations, generalized (61.3 %) and partial (27.4 %) epilepsy are most common (Gibbs et al. 1963; Lagergren 1980; Verrotti et al. 2006). However, some controversy remains. Additional researchers have suggested that partial epilepsy is the most prevalent form of seizure activity observed in CP populations (Carlsson et al. 2003; Hadjipanayis et al. 1997). The observed disagreement may be influenced by multiple factors such as the type of CP present. Researchers have reported differential seizure activity based upon CP manifestation. Wallace (2001) estimated that 70 % of those with hemiplegic CP exhibit partial seizures. Those with spastic tetraplegia and diplegia exhibit seizure activity at earlier points in life when compared to those with hemiplegia (Singhi et al. 2003) and most commonly exhibit generalized tonic–clonic seizures (Hadjipanayis et al. 1997; Kulak and Sobaniec 2003). Despite the efficacy of pharmacotherapy in managing seizures, their presence remains a significant concern for families and caretakers (Verrotti et al. 2006).

Eating and Feeding Deficits

Dysphagia is a common concern and health problem observed in individuals with CP. Dysphagia includes deficits in the oral preparation, oral-pharyngeal, and the esophageal phases of swallowing (Calis et al. 2008). Researchers have suggested that 58–86 % of those with CP evidence signs and symptoms of dysphagia (Dahl et al. 1996; Fung et al. 2002; Stallings et al. 1993). Investigations of individuals with severe and profound ID and comorbid CP reported elevated rates of dysphagia. Researchers estimate that 90–99 % of the individuals with CP and severe or profound ID evidence symptoms of dysphagia (Calis et al. 2008; Reilley et al. 1996). Multiple researchers have hypothesized that malnutrition is partially responsible for the observed retardation in physical growth observed in CP and ID populations given the feeding difficulties present (Krick and Van Duyn 1984; Ruby and Matheny 1962; Shapiro et al. 1986).

Feeding deficits may be further exacerbated by the presence of gastro-oesophageal reflux and food aspiration (Griggs et al. 1989; Rempel et al. 1988). The presence of such difficulties surrounding feeding has resulted in the use enteral feeding strategies (Sleigh and Brocklehurst 2004). Enteral feeding encompasses any procedure used to provide nutrition directly to the gastrointestinal system (Kirby et al. 1995). Researchers have demonstrated the utility and positive benefits (increased nutritional intake, weight gain, and growth) of enteral feeding in children (Brant et al. 1999; Corwin et al. 1996; Patrick et al. 1986; Sullivan et al. 2005). Currently, multiple enteral feeding procedures are available (For an in-depth review see Pearce and Duncan 2002). However, selection may vary depending on the indications and contraindications for tube feeding based upon an individual's needs (Pearce and Duncan 2002).

Despite the observed benefits, the use of enteral feeding options is not without controversy. Researchers have highlighted the need for feeding oversight due to the potential for overfeeding (Sullivan et al. 2006). Complications may occur during the procedures used to introduce percutaneous endoscopic gastrostomy (PEG) placement (e.g., pneumoperitoneum, liver injury, colon injury, and gastro-colo-cutaneous fistula; Schrag et al. 2007). Individuals with feeding tubes are also at a heightened risk for self-injury by pulling on or aggravating the feeding tube or its connection. Further, individuals are at an elevated risk for complications following operation (e.g., fluid aspiration, peristomal pain, infection, gastronintestinal bleeding, and mortality).

Assessment

The initial classification systems used for diagnosing CP were controversial with multiple researchers suggesting different criteria (i.e., neurological and etiological) and dimensions (e.g., mild impairment; Morris 2007). Regardless of classification system used, early and accurate diagnosis of CP is important as it informs treatment and the provision of services (Prechtl et al. 1997; Prechtl 2001). The age of diagnosis for CP is variable and often dependent upon the severity of observed impairment. Researchers suggest that when significant deficits are present, CP may be diagnosed within the first year of life (Palmer 2002); but more mild symptoms may not be identified and accurately diagnosed until 4 years of age (Cans 2000).

With regard to assessment, Aroor (1992) recommended a holistic assessment approach to avoid focusing on a single symptom or dimension. For instance, the author recommended that a small degree of hypotonia does not warrant as much attention as hypotonia and motor development delays combined. It is also important to note that the assessment of individuals with CP should be ongoing after initial identification to monitor symptom manifestation and response to intervention (Aroor 1992).

Spasticity

The early assessment of CP should involve the investigation of muscular spasticity. Methods of measuring spasticity may be organized into three broad categories including clinical, neurophysiologic, and biomechanical methods (Voerman et al. 2007; Voerman et al. 2005).

Clinical Assessments Clinical methods of spasticity assessment include the *Tardieu Scale* (*TS*), which utilizes two velocities of passive muscle stretch to measure muscular spasticity (Boyd and Graham 1999; Scholtes et al. 2006; Tardieu et al. 1953). Initially, the range of motion (ROM) of a muscle group is identified through a slow natural movement. This procedure is then followed by a fast stretch procedure in an attempt to elicit a stretch reflex and detect a catch. Graham et al. (2000) defined a catch as increased muscular resistance or an abrupt stop during a fast passive stretch that occurs prior to completing the individuals ROM. However, there is minimal research regarding the reliability and validity of the *TS* (Haugh et al. 2006).

The *Modified Tardieu Scale* (*MTS*) utilizes both slow and fast speeds to measure resistance to passive movement. Researchers have demonstrated that the *MTS* demonstrates good inter-rater reliability and test–retest reliability for children with CP (Gracies et al. 2010) and adults with ID (Gielen et al. 2008). During an investigation of those with ID and comorbid CP the *MTS* has been observed to demonstrate good inter-rater reliability. However, additional researchers have reported some variation in the reliability of the *MTS* across respondent populations (Anasari et al. 2008b; Mackey et al. 2004; Yam and Leung 2006). However, Waninge et al. (2011) reported that the inter-rater and test–retest reliability of the *MTS* was not acceptable when assessing individuals with profound ID (Waninge et al. 2011). The observed variation in reported reliability for assessment in ID populations warrants further investigation.

In an attempt to standardize the gradation of spasticity, Bohannon and Smith (1987) created the *Modified Ashworth Scale* (*MAS*). It is used to measure resistance to passive movement and muscle tone (Temple et al. 2006). Similar to the *MTS*, there is some disagreement among researchers regarding the reliability of the *MAS*. The *MAS* has been previously evaluated in ID populations with CP and found to demonstrate good inter-rater and test–retest reliability (Waninge et al. 2011). Although some researchers have demonstrated that the *MAS* is unreliable (Mutlu et al. 2008; Anasari et al. 2008a; Yam and Leung 2006), other researchers suggest that it is both a reliable and valid measure of muscular spasticity (Gregson et al. 1999; Waninge et al. 2011).

Neurophysiological Assessment Neurophysiologic approaches focus on the mechanism of stretch reflex by measuring surface electromyography (EMG) latencies and amplitudes to passive muscle movement (Hudders-Algra et al. 1997). EMG procedures rely on surface electrodes to detect the electrical signals that occur prior to muscular activation (Stegeman et al. 2000). Different approaches to the evocation of electrical signals serve to differentiate EMG approaches. EMG methods are variable but may include one of the following techniques to evoke muscle contraction: (a) EMG responses to mechanical stimuli, (b) EMG responses to passive and active movement, and (c) EMG responses to electrical stimuli (Voerman et al. 2005). See Voerman et al. (2005) for a comprehensive review of those procedures commonly utilized. Neurophysiological assessment is useful in the identification of mechanisms underlying spasticity and monitoring the effects of treatment (Barolat-Romana and Davis 1980). Surface EMG may also be used to identify and monitor muscular activation in those areas that surround and are impacted by the presence of muscular spasticity. Abnormalities in interneuronal activity, presynaptic inhibition, and polysynaptic reflexes are some mechanisms that have been linked to the presence of spasticity following neurophysiological evaluations (Ashby et al. 1974; Barolat-Romana and Davis 1980; Delwaide 1973). Given the variability of synaptic pathways involved in EMG analysis, researchers have questioned the reliability and clinical utility of EMG assessment (Uysal et al. 1999; Voerman et al. 2005). Future research is necessary to explore the efficacy of neurophysiological assessment methods of spasticity in ID populations when CP is present.

Biomechanical Assessment A third approach utilizes biomechanical methods to assess for spasticity. Biomechanical methodologies employ direct measures to produce quantifiable data regarding the observed resistance to movement (Pandyan et al. 2001). Most often biomechanical methods are used to assess elbow, knee, and ankle joints (Wood et al. 2005). This approach is often reliant upon a measure of torque such as an isokinetic dynamometer or hand-held dynamometer (Engsberg et al. 1996; Pandyan et al. 2001; Wood et al. 2005). However, researchers have also developed devices for use in specific circumstances and populations (Pandyan et al. 2001). In a review of the literature, Wood et al. (2005) reported that measurement methods commonly assess passive movement (e.g., gravitational, manual, and controlled torque) but may include measuring active movement (voluntary and functional) as well. One challenge to the use of biomechanical measurement in ID populations is the requirements for following specific instructions and muscular demands (Wood et al. 2005). Individuals may not understand the demands necessary to actively participate in the measurement process. Recently, increasing amounts of research have begun to incorporate neurophysiological and biomechanical methodologies concurrently when assessing spasticity (Kim et al. 2005; Malhotra et al. 2008; Wood et al. 2005). The combined approach is suggested to overcome the weaknesses of either method in isolation and lead to an increased understanding of the muscular deficits observed.

Motor Functioning

Due to the previously identified heterogeneity of symptom manifestation observed in CP populations, the development of reliable and standardized assessments has been difficult. This factor is also exacerbated by the multiple classification systems proposed. As such, the following list of assessments is not exhaustive and instead focuses on those assessments with demonstrated psychometric properties. It is important to note that there is currently a paucity of research surrounding the assessment of motor functioning deficits associated with CP in ID populations. Although multiple assessment and classification packages have since developed, the *Gross Motor Function Classification System* (*GMFCS*) was one of the first attempts at creating a standardized measure to classify observed movement impairments in CP populations (Palisano et al. 1997). Prior to the introduction of the *GMFCS* researchers noted that children with CP were often measured with assessments that did not include children with CP in their normative data sets (Campbell 1992; Palisano 1992).

Gross Motor Function Classification System (GMFCS; Palisano et al. 1997) The *GMFCS* organizes children into one of five levels dependent upon their gross motor abilities and limitations across contexts. Levels are most often distinguished by functional limitations observed in level of motor functioning, such as the need for supports (e.g., walkers). Descriptors are arranged according to age, with each age band covering a 2 year period from birth to 12 years of age (e.g., less than 2, 2–4 years of age, etc.). The *GMFCS* included four age bands with descriptors for a child's ability corresponding to a given level of functional impairment (i.e., Level I—Level V, with Level V representing the most severe level of impairment).

The *GMFCS* has recently been expanded and revised (*GMFCS-E&R;* Palisano et al. 2008). This revision included the introduction of an additional age band (a 12–18 year-old group) and the revision of the 6–12 year-old age band (Palisano et al. 2008). Revisions also introduced a distinction between performance and capability regarding motor functioning. The *GMFCS-E&R* also includes a consideration of potential external factors influencing motor function (i.e., environmental and personal).

Inter-rater reliability of the *GMFCS* ranges from 0.55 to 0.93 (Palisano et al. 1997; Wood and Rosenbaum 2000). The lower rate of reliability (0.55) was observed when analyzing a population under 2 years of age. However, reliability increased to 0.75 for the same group of raters in children 2–12 years of age (Palisan et al. 1997). The test–retest reliability of the *GMFCS* was reportedly high (Wood and Rosenbaum 2000). The *GMFCS* has been demonstrated to be a valid predictor of motor functioning (Wood and Rosenbaum 2000). Following the introduction of the *GMFCS* multiple measures of CP and related symptoms have been introduced.

Manual Ability Classification System (MACS; Eliasson et al. 2006) Additional measures such as the *MACS* assess differing areas of CP. The *MACS* is similar to the *GMFCS* but is used to measure the individual's ability to manipulate objects and demonstrates good reliability and validity (Eliasson et al. 2006). Information provided by the *MACS* extends case conceptualization beyond gross motor deficits to incorporate deficiencies in fine motor skills that may also be targeted for intervention. This measure does not discriminate based upon handedness; instead, it measures a child's ability to handle objects in daily living situations (e.g., eating; Eliasson et al. 2006). The classification of impairment is based upon the need for assistance and the quantity and quality of performance.

Functional Mobility Scale (FMS; Graham et al. 2004) Campbell et al. (1990) noted that practitioners often relied on personal experience to monitor treatment and measure outcome. This lack of objective data collection impeded interventions and progress monitoring. In response to the observed deficits researchers have also introduced outcome measures such as the *FMS* which were designed to measure changes in walking ability and the need for assistive devices (e.g., wheelchair) across distances of 5, 50, and 500 m postintervention (Graham et al. 2004). The utility and reliability of the *FMS* in CP populations has been demonstrated (Harvey et al. 2007; Harvey et al. 2010).

Gross Motor Function Measure (GMFM; Russell et al. 1989) An additional outcome measure related to gross motor functioning is the *GMFM*. The *GMFM* is a criterion-based measure which is designed to assess multiple gross motor dimensions: rolling and lying, crawling and kneeling, standing, sitting, walking, running, and jumping (Russell et al. 1993). Consisting of 88 items, the *GMFM* is a direct observation measure that assesses for changes in gross motor functioning capabilities in children with CP (Russell et al. 1989; Russell et al. 1993).

Over 20 articles have investigated the psychometric properties of the *GMFM* (Adair et al. 2012). The *GMFM* is reported to be a reliable and valid measure of change in motor functioning (Josenby et al. 2009). Overall this measure has been reported to demonstrate excellent reliability and internal consistency (Beckung et al. 2007; Bjornson et al. 1998; Russell et al. 2000; Russell et al. 1989). Other researchers have further demonstrated the content, construct, and criterion related validity of the *GMFM* (Bagley et al. 2007; Josenby et al. 2009; Russell et al. 1989; Russell et al. 1998; Russell et al. 2000).

Neuroimaging

Advancements in neuroimaging have renewed interest in the etiological classification of CP by analyzing the correlation between structural impairments in the brain and movement disorders (Accardo et al. 2004). Grant and Barkovich (1997) asserted that the current practice of simply identifying deficits in motor functioning does not provide information relevant to the etiology of CP. Researchers have demonstrated the utility of MRI in providing information relative to the timing and cause of the lesions in the brain (Grant and Barkovich 1997). In comparison to MRIs, Grant and Barkovich (1997) suggest that computed tomography (CT) scanning is less sensitive to acute cerebral damage.

Although neuroimaging is not required for a diagnosis of CP, it is often recommended in cases where the origin is unknown (Ashwal et al. 2004). Based upon a systematic review of the neuroimaging literature, Korzeniewski et al. (2008) suggest that 83 % of individuals with CP evidence abnormal neuroimaging results. The most common irregularity observed is related to damage occurring in the white matter of the brain and is often associated with athetosis, ataxia, and bilateral spasticity (Fedrizzi et al. 1996; Hayakawa et al. 1997; Koeda et al. 1990). But the location and extent of cerebral damage is variable and related to the physiological impairments observed. For instance, those individuals with hemiplegic CP most commonly evidence gray and white matter damage (Korzeniewski et al. 2008).

The utility of MRI research is not limited to investigations of the etiological factors surrounding CP. Researchers have also suggested that an MRI is useful as a prognostic indicator (Grant and Barkovich 1997). Results of MRI scans have previously been used to identify specific pathology associated with CP (Krägeloh-Mann et al. 1995) and it has been used to clarify the occurrence and influence of perinatal asphyxiation in CP populations (Truwit et al. 1992). These investigations are possible through the examination of factors associated with the observed cerebral damage. For instance, researchers are able to evaluate the timing of brain damage with neuroimaging by analyzing glial reactions and/or neuronal migration (Chen 1981; Cioni et al. 1999; Grant and Barkovich 1997; Himmelmann et al. 2005; Yin et al. 2000).

Despite recent advances and the applications noted above, researchers continue to criticize the role of neuroimaging in CP research. A systematic review of the literature identified four common problems observed in neuroimaging research; sample generalizability, correlation between anatomic findings and etiology, inconsistency of timing estimates based upon neuroimaging, and variability in the communication of research results (Cioni et al. 1999; Humphreys et al. 2000). It is also important to note that individuals with ID and CP may exhibit anxiety and apprehension about exposure to neuroimaging procedures and equipment. Anxiety may be reduced by introducing coping mechanisms (e.g., preferred item) or gradually exposing the individual to the procedure. Further, physical and medical restrictions may also impede and restrict those procedures that are available to an individual. These factors should be evaluated and addressed prior to an individual's participation in neuroimaging procedures.

Intervention and Treatment

The provision of care for individuals with developmental disabilities (DDs) is an area that is continuously evolving as researchers and providers strive to identify efficacious and cost-effective interventions for a plethora of disorders. The Centers for Disease Control (CDC) and RTI International (Research Triangle Park, North Carolina) utilized survey, reports, and national health care databases to confirm diagnoses and calculate the estimated average lifetime cost of ID and CP in the USA (CDC 2004). Cost estimates represented both direct and indirect economic costs associated with DDs and did not include those routine medical costs incurred by the general US population. For individuals born with ID in 2000, the estimated total lifetime cost was $ 51.2 billion ($ 1,014,000 per person) and $ 11.5 billion for individuals with CP ($ 921,000 per person; CDC 2004).

Interventions for CP tend to incorporate a multidisciplinary model with individual professionals working in-conjunction with peers to simultaneously treat specific components and deficits. Disciplines often include orthopedic surgery, psychology, special education, spasticity management, occupational, speech, and physical therapy (PT) (Liptak and Accardo 2004). Further, deficits associated with CP produce secondary factors that must be given consideration. For example, severe spasticity is also associated with restrictions in movement and may place the individual at a greater risk for hygienic deficiencies. Spasticity may make movement (e.g., from bed to wheelchair) extremely difficult for individual caregivers (Barnes and Johnson 2008). Specific physical limitations imposed by spasticity may impede bathing attempts in specific areas (e.g., palm of the hand). This increases the need for caregivers to be aware of activities that may be associated with moisture (e.g., swimming or physical activity) as a failure to clean and dry these areas places the individual at an increased risk for illness or infections (Barnes and Johnson 2008).

A large emphasis is placed upon intervention during infancy and toddlerhood because children generally achieve their functional limits in daily living skills and ambulation shortly after they enter school (Molnar 1979; Watt et al. 1989). At this point therapy transitions to the development of self-initiated self-help skill acquisition and increasing motor abilities and endurance (Molnar 1991). Childhood is also associated with increased risk for secondary musculoskeletal deficits (e.g., chronic pain and fatigue, fine motor skills deficits) as children grow (Bax et al. 1988; Tosi et al. 2009). Early interventions include but are not limited to physical, occupational, and speech therapy, orthoses, and nerve blocks. Treatment goals for early intervention include improving: general appearance and posture, speech, feeding, self-help, and locomotion (Phelps 1941). Odding et al. (2006) suggested that children with CP are the single largest group treated through PT. However, the author's literary search indicated that this field publishes significantly less research on the efficacy of interventions for those with CP than other research areas (e.g., neurology and pediatrics).

Physical and Occupational Therapy

The goals of PT often include attempts to enhance self-care, play, motor skill independence, and leisure activities (Scrutton 1984). PT is also suggested to prevent musculoskeletal complication and to enhance motor development (Palmer et al. 1988). Further, PT is used to hedge the effects of inexperience, disuse, and the development of secondary musculoskeletal complications. It is the most common intervention utilized for individuals with CP and is often included as a component of early intervention (Gordon 1987; Mutch et al. 1992). Physical therapists may also aid parents in enhancing their children's quality of life at home by addressing specific deficits (e.g., bathing, dressing, and mobility devices). Despite its prevalence, researchers criticize the relative lack of research investigating the efficacy of PT in CP populations (Bower 1993; Shumway-Cook and Woollacott 1995). The heterogeneity of the CP diagnosis itself is likely a contributing factor to the dearth of available research.

Evidence regarding the efficacy of PT interventions is increasing, but requires additional research. A systematic review of randomized controlled trials (RCTs) evaluating the effects of PT interventions identified moderate evidence for some forms of PT interventions (Anttila et al. 2008). In their review of the available research, the authors noted that the comparison of results was hampered by the identification of as many as eight different intervention categories, each with different target populations and outcome measures (Anttila et al. 2008; Molnar 1991). A moderate amount of evidence for the efficacy of neurodevelopmental therapy in upper extremity interventions was reported (Hallam 1996; Law et al. 1991; Wallen et al. 2007). Anttila et al. (2008) reported that a moderate amount of evidence currently supports the use of strength training to increase walking speed (Liao et al. 2007; Patikas et al. 2006) and stride length in those with CP (Patikas et al. 2006; Unger et al. 2006). In a direct comparison of control conditions to strength training, conflicting evidence was observed regarding the overall effects on gross motor functioning (Dodd et al. 2003; Liao et al. 2007; Patikas et al. 2006). In a study of the efficacy of PT in individuals with severe ID and CP researchers observed no difference in gross motor skills, passive joint motion, and developmental reflexes when comparing a supervised therapy management group, direct PT, and a control group (Sommerfeld et al. 1981).

Occupational therapists often seek to modify a child's environment to enhance quality of life and independence by introducing adaptive components for feeding, communication, and mobility (Bilenker et al. 1983; Finnie 1976). Addressing feeding concerns in CP populations is a significant concern given the propensity for feeding difficulties and malnutrition. Although multiple forms of treatment have been emphasized (e.g., sensory integration therapy, neurodevelopmental treatment; Palmer et al. 1988; Scrutton 1984) and focus on enhancing functional activities and/or improving quality of movement. The provision of occupational therapy resources is flexible and may include occupational therapy home programs (OTHPs; Giller Gajdosik 1991; Hinojosa and Anderson 1991; Schreiber et al. 1995). The efficacy of these interventions has been demonstrated elsewhere (Novak et al. 2009). As a multifaceted intervention, OTHPs often target problems (e.g., fine motor skills and body structure) identified by parents, physicians, and the therapist (Novak et al. 2009). Additional targets may be identified systematically through direct observation and the use of standardized assessment measures.

Function-Based Intervention

An alternative therapeutic approach suggests that motor development is cumulative and evolves from interactions across time and context (Gibson 1986; Thelen 1996). Approaches emphasizing the improvement and quality of the functional use of motor movements are based upon an active intervention view (Anttila et al. 2008; Ketelaar et al. 2001; Thelen 1996). In an active intervention, the therapist shapes the environment to prompt the child and enables them to self-initiate motor movements (Latash and Anson 1996; Leech 1996). This function-based framework is also suggested to increase and support parental involvement (Ketelaar et al. 2001; Palmer et al. 1988). Parents may be better able to identify areas of functioning where their child needs additional support, participate in therapy, and continue providing a structured environment outside of a therapeutic setting to promote generalization.

Assistive Devices

As noted previously, as treatment progresses across time the structure of therapy often shifts with increased emphasis on self-help skills and locomotion (Molnar 1991). This may involve the introduction of devices to improve mobility and/or aid in locomotion and independent movements. Advancements in the construction of assistive devices such as the modification of wheelchair seats have not only enhanced overall mobility, but also the comfort (Bilenker et al. 1983; Molnar 1985; Redford 1986). Molnar (1991) suggested that therapists should incorporate preventative treatments (e.g., splinting, orthotics, and range-of-motion exercises) to prevent secondary insults. For example, orthotics are often employed to enhance joint stability by securing the joint in a functional position and stretching constricted muscle groups (Flett 2003). Fixed and hinged-ankle foot orthotics are also commonly incorporated as an intervention for the management of equinus in those with spastic diplegia and has some demonstrated efficacy in those with spastic hemiplegia (Buckon et al. 2001). However, it is important to consider the biomechanical factors relevant to the observed spasticity prior to the implementation of orthotic intervention (Flett 2003).

Additional assistive devices utilized during treatment may include the use of casting, or constraint-induced (CI) movement therapy. The efficacy and utility of these devices are dependent upon consideration of the individual's condition and the impairment observed. Although the efficacy of casting to prevent muscular contraction and increase muscle length has been demonstrated (Corry et al. 1998; Flett et al. 1999), this procedure is criticized for being inconvenient (multiple cast changes), and is also associated with changes in overall muscle tone (Flett 2003). At present, there are no randomized-control-trials presenting evidence to support the use of casting for equinus in isolation or in combination with Botulinum toxin type A (BTX-A; Blackmore et al. 2007). CI movement therapy used to treat upper limbs in hemiplegic CP is still considered experimental, but preliminary evidence indicates positive effects (Hoare et al. 2007). Researchers have demonstrated that CI therapy produced significant improvement in motor functions for children with CP and that these effects were maintained across time (Taub et al. 2004).

Spasticity Intervention

Prior to spasticity intervention it is necessary to determine if the impairment observed is generalized, focal, or regional (Boyd and Graham 1997; Gormley et al. 2001; Graham et al. 2000). Active intervention for muscular spasticity is necessary to maintain function and prevent secondary insults such as deformities and contractures (O'Shea 2008). Although PT is the most common intervention, other intervention approaches have emerged and been investigated.

Orthopedic Surgery Treatment of CP may include orthopedic surgery when warranted (Bilenker et al. 1983; Bleck 1987; Rethlefsen et al. 1999). Orthopedic surgery procedures may be carried out for multiple reasons. Procedures may be preventative, or carried out to enhance quality of life (i.e., enhancing walking ability or to correct abnormal posture; Molnar 1991). With regard to prevention, researchers have suggested that the use of selective dorsal rhizotomy in pediatric populations may prevent or reduce the need for future surgical procedures (Chicoine et al. 1997). However, there is some disagreement about the appropriate candidates for selective dorsal rhitozomy. Researchers have suggested that children between 4 and 8 years of age who evidence spasticity but are ambulatory and evidence good muscle control and strength are most likely to benefit from this procedure (Gormley 2001). While Flett (2003) suggested that individuals with severe spastic diplegia may be the most ideal candidates for consideration of orthopedic surgery. Research surrounding the general efficacy of orthopedic surgery approaches demonstrated that selective dorsal rhizotomy plus PT has been observed to reduce spasticity but was associated with minimal gains in overall gross motor functioning (McLaughlin et al. 2002). Additionally, Boyd and Graham (1997) cautioned that the long-term efficacy of orthopedic surgery in pediatric populations has not been examined.

Pharmacotherapy The efficacy of oral drug interventions for spasticity has not been sufficiently studied (Flett 2003). This is especially true for pediatric populations (Krach 2001). Barnes and Johnson (2008) cautioned that medication should mainly be used as an additive component to a comprehensive intervention approach and not in isolation. Ward (2008) emphasized that pharmacological treatment should be adjunctive and secondary to physical interventions during the treatment of spasticity. Importantly, although medication may reduce spasticity it is not a precision tool operating in isolation and often produces diffuse muscular weakness in areas other than those inflicted by spasticity and targeted for intervention (Barnes and Johnson 2008). Given the prevalence of comorbid psychological and medical conditions in both ID and CP populations it is also important to consider drug-interaction effects. Aside from interaction effects, it is important to monitor the specific side effects of prescribed medications. In ID populations, those drugs producing sedentary effects may also further decrease cognitive and adaptive functioning.

Examples of oral medications used to treat spasticity include baclofen, dantrolene, and diazepam. Diazepam may be administered for long- and short-term spasticity management, but is associated with sedentary effects (Pentoff 1964). Despite not being labeled as an antispasticity medication (Young et al. 1997); diazepam is one of the most common antispasticity medications, and is the oldest still in use (Krach 2001; Whyte and Robinson 1990). Baclofen is also associated with drowsiness/sedation and there is disagreement in the literature about its ability to cross the blood-brain barrier (i.e., Flett 2003; Krach 2001). Additional side effects of Baclofen include cognitive impairment (Katz and Campagnolo 1994), dizziness, ataxia, and general weakness (Krach 2001). The sedentary effects observed with the use of baclofen (Alonso and Mancall 1991; Whyte and Robinson 1990; Young et al. 1997), but may be reduced with appropriate dose management (Nance and Young 1999).

Dantrolene has limited efficacy for spasticity management (Flett 2003). Although some researchers have presented evidence of subjective improvements in gait, they failed to identify any objective change in muscular spasticity (Ford et al. 1976). Joynt and Leonard (1980) noted that dantrolene did not produce significant alteration in functioning despite producing notable physiological changes. Researchers have highlighted the importance of dose management to decrease side-effects associated with dantrolene (Verrotti et al. 2006). Side effects of dantrolene include drowsiness, tingling sensations, and skin eruptions (Ford et al. 1976).

Emerging medications used in CP populations include tizanidine, clonazepam, and clonidine (Ward and KoKo 2001). However, further research is necessary to clarify their efficacy and to determine appropriate conditions for use. Despite being heavily researched in adult populations, tizanidine has not been researched extensively in children with CP. Verrotti et al. (2006) reported that there are no significant differences between diazepam and tizanidine or tizanidine and baclofen regarding treatment efficacy. Although Clonazepam has been noted to be helpful in pediatric CP populations, it is associated with negative side effects such as drooling and sedation (Flett 2003). Clonidine has been used in CP populations and decreases muscle tone; however, it is associated with hypotension (Nance 1997) and visual hallucinations (Gracies et al. 1997).

A further example of emerging interventions for spasticity in CP includes the use of BTX-A (Ward 2008). BTX-A injections are reportedly painless, easy to administer, and is easily diffused through muscle systems. Notable benefits of BTX-A include that injections are reportedly long-lasting and cause focal paralysis and denervation at the site of injection (Ward 2008). Flett (2003) suggested the use of BTX-A injections alongside traditional therapies as an alternative to orthopedic surgery in young children. Some researchers have associated the early use of non-surgical procedures (BTX-A) with a decreased need for orthopedic surgery at later points in life (Hägglund et al. 2005). Although side effects are reported to be rare they may include localized redness, pain, muscular weakness, incontinence, and bruising (Flett 2003; Ward 2008). The use of BTX-A requires careful consideration of multiple factors including the individualization of dosage, injection site, and drug-interaction effects (Graham et al. 2000). Ward (2008) provided an overview of dosage, injection considerations and additional information regarding the use of BTX-A interventions to treat spasticity in individuals with CP.

To date the efficacy of BTX-A treatments has received mixed reviews. As with other treatment approaches to CP the utility of BTX-A may be limited to specific circumstances and populations, or used in conjunction with additional treatments as a portion of a larger treatment package. Researchers have demonstrated that BTX-A was superior to placebo for improving gait (Cardoso et al. 2006). However, the results of randomized-controlled-trials for BTX-A in treating lower and upper limb spasticity were inconclusive (Ade-hall and Moore 2000; Wasiak et al. 2009). Future research is necessary to analyze drug-interaction effects, and the long-term effects of BTX-A interventions, especially in pediatric populations.

Future Directions

Descriptions of CP have been around since the mid-nineteenth century; however, there are still multiple elements surrounding it that are not understood or agreed upon (Morris 2007). This includes the absence of a single reliable and agreeable definition and description of CP. The identification of diagnostic criteria that accurately describes the heterogeneous presentations associated with CP is paramount in order to streamline future research. The importance of developing a consensus definition is critical to multiple factors surrounding CP including the creation and identification of reliable and valid assessments, and research surrounding treatment efficacy and the provision of services. Clarification and unification of diagnostic criteria for CP may also aid in the identification and treatment of comorbid conditions commonly observed in CP populations. In general, there is a need for research among ID populations with CP to compliment and extend the research that is currently available.

Assessment

Given the suspected prevalence of chronic pain for individuals with CP it is necessary to establish valid and reliable measures of pain occurrence. This is especially true for ID populations with comorbid CP whose communication abilities may be severely impaired. Given the presence of idiosyncratic behaviors commonly observed in ID and CP populations, the use of direct observation to reliably evaluate pain is of limited utility (Fanurik et al. 1999). Accurate identification of chronic pain would facilitate the provision of resources as well as enhance the quality of life of individuals whose pain experiences may be unidentified or under identified. Additionally, this may provide auxiliary goals for treatment and care as alternative sources of discomfort or pain are identified.

The observed variation in the reported reliability of the measurement of spasticity across populations is a topic that warrants further research. Specifically, additional research is necessary for clinical measures of spasticity (*MAS* and *MTS*) to determine their efficacy with regard to specific diagnostic groups (CP and ID), ages (adults and children), comorbidities (e.g., visual impairment), and the degree of impairment observed (e.g., hemiplegic). Multiple limitations surrounding the clinical utility of biomechanical measures of spasticity have been noted. Broadly, future research is necessary to develop protocols for the use of devices developed and employed by individual research groups to determine their sensitivity and specificity in a larger context. To increase research generalizability it will prudent to include a wide range of participants with various levels of spasticity resulting from different etiologies (Wood et al. 2005).

Further research is also necessary to extend the assessment of gross motor functioning. Although multiple measures are available and have demonstrated sound psychometric properties in CP populations, little research is currently available to demonstrate the efficacy of these same measures in populations with ID and comorbid CP.

As researchers and funding sources continue to place emphasis on multidisciplinary research it is likely that neuroimaging research will continue to grow and expand. Future advances in neuroimaging may increase diagnostic accuracy and play a larger role in our understanding of the etiology of CP. This may include the creation of specific neuroimaging approaches for CP or the adoption of methods already in existence for other populations and purposes. Emerging techniques being utilized in CP populations include but are not limited to diffusion tensor imaging (Hoon 2005; Melhem et al. 2002, Neil et al. 2002), functional MRI (Accardo et al. 2004; Novotny et al. 1998), fast spin echoic imaging, and magnetic resonance spectroscopy (Accardo et al. 2004; Hunter and Wang 2001). It will be equally important to monitor the utility of any neuroimaging advancements for individuals with ID as these emerging techniques are developed. It will be important to thoroughly analyze, document, and communicate those modifications and considerations necessary to extend the utility of emerging technology for use with individuals with ID and comorbid CP.

Intervention and Treatment

Intervention for those with CP should extend beyond motor functioning and include a multidisciplinary effort to improve functioning and quality of life while working to prevent additional deficits (Molnar 1991). In general, early therapeutic approaches should emphasize the use of modified play and positioning to enhance posture and motor movement responses that are essential to later fine and gross motor development (Molnar 1991). Researchers have also begun advocating the promotion of activity through rigorous active training as an addition to more traditional PT and occupational therapy approaches (Damiano 2006). The call to activity is based upon the belief that increased activity of individuals with CP has multiple positive effects. These effects include the development and maintenance of neural structures and/or pathways, maximizing physical functioning, and prevention of secondary muscular impairments. Further, increased activity may offset negative side-effects associated with inactivity (e.g., obesity and osteopenia) and simultaneously increase social skills development. As treatment is modified it is necessary to produce research to communicate and support any alterations. This includes a need to evaluate those procedures currently used in PT to identify their efficacy and determine future directions.

The use of evidence-based practice in the field of occupational therapy is growing (Bennett et al. 2003). However, significant room for improvement surrounding research dissemination and utilization remains. A survey by Humphris et al. (2000) indicated that only half of occupational therapists surveyed reported utilizing therapeutic approaches with research support. Barriers to the acceptance of evidence-based practice include time and resource constraints, training, and unfamiliarity with literature navigation (Bennett et al. 2003; Humphris et al. 2000; Upton 1999). It is imperative that emphasis continues to be placed upon the use of evidence-based practices when treating individuals regardless of diagnoses.

Given the prevalence of dysphagia in CP populations and potential negative consequences of difficulties in self-feeding (e.g., malnutrition and aspiration) interventions may also consider the incorporation of oral motor coordination training (Pearson and Williams 1972). Although the benefits of enteral feeding procedures have been presented, future research is necessary to increase our understanding surrounding the use of the various procedures available. For instance, although the use of PEG is common for long-term assistive feeding (i.e., for more than 30 days; Eltami and Sulliran 1997; Gauderer 1999; Kirby et al. 1995) a review of the research literature surrounding their efficacy and utility for long-term use in CP and ID populations is currently limited (Sleigh and Brocklehurt 2004).

Samson-Fang et al. (2003) raised concern surrounding the safety and efficacy of gastrostomy feeding in children with disabilities. Moving forward, it will be important to increase our understanding of the situations surrounding the use of specific enteral feeding techniques in order to maximize their utility while minimizing side effects.

Advancements in identification and treatment have increased the lifespan and quality of life for individuals with DDs. However, despite these remarkable gains there have been only minimal changes made surrounding the provision of resources to adult populations. Multiple researchers have continuously criticized the reduction in services for adults with CP and ID (Bax et al. 1988; Thomas et al. 1989). Instead of a discontinuation of services due to observed improvement, services are often discontinued because they are no longer mandated due to an individual's age. In a longitudinal analysis of motor functioning in adults with CP, Bottos et al. (2001) observed an overall deterioration in functioning following discontinuation of therapy. The authors noted that the effects of CP do not magically subside when an individual reaches adulthood and argued for therapy that focused on the instruction of functional behaviors. This research highlights a phenomenon impacting individuals with a variety of DDs. Future research demonstrating the positive effects of treatments in adults with CP may serve to increase awareness of the benefits of continued treatment and increase communication surrounding the need for additional resources as individuals age.

References

Accardo, J., Kammann, H., & Hoon, A. H. Jr. (2004). Neuroimaging in cerebral palsy. *The Journal of Pediatrics, 145*(2), 19–27.

Adair, B., Said, C. M., Rodda, J., & Morris, M. E. (2012). Psychometric properties of functional mobility tools in hereditary spastic paraplegia and other childhood neurological conditions. *Developmental Medicine and Child Neurology, 54*(7), 596–605.

Ade-Hall, R. A., & Moore, A. P. (2000). Botulinum toxin type A in the treatment of lower limb spasticity in cerebral palsy. *Cochrane Database of Systematic Reviews, 2000*(2), CD001408.

Alonso, R. J., & Mancall, E. L. (1991). The clinical management of spasticity. *Seminars in Neurology, 11*(3), 215–219.

Anasari, N. N., Naghdi, S., Arab, T. K., & Jalaie, S. (2008a). The interrater and intrarater reliability of the modified ashworth scale in the assessment of muscle spasticity: Limb and muscle group effect. *NeuroRehabilitation, 23*(3), 231–237.

Anasari, N. N., Naghdi, S., Hasson, S., Azarsa, M. H., & Azarnia, S. (2008b). The modified tardieu scale for the measurement of elbow flexor spasticity in adult patients with hemiplegia. *Brain Injury, 22*(13–14), 1007–1012.

Anttila, H., Autti-Rämö, I., Suoranta, J., Mäkelä, M., & Malmivaara, A. (2008). Effectiveness of physical therapy interventions for children with cerebral palsy: A systematic review. *BMC Pediatrics, 8*(1), 14.

Aroor, S. R. (1992). Assessment of cerebral palsy. *Indian Journal of Pediatrics, 59*(2), 159–164.

Arvio, M., & Sillanpää, M. (2003). Prevalence, aetiology and comorbidity of severe and profound intellectual disability in Finland. *Journal of Intellectual Disability Research, 47*(2), 108–112.

Ashby, P., Verrier, M., & Lightfoot, E. (1974). Segmental reflex pathways in spinal shock and spinal spasticity in man. *Journal of Neurology, Neurosurgery and Psychiatry, 37*(12), 1352–1360.

Ashwal, S., Russman, B. S., Blasco, P. A., Miller, G., Sandler, A., Shevell, M., & Stevenson, R. (2004). Practice parameter: Diagnostic assessment of the child with cerebral palsy. Report of the quality standards subcommittee of the American academy of neurology and the practice committee of the child neurology society. *Neurology, 62*(6), 851–863.

Bagley, A. M., Gorton, G., Oeffinger, D., Barnes, D., Calmes, J., Nicholson, D., Damiano D., Abel M., Kryscio R., Rogers S., & Tylkowski, C. (2007). Outcome assessments in children with cerebral palsy, part II: Discriminatory ability of outcome tools. *Developmental Medicine and Child Neurology, 49*(3), 181–186.

Barolat-Romana, G., & Davis, R. O. (1980). Neurophysiological mechanisms in abnormal reflex activities in cerebral palsy and spinal spasticity. *Journal of Neurology, Neurosurgery and Psychiatry, 43*(4), 333–342.

Barnes, M. P., & Johnson, G. R. (Eds.). (2008). *Upper motor neuron syndrome and spasticity: Clinical management and neurophysiology*. Cambridge: Cambridge University Press.

Bax, M. C. (1964). Terminology and classification of cerebral palsy. *Developmental Medicine and Child Neurology, 11,* 295–297.

Bax, M., Smyth, D., & Thomas, A. (1988). Health care and physically handicapped young adults. *British Medical Journal, 296,* 1153–1155.

Beckung, E., & Hagberg, G. (2002). Neuroimpairments, activity limitations, and participation restrictions in children with cerebral palsy. *Developmental Medicine and Child Neurology, 44*(5), 309–316.

Beckung, E., Carlsson, G., Carlsdotter, S., & Uvebrant, P. (2007). The natural history of gross motor development in children with cerebral palsy aged 1–15 years. *Developmental Medicine and Child Neurology, 49*(10), 751–756.

Bennett, S., Tooth, L., McKenna, K., Rodger, S., Strong, J., Ziviani, J., Mickan S., & Gibson, L. (2003). Perceptions of evidence-based practice: A survey of Australian occupational therapists. *Australian Occupational Therapy Journal, 50*(1), 13–22.

Bilenker, R. M., Rubin, I., & Thompson, G. H. (Eds.). (1983). *Comprehensive management of cerebral palsy*. Philadelphia: Grune & Stratton.

Bjornson, K. F., Graubert, C. S., McLaughlin, J. F., Kerfeld, C. I., & Clark, E. M. (1998). Test-retest reliability of the gross motor function measure in children with cerebral palsy. *Physical and Occupational Therapy in Pediatrics, 18*(2), 51–61.

Blackmore, A. M., Boettcher-Hunt, E., Jordan, M., & Chan, M. D. Y. (2007). A systematic review of the effects of casting on equinus in children with cerebral palsy: An evidence report of the AACPDM. *Developmental Medicine and Child Neurology, 49*(10), 781–790.

Blair, E., Watson, L., Badawi, N., & Stanley, F. J. (2001). Life expectancy among people with cerebral palsy in Western Australia. *Developmental Medicine and Child Neurology, 43*(8), 508–515.

Bleck, E. E. (1987). *Orthopaedic management in cerebral palsy. Clinics in developmental medicine*. London: Mac Keith Press.

Bohannon, R. W., & Smith, M. B. (1987). Interrater reliability of a modified ashworth scale of muscle spasticity. *Physical Therapy, 67*(2), 206–207.

Bottos, M., Feliciangeli, A., Sciuto, L., Gericke, C., & Vianello, A. (2001). Functional status of adults with cerebral palsy and implications for treatment of children. *Developmental Medicine and Child Neurology, 43*(8), 516–528.

Bower, E. (1993). Physiotherapy for cerebral palsy: A historical review. *Bailliere's Clinical Neurology, 2*(1), 29–54.

Boyd, R. N., & Graham, H. K. (1997). Botulinum toxin A in the management of children with cerebral palsy: Indications and outcome. *European Journal of Neurology, 4*(2), 15–21.

Boyd, R. N., & Graham, H. K. (1999). Objective measurement of clinical findings in the use of botulinum toxin type A for the management of children with cerebral palsy. *European Journal of Neurology, 6*(4), 23–35.

Boyle, C. A., & Lary, J. M. (1996). *Prevalence of selected developmental disabilities in children 3–10 years of age: The metropolitan atlanta developmental disabilities surveillance program, 1991*. US Department of Health and Human Services, Public Health Service, Centers for Disease Control and Prevention (CDC).

Brant, C. Q., Stanich, P., & Ferrari, A. P. Jr. (1999). Improvement of children's nutritional status after enteral feeding by PEG: An interim report. *Gastrointestinal Endoscopy, 50*(2), 183–188.

Brooks-Gunn, J., Klebanov, P. K., & Duncan, G. J. (1996). Ethnic differences in children's intelligence test scores: Role of economic deprivation, home environment, and maternal characteristics. *Child Development, 67*(2), 396–408.

Buckon, C. E., Thomas, S. S., Jakobson-Huston, S., Sussman, M., & Aiona, M. (2001). Comparison of three ankle-foot orthosis configurations for children with spastic hemiplegia. *Developmental Medicine and Child Neurology, 43*(6), 371–378.

Bundey, S., & Brett, E. M. (1985). *Genetics and neurology*. Edinburgh: Churchill Livingstone.

Calis, E. A., Veugelers, R., Sheppard, J. J., Tibboel, D., Evenhuis, H. M., & Penning, C. (2008). Dysphagia in children with severe generalized cerebral palsy and intellectual disability. *Developmental Medicine and Child Neurology, 50*(8), 625–630.

Campbell, S. K. (1992). Measurement of motor performance. In H. Forrsberg & H. Hirschfield (Eds.), *Movement disorders in children* (pp. 264–271). Basel: Karger.

Campbell, S. K., Anderson, J., & Gardner, G. H. (1990). Physicians' beliefs in the efficacy of physical therapy in the management of cerebral palsy. *Pediatric Physical Therapy, 2*(3), 169–173.

Cans, C. (2000). Surveillance of cerebral palsy in Europe: A collaboration of cerebral palsy surveys and registers. *Developmental Medicine and Child Neurology, 42*(12), 816–824.

Cardoso, E. S., Rodrigues, B. M., Barroso, M., Menezes, C. J., Lucena, R. S., Nora, D. B., & Melo, A. (2006). Botulinum toxin type A for the treatment of the spastic equinus foot in cerebral palsy. *Pediatric Neurology, 34*(2), 106–109.

Carlsson, M., Hagberg, G., & Olsson, I. (2003). Clinical and aetiological aspects of epilepsy in children with cerebral palsy. *Developmental Medicine and Child Neurology, 45*(6), 371–376.

Centers for Disease Control and Prevention. (2004). Economic costs associated with mental retardation, cerebral palsy, hearing loss, and vision impairment-United States, 2003. *Morbidity and Mortality Weekly Report, 53*(3), 57.

Chambers, C. T., Reid, G. J., Craig, K. D., McGrath, P. J., & Finley, G. A. (1998). Agreement between child and parent reports of pain. *The Clinical Journal of Pain, 14*(4), 336–342.

Chen, Y. H. (1981). Correlations between computerized tomography of the head and motor developmental disturbances of children with cerebral palsy. *Nihon Seikeigeka Gakkai Zasshi, 55*(1), 85–99.

Chicoine, M. R., Park, T. S., & Kaufman, B. A. (1997). Selective dorsal rhizotomy and rates of orthopedic surgery in children with spastic cerebral palsy. *Journal of Neurosurgery, 86*(1), 34–39.

Christianson, A. L., Zwane, M. E., Manga, P., Rosen, E., Venter, A., Downs, D., & Kromberg, J. G. R. (2002). Children with intellectual disability in rural South Africa: Prevalence and associated disability. *Journal of Intellectual Disability Research, 46*(2), 179–186.

Cioni, G., Sales, B., Paolicelli, P. B., Petacchi, E., Scusa, M. F., & Canapicchi, R. (1999). MRI and clinical characteristics of children with hemiplegic cerebral palsy. *Neuropediatrics, 30*(05), 249–255.

Cohen, M. E., & Duffner, P. K. (1981). Prognostic indicators in hemiparetic cerebral palsy. *Annals of Neurology, 9*(4), 353–357.

Colver, A. F., & Sethumadhavan, T. (2003). The term diplegia should be abandoned. *Archives of Disease in Childhood, 88*(4), 286–290.

Corry, I. S., Cosgrove, A. P., Duffy, C. M., McNeill, S., Taylor, T. C., & Graham, H. K. (1998). Botulinum toxin: A compared with stretching casts in the treatment of spastic equinus: a randomised prospective trial. *Journal of Pediatric Orthopaedics, 18*(3), 304–311.

Cooper, J., Majnemer, A., Rosenblatt, B., & Birnbaum, R. (1995). The determination of sensory deficits in children with hemiplegic cerebral palsy. *Journal of Child Neurology, 10*(4), 300–309.

Corwin, D., Isaacs, J., Georgeson, K., Bartolucci, A. A., Cloud, H. H., & Craig, C. D. (1996). Weight and length increases in children after gastrostomy placement. *Journal of the American Dietetic Association, 96*(9), 874–879.

Craig, J. J., & Van Vuren, J. (1976). The importance of gastrocnemius recession in the correction of equinus deformity in cerebral palsy. *Journal of Bone and Joint Surgery, British Volume, 58*(1), 84–87.

Dahl, M., Thommessen, M., Rasmussen, M., & Selberg, T. (1996). Feeding and nutritional characteristics in children with moderate or severe cerebral palsy. *Acta Paediatrica, 85*(6), 697–701.
Damiano, D. L. (2006). Activity, activity, activity: Rethinking our physical therapy approach to cerebral palsy. *Physical Therapy, 86*(11), 1534–1540.
Darley, F. L., Aronson, A. E., & Brown, J. R. (1969). Differential diagnostic patterns of dysarthria. *Journal of Speech, Language, and Hearing Research, 12*(2), 246–269.
Delwaide, P. J. (1973). Human monosynaptic reflexes and presynaptic inhibition. *New Developments in Electromyography and Clinical Neurophysiology, 3,* 508–522.
Dodd, K. J., Taylor, N. F., & Graham, H. K. (2003). A randomized clinical trial of strength training in young people with cerebral palsy. *Developmental Medicine and Child Neurology, 45*(10), 652–657.
Dolk, H., Pattenden, S., & Johnson, A. (2001). Cerebral palsy, low birth weight and socio-economic deprivation: Inequalities in a major cause of childhood disability. *Pediatric and Perinatal Epidemiology, 15*(4), 359–363.
Dolk, H., Parkes, J., & Hill, N. (2006). Trends in the prevalence of cerebral palsy in Northern Ireland, 1981–1997. *Developmental Medicine and Child Neurology, 48*(6), 406–412.
Douzenis, A., Rizos, E. N., Papadopoulou, A., Papathanasiou, M., & Lykouras, L. (2010). Porencephaly and psychosis: A case report and review of the literature. *BMC psychiatry, 10*(1), 19.
Dowding, V. M., & Barry, C. (1990). Cerebral palsy: Social class differences in prevalence in relation to birth weight and severity of disability. *Journal of Epidemiology and Community Health, 44*(3), 191–195.
Edebol-Tysk, K. (1989). Epidemiology of spastic tetraplegic cerebral palsy in Sweden-I. Impairments and disabilities. *Neuropediatrics, 20*(01), 41–45.
Edebol-Tysk, K., Hagberg, B., & Hagberg, G. (1989). Epidemiology of spastic tetraplegic cerebral palsy in Sweden-II. Prevalence, birth data and origin. *Neuropediatrics, 20*(01), 46–52.
Eliasson, A. C., Krumlinde-Sundholm, L., Rösblad, B., Beckung, E., Arner, M., Öhrvall, A. M., & Rosenbaum, P. (2006). The manual ability classification system (MACS) for children with cerebral palsy: Scale development and evidence of validity and reliability. *Developmental Medicine and Child Neurology, 48*(7), 549–554.
Eltami, M., & Sulliran, P. B. (1997). Nutritional management of the disabled child: The role of percutaneous endoscopic gastrostomy. *Developmental Medicine and Child Neurology, 39*(1), 66–68.
Engel, J. M., Schwartz, L., Jensen, M. P., & Johnson, D. R. (2000). Pain in cerebral palsy: The relation of coping strategies to adjustment. *Pain, 88*(3), 225–230.
Engsberg, J. R., Olree, K. S., Ross, S. A., & Park, T. S. (1996). Quantitative clinical measure of spasticity in children with cerebral palsy. *Archives of Physical Medicine and Rehabilitation, 77*(6), 594–599.
Eyman, R. K., Grossman, H. J., Tarjan, G., & Miller, C. R. (1987). Life expectancy and mental retardation. A longitudinal study in a state residential facility. *Monographs of the American Association on Mental Deficiency, 1982*(7), 1–73.
Eyman, R. K., Borthwick-Duffy, S. A., Call, T. L., & White, J. F. (1988). Prediction of mortality in community and institutional settings. *Journal of Intellectual Disability Research, 32*(3), 203–213.
Eyman, R. K., Call, T. L., & White, J. F. (1989). Mortality of elderly mentally retarded persons in California. *Journal of Applied Gerontology, 8*(2), 203–215.
Eyman, R. K., Grossman, H. J., Chaney, R. H., & Call, T. L. (1990). The life expectancy of profoundly handicapped people with mental retardation. *New England Journal of Medicine, 323*(9), 584–589.
Fanurik, D., Koh, J. L., Schmitz, M. L., Harrison, D. E., & Conrad, T. M. (1999). Children with cognitive impairment: Parent report of pain and coping. *Journal of Developmental and Behavioral Pediatrics, 20*(4), 228–234.
Fedrizzi, E., Inverno, M., Grazia Bruzzone, M., Botteon, G., Saletti, V., & Farinotti, M. (1996). MRI features of cerebral lesions and cognitive functions in preterm spastic diplegic children. *Pediatric Neurology, 15*(3), 207–212.

Fennell, E. B., & Dikel, T. N. (2001). Cognitive and neuropsychological functioning in children with cerebral palsy. *Journal of Child Neurology, 16*(1), 58–63.

Finnie, N. R. (1976). Handling the young cerebral palsied child at home. *The American Journal of Maternal/Child Nursing, 1*(6), 389.

Flett, P. J. (2003). Rehabilitation of spasticity and related problems in childhood cerebral palsy. *Journal of Pediatrics and Child Health, 39*(1), 6–14.

Flett, P., & Saunders, B. (1993). Ophthalmic assessment of physically disabled children attending a rehabilitation centre. *Journal of Pediatrics and Child Health, 29*(2), 132–135.

Flett, P. J., Stern, L. M., Waddy, H., Connell, T. M., Seeger, J. D., & Gibson, S. K. (1999). Botulinum toxin A versus fixed cast stretching for dynamic calf tightness in cerebral palsy. *Journal of Pediatrics and Child Health, 35*(1), 71–77.

Ford, F., Bleck, E. E., Aptekar, R. G., Collins, F. J., & Stevick, D. (1976). Efficacy of dantrolene sodium in the treatment of spastic cerebral palsy. *Developmental Medicine and Child Neurology, 18*(6), 770–783.

Franck, L. S., Greenberg, C. S., & Stevens, B. (2000). Pain assessment in infants and children. *Pediatric Clinics of North America, 47*(3), 487–512.

Fung, E. B., Samson-Fang, L., Stallings, V. A., Conaway, M., Liptak, G., Henderson, R. C., Worley, G., O'Donnell, M., Calvert, R., Rosenbaum, P., Chumlea, W., & Stevenson, R. D. (2002). Feeding dysfunction is associated with poor growth and health status in children with cerebral palsy. *Journal of the American Dietetic Association, 102*(3), 361–373.

Garfinkle, J., & Shevell, M. I. (2011). Cerebral palsy, developmental delay, and epilepsy after neonatal seizures. *Pediatric Neurology, 44*(2), 88–96.

Gauderer, M. (1999). Twenty years of percutaneous endoscopic gastrostomy: Origin and evolution of a concept and its expanded applications. *Gastrointestinal Endoscopy, 50*(6), 879–883.

Gibbs, F. A., Gibbs, E. L., Perlstein, M. A., & Rich, C. L. (1963). Electroencephalographic and clinical aspects of cerebral palsy. *Pediatrics, 32*(1), 73–84.

Gibson, J. J. (1986). *The ecological approach to visual perception*. New York, NY: Psychology Press.

Gielen, E. J. J. M., Elvers, J., & Oostendorp, R. (2008). Measuring spasticity in people with intellectual disabilities: Reliability and validity. *Journal of Intellectual Disability Research, 52*, 749–749.

Giller Gajdosik, C. (1991). Issues of parent compliance: What the clinician and researcher should know. *Physical and Occupational Therapy in Pediatrics, 11*(3), 73–87.

Goldstein, M., & Harper, D. C. (2001). Management of cerebral palsy: Equinus gait. *Developmental Medicine and Child Neurology, 43*(8), 563–569.

Gordon, J. (1987). Assumptions underlying physical therapy intervention: Theoretical and historical perspectives. In J. Carr & R. Sheppard (Eds.), *Movement science: Foundations for physical therapy in rehabilitation*. New York: Aspen Publishers.

Gormley, M. E. G. (2001). Treatment of neuromuscular and musculoskeletal problems in cerebral palsy. *Developmental Neurorehabilitation, 4*(1), 5–16.

Gormley, M. E. Jr., Krach, L. E., & Piccini, L. (2001). Spasticity management in the child with spastic quadriplegia. *European Journal of Neurology, 8*(5), 127–135.

Gracies, J. M., Nance, P., Elovic, E., McGuire, J., & Simpson, D. M. (1997). Traditional pharmacological treatments for spasticity part II: General and regional treatments. *Muscle and Nerve, 20*(6), 92–120.

Gracies, J. M., Burke, K., Clegg, N. J., Browne, R., Rushing, C., Fehlings, D., Matthews, D., Tilton, A., & Delgado, M. R. (2010). Reliability of the Tardieu scale for assessing spasticity in children with cerebral palsy. *Archives of Physical Medicine and Rehabilitation, 91*(3), 421–428.

Graham, H. K., Aoki, K. R., Autti-Rämö, I., Boyd, R. N., Delgado, M. R., Gaebler-Spira, D. J., Gormley, M. E., Guyer, B. M., Heinen, F., Holton, A. F., Matthews, D., Molenaers, G., Motta, F., García Ruiz, P. J., & Wissel, J. (2000). Recommendations for the use of botulinum toxin type A in the management of cerebral palsy. *Gait and Posture, 11*(1), 67–79.

Graham, H. K., Harvey, A., Rodda, J., Nattrass, G. R., & Pirpiris, M. (2004). The functional mobility scale (FMS). *Journal of Pediatric Orthopedics, 24*(5), 514–520.

Grant, P. E., & Barkovich, A. J. (1997). Neuroimaging in CP: Issues in pathogenesis and diagnosis. *Mental Retardation and Developmental Disabilities Research Reviews, 3*(2), 118–128.
Green, L. B., & Hurvitz, E. A. (2007). Cerebral palsy. *Physical and Medical Rehabiltation Clinic of North America, 18*(4), 859–882.
Gregson, J. M., Leathley, M., Moore, A. P., Sharma, A. K., Smith, T. L., & Watkins, C. L. (1999). Reliability of the tone assessment scale and the modified Ashworth scale as clinical tools for assessing poststroke spasticity. *Archives of Physical Medicine and Rehabilitation, 80*(9), 1013–1016.
Griggs, C. A., Jones, P. M., & Lee, R. E. (1989). Videofluoroscopic investigation of feeding disorders of children with multiple handicap. *Developmental Medicine and Child Neurology, 31*(3), 303–308.
Hadjipanayis, A., Hadjichristodoulou, C., & Youroukos, S. (1997). Epilepsy in patients with cerebral palsy. *Developmental Medicine and Child Neurology, 39*(10), 659–663.
Haerer, A. F., Anderson, D. W., & Schoenberg, B. S. (1984). Prevalence of cerebral palsy in the biracial population of Copiah County, Mississippi. *Developmental Medicine and Child Neurology, 26,* 195–199.
Hagberg, B., Hagberg, G., & Zetterstrom, R. (1989). Deceasing perinatal mortality increase in cerebral palsy morbidity? *Acta Paediatrica Scandinavica, 18,* 661–670.
Hägglund, G., Andersson, S., Düppe, H., Pedertsen, H. L., Nordmark, E., & Westbom, L. (2005). Prevention of severe contractures might replace multilevel surgery in cerebral palsy: Results of a population-based health care programme and new techniques to reduce spasticity. *Journal of Pediatric Orthopedics, 14*(4), 269–273.
Hallam, P. M. (1996). *The impact of prehension and fine motor development on gross motor activity in children with cerebral palsy* (Doctoral dissertation, University of Liverpool).
Harbeck, C., & Peterson, L. (1992). Elephants dancing in my head: A developmental approach to children's concepts of specific pains. *Child Development, 63*(1), 138–149.
Harvey, A., Graham, H. K., Morris, M. E., Baker, R., & Wolfe, R. (2007). The functional mobility scale: Ability to detect change following single event multilevel surgery. *Developmental Medicine and Child Neurology, 49*(8), 603–607.
Harvey, A. R., Morris, M. E., Graham, H. K., Wolfe, R., & Baker, R. (2010). Reliability of the functional mobility scale for children with cerebral palsy. *Physical and Occupational Therapy in Pediatrics, 30*(2), 139–149.
Haugh, A. B., Pandyan, A. D., & Johnson, G. R. (2006). A systematic review of the Tardieu scale for the measurement of spasticity. *Disability and Rehabilitation, 28*(15), 899–907.
Hayakawa, K., Kanda, T., Hashimoto, K., Okuno, Y., & Yamori, Y. (1997). MR of spastic tetraplegia. *American Journal of Neuroradiology, 18*(2), 247–253.
Henderson, J. L. (1961). *Cerebral palsy in childhood and adolescence: A medical, psychological, and social study*. London: E. & S. Livingstone.
Himmelmann, K., Hagberg, G., Beckung, E., Hagberg, B., & Uvebrant, P. (2005). The changing panorama of cerebral palsy in Sweden. IX. Prevalence and origin in the birth-year period 1995-1998. *Acta Paediatrica, 94*(3), 287–294.
Himmelmann, K., Beckung, E., Hagberg, G., & Uvebrant, P. (2006). Gross and fine motor function and accompanying impairments in cerebral palsy. *Developmental Medicine and Child Neurology, 48,* 417–423.
Hinojosa, J., & Anderson, J. (1991). Mothers' perceptions of home treatment programs for their preschool children with cerebral palsy. *The American Journal of Occupational Therapy, 45*(3), 273–279.
Hoare, B. J., Wasiak, J., Imms, C., & Carey, L. (2007). Constraint-induced movement therapy in the treatment of the upper limb in children with hemiplegic cerebral palsy. *Cochrane Database of Systematic Reviews, 18*(2), CD004149.
Hodapp, R. M. (1998). *Development and disabilities: Intellectual, sensory and motor impairments*. Cambridge: Cambridge University Press.
Hoon, A. H. (2005). Neuroimaging in cerebral palsy: Patterns of brain dysgenesis and injury. *Journal of Child Neurology, 20*(12), 936–939.

Houlihan, C. M., O'Donnell, M., Conaway, M., & Stevenson, R. D. (2004). Bodily pain and health-related quality of life in children with cerebral palsy. *Developmental Medicine and Child Neurology, 46*(5), 305–310.

Hudders-Algra, M., Nieuwendijk, A. W., Maitijn, A., & Eykern, L. A. (1997). Assessment of general movements: Towards a better understanding of a sensitive method to evaluate brain function in young infants. *Developmental Medicine and Child Neurology, 39*(2), 88–98.

Humphreys, P., Whiting, S., & Pham, B. (2000). Hemiparetic cerebral palsy: Clinical pattern and imaging in prediction of outcome. *Canadian Journal of Neurological Sciences, 27*(3), 210–219.

Humphris, D., Littlejohns, P., Victor, C., O'halloran, P., & Peacock, J. (2000). Implementing evidence-based practice: Factors that influence the use of research evidence by occupational therapists. *The British Journal of Occupational Therapy, 63*(11), 516–522.

Hunter, J. V., & Wang, Z. J. (2001). MR spectroscopy in pediatric neuroradiology. *Magnetic Resonance Imaging Clinics of North America, 9*(1), 165–189.

Jahnsen, R., Villien, L., Aamodt, G., Stanghelle, J., & Holm, I. (2004). Musculoskeletal pain in adults with cerebral palsy compared with the general population. *Journal of Rehabilitation Medicine, 36*(2), 78–84.

Josenby, A. L., Jarnlo, G. B., Gummesson, C., & Nordmark, E. (2009). Longitudinal construct validity of the GMFM-88 total score and goal total score and the GMFM-66 score in a 5-year follow-up study. *Physical Therapy, 89*(4), 342–350.

Joynt, R. L., & Leonard, J. A. (1980). Dantrolene sodium suspension in treatment of spastic cerebral palsy. *Developmental Medicine and Child Neurology, 22*(6), 755–767.

Katz, R. T., & Campagnolo, D. I. (1994). Pharmacologic management of spasticity. *Physical Medicine and Rehabilitation, 8,* 473–473.

Kerr, A. M., McCulloch, D., Oliver, K., McLean, B., Coleman, E., Law, T., Beaton, P., Wallace, S., Newell, E., Eccles, T., & Prescott, R. J. (2003). Medical needs of people with intellectual disability require regular reassessment, and the provision of client-and carer-held reports. *Journal of Intellectual Disability Research, 47*(2), 134–145.

Ketelaar, M., Vermeer, A., Hart, H. T., van Petegem-van Beek, E., & Helders, P. J. (2001). Effects of a functional therapy program on motor abilities of children with cerebral palsy. *Physical Therapy, 81*(9), 1534–1545.

Kim, D. Y., Park, C. I., Chon, J. S., Ohn, S. H., Park, T. H., & Bang, I. K. (2005). Biomechanical assessment with electromyography of post-stroke ankle plantar flexor spasticity. *Yonsei Medical Journal, 46*(4), 546–554.

Kirby, D. F., DeLegge, M. H., & Fleming, C. R. (1995). American Gastroenterological Association technical review on tube feeding for enteral nutrition. *Gastroenterology, 108*(4), 1282–1301.

Koeda, T., Suganuma, I., Kohno, Y., Takamatsu, T., & Takeshita, K. (1990). MR imaging of spastic diplegia. *Neuroradiology, 32*(3), 187–190.

Korzeniewski, S. J., Birbeck, G., DeLano, M. C., Potchen, M. J., & Paneth, N. (2008). A systematic review of neuroimaging for cerebral palsy. *Journal of Child Neurology, 23*(2), 216–227.

Krach, L. E. (2001). Pharmacotherapy of spasticity: Oral medications and intrathecal baclofen. *Journal of Child Neurology, 16*(1), 31–36.

Krägeloh-Mann, I., Petersen, D., Hagberg, G., Vollmer, B., Hagberg, B., & Michaelis, R. (1995). Bilateral spastic cerebral palsy-mri pathology and origin. Analysis from a representative series of 56 cases. *Developmental Medicine and Child Neurology, 37*(5), 379–397.

Krick, J., & Van Duyn, M. A. (1984). The relationship between oral-motor involvement and growth: A pilot study in a pediatric population with cerebral palsy. *Journal of the American Dietetic Association, 84*(5), 555–559.

Kulak, W., & Sobaniec, W. (2003). Risk factors and prognosis of epilepsy in children with cerebral palsy in north-eastern Poland. *Brain and Development, 25*(7), 499–506.

Kwong, K. L., Wong, S. N., & So, K. T. (1998). Epilepsy in children with cerebral palsy. *Pediatric Neurology, 19*(1), 31–36.

Lagergren, J. (1980). Children with motor handicaps. Epidemiological, medical and socio-paediatric aspects of motor handicapped children in a Swedish county. *Acta Paediatrica Scandinavica, Supplement, 289,* 1–71.

Latash, M. L., & Anson, J. G. (1996). What are "normal movements" in atypical populations? *Behavioral and Brain Sciences, 19*(01), 55–68.

Law, M., Cadman, D., Rosenbaum, P., Walter, S., Russell, D., & DeMatteo, C. (1991). Neurodevelopmental therapy and upper-extremity inhibitive casting for children with cerebral palsy. *Developmental Medicine and Child Neurology, 33*(5), 379–387.

Leech, S. K. (1996). Physiotherapy in paediatrics. *Physiotherapy, 82*(1), 69.

Liao, H. F., Liu, Y. C., Liu, W. Y., & Lin, Y. T. (2007). Effectiveness of loaded sit-to-stand resistance exercise for children with mild spastic diplegia: A randomized clinical trial. *Archives of Physical Medicine and Rehabilitation, 88*(1), 25–31.

Liptak, G. S., & Accardo, P. J. (2004). Health and social outcomes of children with cerebral palsy. *The Journal of Pediatrics, 145*(2), S36–S41.

Liu, J. M., Li, S., Lin, Q., & Li, Z. (1999). Prevalence of cerebral palsy in China. *International Journal of Epidemiology, 28*(5), 949–954.

Lorenz, J. M., Wooliever, D. E., Jetton, J. R., & Paneth, N. (1998). A quantitative review of mortality and developmental disability in extremely premature newborns. *Archives of Pediatrics and Adolescent Medicine, 152*(5), 425–435.

Lou, H. C. (1998). Cerebral palsy and hypoxic-hemodynamic brain lesions in the newborn. *Textbook of pediatric Neuropsychiatry, American Psychiatric Association*, Washington, DC, 1073–92.

Mackey, A. H., Walt, S. E., Lobb, G., & Stott, N. S. (2004). Intraobserver reliability of the modified Tardieu scale in the upper limb of children with hemiplegia. *Developmental Medicine and Child Neurology, 46*(4), 267–272.

Malhotra, S., Cousins, E., Ward, A., Day, C., Jones, P., Roffe, C., & Pandyan, A. (2008). An investigation into the agreement between clinical, biomechanical and neurophysiological measures of spasticity. *Clinical Rehabilitation, 22*(12), 1105–1115.

McLaughlin, J., Bjornson, K., Temkin, N., Steinbok, P., Wright, V., Reiner, A., Roberts, T., Drake, J., O'Donnell M., Rosenbaum, P., Barber, J., & Ferrel, A. (2002). Selective dorsal rhizotomy: Meta-analysis of three randomized controlled trials. *Developmental Medicine and Child Neurology, 44*(1), 17–25.

McLellan, D. L. (1991). Excessive and inappropriate muscle activation occurring in association with upper motor neurone syndrome. In M. Swash & J. Oxbury (Eds.), *Functional recovery and the principles of disability medicine. Clinical neurology*. London: Churchill Livingstone.

Melhem, E. R., Mori, S., Mukundan, G., Kraut, M. A., Pomper, M. G., & van Zijl, P. C. (2002). Diffusion tensor MR imaging of the brain and white matter tractography. *American Journal of Roentgenology, 178*(1), 3–16.

Menkes, J. H., & Sarnat, H. B. (2000). Perinatal asphyxia and trauma. In J. H. Menkes & H. B. Sarnat (Eds.), *Child neurology* (pp. 401–466). Philadelphia: Lippincott Williams & Wilkins.

Miller, C., & Eyman, R. (1978). Hospital and community mortality rates among the retarded. *Journal of Intellectual Disability Research, 22*(2), 137–145.

Molnar, G. E. (1979). Cerebral palsy: Prognosis and how to judge it. *Pediatric Annals, 8*(10), 596.

Molnar, G. E. (1985). *Pediatric rehabilitation*. Baltimore: Williams & Wilkins.

Molnar, G. E. (1991). Rehabilitation in cerebral palsy. *Western Journal of Medicine, 154*(5), 569.

Morris, C. (2007). Definition and classification of cerebral palsy: a historical perspective. *Developmental Medicine and Child Neurology, 49*(s109), 3–7.

Moss, S., Goldberg, D., Patel, P., & Wilken, D. (1993). Physical morbidity in older perople with moderate, severe, and profound mental handicap and its relation to psychiatric morbidity. *Social Psychiatry and Psychiatric Epidemiology, 28*, 32–39.

Murphy, C. C., Yeargin-Allsopp, M., Decouflé, P., & Drews, C. D. (1995). The administrative prevalence of mental retardation in 10-year-old children in metropolitan Atlanta, 1985 through 1987. *American Journal of Public Health, 85*(3), 319–323.

Mutch, L., Alberman, E., Hagberg, B., Kodama, K., & Perat, M. V. (1992). Cerebral palsy epidemiology: Where are we now and where are we going? *Developmental Medicine and Child Neurology, 34*(6), 547–551.

Mutlu, A., Livanelioglu, A., & Gunel, M. K. (2008). Reliability of ashworth and modified ashworth scales in children with spastic cerebral palsy. *BMC Musculoskeletal Disorders, 9*(1), 44.

Nance, P. W. (1997). Tizanidine an alpha2 agonist imidazoline with antispasticity effects. *Today's Therapeutic Trends, 15*, 11–25.

Nance, P. W., & Young, R. R. (1999). Antispasticity medications. *Physical Medicine and Rehabilitation Clinics of North America, 10*(2), 337–355.

Neil, J., Miller, J., Mukherjee, P., & Hüppi, P. S. (2002). Diffusion tensor imaging of normal and injured developing human brain-a technical review. *NMR in Biomedicine, 15*(7–8), 543–552.

Nelson, K. B., Dambrosia, J. M., Iovannisci, D. M., Cheng, S., Grether, J. K., & Lammer, E. (2005). Genetic polymorphisms and cerebral palsy in very preterm infants. *Pediatric Research, 57*(4), 494–499.

Nordmark, E., Hagglund, G., & Lagergren, J. (2001). Cerebral palsy in southern Sweden I. Prevalence and clinical features. *Acta Paediatrica, 90*(11), 1271–1276.

Novak, I., Cusick, A., & Lannin, N. (2009). Occupational therapy home programs for cerebral palsy: Double-blind, randomized, controlled trial. *Pediatrics, 124*(4), 606–614.

Novotny, E., Ashwal, S., & Shevell, M. (1998). Proton magnetic resonance spectroscopy: An emerging technology in pediatric neurology research. *Pediatric Research, 44*(1), 1–10.

Oberlander, T. F. (2001). Pain assessment and management in infants and young children with developmental disabilities. *Infants and Young Children, 14*(2), 33–47.

Odding, E., Roebroeck, M. E., & Stam, H. J. (2006). The epidemiology of cerebral palsy: Incidence, impairments and risk factors. *Disability and Rehabilitation, 28*(4), 183–191.

O'Shea, T. M. (2008). Diagnosis, treatment, and prevention of cerebral palsy in near-term/term infants. *Clinical Obstetrics and Gynecology, 51*(4), 816.

Palisano, R. J. (1992). Research on the effectiveness of neurodevelopmental treatment. *Pediatric Physical Therapy, 3*, 143–148.

Palisano, R., Rosenbaum, P., Walter, S., Russell, D., Wood, E., & Galuppi, B. (1997). Development and reliability of a system to classify gross motor function in children with cerebral palsy. *Developmental Medicine and Child Neurology, 39*(4), 214–223.

Palisano, R. J., Rosenbaum, P., Bartlett, D., & Livingston, M. H. (2008). Content validity of the expanded and revised gross motor function classification system. *Developmental Medicine and Child Neurology, 50*(10), 744–750.

Palmer, F. B. (2002). First, observe the patient. *Archives of Pediatrics and Adolescent Medicine, 156*(5), 422–423.

Palmer, F. B., Shapiro, B. K., Wachtel, R. C., Allen, M. C., Hiller, J. E., Harryman, S. E., Mosher, B. S., Meiert, C. L., & Capute, A. J. (1988). The effects of physical therapy on cerebral palsy. *New England Journal of Medicine, 318*(13), 803–808.

Pandyan, A. D., Price, C. I. M., Rodgers, H., Barnes, M. P., & Johnson, G. R. (2001). Biomechanical examination of a commonly used measure of spasticity. *Clinical Biomechanics, 16*(10), 859–865.

Patikas, D., Wolf, S. I., Armbrust, P., Mund, K., Schuster, W., Dreher, T., & Döderlein, L. (2006). Effects of a postoperative resistive exercise program on the knee extension and flexion torque in children with cerebral palsy: A randomized clinical trial. *Archives of Physical Medicine and Rehabilitation, 87*(9), 1161–1169.

Patrick, J., Boland, M., Stoski, D., & Murray, G. E. (1986). Rapid correction of wasting in children with cerebral palsy. *Developmental Medicine and Child Neurology, 28*(6), 734–739.

Pearce, C. B., & Duncan, H. D. (2002). Enteral feeding. Nasogastric, nasojejunal, percutaneous endoscopic gastrostomy, or jejunostomy: Its indications and limitations. *Postgraduate Medical Journal, 78*(918), 198–204.

Pearson, P. H., & Williams, C. E. (1972). *Physical therapy services in the developmental disabilities*. Springfield: Charles C. Thomas Publisher.

Pentoff, E. (1964). Cerebral palsy: A pharmacologic approach. *Clinical Pharmacology and Therapeutics, 5*, 947–954.

Petterson, B., Stanley, F., & Henderson, D. (1990). Cerebral palsy in multiple births in Western Australia: Genetic aspects. *American Journal of Medical Genetics, 37*(3), 346–351.

Pharoah, P. O. D., Cooke, T., Johnson, M. A., King, R., & Mutch, L. (1998). Epidemiology of cerebral palsy in England and Scotland, 1984–9. *Archives of Disease in Childhood-Fetal and Neonatal Edition, 79*(1), F21–25.

Phelps, W. M. (1941). The management of the cerebral palsies. *Journal of the American Medical Association, 117,* 1621–1625.

Pinto, S., Ozsancak, C., Tripoliti, E., Thobois, S., Limousin-Dowsey, P., & Auzou, P. (2004). Treatments for dysarthria in Parkinson's disease. *The Lancet Neurology, 3*(9), 547–556.

Prechtl, H. F. (2001). General movement assessment as a method of developmental neurology: New paradigms and their consequences. *Developmental Medicine and Child Neurology, 43*(12), 836–842.

Prechtl, H. F., Einspieler, C., Cioni, G., Bos, A. F., Ferrari, F., & Sontheimer, D. (1997). An early marker for neurological deficits after perinatal brain lesions. *Lancet, 349*(9062), 1361–1363.

Pruitt, D. W., & Tsai, T. (2009). Common medical comorbidities associated with cerebral palsy. *Physical Medicine and Rehabilitation Clinics of North America, 20*(3), 453–467.

Reddihough, D. S., & Collins, K. J. (2003). The epidemiology and causes of cerebral palsy. Australian. *Journal of Physiotherapy, 49*(1), 7–12.

Redford, J. B. (1986). *Principles of orthotic devices*. Baltimore: Williams and Wilkins.

Reilly, S., Skuse, D., & Poblete, X. (1996). Prevalence of feeding problems and oral motor dysfunction in children with cerebral palsy: A community survey. *The Journal of Pediatrics, 129*(6), 877–882.

Rempel, G. R., Colwell, S. O., & Nelson, R. P. (1988). Growth in children with cerebral palsy fed via gastrostomy. *Pediatrics, 82*(6), 857–862.

Rethlefsen, S., Kay, R., Dennis, S., Forstein, M., & Tolo, V. (1999). The effects of fixed and articulated ankle-foot orthoses on gait patterns in subjects with cerebral palsy. *Journal of Pediatric Orthopaedics, 19*(4), 470–474.

Roboz, P. (1972). Mortality rate in institutionalized mentally retarded children. *The Medical Journal of Australia, 1*(5), 218.

Rodda, J., & Graham, H. K. (2001). Classification of gait patterns in spastic hemiplegia and spastic diplegia: a basis for a management algorithm. *European Journal of Neurology, 8*(s5), 98–108.

Ronen, G. M., Buckley, D., Penney, S., & Streiner, D. L. (2007). Long-term prognosis in children with neonatal seizures: A population-based study. *Neurology, 69*(19), 1816–1822.

Rosenbaum, P., Paneth, N., Leviton, A., Goldstein, M., Bax, M., Damiano, D., Dan, B., & Jacobsson, B. (2007). A report: The definition and classification of cerebral palsy April 2006. *Developmental Medicine and Child Neurology, 109,* 8–14.

Ruby, D. O., & Matheny, W. D. (1962). Comments on growth of cerebral palsied children. *Journal of the American Dietetic Association, 40,* 525.

Russell, D. J., Rosenbaum, P. L., Cadman, D. T., Gowland, C., Hardy, S., & Jarvis, S. (1989). The gross motor function measure: A means to evaluate the effects of physical therapy. *Developmental Medicine and Child Neurology, 31*(3), 341–352.

Russell, D. J., Rosenbaum, P. L., Gowland, C., Hardy, S., Lane, M., Plews, N., & Jarvis, S. (1993). *Manual for the gross motor function measure*. Hamilton, ON: McMaster University.

Russell, D., Palisano, R., Walter, S., Rosenbaum, P., Gemus, M., Gowland, C., Galuppi, B., & Lane, M. (1998). Evaluating motor function in children with Down syndrome: Validity of the GMFM. *Developmental Medicine and Child Neurology, 40*(10), 693–701.

Russell, D. J., Avery, L. M., Rosenbaum, P. L., Raina, P. S., Walter, S. D., & Palisano, R. J. (2000). Improved scaling of the gross motor function measure for children with cerebral palsy: Evidence of reliability and validity. *Physical Therapy, 80*(9), 873–885.

Samson-Fang, L., Butler, C., & O'Donnell, M. (2003). Effects of gastrostomy feeding in children with cerebral palsy: An AACPDM evidence report. *Developmental Medicine and Child Neurology, 45*(6), 415–426.

Schenk-Rootlieb, A. J., van Niewenhuizen, O., van der Graaf, Y., Wittebol-Post, D., & Willmse, J. (1992). The prevalence of cerebral visual disturbance in children with cerebral palsy. *Developmental Medicine and Child Neurology, 34,* 473–480.

Scholtes, V. A., Becher, J. G., Beelen, A., & Lankhorst, G. J. (2006). Clinical assessment of spasticity in children with cerebral palsy: A critical review of available instruments. *Developmental Medicine and Child Neurology, 48*(1), 64–73.

Schrag, S. P., Sharma, R., Jaik, N. P., Seamon, M. J., Lukaszczyk, J. J., Martin, N. D., Hoey, B. A., & Stawicki, S. P. (2007). Complications related to percutaneous endoscopic gastrostomy (PEG) tubes. A comprehensive clinical review. *Journal of Gastrointestinal and Liver Diseases, 16*(4), 407.

Schreiber, J. M., Effgen, S. K., & Palisano, R. J. (1995). Effectiveness of parental collaboration on compliance with a home program. *Pediatric Physical Therapy, 7*(2), 59–64.

Schwartz, L., Engel, J. M., & Jensen, M. P. (1999). Pain in persons with cerebral palsy. *Archives of Physical Medicine and Rehabilitation, 80*(10), 1243–1246.

Scrutton, D. (Ed.). (1984). *Management of the motor disorders of children with cerebral palsy* (No. 90). Cambridge: Cambridge University Press.

Shapiro, B. K., Green, P., Krick, J., Allen, D., & Capute, A. J. (1986). Growth of severely impaired children: Neurological versus nutritional factors. *Developmental Medicine and Child Neurology, 28*(6), 729–733.

Shumway-Cook, A., & Woollacott, M. H. (1995). *Motor control: Theory and practical applications* (Vol. 157). Baltimore: Williams & Wilkins.

Singhi, P., Jagirdar, S., Khandelwal, N., & Malhi, P. (2003). Epilepsy in children with cerebral palsy. *Journal of Child Neurology, 18*(3), 174–179.

Sleigh, G., & Brocklehurst, P. (2004). Gastrostomy feeding in cerebral palsy: A systematic review. *Archives of Disease in Childhood, 89*(6), 534–539.

Sommerfeld, D., Fraser, B. A., Hensinger, R. N., & Beresford, C. V. (1981). Evaluation of physical therapy service for severely mentally impaired students with cerebral palsy. *Physical Therapy, 61*(3), 338–344.

St-Laurent-Gagnon, T., Bernard-Bonnin, A. C., & Villeneuve, E. (1999). Pain evaluation in preschool children and by their parents. *Acta Paediatrica, 88*(4), 422–427.

Stallings, V. A., Charney, E. B., Davies, J. C., & Cronk, C. E. (1993). Nutrition-related growth failure of children with quadriplegic cerebral palsy. *Developmental Medicine and Child Neurology, 35*(2), 126–138.

Stegeman, D. F., Blok, J. H., Hermens, H. J., & Roeleveld, K. (2000). Surface EMG models: Properties and applications. *Journal of Electromyography and Kinesiology, 10*(5), 313–326.

Sullivan, P. B., Juszczak, E., Bachlet, A. M., Lambert, B., Vernon-Roberts, A., Grant, H. W., Eltumi, M., McLean, L., Alder, N., & Thomas, A. G. (2005). Gastrostomy tube feeding in children with cerebral palsy: A prospective, longitudinal study. *Developmental Medicine and Child Neurology, 47*(2), 77–85.

Sullivan, P. B., Alder, N., Grant, H., Juszczak, E., Henry, J., Warner, J., & Wells, J. (2006). Gastrostomy feeding in cerebral palsy: Too much of a good thing? *Developmental Medicine and Child Neurology, 48*(11), 877–882.

Surveillance of Cerebral Palsy in Europe. (2000). Surveillance of cerebral palsy in Europe (SCPE): A collaboration ofcerebral palsy surveys and registers. *Developmental Medicine and Child Neurology, 42,* 816–824.

Sutherland, D. H., & Davids, J. R. (1993). Common gait abnormalities of the knee in cerebral palsy. *Clinical Orthopaedics and Related Research, 288,* 139–147.

Tardieu, G., Shentoub, S., & Delarue, R. (1953). Research on a technic for measurement of spasticity. *Revue neurologique, 91*(2), 143–144.

Tarjan, G., Brooke, C. E., Eyman, R. K., Suyeyasu, A., & Miller, C. R. (1968). Mortality and cause of death in a hospital for the mentally retarded. *American Journal of Public Health and the Nations Health, 58*(10), 1891–1900.

Taub, E., Ramey, S. L., DeLuca, S., & Echols, K. (2004). Efficacy of constraint-induced movement therapy for children with cerebral palsy with asymmetric motor impairment. *Pediatrics, 113*(2), 305–312.

Tekgul, H., Gauvreau, K., Soul, J., Murphy, L., Robertson, R., Stewart, J., Volpe, J., Bourgeois, B., & du Plessis, A. J. (2006). The current etiologic profile and neurodevelopmental outcome of seizures in term newborn infants. *Pediatrics, 117*(4), 1270–1280.

Temple, V. A., Frey, G. C., & Stanish, H. I. (2006). Physical activity of adults with mental retardation: Review and research needs. *American Journal of Health Promotion, 21*(1), 2–12.

Thelen, E. (1996). *A dynamic systems approach to the development of cognition and action*. Cambridge: MIT press.

Thomas, A., Bax, M., Coombers, K., Goldson, E., Smyth, D., & Whitmore, K. (1989). *The health and social needs of young adults with physical disabilities* (No. 106). London: Mac Keith Press.

Tomlin, P. I. (1995). The static encephalopathies. In R. W. Newton (Ed.), *Color atlas of pediatric neurology* (pp. 203–216). London: Times-Wolfe International.

Torfs, C. P., van den Berg, B. J., Oechsli, F. W., & Cummins, S. (1990). Prenatal and perinatal factors in the etiology of cerebral palsy. *The Journal of Pediatrics, 116*(4), 615–619.

Torrey, E. F., Miller, J., Rawlings, R., & Yolken, R. H. (2000). Seasonal birth patterns of neurological disorders. *Neuroepidemiology, 19*(4), 177–185.

Tosi, L. L., Maher, N., Moore, D. W., Goldstein, M., & Aisen, M. L. (2009). Adults with cerebral palsy: A workshop to define the challenges of treating and preventing secondary musculoskeletal and neuromuscular complications in this rapidly growing population. *Developmental Medicine and Child Neurology, 51*(4), 2–11.

Truwit, C., Barkovich, A. J., Koch, T. K., & Ferriero, D. M. (1992). Cerebral palsy: MR findings in 40 patients. *American Journal of Neuroradiology, 13*(1), 67–78.

Turk, M. A., Scandale, J., Rosenbaum, P. F., & Weber, R. J. (2001). The health of women with cerebral palsy. *Physical Medicine and Rehabilitation Clinics of North America, 12*(1), 153–168.

Unger, M., Faure, M., & Frieg, A. (2006). Strength training in adolescent learners with cerebral palsy: A randomized controlled trial. *Clinical Rehabilitation, 20*(6), 469–477.

Upton, D. (1999). Clinical effectiveness and EBP 2: Attitudes of health-care professionals. *International Journal of Therapy and Rehabilitation, 6*(1), 26–30.

Uysal, H., Mogyoros, I., & Burke, D. (1999). Reproducibility of tendon jerk reflexes during a voluntary contraction. *Clinical Neurophysiology, 110*(8), 1481–1487.

van Schrojenstein Lantman-de Valk, H. M., van den Akker, M., Maaskant, M. A., Haveman, M. J., Urlings, H. F., Kessels, A. G., & Crebolder, H. F. (1997). Prevalence and incidence of health problems in people with intellectual disability. *Journal of Intellectual Disability Research, 41*(1), 42–51.

Vargha-Khadem, F., Isaacs, E., vander Werf, S., Robb, S., & Wilson, J. (1992). Development of intelligence and memory in children with hemiplegic cerebral palsy: The deleterious consequences of early seizures. *Brain: A Journal of Neurology, 115*(1), 315–329.

Verrotti, A., Greco, R., Spalice, A., Chiarelli, F., & Iannetti, P. (2006). Pharmacotherapy of spasticity in children with cerebral palsy. *Pediatric Neurology, 34*(1), 1–6.

Voerman, G. E., Gregoric, M., & Hermens, H. J. (2005). Neurophysiological methods for the assessment of spasticity: The Hoffmann reflex, the tendon reflex, and the stretch reflex. *Disability and Rehabilitation, 27*(1–2), 33–68.

Voerman, G. E., Burridge, J. H., Hitchcock, R. A., & Hermens, H. J. (2007). Clinometric properties of a clinical spasticity measurement tool. *Disability and Rehabilitation, 29*(24), 1870–1880.

Wallace, S. J. (2001). Epilepsy in cerebral palsy. *Developmental Medicine and Child Neurology, 43*(10), 713–717.

Wallen, M., O'Flaherty, S. J., & Waugh, M. C. A. (2007). Functional outcomes of intramuscular botulinum toxin type a and occupational therapy in the upper limbs of children with cerebral palsy: A randomized controlled trial. *Archives of Physical Medicine and Rehabilitation, 88*(1), 1–10.

Waninge, A., Rook, R. A., Dijkhuizen, A., Gielen, E., & van der Schans, C. P. (2011). Feasibility, test-retest reliability, and interrater reliability of the modified ashworth scale and modified tardieu scale in persons with profound intellectual and multiple disabilities. *Research in Developmental Disabilities, 32*(2), 613–620.

Ward, A. B. (2008). Spasticity treatment with botulinum toxins. *Journal of Neural Transmission, 115*(4), 607–616.

Ward, A. B., & Koko, C. (2001). *Pharmacological management of spasticity. Upper motor neuron syndrome and spasticity: Clinical management and neurophysiology* (pp. 165–187). Cambridge: Cambridge University Press.

Wasiak, J., Hoare, B. J., & Wallen, M. M. (2009). Botulinum toxin A as an adjunct to treatment in the management of the upper limb in children with spastic cerebral palsy (Review). *The Cochrane Library, 4*, 1–16.

Watt, J. M., Robertson, C. M. T., & Grace, M. G. A. (1989). Early prognosis for ambulation of neonatal intensive care survivors with cerebral palsy. *Developmental Medicine and Child Neurology, 31*(6), 766–773.

Weir, W., Mutch, L., Camerson, M., Cochrane, M., Paterson, M., Thomson, A., … & Renfrew, C. (1992). The Scottish low-birth-weight study. 1. Survival, growth, neuromotor and sensory impairment. *Archives of Disease in Childhood, 67*(6), 675–681.

Whyte, J., & Robinson, K. M. (1990). Pharmacologic management. In M. B. Glenn & J. Whyte (Eds.), *The practical management of spasticity in children and adults* (pp. 201–226). Philadelphia: Lea & Febiger.

Winters, T. F., Gage, J. R., & Hicks, R. (1987). Gait patterns in spastic hemiplegia in children and young adults. *The Journal of Bone and Joint Surgery, 69*(3), 437–441.

Wood, E., & Rosenbaum, P. (2000). The gross motor function classification system for cerebral palsy: A study of reliability and stability over time. *Developmental Medicine and Child Neurology, 42*(5), 292–296.

Wood, D. E., Burridge, J. H., Wijck, F. V., McFadden, C., Hitchcock, R. A., Pandyan, A. D., Haugh, A., Salazar-Torres, J. J., & Swain, I. D. (2005). Biomechanical approaches applied to the lower and upper limb for the measurement of spasticity: A systematic review of the literature. *Disability and Rehabilitation, 27*(1–2), 19–33.

World Health Organization. (2001). *International classification of functioning, disability and health, ICF*. Geneva: World Health Organization.

Yam, W. K. L., & Leung, M. S. M. (2006). Interrater reliability of modified ashworth scale and modified tardieu scale in children with spastic cerebral palsy. *Journal of Child Neurology, 21*(12), 1031–1035.

Yeargin-Allsopp, M., Drews, C. D., Decouflé, P., & Murphy, C. C. (1995). Mild mental retardation in black and white children in metropolitan Atlanta: A case-control study. *American Journal of Public Health, 85*(3), 324–328.

Yeargin-Allsopp, M., Braun, K. V. N., Doernberg, N. S., Benedict, R. E., Kirby, R. S., & Durkin, M. S. (2008). Prevalence of cerebral palsy in 8-year-old children in three areas of the United States in 2002: A multisite collaboration. *Pediatrics, 121*(3), 547–554.

Yekutiel, M., & Jariwala, M. (1994). Sensory deficit in the hands of children with cerebral palsy: A new look at assessment and prevalence. *Developmental Medicine and Child Neurology, 36*(7), 619–624.

Yin, R., Reddihough, D. S., Ditchfield, M. R., & Collins, K. J. (2000). Magnetic resonance imaging findings in cerebral palsy. *Journal of Pediatrics and Child Health, 36*(2), 139–144.

Young, R. R., Emre, M., Nance, P. W., Schapiro, R., & Barnes, M. (1997). Current issues in spasticity management. *The Neurologist, 3*(5), 261.

Zafeiriou, D. I., Kontopoulos, E. E., & Tsikoulas, I. (1999). Characteristics and prognosis of epilepsy in children with cerebral palsy. *Journal of Child Neurology, 14*(5), 289–294.

Wasiak, J., Hoare, B. J., & Wallen, M. M. (2009). Botulinum toxin A as an adjunct to treatment in the management of the upper limb in children with spastic cerebral palsy (Review). *The Cochrane Library, 4*, 1–16.

Watt, J. M., Robertson, C. M. T., & Grace, M. G. A. (1989). Early prognosis for ambulation of neonatal intensive care survivors with cerebral palsy. *Developmental Medicine and Child Neurology, 31*, 766–773.

[illegible]

[illegible]

[illegible]

Wood, E., & Rosenbaum, P. (2000). The gross motor function classification system for cerebral palsy: [illegible] *Developmental Medicine and Child Neurology* [illegible]

[illegible]

Chapter 13
The Relationship of Cerebral Palsy Comorbid Conditions with Participation and Quality of Life

Marta Badia, Begoña Orgaz, Inmaculada Riquelme and Pedro Montoya

Introduction

Recent advances in the study of cerebral palsy (CP) have led to a very relevant change in our knowledge of this disability, which is currently the most frequent cause of physical disability in childhood. The new approach, in which the World Health Organization (WHO) has actively participated, focuses more on health components than on the consequences of the disease. From this perspective, disability is a social construct, implying an interaction between the person and the environment, so that special emphasis is placed on the promotion of quality of life (QOL) and participation in the community of people with disabilities. This chapter will present, on the one hand, the conceptual model proposed for the study of CP, the current definition and classification system, and data about the epidemiology and incidence of the comorbidities. It will also address the importance of participation and QOL in the assessment of the personal outcomes of intervention procedures as well as the role played by the diverse comorbidities associated with CP. To conclude, it will analyze the effects of these changes on our comprehension of CP in order to

M. Badia (✉)
Institute on Community Integration (INICO), Department of Personality, Assessment & Psychological Treatments, University of Salamanca, Salamanca, Spain
e-mail: badia@usal.es

B. Orgaz
Faculty of Psychology, Department of Basic Psychology, Psychobiology, and Methodology of Behavior Sciences, University of Salamanca, Salamanca, Spain

I. Riquelme
Research Institute on Health Sciences—IUNICS, Department of Nursing and Physiotherapy, University of the Balearic Islands, Balearic Islands, Spain

P. Montoya
Research Institute on Health Sciences—IUNICS, University of the Balearic Islands, Balearic Islands, Spain

J. L. Matson, M. L. Matson (eds.), *Comorbid Conditions in Individuals with Intellectual Disabilities,* Autism and Child Psychopathology Series,
DOI 10.1007/978-3-319-15437-4_13

plan and organize support service strategies promoting the participation and QOL of people with CP.

Conceptualizing and Applying the Human Functioning Model to Cerebral Palsy

A Biopsychosocial Model of Cerebral Palsy

Progress in our comprehension of CP has been made possible as a result of the current biopsychosocial conception of disability, emphasizing the relevance of the environment in participation and QOL. The model of human functioning of the International Classification of Functioning, Disability and Health (ICF) (World Health Organization, 2001) includes contextual factors and participation as essential dimensions. They, in turn, include the environmental and personal factors that may affect a person's health. The environmental factors constitute the physical, social, and attitudinal environment in which people live and develop, whereas personal factors are the particular background of a person's life and lifestyle (e.g., sex, age, education, profession, and socioeconomic characteristics). However, according to the ICF, (2001) participation is defined as the act of engaging in a life situation. Some examples of life situations in which people usually participate include relations with family and friends, domestic life, learning and applying knowledge, and community, social, and civic life, including leisure activities.

Hence, the biopsychosocial model of disability, on the one hand, considers participation as an essential dimension related to the person's functioning in society and, on the other, it acknowledges that people with a chronic health condition can enjoy a satisfactory life (Rosenbaum 2008). This perspective underlines the relevance of environment for participation and to achieve optimal levels of QOL in people with CP (Colver 2005; see Fig. 13.1). The ICF (2001) defines the environment as the physical, social, and attitudinal factors that either facilitate or hinder participation. Thus, environmental barriers such as, for example, the lack of adapted transportation or negative attitudes towards children with CP can negatively affect their participation and QOL. Actually, it is important to know not only the negative aspects (barriers) of the environment, because they can worsen the disability and the levels of dependence, but also the positive environmental factors (facilitators), which, when mobilized, can increase levels of participation in the community, in school, or at home.

Definition of Cerebral Palsy from a Biopsychosocial Perspective

Recent advances in the study of CP have led to a very relevant change in our knowledge of this disability. CP has traditionally been considered as a motor disorder, and this conception has marked both research and intervention, which

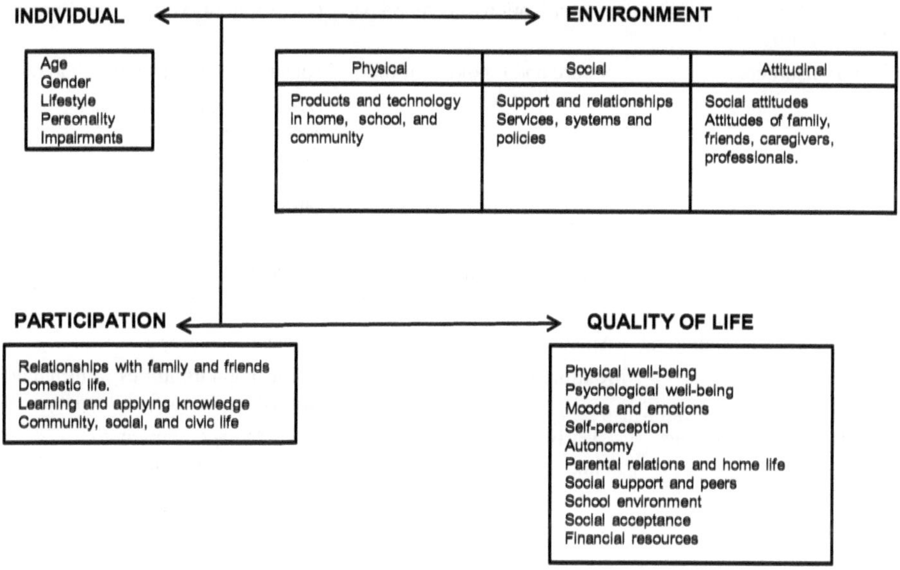

Fig. 13.1 Please insert missing text here

has mainly focused on the motor consequences produced by early brain damage. However, the current perspective of the study of CP, based on an ecological and biopsychosocial model of disability, is fostering important changes in intervention procedures with a clear will to go from an approach focused on persons and limitations to a perspective oriented towards promoting the functional capacities of people in interaction with their environment (home, school, work, community, etc.).

CP is a developmental disability that includes different disorders from heterogeneous etiologies, types, and severity. The *motor* disorders of posture and movement are permanent and not progressive, although changing clinical patterns can manifest, leading to limitations/restrictions of activity (e.g., walking, manipulation, and speech). In addition, CP is usually accompanied by other disorders (e.g., pain, fatigue, and epilepsy), comorbidities to which special attention must be paid.

Rosenbaum et al. (2007) propose the following definition:

> Cerebral palsy describes a group of permanent disorders of the development of movement and posture, causing activity limitation, that are attributed to non-progressive disturbances that occurred in the developing fetal or infant brain. The motor disorders of cerebral palsy are often accompanied by disturbances of sensation, perception, cognition, communication, and behavior, by epilepsy, and by secondary musculoskeletal problems (p. 9).

The strategy adopted for the classification of CP is that described in the Reference and Training Manual of Surveillance of Cerebral Palsy in Europe (SCPE R&TM), available at the website of SCPE (http://www.scpenetwork.eu/en/rtm/), which proposes a classification of CP with four components: (1) motor abnormalities, (2) associated deficiencies, (3) anatomic and radiological findings, and (4) etiology and time of onset of the alteration (see Table 13.1).

Table 13.1 Components of the classification of cerebral palsy (CP) of the surveillance of Cerebral Palsy in Europe

Motor disorders	Nature and typology of the motor disorder	Spastic CP (bilateral or unilateral)
		Dyskinetic CP (dystonic or choreoathetosis CP)
		Ataxic CP
	Functional motor skills	Limited activity
Associated disorders	Presence or absence	Epilepsy
	Impact on functional skills	Intellectual disability
		Sensory disorders
Anatomic and radiological findings	Anatomic distribution	Affected body parts
	Radiological findings	Cortical abnormalities, ventricular elongation, loss of white matter…
Etiology and chronology	Clearly identified cause	Brain damage, meningitis, cerebral malformations…
	Time of onset of the injury	Event that occurred before the affected function developed

Activity Limitations

The current definition of CP within the conceptual biopsychosocial model considers the motor disorder as the cause of the activity limitations. The ICF (2001) refers to activity as the execution of a task or action by a person, and defines limitation of activity as the difficulties a person may have performing that activity. However, one of the problems of the ICF is that it does not present a clear and exclusive division between activity and participation (defined as the act of engaging in a life situation). More specifically, the ICF only provides one classification system of the life areas of the components of activity and participation. Thereby, to solve this problem, the ICF offers four different ways classification forms, leaving the decision to each user of which option to choose in order to differentiate activities from participation. However, since the publication of the ICF, many studies have appeared that are oriented towards achieving a clearer conceptualization of these two components (Badley 2008; Nordenfelt 2003). Thus, Whiteneck and Dijkers (2009) propose considering activity as referring to the performance at the individual level, and participation when referring to outcomes at the social level. Following this suggestion, activities are physical and cognitive tasks carried out by people, whereas participation is the performance of the social role as a member of society.

Thus, the application of the biopsychosocial model of disability in CP contributes to the establishment of individualized functional profiles that become a central aspect in the design and development of intervention programs. Hence, the elaboration of adequate instruments to assess the functional motor skills of people with CP is becoming a priority goal, and there are currently various available measures (see Table 13.2). Although it is important to take activity limitations into account, the way in which motor disorders affect participation—an issue that will be addressed below—should also be considered.

Table 13.2 Measures to assess functional capacity in cerebral palsy (CP)

Instrument	Authors	Purpose of measure	Content
Gross motor function classification system (GMFCS)	Palisano et al. (1997)	Describes the motor performance of children with CP on the basis of their functional abilities and their need for assistive technology and wheeled mobility	Functional levels range from I (independent gross motor function with few limitations) to V (complete dependence for all motor activities)
Manual ability classification system (MACS)	Eliasson et al. (2006)	Describes how children with CP use their hands to manipulate objects in daily activities	It has 5 levels: Level I represents optimal manual skill, and Level V indicates lack of any active function in the hands
Drooling impact scale (DIS)	Reid et al. (2010)	Assesses the effect of interventions to control saliva in the drooling of children with developmental disabilities	It consists of a series of ten items, each one measured on scale ranging from 1 to 10. The total individual scores of the items are calculated to assess the severity and frequency of drooling. A score of 9 or 10 is classified as an excellent to very good reduction, 7 to 8 as a good reduction, and less than 5 as deterioration
Viking speech scale (VSS)	Pennington et al. (2013)	Assesses the functioning of speech in children with CP in daily life	It has 4 levels: no speech disorder (Level 1), imprecise speech but usually comprehensible for strangers (Level II), unclear speech, normally not understood by people who are not familiar or out of context (Level III), incomprehensible speech (Level IV)
Communication function classification system (CFCS)	Hidecker et al. (2011)	Assesses the capacity for communication in daily life situations	It classifies communication in five levels according to the efficacy of current communication: Level I indicates that the emitter and receiver is efficacious with known and unknown interlocutors; Level V indicates that the emitter and receiver is rarely efficacious with known interlocutors
Functional Communication Classification System (FCSS)	The Center for Cerebral Palsy and Cerebral Play League of Queensland (2014)	Assesses the way the child with CP communicates in daily life situations	It has five levels, where Level I indicates a total absence of support to interact, and Level V reflects complete assistance to communicate

Comorbidities in Cerebral Palsy

During the past few years, there has been an increase in the incidence and prevalence of CP, mainly due to the improved documentation of cases recorded in the national registers. Thus, Odding et al. (2006), in a study of a network of CP registers in 14 centers of 8 European countries, called Surveillance of Cerebral Palsy in Europe (SCPE), report the epidemiological data of CP, estimating the prevalence at 2–2.5 per 1000 live newborns. Likewise, the data indicate that each year, about 10,000 new cases of CP are diagnosed in the European Union.

Early brain damage always has motor sequelae but, in many people with CP, there are also other deficiencies that can interfere with their ability to function in daily life and that provoke greater limitations of activities than the motor deficiencies themselves. Baxter (2013) note the relevance of paying more attention to the comorbidities associated with CP because they can have a negative impact on the participation and QOL of children, adolescents, and adults with CP. According to Odding et al. (2006), depending on the type of CP, between 25 and 80 % of people with CP present associated deficiencies.

Somatosensory Deficits

In addition to motor sequelae, people with CP can manifest somatosensory alterations, among which abnormal tactile perception and altered pain sensitivity are noteworthy. For example, people with CP have been observed to present worse levels of tactile discrimination, stereognosis, and proprioception (Cooper et al. 1995; McLaughlin et al. 2005; Riquelme and Montoya 2010; Sanger and Kukke 2007; Wingert et al. 2009), in addition to higher levels of pain than healthy children (Doralp and Bartlett 2010; Malone and Vogtle 2010; Parkinson et al. 2010; Riquelme et al. 2011; Riquelme and Montoya 2010; Vogtle 2009). These somatosensory deficits could be due either to injuries caused by brain damage in the cortical and subcortical sensory areas or to secondary neurophysiological mechanisms provoked by motor limitation (e.g., aberrant feedback of the somatosensory afferences) and which reduce the exploration opportunities of children with CP (Clayton et al. 2003). In this sense, recent neuroimaging studies have revealed alterations in the white matter connecting the motor and somatosensory cortices, suggesting that the motor problems of people with CP could reflect a disruption of both types of connections (Hoon et al. 2002; Hoon et al. 2009; Thomas et al. 2005). Moreover, the developing nervous system is very sensitive to postnatal neural activity, requiring defined patterns of afferences for a normal synaptic organization to occur. Thus, for example, Zwicker et al. (2013) found a relation between neonatal pain and the abnormal development of the corticospinal tract. The patterns of stereotyped and monotonous movements at neonatal age could also produce abnormal afferent feedback that would alter cortical reorganization, producing deficits in somatosensory processing (Coq et al. 2008). Finally, reduced tactile sensitivity has been related to increased pain sensitivity in people with CP (Riquelme and Montoya 2010), suggesting a potential link between abnormal somatosensory experiences in early infancy and long-term changes in somatosensory processing and pain (Schmelzle-Lubiecki et al. 2007).

Pain in Individuals with Cerebral Palsy

People with CP suffer frequent pain at any age, in multiple locations, between moderate and severe intensity. The levels of pain prevalence in adults with CP vary, depending on the studies, between 75 and 25 % (Brattberg 2004; Carter et al. 2002; Hadden and von Baeyer 2002; Hirsh et al. 2011; Hunt et al. 2003; McKearnan et al. 2004; Odding et al. 2006; Parkes et al. 2009; Penner et al. 2013). Pain usually presents constantly or daily in half of the affected individuals and with a pain intensity ranging between 2 and 5 on a 0–10 scale (Hadden and von Baeyer 2002; Hirsh et al. 2011). Pain is mainly due to musculoskeletal causes (Carter et al. 2002) and is located in multiple body areas, with predominance of the cervical and lumbar areas and lower limbs (Brattberg 2004; Carter et al. 2002; Dudgeon et al. 2002; Hadden and von Baeyer 2002; Hirsh et al. 2011; Hunt et al. 2003; Lannin et al. 2007; McKearnan et al. 2004; Arve Opheim et al. 2011; Riquelme et al. 2011; Schmelzle-Lubiecki et al. 2007). It has been observed that the inability to walk does not affect pain intensity, but it does affect the number of body areas affected by pain. Thus, for example, Malone and Vogtle (2010) examined pain and its interference with daily activities in two groups of people with CP, ambulatory and nonambulatory, for 3 months, finding no differences in maximum pain intensity between the two groups, although the walking people presented fewer painful areas than the nonambulatory.

In the pediatric population with CP, pain levels are usually similar to those of adults, with an incidence ranging between 78 and 41 % of the cases, depending on the studies. Pain usually presents with a weekly or daily frequency and with an intensity between moderate and severe (Breau et al. 2003; Engel et al. 2005; Novak et al. 2012; Parkes et al. 2009; Parkinson et al. 2013; Ramstad et al. 2011; Riquelme et al. 2011; Russo et al. 2008; Tervo et al. 2006). The most frequent causes of pain are accidents (especially in children with greater motor disability), gastrointestinal pain, infections, headaches, and musculoskeletal disorders (Breau et al. 2003; Parkinson et al. 2013; Penner et al. 2013; Ramstad et al. 2011). Pain is associated with an increase in children's dependence (Tervo et al. 2006), as well as greater interference in daily activities such as sleeping, physical education programs, or school activity (Engel et al. 2002; Geister et al. 2013; Ramstad et al. 2011; Tervo et al. 2006).

In a disability as complex as CP, with so many associated disorders, pain can be related to multiple variables, such as motor deficit, age, gender, problems with the limbs, chronic fatigue, sleep disorders, and impairment of the physical function (Breau et al. 2003; Carter et al. 2002; McKearnan et al. 2004; Riquelme et al. 2011). One factor that has received particular attention in CP is the relation between pain perception and motor impairment. However, the results obtained to date are contradictory and not very clarifying. Whereas some studies have shown a close association between pain suffered by children with CP and the severity of their motor impairment (children with greater motor impairment present more frequent pain; Barney et al. 2013; Houlihan et al. 2004), other investigations found no significant association between pain and the degree of functional limitation described with the GMFCS. Nevertheless, significant correlations between the GMFCS values and other variables, such as mobility, dexterity, oral expression, sensory deficits, or cognition, have been reported (Kennes et al. 2002). Riquelme et al. (2011) confirmed the presence of pain at early ages of similar intensities to those manifested by adults. With regard to sex, Parkinson et al. (2013) found a higher incidence of pain in young females and in people with emotional problems. Moreover, in one third of the adult population with CP, chronic pain and fatigue are closely related, affecting 16 % of the population (Van Der Slot et al. 2012).

People with CP are not only subject to the same sources of pain as the general population, but also, due to their pathology, to other processes that can cause pain such as spasticity, orthopedic problems, or digestive dysfunctions (Doralp and Bartlett 2010; Engel et al. 2003; Gallien et al. 2007; Intiso et al. 2014; Jahnsen et al. 2004; Jozwiak et al. 2011; Kadhim et al. 2013; Kirstyn et al. 2007; Nolan et al. 2000; Penner et al. 2013; Russo et al. 2008; Schwartz et al. 1999). Painful etiologies, such as spasticity or musculoskeletal problems, can turn daily life activities like standing, walking, or physical activity into sources of pain (Geister et al. 2013; Krigger 2006). In this sense, the study of Riquelme et al. (2011) revealed that people with CP are subject to a greater number of painful health procedures than healthy people. For instance, people with CP repeatedly suffer pain caused by habitual health procedures, such as surgery, injections, stretching, manipulation by other people, immobility, or inadequately adjusted orthotics (Brattberg 2004; Carter et al. 2002; Hadden and von Baeyer 2002; Hunt et al. 2003; Hurvitz et al. 2013; Jaspers et al. 2013; Kadhim et al. 2013; Kibele 1989; Krigger 2006; Lannin et al. 2007; McKearnan et al. 2004; Riquelme et al. 2011). According to a study of Parkinson et al. (2013), 43 % of children with CP experience pain during physiotherapist procedures. Likewise, adults with CP consider habitual physiotherapist activities such as mobilizations, palpations, and supporting weight with the lower limbs to be painful (Krigger 2006). These data reveal the importance of applying techniques to rate, prevent, and relieve pain in habitual clinical practice.

Optimal pain management depends on its accurate rating (Anand and Craig 1996). For this purpose, a series of difficulties should be taken into account beforehand, such as cognitive and communication deficiencies suffered by many people with CP (many of them pediatric patients), as well as multiple painful etiologies (Penner et al. 2013). In this sense, although the direct report by the person with CP is considered the optimal procedure for rating pain (Breau et al. 2003; McGrath et al. 1998), many authors have resorted to rating it by means of reports or questionnaires completed by parents, caregivers, or health professionals, whereas others use combined interviews of the person with CP and his or her parents/caregivers. Nevertheless, in a study carried out by Hadden and von Baeyer (2005) it is suggested that the capacity of children with CP to communicate pain does not influence the way their parents report the observed pain. Parkinson et al. (2010) compared questionnaires administered to communicative children with CP with those completed by parents of communicative and noncommunicative children. The results showed that the frequency of pain perceived in both populations was similar (60 % in the children's questionnaires vs. 73 % in the parents' questionnaires), but the situations related to pain were different. Thus, whereas in the children's questionnaires, pain was associated with age but not with the severity of the pathology, the parents associated greater frequency and intensity of pain with the severity of the pathology and the presence of epileptic crises. However, more recent studies comparing pain ratings of children with CP with those of their parents have found both overrating and underrating of pain by parents (Boling et al. 2013; Ramstad et al. 2011).

Pain Management

As mentioned above, pain of different intensity, frequency, and multiple body locations is one of the most frequent comorbidities in people with CP. Therefore, a goal to improve the well-being of people with CP should be the application of methods or intervention procedures to relieve pain. In this sense, Hadden and von Baeyer (2002) estimated that almost one third of adults with CP expressed dissatisfaction with the care and treatment they receive for their problems of pain. Likewise, Krigger (2006) stated than only 13.6 % of the adolescents and adults with CP and without ambulatory ability who feel pain receive specific pain treatment, despite the relation between pain and the rehabilitation procedures (e.g., mobilizations or palpations). In turn, health professionals do not always monitor pain systematically and they also confer little relevance to pain in children with CP with cognitive deficits (Dudgeon et al. 2002; Massaro et al. 2013). In contrast, according to Vargus-Adams and Martin (2011) pain was revealed to be one of the main treatment goals for health professionals who work with people with CP. From this perspective, Swiggum et al. (2010) stated that 80 % of the physiotherapists attending children with neurological problems apply subjective measures to rate pain. Of them, 70 % use scales completed by the child, and 48 % use behavioral and physiological measures. In addition, they usually use distraction, praise, information, and conversation to decrease pain and stress during painful procedures. In this sense, the literature also presents institutionally established protocols to reduce anxiety associated with painful health procedures, for example, explaining through play the procedure of injecting botulinum toxin in a prior nursing consultation (Gosset et al. 2012). Another procedure such as the presence of clowns during the botulinum toxin injections was efficacious in some cases (girls after several visits), but it was harmful in others (children younger than 8 years) (Hansen et al. 2011).

A decrease is noted in the use of health services by people with CP when they reach adulthood (Hilberink et al. 2007). Engel et al. (2002) have shown that fewer than 25 % of adults with CP requested help from health services for pain management. When they did so, they went to various health professionals (doctors, nurses, physiotherapists, and occupational therapists) (Engel et al. 2002; Hirsh et al. 2011).

Physiotherapy interventions seem to be the most frequently used technique to relieve pain and are considered moderately effective by adults with CP (Engel et al. 2002; Hirsh et al. 2011; Opheim et al. 2011). Also, the study of Engel et al. (2002) showed the scarce use of a single treatment and that passive interventions were preferred to those requiring the subject's active intervention. Thus, for example, analgesic medication was used by 72 % of the subjects, whereas psychological intervention was used by 16 %, and physical exercise only by 3 %, although this was one of the interventions considered the most effective by the subjects themselves. More invasive interventions, such as surgery, are not received due to lack of access, lack of interest, or because they are considered inadequate for the specific case. Although people with CP perceive that most analgesic treatments were at least moderately useful, they were used by a relatively small part of the sample and only for a short period of time. A 2-year longitudinal study revealed an increase in the frequency of treatments used by adults with CP, who considered that most treatments were moderately helpful (Jensen et al. 2004). However, at the end of the study, the only treatments showing a perceived decrease in pain intensity were whirlpool baths, ultrasound, and transcutaneous electrical nerve stimulation (TENS). The remaining treatments seem to produce some pain relief for a short time after their administration; however, the relief was subjectively rated by the subjects as "better than nothing." Engel et al. (2003) showed low levels of satisfaction with the general procedures of pain relief, with 32.8 % of the interviewees referring to dissatisfaction, which was positively related to the subject's degree of pain intensity.

The use of antispastic drugs has shown beneficial effects in pain relief in people with CP (Chaleat-Valayer et al. 2011; Intiso et al. 2014). Orthopedic surgery can produce a decrease in pain associated with musculoskeletal deformities (Hasler 2013; Vles et al. 2013). Multimodal analgesia and epidural analgesia associated with surgery have been shown to be effective to control perioperative pain in children with CP (Moore et al. 2013), as well as local analgesic products used during the injections of botulinum toxin (Brochard et al. 2011). However, Vogtle et al. (2013) showed that physical exercise decreased pain and fatigue in adults with CP. The use of somatosensory therapy has been shown to increase pain thresholds in adults with CP (Riquelme et al. 2013). Other authors are investigating the efficacy of less conventional treatments such as techniques to modulate pain by means of virtual reality (Steele et al. 2003). Caregivers' attention to positioning and in the daily care activities could improve pain in nonambulatory people with CP (Bischof and Chirwa 2011).

People with CP seem to use many pain coping strategies spontaneously, which allow them to adapt to their chronic pain by means of pain management programs (exercise sets, distraction, persistence in tasks, ignoring pain, relaxation or seeking social support) (Dudgeon et al. 2002). Jensen et al. (2006, 2011) associated pain in people with CP with psychosocial factors such as catastrophism, strategies for resting and persisting at a task, and seeking social support. These authors confirmed that changes in coping strategies were related to changes in functionality (for example, a decrease in catastrophism and an increase in perseverance in the activity were associated with decreases in the levels of interference due to pain and the levels of depression at 6 months). According to these studies, the most efficient strategies to increase functionality were decreasing catastrophism and persevering in the task, so prioritizing these strategies could increase the levels of participation of people with CP. Engel et al. (2002) proposed the existence of a cognitive-behavioral model of chronic pain that is applicable to people with CP, so cognitive-behavioral interventions could train coping responses to reduce depression and increase participation. Brunton and Bartlett (2013) proposed the use of strategies to promote awareness of one's body, thereby facilitating recognition of the painful effects produced by diverse activities as a way of improving pain management and fostering responsibility for health needs in adolescents with CP. Chong et al. (2012) found a relationship between the size of drawings of their own body and pain perception in children with CP, and recommend its use as a therapeutic strategy in clinical practice to help the children discuss their condition.

Other Comorbidities

Brain damage is usually accompanied by other deficiencies, so that, due to their high prevalence, the extent to which they interfere with the person's skills to participate in desired activities and roles should be analyzed. Different disorders that usually coexist with CP are described below:

- *Intellectual disability (ID).* It is estimated that 23–44 % of the people with CP present ID. The prevalence of cognitive alterations varies as a function of the type of CP, and it increases especially in the presence of epilepsy (Odding et al. 2006).
- *Behavior problems and psychiatric disorders.* Parkes et al. (2008) and Brossard-Racine et al. (2012) note that approximately 40 % of the children with CP present behavior problems. The problems most frequently found have been difficulties with classmates, hyperactivity, attention deficit, emotional symptoms, and absence of prosocial behaviors (Bjorgaas et al. 2013; Bjorgaas et al. 2012; Brossard-Racine et al. 2012; Parkes et al. 2008; Sigurdardottir et al. 2010). More than one half of the children with CP meet the diagnostic criterion for Attention Deficit with Hyperactivity Disorder/Attention Deficit Disorder (ADHD) (Bjorgaas et al. 2012; Parkes et al. 2008).
- *Sensory deficiencies.* Vision, hearing, and other sensory pathways may be affected, although they are more frequent in CP with hemiplegia. Sixty-two percent of the children present ophthalmologic problems (Odding et al. 2006).
- *Endocrinological disorders.* Most children with CP suffer from gastrointestinal and feeding problems. Thus, for example, suction (57 %) and salivation problems (38 %) are very common in the first 12 months of life. Children with CP also present retarded growth and weight problems (Odding et al. 2006).
- *Urogenital disorders.* At least 25 % of the children and adolescents with CP have primary urinary incontinence, which is more frequent in quadriplegic CP accompanied by ID (Odding et al. 2006).
- *Communication.* CP can present a great diversity of language and communication problems. Estimations of these alterations vary very much depending on the

authors, but it can be stated that about 60 % of the cases of CP present language problems. These alterations vary considerably in each person and refer to problems in language acquisition and expressive language (80 %). In this sense, these people usually present a communicative deficit that may be due to ID or to a speech disorder (dysarthria) or to both (Odding et al. 2006).

- *Epilepsy*. People with CP can present diverse epileptic syndromes. It is present in about 20–40 % of the children and is more common in hemiplegic and quadriplegic CP (Odding et al. 2006).
- *Secondary musculoskeletal problems*. Muscular contractions (73 %), hip dislocations (75 %), and scoliosis (72 %) are very frequent (Odding et al. 2006).
- *Fatigue*. The experience of physical fatigue is significant in people with CP and it has an impact on the maintenance of functional skills and on the perception of life satisfaction (Brunton and Rice 2012; Jahnsen et al. 2003; Opheim et al. 2009).

Participation and Quality of Life

The new approach, in which the WHO has actively participated, focuses more on health components rather than on the consequences of the disease. From this perspective, disability is a social construct, implying an interaction between the person and the environment, so that special emphasis is granted to promoting participation and QOL of people with disabilities.

The right to participation of people with disabilities, like any other citizen, is reflected in the Convention of Rights of People with Disabilities (United Nations 2006), has the goal of "promoting, protecting, and ensuring the full enjoyment and in conditions of equality of all the essential rights and liberties of all people with disabilities, and to promote the respect of their inherent dignity" (p. 4). More specifically, in Article 3, the commitment of the member states is to "guarantee full and effective participation and inclusion in society" (p. 5).

From the biopsychosocial perspective of the model of human functioning, participation is understood as the person's capacity to engage in different life situations (related to family, education, life at home, etc.). Moreover, participation is considered an essential part of the person's development and is related to the outcomes of QOL. The current explanatory models of participation do not focus exclusively on the child's factors, describing it instead from many perspectives or levels. Thus, for example, King et al. (2003) propose a conceptual model with 11 environmental, family, and children's factors, which can influence their participation in leisure activities, and serves as a tool to guide research and to plan social policies and programs for children with disabilities and for their families. The model adopts an integral, socioecological perspective, focusing on children's strengths, the family, and the community. According to the authors, some factors directly predict participation, such the child's functional ability (cognitive, communicative, and motor), the family's participation in recreational and leisure activities, and values regarding cultural and intellectual aspects and, finally, the child's preference for activities.

The factors that indirectly predict participation are the parents' perception of environmental barriers, family cohesion, supportive relations toward the child, as well as the family income. Basically, the model attempts to analyze the complex relations between the child and the family and community contexts (King et al. 2003).

Currently, there is growing interest in the study of the construct of participation and in the development of assessment instruments. The available literature on the topic indicates that there are many dimensions to participation. Most of them consider the number of activities carried out (diversity), the frequency of participation in the activities (intensity), enjoyment, and preference for activities. In fact, it is important to assess all the dimensions of participation to further our comprehension of the phenomenon and, especially, to know which activities the children and adolescents perform, with whom, and the degree of enjoyment of the activities, regardless of the degree of difficulty or help needed to perform them (Law et al. 2006; Michelsen et al. 2009). Actually, participation is a complex phenomenon and it includes objective and subjective aspects (Imms et al. 2008). Table 13.3 presents some of the most extensively used assessment instruments according to the definition of participation of the ICF (2001).

Interest in QOL in educational, health, and social service settings has grown in the past three decades. This has led to a better comprehension of the construct of QOL in its conceptualization, measurement, and application. Currently, a consensus

Table 13.3 Assessment instruments of participation according to the ICF model

Instrument	Authors/Year	Contents
Children's assessment of participation and enjoyment (CAPE/PAC)	(King et al. 2007)	It assesses participation in the leisure activities outside the school setting
Child and adolescent scale of participation (CASP)	(Bedell 2004)	It appraises participation at home, at school, and in the community
Frequency of participation questionnaire (FPQ)	(Michelsen et al. 2009)	It assesses participation frequency in activities related to the social context
Lifestyle assessment questionnaire) LAQ-CP	(Mackie et al. 1998)	It appraises restrictions to participate in the activities
Assessment of life habits for children (LIFE-H)	(Noreau et al. 2007)	It assesses participation in the areas described by the ICF
Assessment of life habits for adults (LIFE-H)	(Noreau et al. 2004)	It assesses participation of older persons in significant social roles such as leisure and community life
Questionnaire of young people's participation (QYPP)	(Tuffrey et al. 2013)	It assesses participation frequency during leisure time at home, at school, or at work
Community participation indicators (CPI)	(Heinemann et al. 2011)	It has 20 engagement items: frequency of the activity, and importance of the activity and assessment of the feelings of people who do the activity enough, too much or not enough. It also has 48 items measuring independence

has been reached about four guidelines that can serve as a basis to use QOL outcomes for personal development. These four guidelines are the following: (1) QOL is multidimensional and has the same components for everyone; (2) its measurement consists of the degree to which people are satisfied with life; (3) it improves with self-determination, resources, a life purpose, and a feeling of belonging; and (4) the predictors of quality outcomes should be the focus (Schalock et al. 2008; Verdugo et al. 2005). Likewise, the application of the concept of QOL has become an agent of change, because it allows us to understand people with disabilities and it facilitates establishing practical changes and changes in the social policies in order to improve QOL outcomes (Schalock et al. 2008).

However, QOL is related to the concept of health of the WHO—physical, mental, and social well-being—rated from individuals' perception of health, attending to their cultural demands, systems of values, goals, expectations, and concerns. According to the model proposed by Schalock and Verdugo (2002), QOL is a concept that reflects the desired conditions in eight essential needs that represent the core of a person's life dimensions: emotional well-being, interpersonal relationships, material well-being, personal development, physical well-being, self-determination, social inclusion, and rights. These eight domains have been described as quality indicators through the analysis of the scientific literature on QOL (Schalock et al. 2005; Schalock and Verdugo 2002). These dimensions are affected by environmental and personal factors and they are the same for everyone although they can vary depending on the value and importance attributed to them by each person. Summing up, QOL is a multidimensional construct, which incorporates objective and subjective accounts of personal feelings, social relationships, local environment, societal values, political institutions, economic conditions, and international relations (Bjornson and McLaughlin 2001; Colver 2009).

The current model to understand disability has led to a change in the intervention procedures aimed towards the improvement of QOL outcomes in people with CP. As a result, extensive research has been carried out in order to develop assessment instruments for QOL. Verdugo et al. (2005) propose the following guidelines for the measurement of QOL: (1) it should reflect the dimensions of QOL and the perceptions of personal satisfaction, (2) it should include the dimensions and indicators, (3) it should include objective and subjective aspects, (4) it should include the use of consumers as interviewers, and (5) it should relate it to natural behavior and everyday settings.

Thus, the comprehension model, based on the biopsychosocial approach to disability, has promoted the development of intervention procedures oriented towards improving QOL outcomes in people with CP. As a result, extensive research has been carried out in order to design and validate assessment instruments for QOL. For example, within the European Community framework, two projects were carried out with the goal of constructing assessment instruments of QOL. The first project is the KIDSCREEN, which led to three generic QOL instruments: KIDSCREEN-52, KIDSCREEN-27, and the KIDSCREEN-10 Index. These assessment instruments rate self-perceived QOL in healthy children and adolescents and in those who have chronic diseases. As they were developed conjointly and simultaneously in 13 European countries, these are cross-cultural QOL instruments

(Ravens-Sieberer et al. 2008; Ravens-Sieberer et al. 2013). The KIDSCREEN-52 provides detailed information about the health profile for ten QOL dimensions and it has 52 items. It contains the following dimensions: physical well-being, psychological well-being, mood, self-perception, autonomy, relation with parents and family life, economic resources, friends and social support, school setting, and social acceptance. The KIDSCREEN-52 is available in versions for children and adolescents, as well as a version for mothers, fathers, or informers, and it has been translated and adapted to different languages.

The second project is DISABKIDS, which has provided two questionnaire modules. The first one consists of the construction of a generic questionnaire for children and adolescents who suffer from any chronic medical condition. The second one is a group of specific questionnaires, one for each chronic health condition, among them, one for children and adolescents with CP (Baars et al. 2005).

Participation Outcomes

People with CP have fewer opportunities to participate in different relevant life areas, such as social life, education, work, etc., which can negatively affect their perceived levels of QOL (Fauconnier et al. 2009; Law et al. 2006; Parkes et al. 2010). Diverse studies have shown that children and adolescents with CP present low diversity and intensity of extracurricular activities, they participate in few formal activities, although they display high levels of enjoyment (Bult et al. 2010; Bult et al. 2011; Engel-Yeger et al. 2009; Fauconnier et al. 2009; Imms et al. 2008; Longo et al. 2013; Shikako-Thomas et al. 2012; Shikako-Thomas et al. 2013). When analyzing the type of activities in which children and adolescents with CP engage, the results show that they participate more frequently in social and recreational activities (Longo et al. 2013; Shikako-Thomas et al. 2013) in comparison with physical and self-improvement activities (Bult et al. 2010; Imms et al. 2008; Law et al. 2006; Orlin et al. 2010; Shikako-Thomas et al. 2013).

However, although there has been a relevant advance in the study of the participation of children and adolescents with CP, most studies have focused on leisure and physical activity; it is, therefore, necessary to determine their participation in the diverse categories of ICF (2001). From this more extensive perspective of the concept of participation, Michelsen et al. (2013) recently analyzed the participation frequency of adolescents living in Europe, using the Questionnaire of Young People's Participation (QYPP), an instrument that assesses engagement across different life situations (family life, education, work, recreation and leisure, autonomy, etc.) in young people with disability. The results of the study showed that adolescents with CP spent less time with friends, practiced sports with lower frequency, were more sedentary, and felt less autonomous in daily life. Nevertheless, as participation is a multidimensional construct that includes objective and subjective aspects and is made up of diverse dimensions (e.g., diversity, frequency, preference, satisfaction, etc.), it is important to advance in its study, taking into account all its dimensions to further our comprehension of the phenomenon.

Although there is currently greater interest in participation, there are few studies analyzing the engagement of adults with CP in diverse life situations. Levasseur et al. (2004) indicate that older people with physical disabilities present moderate alterations in social participation and restrictions in the social roles of daily life. In the sphere of engagement of people with CP in leisure time, Badia et al. (2013), in a study with youngsters and adults with developmental disabilities (16 % CP), found that the activities with the highest participation were social activities (70 %), followed by recreational activities at home (58.5 %) and, in a much lower percentage, physical activities (27.5 %). However, they also found that the participants preferred social (63.7 %) and physical activities (63.7 %) more frequently than recreational activities at home (51.3 %). Regarding their interest in new leisure activities, they showed greater interest in participating in physical activities (33 %) (Badia et al. 2013). Nevertheless, the scarce information currently available about the engagement of adults with CP in different life areas reflects the need to advance in the study of participation, as it is considered as a determinant of a person's QOL.

The Impact of Disability Factors on Participation

From the perspective of human functioning, motor and communication limitations and other restrictions in the activity usually presented by people with CP can have a negative impact on their participation. Thus, for example, diverse studies have shown that the levels of gross motor function and of ID influence the diversity and intensity of participation in leisure activities (Fauconnier et al. 2009; Kerr et al. 2007; Maher et al. 2007; Majnemer et al. 2008; Morris and Bartlett 2004; Morris et al. 2006). Likewise, Michelsen et al. (2013) have shown that adolescents with CP with greater motor, cognitive, and communicative impairment had fewer social contacts and scarce opportunities for decision making. For example, it has also been observed that communication skills are one of the functional characteristics that has more predictive value for participation in self-overcoming activities (e.g., shopping, doing homework, reading, etc.) (Clarke et al. 2011). It has also been shown that pain interferes with daily activities, contributing to deterioration of the capacity to walk, balance, and increasing physical fatigue (Carter et al. 2002; Odding et al. 2006) and in general, interfering with the independence and capacity to participate in a person with CP (McKearnan et al. 2004; Penner et al. 2013). Diverse studies have shown a positive correlation between the number of painful areas or pain duration and the capacity to carry out daily activities (Barney et al. 2013; Malone and Vogtle 2010). Moreover, Ramstad et al. (2012) associated recurrent musculoskeletal pain with parents' lower satisfaction with the social role fulfillment of their children with CP.

Quality of Life Outcomes

The application of the concept of QOL has become an important measurement of the outcomes of intervention procedures, as it allows us to understand that people with CP, despite the presence of deficiencies, can lead a satisfactory life and, in addition, it promotes changes in the professional practices in order to improve QOL outcomes.

Some investigations indicate that children with CP have worse QOL outcomes. For example, Majnemer et al. (2007) reported that approximately one half of the children with CP of their study obtained worse QOL outcomes, indicating that motor limitations, behavior problems, and family functioning were determinants of QOL. However, the study carried out by the SPARCLE group, in which six European countries participated, has shown that the self-reports of QOL in children with CP are similar to those of children from the general population, and children with CP even obtained better results in the school setting domain, where they reported a significantly higher QOL (Dickinson et al. 2007).

Therefore, recent research shows that children with CP perceive satisfactory well-being in spite of the limitations in their functioning, which means that they adapt well to their limited activity. As noted by Rosenbaum (2008), it is surprising that the subjective QOL of children with CP is similar to that of the general population. However, although an adult without disability may not perceive it this way, from the viewpoint of a child with CP who was born and grew up with that disability, life has the same intensity as it does for most children (Rosenbaum 2008). That is, these results reveal that there are differences in the perceptions of children with CP and those of their parents with regard to their QOL. Thus, some studies comparing the perceptions of QOL of children and adolescents CP with those of their parents confirm that the parents tend to underestimate their children's QOL in most domains (physical and emotional well-being, mood and emotions, self-perception, social support, social acceptance, and bullying) (Davis et al. 2007; White-Koning et al. 2007).

Currently, there is no available extensive research on QOL of adults with CP, so we do not know their degree of satisfaction with the diverse life spheres, including physical, social, economic, and psychological well-being. A recent study of Badia et al. (2013) has shown that, analyzed from the perspective of professionals, the QOL of adults with CP is good. However, the analysis of the participants' QOL profile revealed poorer results in self-determination, rights, and social inclusion. These findings agree with some prior studies showing that people with developmental disabilities do not enjoy high levels of self-determination (Wehmeyer and Garner 2003) and obtain worse results in the dimensions related to social inclusion and rights (Jenaro et al. 2013).

Comorbidities and Quality of Life

People with CP may perceive satisfactory well-being in spite of the presence of other deficits (Dickinson et al. 2007; Majnemer et al. 2007). Dickinson et al. (2007) in the SPARCLE study, showed that, in many aspects, QOL is not associated with deficiencies, suggesting that it is probably determined by social and environmental factors. Nevertheless, when they attempted to identify which factors influenced worse QOL outcomes, they found that children with worse motor impairment obtained a low level of physical well-being, and that the presence of ID was related to poorer scores in mood and autonomy (Dickinson et al. 2007). It seems confirmed that the presence of pain has an impact on QOL, not only on the physical domains, but also on the emotional and social domains (Arnaud et al. 2008; Dickinson et al. 2007; Riquelme et al. 2011; Swiggum et al. 2010). Finally, according to Majnemer et al. (2007), children with behavior problems may have more difficulties adapting to daily tasks and integrating socially, and this can affect their emotional well-being and relations with their classmates.

In ageing adults with CP, it was found that their level of motor function measured by means of the GFMCS does not influence their QOL (Badia-Corbella et al. 2013; Tarsuslu and Livanelioglu 2010). Nevertheless, Badia-Corbella et al. (2013) found that, when analyzing the different dimensions of QOL, adults who need physical assistance to walk (level III of the GMFCS) obtained lower levels of material and physical well-being. This outcome shows that the ageing process affects QOL in people with ambulatory limitations and is one of the causes of the presence of pain (Andersson and Mattsson 2001). In fact, pain is indicated as a significant concern in adults with CP, related to increasing age, decrease in functionality, and inactivity (Murphy 2010; Tarsuslu and Livanelioglu 2010; Turk 2009).

Investigations like those de Engel et al. (2003) and Jahnsen et al. (2004) focused on the intensity and location of pain, finding that 67% of adults with CP present chronic pain in one or more body parts (back, hips, and lower limbs). Orthopedic problems, poor bone density, fractures, and mandibular, dental, and feeding problems are also sources of pain in adults with CP (Vogtle 2009). Moreover, it has been confirmed that pain increases with age (Vogtle 2009) and can negatively affect QOL (Riquelme et al. 2011). In a study of Engel et al. (2003) revealed that people with CP who suffered pain indicated high levels of psychological stress and moderate life satisfaction, although the interference of pain in their daily activities was rated as low (2.5–3 on a scale ranging from 0 to 10). Other authors have shown that pain is associated with depression, frustration, and feelings of loneliness (McKearnan et al. 2004; Van Der Slot et al. 2012). However, Badia-Corbella et al. (2013) also showed that the level of self-determination, an essential dimension of QOL for people to cope with situations independently, decreases as the degree ID increases. Finally, it has been confirmed that adults with CP with problems of social communication have fewer social interactions and they suffer from loneliness (Ballin and Balandin 2007), which negatively affects QOL in all its dimensions, except for the dimension of physical well-being (Badia-Corbella et al. 2013).

Basically, these findings suggest that health problems—such as the presence of chronic pain and the difficulty to obtain adequate mobility devices—negatively affect the QOL outcomes in adults with CP who need mobility aids.

Intervention Approach to Enhance Personal Outcomes

The current definition of CP based on the socioecological comprehension of human functioning is promoting a change in the organization and planning of support services for people with CP and their families in different countries. These services have the purpose of guaranteeing their inclusion in the community, favoring their participation, and improving their QOL.

Consequently, the current orientation of interventions is aimed at the development of procedures to promote the achievement of functional skills that facilitate autonomy and participation. Thereby, by means of an adaptation to a task (for example, a technical aid for communication) or a modification of the environment (for example, the availability or ramps in public spaces), functional independence (for example, autonomous mobility in the community using a wheelchair) and good QOL can be achieved in spite of the presence of functioning limitations (Majnemer and Mazer 2004). There are basically two notable aspects that are necessary to assess the services targeting people with CP. The first should be "what does the child or adolescent do?" (participation), and the second, "how does the child or adolescent feel?" (QOL) (Colver and Sparcle group 2006).

Summary

The current perspective of the study of CP, based on the biopsychosocial model of disability, promotes the planning of intervention procedures that represent an important change in the care practices carried out till not very long ago. The current concept of CP is based on a multidimensional and individual perspective of human functioning, and on a definition that includes the diverse associated comorbidities. People with CP present a motor disorder, but the impact that other very common disorders may have on their participation and QOL is also acknowledged. Finally, in the past two decades, more interest has been awakened by multidisciplinary intervention programs aimed at achieving better participation and QOL outcomes for people with CP.

References

Anand, K. J., & Craig, K. D. (1996). New perspectives on the definition of pain. *Pain, 67,* 3–6.

Andersson, C., & Mattsson, E. (2001). Adults with cerebral palsy: A survey describing problems, needs, and resources, with special emphasis on locomotion. *Developmental Medicine and Child Neurology, 43*(2), 76–82.

Arnaud, C., White-Koning, M., Michelsen, S. I., Parkes, J., Parkinson, K., Thyen, U., Beckung, E., Dickinson, H. O., Fauconnier, J., Marcelli, M., McManus, V., & Colver, A. (2008). Parent-reported quality of life of children with cerebral palsy in Europe. *Pediatrics, 121*(1), 54–64.

Baars, R. M., Atherton, C. I., Koopman, H. M., Bullinger, M., & Power, M. (2005). The European DISABKIDS project: Development of seven condition-specific modules to measure health-related quality of life in children and adolescents. *Health Quality of Life Outcomes, 3,* 70.

Badia, M., Orgaz, M. B., Verdugo, M. Á., & Ullán, A. M. (2013). Patterns and determinants of leisure participation of youth and adults with developmental disabilities. *Journal of Intellectual Disability Research, 57*(4), 319–332.

Badia-Corbella, M., Rodríguez-Pedraza, P., Orgaz-Baz, M. B., & Blanco-Pedraz, J. M. (2013). Quality of life in patients with cerebral palsy during aging process. [Calidad de vida en los pacientes con parálisis cerebral en proceso de envejecimiento]. *Rehabilitación, 47,* 194–199.

Badley, E. M. (2008). Enhancing the conceptual clarity of the activity and participation components of the international classification of functioning, disability, and health. *Social Science Medicine, 66*(11), 2335–2345.

Ballin, L., & Balandin, S. (2007). An exploration of loneliness: Communication and the social networks of older people with cerebral palsy. *Journal of Intellectual & Developmental Disabilities, 32*(4), 315–326.

Barney, C. C., Krach, L. E., Rivard, P. F., Belew, J. L., & Symons, F. J. (2013). Motor function predicts parent-reported musculoskeletal pain in children with cerebral palsy. *Pain Research & Management, 18*(6), 323–327.

Baxter, P. (2013). Comorbidities of cerebral palsy need more emphasis—especially pain. *Developmental Medicine and Child Neurology, 55*(5), 396.

Bedell, G. M. (2004). Developing a follow-up survey focused on participation of children and youth with acquired brain injuries after discharge from inpatient rehabilitation. *NeuroRehabilitation, 19*(3), 191–205.

Bischof, F. M., & Chirwa, T. F. (2011). Daily care activities and hip pain in non-ambulatory children and young adults with cerebral palsy. *Journal of Pediatric Rehabilitation Medicine, 4*(3), 219–223.

Bjornson, K. F., & McLaughlin, J. F. (2001). The measurement of health-related quality of life (HRQL) in children with cerebral palsy. *European Journal of Neurology, 8,* 183–193.

Bjorgaas, H. M., Hysing, M., & Elgen, I. (2012). Psychiatric disorders among children with cerebral palsy at school starting age. *Research in Developmental Disabilities, 33*(4), 1287–1293.

Bjorgaas, H. M., Elgen, I., Boe, T., & Hysing, M. (2013). Mental health in children with cerebral palsy: Does screening capture the complexity? *The Scientific World Journal, 2013,* 468402. doi:10.1155/2013/468402

Boling, S., Tarja, V., Helena, M., Wivi, F., Ilona, A. R., & Leena, H. (2013). Measuring quality of life of Finnish children with cerebral palsy. *Journal of Pediatric Rehabilitation Medicine, 6*(3), 121–127.

Brattberg, G. (2004). Do pain problems in young school children persist into early adulthood? A 13-year follow-up. *European Journal of Pain, 8*(3), 187–199.

Breau, L. M., Camfield, C. S., McGrath, P. J., & Finley, G. A. (2003). The incidence of pain in children with severe cognitive impairments. *Archives of Pediatrics & Adolescents Medicine, 157*(12), 1219–1226.

Brochard, S., Blajan, V., Lempereur, M., Garlantezec, R., Houx, L., Le Moine, P., Peudenier, S., Lefranc, J., & Rémy-Néris, O. (2011). Determining the technical and clinical factors associated with pain for children undergoing botulinum toxin injections under nitrous oxide and anesthetic cream. *European Journal of Paediatric Neurology, 15*(4), 310–315.

Brossard-Racine, M., Hall, N., Majnemer, A., Shevell, M. I., Law, M., Poulin, C., & Rosenbaum, P. (2012). Behavioural problems in school age children with cerebral palsy. *European Journal of Paediatric Neurology, 16*(1), 35–41.

Brunton, L. K., & Bartlett, D. J. (2013). The bodily experience of cerebral palsy: A journey to self-awareness. *Disability and Rehabilitation, 35*(23), 1981–1990.

Brunton, L. K., & Rice, C. L. (2012). Fatigue in cerebral palsy: A critical review. *Developmental Neurorehabilitation, 15*(1), 54–62.

Bult, M. K., Verschuren, O., Gorter, J. W., Jongmans, M. J., Piskur, B., & Ketelaar, M. (2010). Cross-cultural validation and psychometric evaluation of the Dutch language version of the children's assessment of participation and enjoyment (CAPE) in children with and without physical disabilities. *Clinical Rehabilitation, 24*(9), 843–853.

Bult, M. K., Verschuren, O., Jongmans, M. J., Lindeman, E., & Ketelaar, M. (2011). What influences participation in leisure activities of children and youth with physical disabilities? A systematic review. *Research in Developmental Disabilities, 32*(5), 1521–1529.

Carter, B., McArthur, E., & Cunliffe, M. (2002). Dealing with uncertainty: Parental assessment of pain in their children with profound special needs. *Journal of Advanced Nursing, 38*(5), 449–457.

Chaleat-Valayer, E., Parratte, B., Colin, C., Denis, A., Oudin, S., Berard, C., Bernard, J. C., Bourg, V., Deleplanque, B., Dulieu, I., Evrard, P., Filipetti, P., Flurin, V., Gallien, P., Héron-Long, B., Hodgkinson, I., Husson, I., Jaisson-Hot, I., Maupas, E., Meurin, F., Monnier, G., Pérennou, D., Pialoux, B., Quentin, V., Moreau, M. S., Schneider, M., Yelnik, A., & Marque, P. (2011). A French observational study of botulinum toxin use in the management of children with cerebral palsy: BOTULOSCOPE. *European Journal of Paediatric Neurology, 15*(5), 439–448.

Chong, J., Mackey, A. H., Broadbent, E., & Stott, N. S. (2012). Children's perceptions of their cerebral palsy and their impact on life satisfaction. *Disability and Rehabilitation, 34*(24), 2053–2060.

Clarke, M. T., Newton, C., Griffiths, T., Price, K., Lysley, A., & Petrides, K. V. (2011). Factors associated with the participation of children with complex communication needs. *Research in Developmental Disabilities, 32*(2), 774–780.

Clayton, K., Fleming, J. M., & Copley, J. (2003). Behavioral responses to tactile stimuli in children with cerebral palsy. *Physical & Occupational Therapy in Pediatrics, 23*(1), 43–62.

Colver, A. (2005). A shared framework and language for childhood disability. *Developmental Medicine and Child Neurology, 47*(11), 780–784.

Colver, A. (2009). Quality of life and participation. *Developmental Medicine and Child Neurology, 51*(8), 656–659.

Colver, A., & SPARCLE group. (2006). Study protocol: SPARCLE—a multi-centre European study of the relationship of environment to participation and quality of life in children with cerebral palsy. *BMC Public Health, 6*(1), 105.

Cooper, J., Majnemer, A., Rosenblatt, B., & Birnbaum, R. (1995). The determination of sensory deficits in children with hemiplegic cerebral palsy. *Journal of Child Neurology, 10*(4), 300–309.

Coq, J. O., Strata, F., Russier, M., Safadi, F. F., Merzenich, M. M., Byl, N. N., & Barbe, M. F. (2008). Impact of neonatal asphyxia and hind limb immobilization on musculoskeletal tissues and S1 map organization: Implications for cerebral palsy. *Experimental Neurology, 210*(1), 95–108.

Davis, E., Nicolas, C., Waters, E., Cook, K., Gibbs, L., Gosch, A., & Ravens-Sieberer, U. (2007). Parent-proxy and child self-reported health-related quality of life: Using qualitative methods to explain the discordance. *Quality of Life Research, 16*(5), 863–871.

Dickinson, H. O., Parkinson, K. N., Ravens-Sieberer, U., Schirripa, G., Thyen, U., Arnaud, C., Beckung, E., Fauconnier, J., McManus, V., Michelsen, S. I., Parkes, J., & Colver, A. F. (2007). Self-reported quality of life of 8–12-year-old children with cerebral palsy: A cross-sectional European study. *Lancet, 369*(9580), 2171–2178.

Doralp, S., & Bartlett, D. J. (2010). The prevalence, distribution, and effect of pain among adolescents with cerebral palsy. *Pediatric Physical Therapy, 22*(1), 26–33.

Dudgeon, B. J., Gerrard, B. C., Jensen, M. P., Rhodes, L. A., & Tyler, E. J. (2002). Physical disability and the experience of chronic pain. *Archives of Physical Medicine and Rehabilitation, 83*(2), 229–235.

Eliasson, A. C., Krumlinde-Sundholm, L., Rosblad, B., Beckung, E., Arner, M., Ohrvall, A. M., & Rosenbaum, P. (2006). The manual ability classification system (MACS) for children with cerebral palsy: Scale development and evidence of validity and reliability. *Developmental Medicine and Child Neurology, 48*(7), 549–554.

Engel, J. M., Kartin, D., & Jensen, M. P. (2002). Pain treatment in persons with cerebral palsy: Frequency and helpfulness. *American Journal of Physical Medicine & Rehabilitation, 81*(4), 291–296.

Engel, J. M., Jensen, M. P., Hoffman, A. J., & Kartin, D. (2003). Pain in persons with cerebral palsy: Extension and cross validation. *Archives of Physical Medicine and Rehabilitation, 84*(8), 1125–1128.

Engel, J. M., Petrina, T. J., Dudgeon, B. J., & McKearnan, K. A. (2005). Cerebral palsy and chronic pain: A descriptive study of children and adolescents. *Physical & Occupational Therapy in Pediatrics, 25*(4), 73–84.

Engel-Yeger, B., Jarus, T., Anaby, D., & Law, M. (2009). Differences in patterns of participation between youths with cerebral palsy and typically developing peers. *American Journal of Occupational Therapy, 63*(1), 96–104.

Fauconnier, J., Dickinson, H. O., Beckung, E., Marcelli, M., McManus, V., Michelsen, S. I., Parkes, J., Parkinson, K. N., Thyen, U., Arnaud, C., & Colver, A. (2009). Participation in life situations of 8–12 year old children with cerebral palsy: Cross-sectional European study. *British Medical Journal, 338,* b1458.

Gallien, P., Nicolas, B., Dauvergne, F., Petrilli, S., Houedakor, J., Roy, D., & Durufle, A. (2007). La douleur chez le sujet adulte infirme moteur cerebral [Pain in adults with cerebral palsy]. *Annales de Readaptation et de Medecine Physique, 50*(7), 558–563.

Geister, T. L., Quintanar-Solares, M., Martin, M., Aufhammer, S., & Asmus, F. (2013). Qualitative development of the 'Questionnaire on Pain caused by Spasticity (QPS),' a pediatric patient-reported outcome for spasticity-related pain in cerebral palsy. *Quality of Life Research.* doi:10.1007/s11136–013-0526–2

Gosset, B., Dufour, E., Jonas, M. V., Hiriart, B., Morelle, S., Keirel, I., Longue, V, & Lamy, V. (2012). The prevention of pain during botulinum toxin injections in children. *Soins, 764,* 21–24.

Hadden, K. L., & von Baeyer, C. L. (2002). Pain in children with cerebral palsy: Common triggers and expressive behaviors. *Pain, 99*(1–2), 281–288.

Hadden, K. L., & von Baeyer, C. L. (2005). Global and specific behavioral measures of pain in children with cerebral palsy. *The Clinical Journal of Pain, 21*(2), 140–146.

Hansen, L. K., Kibaek, M., Martinussen, T., Kragh, L., & Hejl, M. (2011). Effect of a clown's presence at botulinum toxin injections in children: A randomized, prospective study. *Journal of Pain Research, 4,* 297–300.

Hasler, C. C. (2013). Operative treatment for spinal deformities in cerebral palsy. *Journal of Children's Orthopaedics, 7*(5), 419–423.

Heinemann, A. W., Lai, J. S., Magasi, S., Hammel, J., Corrigan, J. D., Bogner, J. A., & Whiteneck, G. G. (2011). Measuring participation enfranchisement. *Archives of Physical Medicine and Rehabilitation, 92*(4), 564–571.

Hidecker, M. J. C., Paneth, N., Rosenbaum, P. L., Kent, R. D., Lillie, J., Eulenberg, J. B., Chester, K. Jr., Johnson, B., Michalsen, L., Evatt, M., & Taylor, K. (2011). Developing and validating the communication function classification system for individuals with cerebral palsy. *Developmental Medicine and Child Neurology, 53*(8), 704–710.

Hilberink, S. R., Roebroeck, M. E., Nieuwstraten, W., Jalink, L., Verheijden, J. M., & Stam, H. J. (2007). Health issues in young adults with cerebral palsy: Towards a life-span perspective. *Journal of Rehabilitation Medicine, 39*(8), 605–611.

Hirsh, A. T., Kratz, A. L., Engel, J. M., & Jensen, M. P. (2011). Survey results of pain treatments in adults with cerebral palsy. *American Journal of Physical Medicine & Rehabilitation, 90*(3), 207–216.

Hoon, A. H., Jr., Lawrie, W. T., Jr., Melhem, E. R., Reinhardt, E. M., Van Zijl, P. C., Solaiyappan, M., Jiang, H., Johnston, M. V., & Mori, S. (2002). Diffusion tensor imaging of periventricular leukomalacia shows affected sensory cortex white matter pathways. *Neurology, 59*(5), 752–756.

Hoon, A. H., Jr., Stashinko, E. E., Nagae, L. M., Lin, D. D., Keller, J., Bastian, A., Campbell, M. L., Levey, E., Mori, S., & Johnston, M. V. (2009). Sensory and motor deficits in children with cerebral palsy born preterm correlate with diffusion tensor imaging abnormalities in thalamocortical pathways. *Developmental Medicine and Child Neurology, 51*(9), 697–704.

Houlihan, C. M., O'Donnell, M., Conaway, M., & Stevenson, R. D. (2004). Bodily pain and health-related quality of life in children with cerebral palsy. *Developmental Medicine and Child Neurology, 46*(5), 305–310.

Hunt, A., Mastroyannopoulou, K., Goldman, A., & Seers, K. (2003). Not knowing—the problem of pain in children with severe neurological impairment. *International Journal of Nursing Studies, 40*(2), 171–183.

Hurvitz, E. A., Marciniak, C. M., Daunter, A. K., Haapala, H. J., Stibb, S. M., McCormick, S. F., Muraszko, K. M., & Gaebler-Spira, D. (2013). Functional outcomes of childhood dorsal rhizotomy in adults and adolescents with cerebral palsy. *Journal of Neurosurgery: Pediatrics, 11*(4), 380–388.

Imms, C., Reilly, S., Carlin, J., & Dodd, K. (2008). Diversity of participation in children with cerebral palsy. *Developmental Medicine and Child Neurology, 50*(5), 363–369.
Intiso, D., Simone, V., Di Rienzo, F., Iarossi, A., Pazienza, L., Santamato, A., Maruzzi, G., & Basciani, M. (2014). High doses of a new botulinum toxin type A (NT-201) in adult patients with severe spasticity following brain injury and cerebral palsy. *NeuroRehabilitation, 34*(3), 515–522.
Jahnsen, R., Villien, L., Stanghelle, J. K., & Holm, I. (2003). Fatigue in adults with cerebral palsy in Norway compared with the general population. *Developmental Medicine and Child Neurology, 45*(5), 296–303.
Jahnsen, R., Villien, L., Aamodt, G., Stanghelle, J. K., & Holm, I. (2004). Musculoskeletal pain in adults with cerebral palsy compared with the general population. *Journal of Rehabilitation Medicine, 36*(2), 78–84.
Jaspers, E., Verhaegen, A., Geens, F., Van Campenhout, A., Desloovere, K., & Molenaers, G. (2013). Lower limb functioning and its impact on quality of life in ambulatory children with cerebral palsy. *European Journal of Paediatric Neurology, 17*(6), 561–567.
Jenaro, C., Vega, V., Flores, N., & Cruz, M. (2013). Quality of services and quality of life from service providers' perspectives: Analysis with focus groups. *Journal of Intellectual Disability Research, 57*(6), 489–499.
Jensen, M. P., Engel, J. M., Hoffman, A. J., & Schwartz, L. (2004). Natural history of chronic pain and pain treatment in adults with cerebral palsy. *American Journal of Physical Medicine & Rehabilitation, 83*(6), 439–445.
Jensen, M. P., Engel, J. M., & Schwartz, L. (2006). Coping with cerebral palsy pain: A preliminary longitudinal study. *Pain Medicine, 7*(1), 30–37.
Jensen, M. P., Moore, M. R., Bockow, T. B., Ehde, D. M., & Engel, J. M. (2011). Psychosocial factors and adjustment to chronic pain in persons with physical disabilities: A systematic review. *Archives of Physical Medicine and Rehabilitation, 92*(1), 146–160.
Jozwiak, M., Harasymczuk, P., Koch, A., & Kotwicki, T. (2011). Incidence and risk factors of hip joint pain in children with severe cerebral palsy. *Disabililty and Rehabilitation, 33*(15–16), 1367–1372.
Kadhim, M., Holmes, L., Jr., & Miller, F. (2013). Long-term outcome of planovalgus foot surgical correction in children with cerebral palsy. *Journal of Foot and Ankle Surgery, 52*(6), 697–703.
Kennes, J., Rosenbaum, P., Hanna, S. E., Walter, S., Russell, D., Raina, P., Bartlett, D., & Galuppi, B. (2002). Health status of school-aged children with cerebral palsy: Information from a population-based sample. *Developmental Medicine and Child Neurology, 44*(4), 240–247.
Kerr, C., McDowell, B., & McDonough, S. (2007). The relationship between gross motor function and participation restriction in children with cerebral palsy: An exploratory analysis. *Child: Care, Health and Development, 33*(1), 22–27.
Kibele, A. (1989). Occupational therapy's role in improving the quality of life for persons with cerebral palsy. *American Journal of Occupational Therapy, 43*(6), 371–377.
King, G. A., Law, M., King, S., Rosenbaum, P., Kertoy, M. K., & Young, N. L. (2003). A conceptual model of the factors affecting the recreation and leisure participation of children with disabilities. *Physical & Occupational Therapy in Pediatrics, 23*(1), 63–90.
King, G. A., Law, M., King, S., Hurley, P., Hanna, S., Kertoy, M., & Rosenbaum, P. (2007). Measuring children's participation in recreation and leisure activities: Construct validation of the CAPE and PAC. *Child: Care, Health and Development, 33*(1), 28–39.
Kirstyn, C., Christine, I., & Linsey, H. (2007). Being in pain: A phenomenological study of young people with cerebral palsy. *Developmental Medicine and Child Neurology, 49*(6), 445–449.
Krigger, K. W. (2006). Cerebral palsy: An overview. *American Family Physician, 73*(1), 91–100.
Lannin, N. A., Novak, I., & Cusick, A. (2007). A systematic review of upper extremity casting for children and adults with central nervous system motor disorders. *Clinical Rehabilitation, 21*(11), 963–976.
Law, M., King, G., King, S., Kertoy, M., Hurley, P., Rosenbaum, P., Young, N., & Hanna, S. (2006). Patterns of participation in recreational and leisure activities among children with complex physical disabilities. *Developmental Medicine and Child Neurology, 48*(5), 337–342.
Levasseur, M., Desrosiers, J., & Noreau, L. (2004). Is social participation associated with quality of life of older adults with physical disabilities? *Disability and Rehabilitation, 26*(20), 1206–1213.

Longo, E., Badia, M., & Orgaz, B. M. (2013). Patterns and predictors of participation in leisure activities outside of school in children and adolescents with cerebral palsy. *Research in Developmental Disabilities, 34*(1), 266–275.

Mackie, P. C., Jessen, E. C., & Jarvis, S. N. (1998). The lifestyle assessment questionnaire: An instrument to measure the impact of disability on the lives of children with cerebral palsy and their families. *Child: Care, Health and Development, 24*(6), 473–486.

Maher, C. A., Williams, M. T., Olds, T., & Lane, A. E. (2007). Physical and sedentary activity in adolescents with cerebral palsy. *Developmental Medicine and Child Neurology, 49*(6), 450–457.

Majnemer, A., & Mazer, B. (2004). New directions in the outcome evaluation of children with cerebral palsy. *Seminars in Pediatric Neurology, 11*(1), 11–17.

Majnemer, A., Shevell, M., Rosenbaum, P., Law, M., & Poulin, C. (2007). Determinants of life quality in school-age children with cerebral palsy. *The Journal of Pediatrics, 151*(5), 470–475.

Majnemer, A., Shevell, M., Law, M., Birnbaum, R., Chilingaryan, G., Rosenbaum, P., & Poulin, C. (2008). Participation and enjoyment of leisure activities in school-aged children with cerebral palsy. *Developmental Medicine and Child Neurology, 50*(10), 751–758.

Malone, L. A., & Vogtle, L. K. (2010). Pain and fatigue consistency in adults with cerebral palsy. *Disability and Rehabilitation, 32*(5), 385–391.

Massaro, M., Pastore, S., Ventura, A., & Barbi, E. (2013). Pain in cognitively impaired children: A focus for general pediatricians. *European Journal of Pediatrics, 172*(1), 9–14.

McGrath, P. J., Rosmus, C., Canfield, C., Campbell, M. A., & Hennigar, A. (1998). Behaviours caregivers use to determine pain in non-verbal, cognitively impaired individuals. *Developmental Medicine and Child Neurology, 40*(5), 340–343.

McKearnan, K. A., Kieckhefer, G. M., Engel, J. M., Jensen, M. P., & Labyak, S. (2004). Pain in children with cerebral palsy: A review. *Journal of Neuroscience Nursing, 36*(5), 252–259.

McLaughlin, J. F., Felix, S. D., Nowbar, S., Ferrel, A., Bjornson, K., & Hays, R. M. (2005). Lower extremity sensory function in children with cerebral palsy. *Pediatric Rehabilitation, 8*(1), 45–52.

Michelsen, S. I., Flachs, E. M., Uldall, P., Eriksen, E. L., McManus, V., Parkes, J., Parkinson, K. N., Thyen, U., Arnaud, C., Beckung, E., Dickinson, H. O., Fauconnier, J., Marcelli, M., & Colver, A. (2009). Frequency of participation of 8–12-year-old children with cerebral palsy: A multi-centre cross-sectional European study. *European Journal of Paediatric Neurology, 13*(2), 165–177.

Michelsen, S. I., Flachs, E. M., Damsgaard, M. T., Parkes, J., Parkinson, K., Rapp, M., Arnaud, C., Nystrand, M., Colver, A., Fauconnier, J., Dickinson, H. O., Marcelli, M., & Uldall, P. (2013). European study of frequency of participation of adolescents with and without cerebral palsy. *European Journal of Paediatric Neurology*. doi:10.1016/j.ejpn.2013.12.003.

Moore, R. P., Wester, T., Sunder, R., Schrock, C., & Park, T. S. (2013). Peri-operative pain management in children with cerebral palsy: Comparative efficacy of epidural vs. systemic analgesia protocols. *Paediatric Anaesthesia, 23*(8), 720–725.

Morris, C., & Bartlett, D. (2004). Gross motor function classification system: Impact and utility. *Developmental Medicine and Child Neurology, 46*(1), 60–65.

Morris, C., Kurinczuk, J. J., Fitzpatrick, R., & Rosenbaum, P. L. (2006). Do the abilities of children with cerebral palsy explain their activities and participation? *Developmental Medicine and Child Neurology, 48*(12), 954–961.

Murphy, K. P. (2010). The adult with cerebral palsy. *The Orthopedic Clinics of North America, 41*(4), 595–605.

Nolan, J., Chalkiadis, G. A., Low, J., Olesch, C. A., & Brown, T. C. (2000). Anaesthesia and pain management in cerebral palsy. *Anaesthesia, 55*(1), 32–41.

Nordenfelt, L. (2003). Action theory, disability and ICF. *Disability and Rehabilitation, 25*(18), 1075–1079.

Noreau, L., Desrosiers, J., Robichaud, L., Fougeyrollas, P., Rochette, A., & Viscogliosi, C. (2004). Measuring social participation: Reliability of the LIFE-H in older adults with disabilities. *Disability and Rehabilitation, 26*(6), 346–352.

Noreau, L., Lepage, C., Boissiere, L., Picard, R., Fougeyrollas, P., Mathieu, J., Desmarais, G., & Nadeau, L. (2007). Measuring participation in children with disabilities using the Assessment of Life Habits. *Developmental Medicine and Child Neurology, 49*(9), 666–671.

Novak, I., Hines, M., Goldsmith, S., & Barclay, R. (2012). Clinical prognostic messages from a systematic review on cerebral palsy. *Pediatrics, 130*(5), 1285–1312.

Odding, E., Roebroeck, M. E., & Stam, H. J. (2006). The epidemiology of cerebral palsy: Incidence, impairments and risk factors. *Disability and Rehabilitation, 28*(4), 183–191.

Opheim, A., Jahnsen, R., Olsson, E., & Stanghelle, J. K. (2009). Walking function, pain, and fatigue in adults with cerebral palsy: A 7-year follow-up study. *Developmental Medicine and Child Neurology, 51*(5), 381–388.

Opheim, A., Jahnsen, R., Olsson, E., & Stanghelle, J. K. (2011). Physical and mental components of health-related quality of life and musculoskeletal pain sites over seven years in adults with spastic cerebral palsy. *Journal of Rehabilitation Medicine, 43*(5), 382–387.

Orlin, M. N., Palisano, R. J., Chiarello, L. A., Kang, L.-J., Polansky, M., Almasri, N., & Maggs, J. (2010). Participation in home, extracurricular, and community activities among children and young people with cerebral palsy. *Developmental Medicine and Child Neurology, 52*(2), 160–166.

Palisano, R., Rosenbaum, P., Walter, S., Russell, D., Wood, E., & Galuppi, B. (1997). Development and reliability of a system to classify gross motor function in children with cerebral palsy. *Developmental Medicine and Child Neurology, 39*(4), 214–223.

Parkes, J., White-Koning, M., Dickinson, H. O., Thyen, U., Arnaud, C., Beckung, E., Fauconnier, J., Marcelli, M., McManus, V., Michelsen, S. I., Parkinson, K., & Colver, A. (2008). Psychological problems in children with cerebral palsy: A cross-sectional European study. *Journal of Child Psychology and Psychiatry, and Allied Disciplines, 49*(4), 405–413.

Parkes, J., McCullough, N., Madden, A., & McCahey, E. (2009). The health of children with cerebral palsy and stress in their parents. *Journal of Advanced Nursing, 65*(11), 2311–2323.

Parkes, J., McCullough, N., & Madden, A. (2010). To what extent do children with cerebral palsy participate in everyday life situations? *Health and Social Care in the Community, 18*(3), 304–315.

Parkinson, K. N., Gibson, L., Dickinson, H. O., & Colver, A. F. (2010). Pain in children with cerebral palsy: A cross-sectional multicentre European study. *Acta Paediatrica, 99*(3), 446–451.

Parkinson, K. N., Dickinson, H. O., Arnaud, C., Lyons, A., & Colver, A. (2013). Pain in young people aged 13–17 years with cerebral palsy: Cross-sectional, multicentre European study. *Archives of Disease Childhood, 98*(6), 434–440.

Penner, M., Xie, W. Y., Binepal, N., Switzer, L., & Fehlings, D. (2013). Characteristics of pain in children and youth with cerebral palsy. *Pediatrics, 132*(2), e407–413.

Pennington, L., Virella, D., Mjoen, T., da Graca Andrada, M., Murray, J., Colver, A., Himmelmann, K., Rackauskaite, G., Greitane, A., Prasauskiene, A., Andersen, G., & de la Cruz, J. (2013). Development of the Viking speech Scale to classify the speech of children with cerebral palsy. *Research in Developmental Disabilities, 34*(10), 3202–3210.

Ramstad, K., Jahnsen, R., Skjeldal, O. H., & Diseth, T. H. (2011). Characteristics of recurrent musculoskeletal pain in children with cerebral palsy aged 8–18 years. *Developmental Medicine and Child Neurology, 53*(11), 1013–1018.

Ramstad, K., Jahnsen, R., Skjeldal, O. H., & Diseth, T. H. (2012). Parent-reported participation in children with cerebral palsy: The contribution of recurrent musculoskeletal pain and child mental health problems. *Developmental Medicine and Child Neurology, 54*(9), 829–835.

Ravens-Sieberer, U., Gosch, A., Rajmil, L., Erhart, M., Bruil, J., Power, M., Duer, W., Auquier, P., Cloetta, B., Czemy, L., Mazur, J., Czimbalmos, A., Tountas, Y., Hagquist, C., & Kilroe, J. (2008). The KIDSCREEN-52 quality of life measure for children and adolescents: Psychometric results from a cross-cultural survey in 13 European countries. *Value Health, 11*(4), 645–658.

Ravens-Sieberer, U., Herdman, M., Devine, J., Otto, C., Bullinger, M., Rose, M., & Klasen, F. (2013). The European KIDSCREEN approach to measure quality of life and well-being in children: Development, current application, and future advances. *Quality of Life Research.* doi:10.1007/s11136–013-0428-3

Reid, S. M., Johnson, H. M., & Reddihough, D. S. (2010). The Drooling Impact Scale: A measure of the impact of drooling in children with developmental disabilities. *Developmental Medicine and Child Neurology, 52*(2), 23–28.

Riquelme, I., & Montoya, P. (2010). Developmental changes in somatosensory processing in cerebral palsy and healthy individuals. *Clinical Neurophysiology, 121*(8), 1314–1320.

Riquelme, I., Cifre, I., & Montoya, P. (2011). Age-related changes of pain experience in cerebral palsy and healthy individuals. *Pain Medicine, 12*(4), 535–545.

Riquelme, I., Zamorano, A., & Montoya, P. (2013). Reduction of pain sensitivity after somatosensory therapy in adults with cerebral palsy. *Frontiers in Human Neuroscience, 7,* 276. doi:10.3389/fnhum.2013.00276.

Rosenbaum, P. (2008). Children's quality of life: Separating the person from the disorder. *Archives of Disease in Childhood, 93*(2), 100–101.

Rosenbaum, P., Paneth, N., Leviton, A., Goldstein, M., Bax, M., Damiano, D., Dan, B., & Jacobsson, B. (2007). A report: The definition and classification of cerebral palsy April 2006. *Developmental Medicine and Child Neurology, 49*(109), 8–14.

Russo, R. N., Miller, M. D., Haan, E., Cameron, I. D., & Crotty, M. (2008). Pain characteristics and their association with quality of life and self-concept in children with hemiplegic cerebral palsy identified from a population register. *The Clinical Journal of Pain, 24*(4), 335–342.

Sanger, T. D., & Kukke, S. N. (2007). Abnormalities of tactile sensory function in children with dystonic and diplegic cerebral palsy. *Journal of Child Neurology, 22*(3), 289–293.

Schalock, R. L., & Verdugo, M. A. (2002). *Handbook on quality of life for human service practitioners*. Washington, DC: American Association on Mental Retardation.

Schalock, R. L., Verdugo, M. A., Jenaro, C., Wang, M., Wehmeyer, M., Jiancheng, X., & Lachapelle, Y. (2005). Cross-cultural study of quality of life indicators. *American Journal of Mental Retardation, 110*(4), 298–311.

Schalock, R. L., Verdugo, M. A., Bonham, G. S., Fantova, F., & Van Loon, J. (2008). Enhancing personal outcomes: Organizational strategies, guidelines, and examples. *Journal of Policy and Practice in Intellectual Disabilities, 5*(4), 276–285.

Schmelzle-Lubiecki, B. M., Campbell, K. A., Howard, R. H., Franck, L., & Fitzgerald, M. (2007). Long-term consequences of early infant injury and trauma upon somatosensory processing. *European Journal of Pain, 11*(7), 799–809.

Schwartz, L., Engel, J. M., & Jensen, M. P. (1999). Pain in persons with cerebral palsy. *Archives of Physical Medicine and Rehabilitation, 80*(10), 1243–1246.

Shikako-Thomas, K., Dahan-Oliel, N., Shevell, M., Law, M., Birnbaum, R., Rosenbaum, P., Poulin, C., & Majnemer, A. (2012). Play and be happy? Leisure participation and quality of life in school-aged children with cerebral palsy. *International Journal of Pediatrics, 2012,* 387280. doi:10.1155/2012/387280

Shikako-Thomas, K., Shevell, M., Schmitz, N., Lach, L., Law, M., Poulin, C., & Majnemer, A. (2013). Determinants of participation in leisure activities among adolescents with cerebral palsy. *Research in Developmental Disabilities, 34*(9), 2621–2634.

Sigurdardottir, S., Indredavik, M. S., Eiriksdottir, A., Einarsdottir, K., Gudmundsson, H. S., & Vik, T. (2010). Behavioural and emotional symptoms of preschool children with cerebral palsy: A population-based study. *Developmental Medicine and Child Neurology, 52*(11), 1056–1061.

Steele, E., Grimmer, K., Thomas, B., Mulley, B., Fulton, I., & Hoffman, H. (2003). Virtual reality as a pediatric pain modulation technique: A case study. *Cyberpsychology & Behavior, 6*(6), 633–638.

Swiggum, M., Hamilton, M. L., Gleeson, P., & Roddey, T. (2010). Pain in children with cerebral palsy: Implications for pediatric physical therapy. *Pediatric Physical Therapy, 22*(1), 86–92.

Tarsuslu, T., & Livanelioglu, A. (2010). Relationship between quality of life and functional status of young adults and adults with cerebral palsy. *Disability and Rehabilitation, 32*(20), 1658–1665.

Tervo, R. C., Symons, F., Stout, J., & Novacheck, T. (2006). Parental report of pain and associated limitations in ambulatory children with cerebral palsy. *Archives of Physical Medicine and Rehabilitation, 87*(7), 928–934.

The Centre for Cerebral Palsy and Cerebral Palsy League of Queensland. (2014) *Functional Communication Classification System*. http://www.tccp.com.au/docs/documents/FCCS%20and%20Prompt%20Questions.pdf. Accessed Jan 2014.

Thomas, B., Eyssen, M., Peeters, R., Molenaers, G., Van Hecke, P., De Cock, P., & Sunaert, S. (2005). Quantitative diffusion tensor imaging in cerebral palsy due to periventricular white matter injury. *Brain, 128,* 2562–2577.

Tuffrey, C., Bateman, B. J., & Colver, A. C. (2013). The Questionnaire of young people's participation (QYPP): A new measure of participation frequency for disabled young people. *Child: Care, Health and Development, 39*(4), 500–511.

Turk, M. A. (2009). Health, mortality, and wellness issues in adults with cerebral palsy. *Developmental Medicine and Child Neurology, 51,* 24–29.

United Nations. (2006). *Convention on rights of persons with disability*. http://www.otg/disabilities/convention. Accessed 14 March 2014.

Van Der Slot, W. M., Nieuwenhuijsen, C., Van Den Berg-Emons, R. J., Bergen, M. P., Hilberink, S. R., Stam, H. J., & Roebroeck, M. E. (2012). Chronic pain, fatigue, and depressive symptoms in adults with spastic bilateral cerebral palsy. *Developmental Medicine and Child Neurology, 54*(9), 836–842.

Vargus-Adams, J. N., & Martin, L. K. (2011). Domains of importance for parents, medical professionals and youth with cerebral palsy considering treatment outcomes. *Child: Care, Health and Development, 37*(2), 276–281.

Verdugo, M. A., Schalock, R. L., Keith, K. D., & Stancliffe, R. J. (2005). Quality of life and its measurement: Important principles and guidelines. *Journal of Intellectual Disability Research, 49,* 707–717.

Vles, G. F., Soudant, D. L., Hoving, M. A., Vermeulen, R. J., Bonouvrie, L. A., van Oostenbrugge, R. J., & Vles, J. S. (2013). Long-term follow-up on continuous intrathecal Baclofen therapy in non-ambulant children with intractable spastic cerebral palsy. *European Journal of Paediatric Neurology, 17*(6), 639–644.

Vogtle, L. K. (2009). Pain in adults with cerebral palsy: Impact and solutions. *Developmental Medicine and Child Neurology, 51,* 113–121.

Vogtle, L. K., Malone, L. A., & Azuero, A. (2013). Outcomes of an exercise program for pain and fatigue management in adults with cerebral palsy. *Disability and Rehabilitation*. doi:10.3109/09638288.2013.821181

Wehmeyer, M. L., & Garner, N. W. (2003). The impact of personal characteristics of people with intellectual and developmental disability on self determination and autonomous functioning. *Journal of Applied Research in Intellectual Disabilities, 16*(4), 255–265.

White-Koning, M., Arnaud, C., Dickinson, H. O., Thyen, U., Beckung, E., Fauconnier, J., McManus, V., Michelsen, S. I., Parkes, J., Parkinson, K., Schirripa, G., & Colver, A. (2007). Determinants of child-parent agreement in quality-of-life reports: A European study of children with cerebral palsy. *Pediatrics, 120*(4), 804–814.

Whiteneck, G., & Dijkers, M. P. (2009). Difficult to measure constructs: Conceptual and methodological issues concerning participation and environmental factors. *Archives of Physical Medicine and Rehabilitation, 90*(11 Suppl.), S22–S35.

Wingert, J. R., Burton, H., Sinclair, R. J., Brunstrom, J. E., & Damiano, D. L. (2009). Joint-position sense and kinesthesia in cerebral palsy. *Archives of Physical Medicine and Rehabilitation, 90*(3), 447–453.

World Health Organization. (2001). *International classification of functioning, disability and health* (*ICF*). Geneva: World Health Organization.

Zwicker, J. G., Grunau, R. E., Adams, E., Chau, V., Brant, R., Poskitt, K. J., Synnes, A., & Miller, S. P. (2013). Score for neonatal acute physiology-II and neonatal pain predict corticospinal tract development in premature newborns. *Pediatric Neurology, 48*(2), 123–129.

Part V
Conclusion

Chapter 14
Current Status and Future Directions

Rachel L. Goldin and Johnny L. Matson

Introduction

The ability of professionals to comprehensively assess and treat individuals with intellectual disabilities (ID) has improved immensely in recent years. Advances in the understanding of developmental and psychological processes and techniques to study them, such as neuroimaging and genetic testing, have allowed researchers to expand the current knowledge base about both typical and atypical functioning. Implications of this progress have led to positive developments in how society views those with ID and how we care for this population. However, much is still unknown about ID, especially when it co-occurs with other psychopathologies.

Individually, ID and the conditions that commonly co-occur with it are well defined. However, due to the complexity of symptom interactions, symptom presentations, and course of ID and co-occurring disorders, further exploration is required. Accurate diagnosis is critical for planning and implementing comprehensive interventions that address both the diagnosis of ID and comorbid conditions (Matson et al. 2005; Matson and Williams 2014; Rojahn et al. 2003).

Fortunately, the study of comorbid conditions among persons with ID is growing exponentially. In order to aid professionals in better understanding how to effectively treat people with disabilities, this chapter provides an overview of the current status of research on comorbid conditions among person with ID and the future directions of research on this topic. Topics covered include the assessment of comorbid psychopathologies, symptom interaction, children with ID and comorbid

J. L. Matson (✉) · R. L. Goldin
Department of Psychology, Louisiana State University, Baton Rouge, LA, USA
e-mail: johnmatson@aol.com

R. L. Goldin
e-mail: rgoldi3@lsu.edu

J. L. Matson, M. L. Matson (eds.), *Comorbid Conditions in Individuals with Intellectual Disabilities,* Autism and Child Psychopathology Series,
DOI 10.1007/978-3-319-15437-4_14

psychopathologies, methods of treatment, and the use of neuroimaging and genetic testing to better understand the etiology of ID. Before discussing recent findings and areas in need of further research, the current state of assessing comorbid conditions is reviewed. The development of measures to accurately assess comorbid conditions in person with ID was a crucial step in advancing the field.

Assessment of Comorbid Disorders

It is well established that not only do individuals with ID present with a full range of psychopathologies, but that they are at higher risk for psychopathologies than individuals with normal intelligence (Cherry et al. 1997; Cherry et al. 2000; Dekker and Koot 2003; Dekker et al. 2002; Di Nuovo and Buono 2007; Emerson 2003; Matson and Smiroldo 1997; Matson et al. 1997b; Paclawskyj et al. 1997; Rojahn and Tasse 1996; Szymanski and Tanquay 1980). This knowledge is the result of work that began in the 1980s to develop comorbid psychopathology screening measures specific to those with ID. Researchers continue to modify and revise these measures in accordance with a growing body of knowledge on persons with ID. The ability to accurately assess comorbid conditions has been critical to the evolution of the field and continues to be of the upmost importance, as it informs research methodologies, treatment planning and implementation, prognosis predictions, and access to services and supports. Due to the significant impact of these assessment measures, the first section of this chapter reviews commonly used measures, current research on assessment, and areas where additional research is needed.

Measure Design

Researchers have developed multiple scales designed to measure the presence and severity of comorbid conditions in individuals with ID. The strength of these measures over those commonly used in assessing typically developing individuals is that they were developed with an eye to how symptom presentation of a disorder may differ in someone who has ID versus someone with higher cognitive functioning. Additionally, many of the behaviors and abilities of individuals with ID are already considered atypical compared to the general population; thus, measures to assessing comorbidity in this population were designed to take this into account, and measure deviations in behavior that are beyond those typically seen in the context of ID. General measures of anxiety disorders or personality disorders, for example, do not include these considerations and may not capture a disorder or misdiagnose a disorder. Errors of this sort can thus lead to inappropriate services or complete lack of necessary services. For example, behavior problems are often treated with antipsychotic medications when in reality, the root of the behavior problem is environmentally maintained and would be more appropriately treated through functional analysis (FA) and a behavior modification plan.

The most commonly used measures for this purpose include the *Psychopathology Instrument for Mentally Retarded Adults* (*PIMRA*; Kazdin et al. 1983; Matson 1988; Matson et al. 2012), the *Aberrant Behavior Checklist* (*ABC*; Aman et al. 1985), the *Psychiatric Assessment Schedule for Adults with Developmental Disabilities* (*PAS-ADD*; Moss et al. 1993), *Reiss Screen for Maladaptive Behavior* (*RSMB*; Reiss 1988), the *Diagnostic Assessment for the Severely Handicapped revised* (*DASH-II*; Matson et al. 1997a), and the *Assessment for Dual Diagnosis* (*ADD*; Matson and Bamburg 1998). Characteristics of these measures that make them better suited for individuals with ID include forms for multiple reporters (e.g., self-report and informant report), screening questions for a range of comorbid conditions, and a design supported for repeated use. To illustrate these characteristics, the *PIMRA* will be discussed in depth as it was the first empirically validated scale solely for this purpose.

The Psychopathology Instrument for Mentally Retarded Adults

The *PIMRA* is a structured interview designed as a screening instrument to aid in the differential diagnosis of individuals with ID. To accommodate possible communication impairments, an informant version and self-report version of the *PIMRA* exist. The informant version is administered by an interviewer to an informant with at least 6 months experience working with the individual being assessed. The measure consists of 56 items and 8 subscales; schizophrenia, affective disorder, psychosexual disorder, adjustment disorder, anxiety disorder, somatoform disorder, personality disorder, and inappropriate adjustment. Item responses are recorded a "yes" or "no" format with regard to whether the item is true or false for the individual being assessed. Responses to items are added up for each subscale and for a total score. Interpretation of the scores is made by an appropriate professional. For the self-report version of the *PIMRA*, the interviewer asks the individual each item directly and records the individual's responses. The scoring and interpretation of the self-report version is done in the same as the informant version.

Researchers have found good reliability of both versions of the *PIMRA* (Matson et al. 1984; Senatore et al. 1985; Swiezy et al. 1995; Watson et al. 1988). Internal consistency as assessed using coefficient alpha was 0.83 for the informant version and 0.85 for the self-report version (Matson et al. 1984). Numerous studies have also examined the validity of the measure (Balboni et al. 2000; Gustafsson and Sonnander 2005; Linaker 1991; Linaker and Helle 1994; Swiezy et al. 1995; van Minnen et al. 1994). Linaker (1991) evaluated the psychometric properties of the *PIMRA* with a Norwegian sample of 163 individuals with ID. Results of the study indicated a correct classification of 69 % for the factors of the *PIMRA*. Intermethod agreement was found to be 88 % and a kappa of 0.62.

The *PIMRA* is just one example of a measure to screen for comorbid psychopathologies in individuals with ID. The other measures mentioned above differ in design with some utilizing checklist or rating scale formats. An important note about all of these scales is that they cannot be used to make a diagnosis of a psychiatric disorder on their own. As with psychological assessment in typically developing individuals, the diagnostic process is complex and requires convergence across multiple means of assessment. Researchers have concluded that rating scales and checklists, while an important part of assessment, are best used to indicate areas in need of a more comprehensive assessment, and/or as a means of tracking symptom change over time (Mohr and Costello 2007). Further limitations practically, theoretically, and statistically exist, which do not negate the significant impact of these measures, but highlight that work in the area of assessing comorbid psychopathologies in persons with ID is still needed.

Assessment Limitations

One area that warrants continued consideration is the development of within population specific designs. For instance, there is a lack of measures that are specific to children versus adults, or those with mild or moderate ID versus those with severe or profound ID. Discussed later in the chapter are differences in prevalence of comorbid conditions and symptom presentation of comorbid conditions depending on level of ID. Most of the scales in existence today do not take into account varying levels of ID. As research on the presentation of comorbid psychopathologies advances, and we gain greater understanding of how symptoms may vary based on demographic factors, the field would benefit from incorporating this information into the assessment process by developing new measures or modifying existing measures accordingly. Beyond more accurate diagnosis, within population specific measures (e.g., level of ID, children, and adults) would provide advantages for research and treatment procedures.

Four other areas also warrant future research. First, attention also should be paid to understanding the parameters that define individuals who are able to reliably self-report and those who cannot. Accurate diagnosis is dependent on accurate reporting. Second, though major advancements have been made in the development of measures for individuals with ID, a high level of comorbid disorders still go undetected, and therefore untreated (Deb et al. 2001). Researchers should focus on improving the sensitivity and accuracy of identifying comorbid conditions in individuals with ID, and referring them for follow-up evaluations. Third, the development of follow-up scales for specific psychopathologies is warranted. Most scales currently assess a range of psychopathologies. Creating disorder-specific scales will lead to improved treatment planning. Finally, with the recent publication of the *Diagnostic and Statistical Manual of Mental Disorders, Fifth Edition* (American Psychiatric Association 2013), the field would benefit from modifying existing measures and validating them against diagnostic criteria changes.

Severe and Profound ID

Much of the current research on ID is focused on those with mild and moderate ID. This trend is not surprising as most assessment measures require verbal communication, and a certain level of understanding. Those with severe and profound ID may lack the ability to answer questions in the manner necessary to complete these measures, or may be unable to answer questions due to the wording of questions that may require a certain level of understanding. Additionally, persons with mild to moderate ID tend to have a greater behavioral repertoire in which to evince excesses or deficits in normal behavior, for those with severe and profound ID, it can often be harder to differentiate behaviors that are indicative of additional problems when completing assessment measures. As a result, research is lacking with regard to how to best assess for comorbid psychopathology in individuals with severe and profound ID (Campo et al. 1997; Ross and Oliver 2003). This section will discuss some issues with regard to assessment and research specific to individuals with severe and profound ID.

Limitations of Assessment

Often in order to study those with severe and profound ID, researchers are limited to informant reports (Felce and Perry 1995; McVilly and Rawlinson 1998). However, informant reporting poses many challenges such as accuracy of reporting and agreement between multiple informants (Ross and Oliver 2003). Ross and Oliver (2003) noted that when assessing certain variables, such as quality of life, relying on informant report is inadequate "since the concept of quality of life is, in essence, 'deeply personal'" (McVilly and Rawlinson 1998; Parmenter 1992). This point is especially pertinent when studying individuals with severe or profound ID and comorbid conditions.

Some techniques have been suggested to address assessment limitations for persons with severe or profound ID. One technique suggested for assessing mood and affect in those with severe and profound ID is through behavioral approaches. Focusing research on understanding how positive and negative affective states may be expressed by those with no or limited expressive language may reduce the dependence on informant reporting (Ross and Oliver 2003). Applied behavioral analysis (ABA) has been proposed as a reliable way to measure positive and negative affective states (Favell et al. 1996; Green and Reid 1996). Favell et al. (1996) and Green and Reid (1996) have asserted that it may be possible to operationally define behaviors that are equated to happiness. Once these behaviors are operationally defined, the individual should be observed, the behaviors should be quantified, intervention should be implemented, and intervention effects should be examined. However, this technique does pose some issues such as, can we reliably denote behaviors that indicate happiness or unhappiness? Regardless, this line a research should be further explored as it may prove informative for other areas of assessment.

Barriers for Research

Lack of appropriate assessment procedure for individuals with ID poses problems for research. The assessment of co-occurring depression will be discussed as an example to illustrate this issue. Individuals with mild or moderate ID and comorbid depression have been found to exhibit a range of symptoms of depression consistent with those included in the ICD-10 criteria (Marston et al. 1997; Pawlarcyzk and Beckwith 1997). These findings, however, have not been replicated for individuals with severe or profound ID. One reason is that the diagnostic criteria require the use of expressive language to convey the presences or absence of symptoms. For example, criteria include statements such as "suicidal thoughts," "guilt or self-blame," and "ideas of worthlessness" (World Health Organization 1992). With limited or no expressive language, determining presence of these symptoms is nearly impossible. Consequently, this provides methodological challenges for researchers examining comorbid depression in this population (Ross and Oliver 2003).

In order to better assess for and understand the symptoms of depression in those with severe or profound ID, researchers must focus on creating techniques for determining the presence of these symptoms. Most importantly, measures must address the communication difficulties that are common in those with severe or profound ID. It must also be determined if typical symptoms of depression are even applicable to this population. The profile of depression in this population may not be consistent with that in individuals with mild or moderate ID. In order to treat depression in individuals with severe or profound ID, symptoms must be defined to create a picture of the disorder. The need for more knowledge on symptom presentation in individuals with severe or profound ID is not limited to depression. Research of this type is necessary for many other co-occurring disorders.

To address the limitations of assessment, some research has been devoted to examining the effectiveness of using observational techniques (Lowry 1993, 1994, 1998). An observational technique eliminates the need for self-report measures, and utilizes objective daily tracking of behaviors (Ross and Oliver 2003). Research of this kind may lead to the development of informant-based measures which are based on clearly defined behaviors associated with certain psychopathologies.

Symptom Presentation

Briefly mentioned earlier, symptoms of comorbid conditions may present differently in individuals with ID compared to those without; however, evidence regarding this is not conclusive. The interaction between ID and comorbid conditions is complex and can present a clinical profile that is not easily distinguishable. The symptoms of comorbid conditions and ID can reciprocally influence one another making diagnosis challenging. This section will review instances where the presence of ID results in a clinical presentation that differs from that of the general population and where it does not.

Marston et al. (1997) examined the symptom presentation of depressive disorder in persons with varying levels of ID, finding both common and distinctive symptoms. Symptoms common to those with mild ID, moderate ID, and severe ID were depressed affect and sleep disturbance. Depressive symptoms distinct to persons with mild ID included tearfulness, loss of interest and energy, low self-esteem, and diurnal mood variation. For participants with moderate ID, distinctive symptoms included weight loss, social isolation, and self-injurious behavior. In those with severe ID, distinctive depressive symptoms included aggression, screaming, and self-injurious behavior. Participants with mild ID exhibited symptoms of depression closest to those of the general population, while those with severe ID exhibited depressive symptoms that more closely resembled problem behaviors (e.g., aggression and tantrums; Marston et al. 1997). For those with more severe ID, a phenomenon called "diagnostic overshadowing" often occurs. Diagnostic overshadowing is when a professional attributes behavior problems to ID rather than a psychiatric disorder (Reiss et al. 1982; Reiss and Szyszko 1983; Smith and Matson 2010). Certain behaviors may be mistakenly ascribed to lower cognitive functioning, but in reality the behavior may be indicating a comorbid condition (Neece et al. 2013). In these cases, of diagnostic overshadowing, further assessment is generally disregarded and comorbid disorders may be left undiagnosed and untreated because symptoms do not closely resemble a classical presentation of a disorder.

In some cases, comorbid conditions have been found to present similarly in those with ID versus those without. For example, Neece et al. (2013) examined the validity of the attention-deficit hyperactivity disorder (ADHD) diagnosis for adolescents with ID. Presentation of ADHD within participants with ID and those without was examined in relation to sex, comorbidity of disorders, clinical presentation, and level of impairment. Findings indicated no difference in the diagnosis ratio of males to females, presentation of symptoms, or number of diagnostic criteria met between the groups. With regard to impairment, Neece and colleagues found that ADHD diagnosis predicted level of impairment greater than would be expected given the participant's intellectual functioning. Meaning that those with ID and ADHD were more impaired as they had a higher rate of clinical diagnoses, and higher level of symptoms over time (Neece et al. 2013).

The symptom presentation or clinical profile of comorbid conditions in persons with ID should not be expected to appear as those do in typically developing persons; on the other hand, it is probable that some similarities in presentation exist. In order to understand which comorbid conditions present similarly, which do not, and where discrepancies lay, the study of interactions between ID and the most commonly co-occurring conditions is needed. Benefits from greater knowledge in this area include more accurate diagnosis, better treatment planning, and better prediction of prognosis over time.

Children with ID

Children are not immune to psychopathological disorders, and can suffer from the full range of psychopathological disorders experienced by adults. Up until recently, research on comorbid psychopathology in persons with ID generally focused on adults. With an increased focus on the importance of early intervention, researchers have begun to pay greater attention to children with ID. This section discusses recent findings on comorbid conditions in children with ID and areas where additional research is needed.

Children with ID have been found to be at greater risk of psychiatric disorders compared to children with normal intelligence (Dykens 2000). Researchers have estimated that children with ID are three to seven times more likely to experience psychiatric disturbance as children without ID (Baker et al. 2003; Baker et al. 2005; Emerson 2003; Linna et al. 1999). A population-based study of children with ID in Australia found that 40 % of the sample exhibited psychopathology (Einfeld and Tonge 1996), while a similar study in Scotland found that 38 % of their sample of children with ID presented with psychopathologies (Hoare et al. 1998). Emerson (2003) compared the rate of overall psychiatric disorders and specific psychiatric disorders in a sample of 245 children with ID to those without ID. Presence of comorbid psychiatric disorders was found to be consistent with previous research at 39 %. The prevalence of conduct disorder, anxiety disorder, hyperkinesis, and pervasive developmental disorder were significantly greater among children with ID compared to children without ID (Emerson 2003). Similar research by Tonge and Einfeld (2003) concluded that ADHD, anxiety, and depression were four to five times more prevalent in children with ID than children without ID.

Similar to adults with ID, differences have been found with regard to level of ID and presence of psychopathologies. Einfeld and Tonge (1996) compared the prevalence of psychopathology in a sample of 454 children with varying levels of ID. With regard to prevalence of psychiatric disorders, no significant differences were found for level of ID, age, or gender. However, significant differences were found with regard to type of psychiatric disorder and level of ID. Rates of disruptive behavior and anxiety were found to increase with level of IQ, while autistic disorder rates were found to be the highest in those with severe ID (Einfeld and Tonge 1996).

Children with profound ID were found to overall have the lowest scores in the psychopathologies assessed (Einfeld and Tonge 1996).

Einfeld and Tonge also assessed what percent of their sample with a psychiatric disorder or major emotional/behavioral disturbance received assistance from specialist professionals. Only 9 % of their sample received assistance from a professional with expertise in both mental health and ID. Another 31 % received assistance from a professional working in either mental health or ID (Einfeld and Tonge 1996). These findings are concerning as the literature clearly evinces that child with ID are at high risk for comorbid psychopathology. Future research should explore reasons for which children with ID and comorbid psychopathologies are not receiving services from specialized professionals and what barriers might be contributing these disconcerting findings.

This line of research is important for multiple reasons. First and most obvious, appropriate treatment is fundamental to increasing positive outcomes for children with ID and comorbid psychopathology. Second, lack of treatment or inappropriate treatment of comorbid psychopathologies in children with ID can add further stress to the child's caregivers, and consequently have a negative impact on their well-being (Baker et al. 2003; Einfeld et al. 2006). Research examining parental stress in regard to having a child with ID and comorbid psychopathology has demonstrated that parental stress is more strongly associated with the child's behavior problems than cognitive functioning (Baker et al. 2003). Thus, appropriate treatment of such behaviors in children with ID can consequently reduce parental stress and their ability to provide the best care for their child. These findings are encouraging and emphasize the importance of aiding families of children with ID and comorbid psychopathologies to specialized professionals for treatment.

A final area of research concerning this population that would benefit from further exploration is course of comorbid psychopathologies over time. Little research attention has been paid to this topic; however, understanding if and how comorbid psychopathologies evolve through development is crucial to providing continued effective care for this population. Understanding comorbid conditions in children with ID is a line of research that is expected to grow exponentially in the future.

Understanding the Etiology of ID

Researchers are getting closer and closer to understanding the etiology of ID with technological advances in techniques such as neuroimaging and genetic testing. Gaining an etiological understanding has the possibility of improving prognosis predictions, accessing appropriate supports, informing the course of assessment and appropriate treatment, and avoiding unnecessary testing. The use of more complex research techniques and how their findings can be translated to clinical practice will be an emerging trend in the field of individuals with ID and comorbid conditions. This section reviews recent findings on the etiology of ID using neuroimaging and genetic testing.

Neuroimaging

Neuroimaging is increasingly being utilized to investigate the exact etiology of ID, which is currently still unknown and probably varies widely from person to person depending on a number of factors. Most neuroimaging research has focused on individuals with ID only and has not included individuals with additional conditions. This is not surprising as an understanding of the abnormal circuitry and how it relates to ID is still uncertain.

Magnetic resonance imaging (MRI) is currently the most widely used means of neurologically studying ID (Moeschler 2008). In a review of nine studies that used MRI, the average rate of abnormalities found in individuals with ID was 30 % (range, 6.2–48.7 %). Mannerkoski et al. (2009) found that compared to controls, participants with ID had significantly more abnormalities. Commonly found abnormalities in individuals with ID include ventricular enlargements, subtle corpus callosum abnormalities, cerebral cortical anomalies, white matter signal intensity abnormalities, and mild cerebellar fissure enlargements (Decobert et al. 2005; Mannerkoski et al. 2009; Spencer et al. 2005; Soto-Ares et al. 2003; Widjaja et al. 2008). Further, IQ has been found to correlate negatively with total number of abnormalities in participants with ID (Mannerkoski et al. 2009; Spencer et al. 2005). A greater number of abnormalities were found with moderate to profound ID compared to borderline to mild ID (van Karnebeek et al. 2005). Despite these findings, multiple studies have found that though MRI is able to identify abnormalities, the abnormalities identified are not ID specific and the sensitivity in revealing etiological causes are low (Mannerkoski et al. 2009; Moeschler 2008; van Karnebeek et al. 2005).

Research that utilizes neuroimaging is a trend that will continue in this field as technology in the area advances. For those with ID and comorbid psychopathology, where diagnosis is more difficult, neuroimaging can be useful in ruling-out an organic etiology for psychiatric symptoms (Pickard and Robertson 2007). This may be especially important in individuals with severe ID, who have impaired communication. Along with exploring the etiology of ID, neuroimaging may be useful in treatment planning. When neuropsychological functioning is highly impaired, certain forms of treatment may be inappropriate (Pickard and Robertson 2007). Identifying where structural abnormalities exist can aid professionals in better designing treatments for individuals with ID and comorbid psychopathology.

Genetic Testing

Most cases of ID are thought to have a genetic etiology (Habela and Hamosh 2013). Research examining genetic abnormalities that may be associated with ID is not entirely new to the field; however, techniques to explore the genetics involved in ID are continuing to evolve. Array-based chromosomal analysis is used to identify common causative duplications or deletions that are below the detection level of conventional karyotyping in individuals with ID (Tallantyre and Robertson 2013). Another technique, exome-wide sequencing, can be used at a relatively low cost to sequence the entire coding portion of the genome to detect de novo mutations. De novo mutations are genetic mutations that are neither parent possessed or transmitted. Using exome-wide sequencing, de Ligt et al. (2012) found the presence of de novo mutations in 53 % of their sample of adults with ID. De novo mutations were found to provide a conclusive genetic diagnosis in at least 13 % of the sample, with an additional 3 % of X-linked inherited mutations in known ID genes. These findings highlight the potential importance of de novo mutations as a cause of ID and signal an important area of continued research (de Ligt et al. 2012).

Still though, problems arise using genetic testing techniques. Predicting which de novo mutation will likely be pathogenic remains a challenge, as newborns typically acquire 50–100 de novo mutations in his/her genome, most of which are benign (Tallantyre and Robertson 2013). With constant improvement in genetic testing techniques, this line of research will continue to grow and shed light on the causes of ID. In the future, these techniques will hopefully no longer be limited to research laboratories any may be employed in clinical settings. Once more genetic knowledge is attained on those with ID only, researchers should attend to those with ID and comorbid conditions. Interesting findings may lie in the comparison of those with ID and comorbid conditions and those without.

Behavioral Phenotypes

The relationship between behavioral phenotypes and related genotypes is another area where knowledge is advancing rapidly. Behavioral phenotype denotes the social, cognitive, and linguistic characteristic patterns associated with a biological or genetic disorder (O'Brian and Bevan 2011). Attaining knowledge about the specific genotype related to behavioral phenotypes can greatly inform future prognosis, and best options for treatment. Research to date has begun to unravel the complex relationship between behavioral phenotypes, genotypes, and other genetic modifiers which complicate the picture.

Angelman syndrome (AS), for instance, is characterized by severe ID, jerky movements, unique facial appearance (e.g., deep set-eyes and prominent chin), seizures, and unstable gait. Most individuals with AS also exhibit significant speech and language impairments, a happy demeanor, a short attention span, sleep difficulties, and anxiety. Prevalence of AS is estimated to be 1 in 12,000 births (Clayton-Smith and Lann 2003). AS is known to be caused by genetic abnormalities affecting the expression of the gene UBE3A at chromosome 15q11–13 (Greer et al. 2010; Panda et al. 2013). The protein ubiquitin-protein ligase which is encoded at the UBE3A gene regulates excitatory synapse development by controlling the degradation of proteins involved in the function of glutamate receptors. The neurological picture and ID present in AS is thought to be caused by the disruption in this pathway (Greer et al. 2010).

Understanding the association between behavioral phenotypes and genotypes has a huge impact on accurate diagnosis and treatment. Presentation of a certain pattern of symptoms can lead professionals to refer families to genetic testing. If we are able to know from a genetic test the definite cause of ID and that comorbid symptoms are a result of a certain disorder, professionals can better prepare families for future challenges that may arise, direct them to interventions that have been empirically supported to work with that disorder, and avoid unnecessary and further testing. Research in this area is heading towards translating what we are learning about the genetics of ID into targeted treatment interventions.

Treatment

Treating comorbid conditions in persons with ID has received considerable attention in recent years. Effectively treating comorbid conditions has been hindered in certain aspects with regard to limitations in accurate assessment mentioned earlier. Modifications of standard treatments are often required when working with this population. Treatment of challenging behaviors, for instance, must be modified to effectively accommodate the lower level of cognitive function of individuals with ID. Commonly used treatments such as CBT require that the individual have a certain level of cognitive awareness. Individuals with ID often do not possess a level of cognitive functioning high enough to participate in a therapy such as CBT. Thus, researchers have devoted attention to the development of new interventions, and modification of existing interventions to treat comorbid conditions in persons with ID that either do not respond or do not possess the abilities to receive standard interventions. This section reviews commonly used interventions for treating comorbid conditions in individuals with ID, along with highlighting a few areas where further research attention is merited.

Functional Assessment

The treatment of challenging behaviors in persons with ID is critical to their well-being, and the well-being of those around them. In order to properly treat challenging behaviors, setting events and the factors which maintain the behavior must first be identified. A commonly used and empirically supported assessment technique to this end is functional assessment. Functional assessment is the process of identifying the function of a behavior. The function of the behavior is the variable(s) maintaining the occurrence of the target behavior. Functional assessment can be conducted through natural observation, in a structured setting, or with the use of a functional assessment rating scale such as the *Questions About Behavior Function* (Matson and Vollmer 1995).

FA was popularized by Iwata et al. (1982) as means of assessing the functional relationship between a challenging behavior and reinforcer. Through repeated exposure, the goal is to determine whether challenging behavior is maintained by sensory stimulation, escape from demand, social attention, or tangible reinforcement. FA has garnered considerable empirical support and is often a starting point for determining appropriate treatment approaches (Horner 1989; Iwata et al. 1994; Repp et al. 1988). The nature of FA makes it extremely useful when working with individuals with ID and comorbid conditions because of the simplicity of the design. From the result of FA, appropriate treatment methods can be selected and implemented.

Behavioral Therapy

ABA is one of the most commonly used and empirically supported behavioral interventions to change socially significant behavior. ABA relies on the principles established in learning to modify behavior (Baer et al. 1968). Most often used in treating symptoms of autism spectrum disorder, researchers have found that ABA is also effective in treating psychiatric disorders, maladaptive behaviors, self-injurious behaviors, pica, and phobic avoidance (Didden et al. 1997, 2006; Mafifei-Almodovar and Sturmey 2012; McAdam 2012; Sturmey 2012; Sturmey et al. 2012).

ABA focuses on operant behavior and environmental factors that control behavior. Through FA, antecedents and consequences of behavior are identified to employ methods of ABA to control behavior. Reinforcement is a key component of ABA. Principles of ABA suggest that a behavior is strengthened if it is closely followed by a rewarding stimulus, resulting in an increase in the future frequency of that behavior. The addition of a stimulus following a behavior is called a positive reinforcer, and the removal of a stimulus following a behavior is called a negative reinforcer (Flora 2004). ABA can also be used to decrease the frequency of a behavior through a process called punishment. Similar to reinforcement, a stimulus follows closely after a maladaptive behavior and is aimed at reducing the behavior. Punishment is generally administered in three techniques: presentation of aversive stimuli; response cost, which is the removal of desirable stimuli; and restriction of freedom, such as time outs (Cooper et al. 2007; Reese 1966). Techniques of ABA can be used for a variety of behaviors and can be generalized to a variety of environments (Cooper et al. 2007).

Researchers have devoted much attention to the use of ABA and other behavioral interventions for treating both maladaptive behavior and psychiatric disorders in individuals with ID (Aman et al. 2004; Rush and Frances 2000). A review of empirically supported treatments for phobic avoidance in persons with ID found that most treatment packages examined included in vivo exposure to the avoided stimulus and reinforcement for appropriate behavior during the exposure. Other features of the treatment packages used in some but not all studies include structured graduated exposure, modeling, prompting, use of distracting stimuli, and escape extinction

(Jennett and Hagopian 2008). Behavioral treatment packages for individuals with ID and comorbid phobic avoidance are empirically supported for the behavioral components of phobic avoidance. However, most of these studies did not measure the effectiveness of behavioral interventions on the physiological and cognitive components of phobic awareness (Jennett and Hagopian 2008). Future research would benefit from looking further into these components of phobic awareness as they may be predictors of treatment outcomes and maintenance.

Treating challenging behaviors and anxiety disorders have received the most focus with regard to behavioral interventions. The effectiveness of behavioral therapies in other psychiatric disorders such as obsessive–compulsive disorder (OCD) and post-traumatic stress disorder (PTSD) have been studied less (Chambless and Hollon 1998). Lew (1995) suggested three types of behavioral interventions to treat OCD in persons with ID. First, preventative interventions such as manipulating the antecedent variables to reduce the likelihood of the OCD behavior were purposed. Second, proactive or skill-building methods were suggested to teach alternative responses to antecedent variables. The third intervention addressed introducing consequences contingent upon an effort to reduce OCD behaviors. Unlike challenging behaviors and anxiety disorders, few follow-up studies have been conducted to examine the efficacy of these proposed behavioral interventions (Kostinas et al. 2001; Matson 1982).

Due to the established efficacy of behavioral treatments in persons without ID, and the limited but promising results of efficacy in person with ID, researchers in this field should continue to examine the application of behavioral treatments with this population. A major benefit of behavioral treatments is that they can be conducted with individuals with all levels of ID. Unlike CBT, the behavioral techniques do not require a certain level of cognitive function and behavioral treatments can be modified extensively depending on the individual's level of functioning. Focusing resources on studying behavioral interventions for the treatment of a variety of comorbid disorders in persons with ID is of the upmost importance for improving the well-being of this population.

Pharmacological

The use of medication is an emerging trend in the study of ID and comorbid disorders. Until recently, few randomized controlled treatments (RCT) using medication to treat comorbid conditions in individuals with ID had been conducted (Jesner et al. 2007). Sohanpal et al. (2007) conducted a systematic review of studies examining the effectiveness of antidepressant medication in the management of behavior problems in adults with ID. The authors found that the research conducted on this topic was lacking. The studies reviewed were primarily based on small sample sizes and often used nonvalidated outcome measures (Sohanpal et al. 2007).

Selective serotonin reuptake inhibitors (SSRIs) were the most common class of medication studied, though one study examined the effectiveness of clomipramine.

Findings on the effectiveness of SSRIs were not consistent; therefore, Sohanpal et al. noted that drawing definite conclusions from the findings is difficult 2007. Similar conclusions were drawn in a systematic review of the effectiveness of antipsychotic medication in the management of behavior problems in adults with ID by Deb and colleagues (2007). Deb et al. found risperidone to be the most effective in both child and adults (Deb et al. 2007). Results from these reviews suggest methodological weaknesses as a major concern in most of the studies reviewed. Thus, the lack of evidence for pharmacological treatments does not mean that medications are ineffective; instead, methodological techniques need to be better refined to appropriately assess the effects of medication (Deb et al. 2008; Deb and Unwin 2007; Singh et al. 2005, 2010).

In order to best evaluate whether medication should be considered an option in treating comorbid conditions, it is absolutely essential that a thorough and precise assessment be conducted. Misdiagnosis can easily occur since a large amount of symptom overlap exists. For instance, self-injurious behaviors may be a symptom of anxiety, depression or even as a means to be oppositional, or to escape an undesired task. Targeting self-injurious behaviors therefore will be ineffective as the behaviors are symptom of a bigger issue. Treatment can only be as good as the assessment preceding it so it is crucial that an accurate diagnosis is made through a comprehensive battery of assessments and clinical observation. It is recommended that screening measures such as rating scales be used along with interviews, observations, and review of medical history and tests before medication is prescribed.

Limitations of Treatment Research

Much more work is needed in the area of treating comorbid conditions in person with ID. Promising findings with regard to behavioral interventions and pharmacological treatments suggest that research is likely to continue in this direction. Other areas where further research would be beneficial include reliable diagnosis of psychiatry disorders in person with ID, combined psychopharmacological and psychosocial treatment, and social validation of behavioral changes. First, the reason that research to examine medication to treat comorbid conditions in persons with ID is limited is because of the difficulty of making reliable psychiatric diagnoses in individuals with ID (Sturmey 2012). Thus, as touched on previously, researchers must continue focusing on studying the symptom presentation of comorbid conditions in individuals with ID to support better research. Second, the combination of behavioral therapy and pharmacology would be a promising direction for the field to study. Researchers have found that combination therapy can be very beneficial in treating disorders in those without ID, therefore, exploring combination therapy in individuals with ID is promising (Keeton et al. 2009; Walkup et al. 2008). Finally, little attention has been paid to evaluating the social validity of behavioral changes from pharmacological treatments (Sturmey 2012). Researchers must weigh the pros and cons of pharmacological treatments and determine if the effects of treatment significantly improve quality of life (Sturmey 2012). The development of treatments that are more suitable is a critical trend the field must further perused.

Discussion

What We Know

This chapter has reviewed recent research findings pertaining to individuals with ID and comorbid conditions. What we currently know is that the assessment of comorbid condition in person with ID is possible. Measures have been developed and validated that can screen for the presence of a variety of psychopathologies in those with ID. The development of the measures has allowed researcher to begin to examine comorbid symptomology and whether the clinical presentation is similar or different compared to those without ID. By better understand the presentation of comorbid conditions, researchers have been able to explore symptom profiles compared to individuals without ID, but also within the ID population by level of ID and age. Level of cognitive functioning can impact the prevalence of specific comorbid conditions but also the severity. Further, comorbid psychopathologies are not limited to adults, and recent findings have indicated that children can possess a wide range of psychopathologies.

Confirmation of the presence and high prevalence of comorbid conditions in person with ID has lead researchers to explore the etiology of ID through neuroimaging and genetic testing. Though the etiology of ID is still unknown, researchers have discovered brain abnormalities and de novo gene mutations that with further exploration may shed light on the etiology of ID. A better understanding of the etiology of ID can benefit assessment methodologies, treatment selection, and treatment methods. Despite a full understanding of the possible causes of ID, many empirically supported treatments for comorbid conditions in persons with ID have emerged. Behavioral methods along with medications have been recognized as being effective in treating some comorbid conditions experienced by individuals with ID. Though great advancements have been made in this field, much is still unknown or needs further attention.

Where We Are Headed

A strong foundation in the study of comorbid conditions in persons with ID exists, but the details with regard to the population require further research attention. Assessment methods must be expanded to accurately assess those with differing levels of ID, as well as children who may evince the condition. Methods of assessment often are self-report which is problematic when working with individuals who have severe or profound ID, and may not possess a level of understanding necessary to answer the items or the skills to effectively communicate. Additionally, the development of follow-up scales is crucial to gaining a better understanding of the symptom presentation of comorbid in person with ID. A more informed understand of symptom presentation and how it may or may not differ from those without ID or those with varying levels of ID is needed to accurately define comorbid conditions.

Without a clear picture of how comorbid conditions are exhibited in persons with ID, psychopathologies can often go undetected, be misdiagnosed, and/or inappropriately treated. The acceptance of comorbid conditions and the ability to differentiate them from symptoms of ID was a huge step in the field. However, now research attention must be focused on enhancing diagnostic accuracy and creating clear diagnostic criteria for comorbid conditions in this population. Along these lines, the focus on understanding and gaining knowledge on comorbid psychopathology in children with ID has grown exponentially recently. Researchers have established that children with ID can exhibit the full range of psychopathologies as adults and the prevalence rates of specific disorders. Research is lacking however, on the course of comorbid conditions in children and the effect on prognosis. Longitudinal research is of much need as it can have a significant impact on choice of treatment, implementation, and it can provide professionals and parents with a predication of future prognosis and what services and needs may be required in the future. While advances in health care are allowing people to live longer lives, this line of research is critical and over time will take on even greater significance (Matson and Cervantes 2013). As individuals with ID live longer, the likelihood of outliving their parents increases, highlighting the need to develop long-term social supports that go beyond the immediate family.

Research understanding the etiology of ID is still in the beginning stages, but with the development of better neuroimaging techniques, and genetic testing, researchers are getting closer to identifying possible causes. Determining the etiology of ID will have an enormous impact on all areas of the field. The next step will be determining how neuroimaging and genetic testing can be incorporated into clinical practice. Additionally, once ID alone is better understood, researchers should explore the use of these technologies in studying the interaction between ID and comorbid psychopathologies.

Finally, the treatment of comorbid conditions in persons with ID has made significant progress of late. However, most attention has been paid to the treatment of only a few comorbid conditions. Research on empirically supported behavioral treatments must be expanded to a variety of commonly co-occurring psychopathologies. With regard to the use of medications in the treatment of comorbid conditions, an increased number of RCT with large samples sizes are needed to further examine the effectiveness of medication, and safety of short-term and long-term use of medications. Further, the use of medications in children has received limited attention. Due to the rapid development of children, the safety of medication use, as well as the pros and cons of medication requires considerable attention. Treating comorbid conditions in persons with ID is of the upmost importance and requires continued attention from researchers.

References

Aman, M. G., Singh, N. N., Stewart, A. W., & Field, C. J. (1985). Psychometric characteristics of the aberrant behavior checklist. *American Journal of Mental Deficiency, 89*(5), 492–502.

Aman, M. G., Crismon, M. L., Frances, A., King, B. H., & Rojahn, J. (Eds.). (2004). *Treatment of psychiatric and behavioral problems in individuals with mental retardation: An update of the expert consensus guidelines*. Englewood: Postgraduate Institute for Medicine.

American Psychiatric Association. (2013). *Diagnostic and statistical manual of mental disorders* (5th ed.). Washington, DC: Author.

Baer, D. M., Wolf, M. M., & Risely, T. R. (1968). Some current dimensions of applied behavior analysis. *Journal of Applied Behavior Analysis, 1,* 91–97.

Baker, B. L., McIntyre, L. L., Blacher, J. J., Crnic, K. K., Edelbrock, C. C., & Low, C. C. (2003). Pre-school children with and without developmental delay: Behaviour problems and parenting stress over time. *Journal of Intellectual Disability Research, 47*(4/5), 217–230.

Baker, B. L., Blacher, J. J., & Olsson, M. B. (2005). Preschool Children with and without Developmental Delay: Behaviour Problems, Parents Optimism and Well-Being. *Journal of Intellectual Disability Research, 49*(8), 575–590.

Balboni, G., Battagliese, G., & Pedrabissi, L. (2000). The pscyhopathology inventory for mentally retarded adults: Factor structure and comparisons between subjects with or without dual diagnosis. *Research in Developmental Disabilities, 21,* 311–321.

Campo, S. F., Sharpton, W. R., Thompson, B., & Sexton, D. (1997). Correlates of the quality of life of adults with severe or profound mental retardation. *Mental Retardation, 35,* 329–337.

Chambless, D. L., & Hollon, S. D. (1998). Defining empirically supported therapies. *Journal of Consulting and Clinical Psychology, 66*(1), 7–18.

Cherry, K. E., Paclawskyj, T., & Matson, J. L. (1997). Psychopathology in older adults with severe and profound mental retardation. *American Journal of Mental Retardation, 101,* 445–458.

Cherry, K. E., Penn, D., Matson, J. L., & Bamburg, J. W. (2000). Characteristics of schizophrenia in persons with severe and profound mental retardation. *Psychiatric Services, 51,* 422–423.

Clayton-Smith, J., & Laan, L. (2003). Angelman syndrome: A review of the clinical and genetic aspects. *Journal of Medical Genetics, 40,* 87–95.

Cooper, J. O., Heron, T. E., & Heward, W. L. (2007). *Applied behavior analysis* (2nd ed.). Englewood Cliffs: Pearson.

de Ligt, J., Willemsen, M. H., van Bon, B. M., Kleefstra, T., Yntema, H. G., Kroes, T., Vulto-van Silfhout, A. T., Koolen, D. A., de Vries, P., Gilissen, C., del Rosario, M., Hoischen, A., Scheffer, H., de Vries, B. B., Brunner, H. G., Veltman, J. A., & Vissers, L. M. (2012). Diagnostic exome sequencing in persons with severe intellectual disability. *New England Journal of Medicine, 367*(20), 1921–1929.

Deb, S., & Unwin, G. (2007). Psychotropic medication for behaviour problems in people with intellectual disability: A review of the current literature. *Current Opinion in Psychiatry, 20*(5), 461–466.

Deb, S., Thomas, M., & Bright, C. (2001). Mental disorder in adults with intellectual disability. 1: Prevalence of functional psychiatric illness among community-based population aged between 16 and 64 years. *Journal of Intellectual Disability Research, 45,* 495–505.

Deb, S., Sohanpal, S., Soni, R., Lenôtre, L., & Unwin, G. (2007). The effectiveness of antipsychotic medication in the management of behaviour problems in adults with intellectual disabilities. *Journal of Intellectual Disability Research, 51,* 766–777.

Deb, S. S., Chaplin, R. R., Sohanpal, S. S., Unwin, G. G., Soni, R. R., & Lenôtre, L. L. (2008). The effectiveness of mood stabilizers and antiepileptic medication for the management of behaviour problems in adults with intellectual disability: A systematic review. *Journal of Intellectual Disability Research, 52*(2), 107–113.

Decobert, F., Grabar, S., Merzoug, V., Kalifa, G., Ponsot, G., Adamsbaum, C., & des Portes, V. (2005). Unexplained mental retardation: Is brain MRI useful? *Pediatric radiology, 35*(6), 587–596.

Dekker, M. C., & Koot, H. M. (2003). DSM-IV disorders in children with borderline to moderate intellectual disability. I: Prevalence and impact. *Journal of the American Academy of Child and Adolescent Psychiatry, 42,* 915–922.

Dekker, M. C., Koot, H. M., van der Ende, J., & Verhulst, F. C. (2002). Emotional and behavioral problems in children and adolescents with and without intellectual disability. *Journal of Child Psychology and Psychiatry, 43,* 1087–1098.

Di Nuovo, S. F., & Buono, S. (2007). Psychiatric syndromes comborbid with mental retardation: Differences in cognitive and adaptive skills. *Journal of Psychiatric Research, 41,* 795–800.

Didden, R., Duker, P. C., & Korzilius, H. (1997). Meta-analytic study on treatment effectiveness for problem behaviors with individuals who have mental retardation. *American Journal of Mental Retardation, 101,* 387–399.

Didden, R., Korzilius, H., van Oorsouw, W., & Sturmey, P. (2006). Behavioral treatment of challenging behaviors in individuals with mild mental retardation: Meta-analysis of single-subject research. *American Journal on. Mental Retardation, 111*(4), 290–298.

Dykens, E. M. (2000). Psychopathology in children with intellectual disability. *Journal of Child Psychology and Psychiatry, 41,* 407–417.

Einfeld, S. L., & Tonge, J. J. (1996). Population prevalence of psychopathology in children and adolescents with intellectual disability: II. Epidemiological findings. *Journal of Intellectual Disability Research, 40*(2), 99–109.

Einfeld, S. L., Piccinin, A. M., Mackinnon, A., Hofer, S. M., Taffe, J., Gray, K. M., Bontempo, D. E., Hoffman, L. R., Parmenter, T., & Tonge, B. J. (2006). Psychopathology in young people with intellectual disability. *Journal of the American Medical Association, 296*(16), 1981–1989.

Emerson, E. (2003). Prevalence of psychiatric disorders in children and adolescents with and without intellectual disability. *Journal of Intellectual Disability Research, 47,* 51–58.

Favell, J. E., Realon, R. E., & Sutton, K. A. (1996). Measuring and increasing the happiness of people with profound mental retardation and physical handicaps. *Behavioral Interventions, 11,* 47–58.

Felce, D., & Perry, J. (1995). Quality of life: Its definition and measurement. *Research in Mental Retardation, 16,* 51–74.

Flora, S. R. (2004). *The power of reinforcement.* Albany: State University of New York Press.

Green, C. W., & Reid, D. H. (1996). Defining, validating and increasing indices of happiness among people with profound multiple disabilities. *Journal of Applied Behavior Analysis, 29,* 67–78.

Greer, P. L., Hanayama, R., Bloodgood, B. L., Mardinly, A. R., Lipton, D. M., Flavell, S. W., Kim, T. K., Griffith, E. C., Waldon, Z., Maehr, R., Ploegh, H. L., Chowdhury, S., Worley, P. F., Steen, J., & Greenberg, M. E. (2010). The Angelman Syndrome protein Ube3A regulates synapse development by ubiquitinating arc. *Cell, 140*(5), 704–716.

Gustafsson, C., & Sonnander, K. (2005). A psychometric evaluation of a Swedish version of the psychopathology inventory for mentally retarded adults (PIMRA). *Research in Developmental Disabilities, 26,* 183–201.

Habela, C. W., & Hamosh, A. (2013). Genetic testing for intellectual disability. *Contemporary Pediatrics, 30*(6), 21–30.

Hoare, P., Harris, M., Jackson, P., & Kerley, S. (1998). A community survey of children with severe intellectual disability and their families: Psychological adjustment, carer distress and the effect of respite care. *Journal of Intellectual Disability Research, 42,* 218–227.

Horner, R. H. (1989). Recommendations based on community support for people with developmental disabilities and destructive behavior. In Treatment of destructive behaviors in persons with developmental disabilities (NIH Publication No. 91-2410, pp. 64–69). Bethesda: National Institutes of Health.

Iwata, B. A., Dorsey, M. F., Slifer, K. J., Bauman, K. E., & Richman, G. S. (1982). Toward a functional analysis of self-injury. *Journal of Applied Behavior Analysis, 2*7(2), 197–209.

Iwata, B. A., Pace, G. M., Dorsey, M. F., Zarcone, J. R., Vollmer, T. R., Smith, R. G., & Willis, K. D. (1994). The functions of self-injurious behavior: An experimental-epidemiological analysis. *Journal of Applied Behavior Analysis, 27*(2), 215–240. doi:10.1901/jaba.1994.27-215

Jennett, H. K., & Hagopian, L. P. (2008). Identifying empirically supported treatments for phobic avoidance in individuals with intellectual disabilities. *Behavior Therapy, 39*(2), 151–161.

Jesner, O. S., Aref-Adib, M., & Coren, E. (2007). Risperidone for autism spectrum disorder. *Cochrane Database of Systematic Reviews,* 1–28.

Kazdin, A. E., Matson, J. L., & Senatore, V. (1983). Assessment of depression in mentally retarded adults. *American Journal of Psychiatry, 140,* 1040–1043.

Keeton, C., Kolos, A. C., & Walkup, J. T. (2009). Pediatric generalized anxiety disorder. *Pediatric Drugs, 11*(3), 171–183.

Kostinas, G., Scandlen, A., & Luiselli, J. K. (2001). Effects of DRL and DRL combined with response cost on perseverative verbal behavior on an adult with mental retardation and obsessive compulsive disorder. *Behavioral Interventions, 16*(1), 27–37.

Lew, M. (1995). Behavioral approaches to working with obsessive-compulsive disorder in persons with mental retardation. *The Habilitative Mental Healthcare Newsletter, 14,* 83–89.

Linaker, O. (1991). DSM-III diagnosis compared with factor structure of the Psychopathology Instrument for Mentally Retarded Adults (PIMRA) in an institutionalized, mostly severely retarded population. *Research in Developmental Disabilities, 12,* 143–153.

Linaker, O. M., & Helle, J. (1994). Validity of the schizophrenia diagnosis of the Psychopathology Instrument for Mentally Retarded Adults (PIMRA): A comparison of Schizophrenic patients with and without mental retardation. *Research in Developmental Disabilities, 15,* 473–486.

Linna, S. L., Moilanen, I., Ebeling, H., Piha, J., Kumpulainen, K., Tamminen, T., & Almqvist, F. (1999). Psychiatric symptoms in children with intellectual disability. *European Child and Adolescent Psychiatry, 8*(Suppl. 4, IV), 77–82.

Lowry, M. A. (1993). A clear link between problem behaviors and mood disorders. *Habilitative Mental Healthcare Newsletter, 12,* 105–110.

Lowry, M. A. (1994). Functional assessment of problem behaviors associated with mood disorders. *Habilitative Mental Healthcare Newsletter, 13,* 79–83.

Lowry, M. A. (1998). Assessment and treatment of mood disorders in persons with mental retardation. *Journal of Mental Retardation, 10,* 387–405.

Mafifei-Almodovar, L., & Sturmey, P. (2012). Evidence-based practice and crisis intervention. In D. D. Reed, F. D. DiGennaro Reed & J. K. Luiselli (Eds.), *Handbook of crisis intervention for individuals with developmental disabilities*. New York: Springer.

Mannerkoski, M. M., Heiskala, H. H., Raininko, R. R., Åberg, L. L., Sarna, S. S., Wirtavuori, K. K., & Autti, T. T. (2009). Brain magnetic resonance imaging of siblings from families with two or more children with learning or intellectual disabilities and need for full-time special education. *Acta Radiologica, 50*(4), 437–445.

Marston, G. M., Perry, D. W., & Roy, A. (1997). Manifestations of depression in people with developmental disability. *Journal of Intellectual Disability Research, 41,* 476–480.

Matson, J. L. (1982). Treating obsessive-compulsive behavior in mentally retarded adults. *Behavior Modification, 6,* 551–567.

Matson, J. L. (1988). *Psychopathology Instrument for Mentally Retarded Adults* (*PIMRA*). Worthington: International Diagnostic Systems.

Matson, J. L., & Bamburg, J. W. (1998). Reliability of the assessment of dual diagnosis (ADD). *Research in Developmental Disabilities, 19*(1), 89–95.

Matson, J. L., & Cervantes, P. E. (2013). Comorbidity among persons with intellectual disabilities. *Research in Autism Spectrum Disorders, 7*(11), 1318–1322.

Matson, J. L., & Smiroldo, B. B. (1997). Validity of the mania subscale of the Diagnostic Assessment for the Severely Handicapped-II (DASH-II). *Research in Developmental Disabilities, 18,* 221–225.

Matson, J. L., & Vollmer, T. R. (1995). *User's guide: Questions About Behavioral Function* (*QABF*). Baton Rouge: Scientific Publishers, Inc.

Matson, J. L., & Williams, L. (2014). The making of a field: The development of comorbid psychopathology research for persons with intellectual disabilities and autism. *Research in Developmental Disabilities, 35,* 234–238.

Matson, J. L., Kazdin, A. E., & Senatore, V. (1984). Psychometric properties of the psychopathology instrument for mentally retarded adults. *Applied Research in Mental Retardation, 5,* 81–90.
Matson, J. L., Kiely, S. L., & Bamburg, J. W. (1997a). The effect of stereotypies on adaptive skills as assessed with the DASH-II and Vineland Adaptive Behavior Scales. *Research in Developmental Disabilities, 18*(6), 471–476.
Matson, J. L., Simroldo, B. B., Hamilton, M., & Baglio, C. S. (1997b). Do anxiety disorders exist in persons with severe and profound mental retardation? *Research in Developmental Disabilities, 18,* 39–44.
Matson, J. L., Mayville, S. B., Kuhn, D. E., Sturmey, P., Laud, R., & Cooper, C. (2005). The behavioral function of feeding problems as assessed by the Questions About Behavioral Function (QABF). *Research in Developmental Disabilities, 26*(4), 399–408.
Matson, J. L., Belva, B. C., Hattier, M. A., & Matson, M. L. (2012). Scaling methods to measure psychopathology in persons with intellectual disabilities. *Research in Developmental Disabilities, 33*(2), 549–562.
McAdam, D., Breidbord, J., Levine, A., & Williams, D. E. (2012). Pica. In M. Hersen & P. Sturmey (Eds.), *Handbook of evidence-based practice in clinical psychology. Vol. 1, Children and adolescents*. New York: John Wiley & Sons, Ltd.
McVilly, K. R., & Rawlinson, R. B. (1998). Quality of life issues in the development and evaluation of services for people with developmental disability. *Journal of Intellectual and Developmental Disability, 23,* 199–218.
Moeschler, J. (2008). Genetic evaluation of intellectual disabilities. *Seminars in Pediatric Neurology, 15*(1), 2–9.
Mohr, C., & Costello, H. (2007). Mental health assessment and monitoring tools. In N. Bouras & G. Holt (Eds.), *Psychiatric and behavioural disorders in intellectual and developmental disabilities, second edition*. New York: Cambridge University Press.
Moss, S., Patel, P., Prosser, H., Goldberg, D., Simpson, N. E. I. L. L., Rowe, S. T. E., et al. (1993). Psychiatric morbidity in older people with moderate and severe learning disability. I: Development and reliability of the patient interview (PAS-ADD). *British Journal of Psychiatry, 163*(4), 471–480.
Neece, C. L., Baker, B. L., Crnic, K., & Blacher, J. (2013). Examining the validity of ADHD as a diagnosis for adolescents with intellectual disabilities: Clinical presentation. *Journal of Abnormal Child Psychology, 41*(4), 597–612.
O'Brien, G., & Bevan, R. (2011). Recent advances in behavioral phenotypes as they affect adults. *Advances in Mental Health and Intellectual Disabilities, 5*(4), 5–14.
Paclawskyj, T. R., Matson, J. L., Bamburg, J. W., & Baglio, C. S. (1997). A comparison of the Diagnostic Assessment for the Severely Handicapped-II (DASH-II) and the Aberrant Behavior Checklist (ABC). *Research in Developmental Disabilities, 18,* 289–298.
Panda, A., Kar, S., & Gopinath, G. G. (2013). Angelman syndrome in three biological siblings: Focusing on the neuropsychiatric domain. *Journal Of Pediatric Neurosciences, 8*(3), 213–216.
Parmenter, T. R. (1992). Quality of life of people with mental retardation. *International Review of Research in Mental Retardation, 18,* 247–287.
Pawlarcyzk, D., & Beckwith, B. (1997). Depressive symptoms displayed by persons with mental retardation: A review. *Mental Retardation, 25,* 325–330.
Pickard, M., & Robertson, D. (2007). Neuroimaging and intellectual disabilities. In N. Bouras & G. Holt (Eds.), *Psychiatric and behavioural disorders in intellectual and developmental disabilities, second edition*. New York: Cambridge University Press.
Reese, E. P. (1966). *The analysis of human operant behavior*. Dubuque IA: Brown.
Reiss, S. (1988). *The reiss screen for maladaptive behavior test manual*. Worthington: IDS Publishing Corporation.
Reiss, S., & Szyszko, J. (1983). Diagnostic overshadowing and professional experience with mentally retarded persons. *American Journal of Mental Deficiency, 87,* 396–402.
Reiss, S., Levitan, G. W., & Szyszko, J. (1982). Emotional disturbance and mental retardation: Diagnostic overshadowing. *American Journal on Mental Deficiency, 86,* 567–574.

Repp, A. C., Felce, D., & Barton, L. E. (1988). Basing the treatment of stereotypic and self-injurious behaviors on hypotheses of their causes. *Journal of Applied Behavior Analysis, 21,* 281–289.
Rojahn, J., & Tasse, M. J. (1996). Psychopathology in mental retardation. In J. W. Jacobson & J. A. Mulick (Eds.), *Manual of diagnosis and professional practice in mental retardation.* Washington DC: American Psychological Association.
Rojahn, J., Aman, M. G., Matson, J. L., & Mayville, E. (2003). The aberrant behavior checklist and the behavior problems inventory: Convergent and divergent validity. *Research in Developmental Disabilities, 24*(5), 391–404.
Ross, E., & Oliver, C. (2003). The assessment of mood in adults who have severe or profound mental retardation. *Clinical Psychology Review, 23*(2), 225.
Rush, A., & Frances, A. E. (2000). Expert consensus guideline series: Treatment of psychiatric and behavioral problems in mental retardation. *American Journal on Mental Retardation, 105,* 159–228.
Senatore, V., Matson, J. L., & Kazdin, A. E. (1985). An inventory to assess psychopathology of mentally retarded adults. *American Journal of Mental Deficiency, 89,* 459–466.
Singh, A. N., Matson, J. L., Cooper, C. L., Dixon, D., & Sturmey, P. (2005). The use of risperidone among individuals with mental retardation: Clinically supported or not? *Research in Developmental Disabilities: A Multidisciplinary Journal, 26*(3), 203–218.
Singh, A., Matson, J., Hill, B., Pella, R., Cooper, C., & Adkins, A. (2010). The use of clozapine among individuals with intellectual disability: A review. *Research in Developmental Disabilities, 31*(6), 1135–1141.
Smith, K. R. M., & Matson, J. L. (2010). Psychopathology: Differences among adults with intellectual disability, and comorbid autism spectrum disorders, and epilepsy. *Research in Developmental Disabilities, 31,* 743–749.
Sohanpal, S., Deb, S., Thomas, C., Soni, R., Lenôtre, L., & Unwin, G. (2007). The effectiveness of antidepressant medication in the management of behaviour problems in adults with intellectual disabilities: A systematic review. *Journal of Intellectual Disability Research, 51,* 750–765.
Soto-Ares, G., Joyes, B., Lemaître, M. P., Vallée, L., & Pruvo, J. P. (2003). MRI in children with mental retardation. *Pediatric radiology, 33*(5), 334–345.
Spencer, M. D., Gibson, R. J., Moorhead, T. W. J., Keston, P. M., Hoare, P., Best, J. J., Lawrie, S. M., & Johnstone, E. C. (2005). Qualitative assessment of brain anomalies in adolescents with mental retardation. *American Journal of Neuroradiology, 26*(10), 2691–2697.
Sturmey, P. (2012). Treatment of Psychopathology in People with Intellectual and Other Disabilities. *Canadian Journal of Psychiatry, 57*(10), 593–600.
Sturmey, P., Maffei-Almodovar, L., Madzharova, M. S., & Cooper, J. (2012). Self injurious behavior. In P. Sturmey & M. Hersen (Eds.)., *Handbook of evidence-based practice in clinical psychology. Vol. 2, Adults.* New York: John Wiley & Sons, Ltd.
Swiezy, N. B., Matson, J. L., Kirkpatrick-Sanchez, S., & Williams, D. E. (1995). A criterion validity study of the schizophrenia subscale of the Psychopathology Instrument for Mentally Retarded Adults (PIMRA). *Research in Developmental Disabilities, 16*(1), 75–80.
Szymanski, L. S., & Tanquay, P. E. (1980). *Emotional disorders of mentally retarded people.* Baltimore: University Park Press.
Tallantyre, E., & Robertson, N. (2013). Autism and intellectual disability. *Journal of Neurology, 260*(3), 936–939.
Tonge, B. J., & Einfeld, S. L. (2003). Psychopathology and intellectual disability: The Australian child to adult longitudinal study. In L. Glidden (Ed.), International review of research in mental retardation, Vol. 26 (pp. 61–91). San Diego Academic Press.
van Karnebeek, C. M., Jansweijer, M. E., Leenders, A. E., Offringa, M., & Hennekam, R. M. (2005). Diagnostic investigations in individuals with mental retardation: A systematic literature review of their usefulness. *European Journal of Human Genetics, 13*(1), 6–25.
van Minnen, A., Savelsberg, P. M., & Hoogduin, K. A. (1994). A Dutch version of the Psychopathology Inventory for Mentally Retarded Adults (PIMRA). *Research in Developmental Disabilities, 15,* 269–278.

Walkup, J. T., Albano, A. M., Piacentini, J., Birmaher, B., Compton, S. N., Sherrill, J. T., Ginsburg, G. S., Rynn, M. A., McCracken, J., Waslick, B., Iyengar, S., March, J. S., & Kendall, P. C. (2008). Cognitive behavioral therapy, sertraline, or a combination in childhood anxiety. *New England Journal of Medicine, 359*(26), 2753–2766.

Watson, J. E., Aman, M. G., & Singh, N. N. (1988). The Psychopathology Instrument for Mentally Retarded Adults: Psychometric characteristics, factor structure, and relationship to subject characteristics. *Research in developmental disabilities, 9*(3), 277–290.

Widjaja, E., Nilsson, D., Blaser, S., & Raybaud, C. (2008). White matter abnormalities in children with idiopathic developmental delay. *Acta Radiologica, 49*(5), 589–595.

World Health Organisation. (1992). *The ICD-10 classification of mental and behavioral disorders: Clinical descriptions and diagnostic guidelines*. Geneva: World Health Organization.

Erratum to: Gait and Balance

Dimitrios Patikas

Chapter 11: *Gait and Balance,* which appears in Comorbid Conditions in Individuals with Intellectual Disabilities, J.L. Matson and M.L. Matson (eds.), DOI 10.1007/978-3-319-15437-4_11, contained an error in the author name in both printed and electronic versions. The error has been corrected and is reflected in both print and electronic versions.

The online version of the original chapter can be found under:
http://dx.doi.org/10.1007/10.1007/978-3-319-15437-4_11

D. Patikas (✉)
Department of Physical Education and Sport Science at Serres, Aristotle University, Thessaloniki, Greece
e-Mail: dpatikas@auth.gr

J. L. Matson, M. L. Matson (eds.), *Comorbid Conditions in Individuals with Intellectual Disabilities,* Autism and Child Psychopathology Series,
DOI 10.1007/978-3-319-15437-4_15

Index

J. L. Matson, M. L. Matson (eds.), *Comorbid Conditions in Individuals with Intellectual Disabilities,* Autism and Child Psychopathology Series,
DOI 10.1007/978-3-319-15437-4

MIX
Papier aus verantwortungsvollen Quellen
Paper from responsible sources
FSC® C105338

If you have any concerns about our products,
you can contact us on
ProductSafety@springernature.com

In case Publisher is established outside the EU,
the EU authorized representative is:
Springer Nature Customer Service Center GmbH
Europaplatz 3, 69115 Heidelberg, Germany

Printed by Libri Plureos GmbH
in Hamburg, Germany